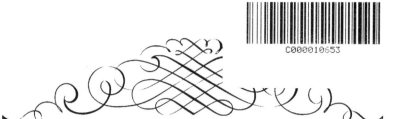
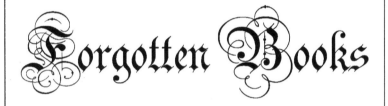

ISBN 978-1-5280-0824-2
PIBN 10912862

1 MONTH OF
FREE
READING

at

www.ForgottenBooks.com

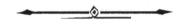

By purchasing this book you are eligible for one month membership to ForgottenBooks.com, giving you unlimited access to our entire collection of over 1,000,000 titles via our web site and mobile apps.

To claim your free month visit:

www.forgottenbooks.com/free912862

English
Français
Deutsche
Italiano
Español
Português

www.forgottenbooks.com

Mythology Photography **Fiction**
Fishing Christianity **Art** Cooking
Essays Buddhism Freemasonry
Medicine **Biology** Music **Ancient**
Egypt Evolution Carpentry Physics
Dance Geology **Mathematics** Fitness
Shakespeare **Folklore** Yoga Marketing
Confidence Immortality Biographies
Poetry **Psychology** Witchcraft
Electronics Chemistry History **Law**
Accounting **Philosophy** Anthropology
Alchemy Drama Quantum Mechanics
Atheism Sexual Health **Ancient History**
Entrepreneurship Languages Sport
Paleontology Needlework Islam
Metaphysics Investment Archaeology
Parenting Statistics Criminology
Motivational

DISEASES
OF THE INTESTINES

THEIR SPECIAL PATHOLOGY, DIAGNOSIS,
AND TREATMENT

WITH

SECTIONS ON ANATOMY AND PHYSIOLOGY, MICROSCOPIC AND CHEMIC
EXAMINATION OF THE INTESTINAL CONTENTS, SECRETIONS, FECES,
AND URINE. INTESTINAL BACTERIA AND PARASITES; SUR-
GERY OF THE INTESTINES; DIETETICS,
DISEASES OF THE RECTUM, ETC.

BY

JOHN C. HEMMETER, M.D., PHILOS.D.

PROFESSOR IN THE MEDICAL DEPARTMENT OF THE UNIVERSITY OF MARYLAND, CONSULTANT TO THE
UNIVERSITY HOSPITAL AND DIRECTOR OF THE CLINICAL LABORATORY;
AUTHOR OF A TREATISE ON "DISEASES OF THE STOMACH," ETC.

IN TWO VOLUMES

VOLUME II

APPENDICITIS, TUBERCULOSIS, SYPHILIS, ACTINOMYCOSIS OF INTESTINE, THE
OCCLUSIONS, CONTUSIONS, RUPTURE, ENTERORRHAGIA, INTESTINAL
SURGERY, ATROPHY, ABNORMALITIES OF FORM AND POSI-
TION, THROMBOSIS, EMBOLISM, AMYLOIDOSIS,
NEUROSES OF THE INTESTINES, INTES-
TINAL PARASITES, DISEASES
OF RECTUM

With Plates and many Other Original Illustrations

PHILADELPHIA
P. BLAKISTON'S SON & CO.
1012 WALNUT STREET

I 2

WM. F. FELL & CO.,
ELECTROTYPERS AND PRINTERS
1220-24 SANSOM STREET,
PHILADELPHIA.

TO

Edward G. Janeway, M.D., LL.D.,

DEAN, AND PROFESSOR OF MEDICINE,
THE UNIVERSITY AND BELLEVUE HOSPITAL MEDICAL COLLEGE,
NEW YORK CITY,   .

THIS VOLUME IS RESPECTFULLY DEDICATED.

" Integra mens augustissima possessio."

February, 1902.   THE AUTHOR.

PREFACE.

In the second volume of "Diseases of the Intestines" are embraced those pathological conditions that occupy the border-land between internal medicine and surgery. The modern evolution of the exact methods of clinical diagnosis, relating to many diseases of the human body, can not but command universal admiration; but the technics of the microscope, and chemical as well as physiological investigation, have as yet left large vacancies in the pathology of the intestinal function; and where these exact methods desert us, there is but one beacon light for the general practitioner, and that is *clinical experience*.

The comprehensive subject of Intestinal Obstruction has been presented mainly under two headings: (1) the enterostenoses, and (2) the obstructions. Under the latter there are many sub-types, which it was necessary to consider separately. Clinically, the enterostenoses are quite distinctive from the obstructions, although pathologically and anatomically the obstruction and the stenosis may be due to the same cause. In the introduction to the chapter on Intestinal Obstruction will be found a special consideration of the pathogenesis and the mechanism whereby they are brought about.

In this connection it is often difficult to emphasize the difference between truth and mere facts. These two are often, unfortunately, considered synonymous. Facts are the little truths that our senses are capable for the present of comprehending; but back of and beyond these facts later experience often reveals the higher and greater truth. Accordingly, it was not considered advisable to argue in all cases of doubtful pathogenesis and diagnosis. The reader will, however, find that the facts and truths are presented for his consideration as thoroughly as possible in the light of our present knowledge, when it is not safe to be dogmatic in conclusions pertaining to clinical or pathological questions. The author has endeavored, when the discussion is in debatable territory, to suggest to the reader the proper solution of a given diagnostic problem.

To a large number of American surgeons and clinicians mentioned in the text I am under obligations for personal expression of their opinions concerning the treatment to be pursued in the conditions embraced in the border-land between medicine and surgery. More especially it becomes my duty to express my thanks to Dr. Charles Wardell Stiles, of the Bureau of Animal Industry, U. S. Department of Agriculture, for reading the proof of the chapter on Intestinal Parasites, and for making numerous valuable suggestions thereto. Also to Dr. William Sydney Thayer for his generous aid given to the section devoted to *Strongyloides intestinalis.*

If this work, in addition to being an aid to the practitioner, as well as the specialist, will prove an inspiration to exact and objective clinical observation, as well as experimental investigation, the most heartfelt wish of the author will be fulfilled. Many masterly minds have concentrated their energies upon the solution of problems concerning intestinal pathology, and with a more enlightened understanding will come a more effective treatment.

'Ομὲν βίος βραχύς ἡ δὲ τέχνη μακρά. ("*Life is short, but Art is long.*")
—HIPPOCRATES.

JOHN C. HEMMETER.

February, 1902.

TABLE OF CONTENTS.—VOL. II.

xi

CHAPTER IV.

CHAPTER V.

LIST OF ILLUSTRATIONS.

Diseases of the Intestines.
Volume II.

CHAPTER I.

APPENDICITIS.

Synonym.—Simple catarrhal inflammation of the vermiform process.

The designation typhlitis comes from the Greek word τυφλός, meaning "cecum," and ιτις, meaning "inflammation." The word appendicitis was first suggested by Reginald H. Fitz to cover a large number of pathological conditions in the right iliac fossa, known prior to his masterly article (" Amer. Jour. of the Med. Sciences," 1886) under the most varied terms—viz., iliac abscess, iliac phlegmon, typhlitis, peri-, para-, and epityphlitis, typhloenteritis. The term "appendicitis" was offered to indicate the primary disease, the results of which were so variously named. Wood and Fitz (" Practice of Medicine," p. 876) state that the practical importance of the term has made it welcome in spite of the barbarism contained in it, for it is a Latin word with a Greek ending. Nothnagel (*l. c.*, p. 611), for orthological reasons, has suggested the name "*skolikoiditis.*" In Greek anatomy the vermiform process is called σκωληκοειδὴς ἀποφυσις, σκωλης meaning worm. "*Apophysitis*" would be linguistically correct, but as there are a great many apophyses in anatomical nomenclature, we would not be able to designate the particular one which is inflamed by this term alone. Küster has suggested the name "*epityphlitis*" (from ἐπιτυφλόν, meaning something "superimposed upon the cecum "). The word appendicitis, however, has become so familiar and wide-spread a term that it will be practically impossible to replace it; and so long as we all understand what is meant by the term, it is as serviceable as any other, though it is conceded it would have been preferable to comply with orthological demands in the beginning.

Painful swellings in the ileocecal region have been described in medical literature from the remotest times. One of the earliest references of ileocecal pain is found in Celsus. The early history of appendicitis typhlitis is merged with that of iliac phlegmon and peri- and paratyphlitis. The history since 1642 is given in a scholarly contribution to the history and literature of appendicitis by George M. Edebohls, "New York Medical Record," November 25, 1899.

At the beginning of the nineteenth century the importance and rôle of the vermiform process and its perforation in the generaation of typhlitis and perityphlitis began to be the object of medical interest. The accumulation of fecal matter in the cecum was still considered the cause of severe disease changes in the environment of the cecum. Emphasis was laid on the "typhlitis stercoralis."

The existence of the appendix was not recognized anatomically previous to the sixteenth century (Kelynack, "The Pathology of the Vermiform Appendix," London, 1893). During the sixteenth century descriptions of it were given by Carpi, Estienne, and Vidus Vidius, the latter designating it for the first time as "vermiform." In 1739 Lieberkühn ("De Valvula Coli usu Processus Vermicularis," Ludg. Bat., 1739) contributed the most accurate and thorough description of the appendix to anatomical knowledge that had been published up to that date. Ten years later J. Vosse followed with an equally exact anatomical account of this rudimentary organ ("De intestino cæco ejusque appendice vermiformi," sm. 4to, Goettingæ, 1749). In 1759 Mestivier recognized appendicitis as a distinct morbid entity ("Journ. de med. chir.", "Proc. verb.", etc., Paris, 1759, x, p. 442). The end of the eighteenth and the beginning of the nineteenth century gave birth to many publications on appendicitis with perforation and abscess formation, based on surgical observation as well as on records of necropsies.

Albers (T. F. H. Albers, "Beobacht. a. d. Gebiet d. Pathol.," Bonn, 1838) noted the possibility of disease of the right iliac fossa occurring as the result of inflammation of the vermiform appendix, but he thought that it was more frequently caused by disease of the cecum.

Since 1880 the significance of the vermiform process for pathological conditions that may develop in the right iliac fossa had been
emphasized in the literature on this subject. This new era, bringing
with it a correct knowledge of the state of affairs, is largely due to
the work of American surgeons, which was promptly imitated in
Europe and led to the early operation for diseases occurring in the
right iliac fossa. Under these conditions it was possible to recognize the pathological and anatomical relations in the living
patient, and the important rôle of the appendix in the origin of the
disease of the cecal region has been so much emphasized that the
assertion was made that the cecum itself was never primarily diseased,
but only secondarily as a consequence of disease in the appendix.
One of the most scholarly articles on the subject of appendicitis was
that of R. H. Fitz, which appeared in the "American Journal of the
Medical Sciences," in 1886. Much of the inspiration leading to the
thorough study of appendicitis is due to this valuable contribution,
which has since been looked upon as a landmark in the literature of
the subject (Talamon, *l. c.*). Since then numerous publications have
given evidence to the fact that the cecum may really be primarily
affected and be the seat of ulceration and perforation whilst the appendix is apparently normal. These are instances of genuine typhlitis, pure and simple. I have observed two cases in my experience in which perityphlitis was due to the perforation of a
cecal ulcer and the appendix was found normal at necropsy. The
great scarcity, however, of such cases is evident from the fact that
Fitz was able to collect only three cases of perforating cecal ulcers.
The exact relation as to how many cases of cecal and pericecal
inflammations are primary in the cecum itself, and how many have
originated from the appendix, will always be more or less conjectural.
According to Maurin, who studied 136 cases of suppuration of the
cecal region, 95 were exclusively lesions of the appendix, 6 had
started from the cecum and appendix, and 35 had involved the
cecum alone. Einhorn describes perityphlitis as due to the perforation of the appendix in 90 per cent. of the cases, and perforation of
the cecum in 9 per cent. In the memorable work of Fitz, both in
the first publication in the "American Journal of the Medical
Sciences," 1886, as well as in the second, published in 1888, he
emphasizes that the symptoms of typhlitis and perityphlitis, of which

he collected in the first paper 209 cases, and those of perforating appendicitis, of which he collected 257 cases, were almost identical. I shall speak more fully of this publication under the heading Perforating Appendicitis.   In the second report of 1888, Fitz advanced the radical theory that typhlitis, perityphlitis, appendicular peritonitis, and perityphlitic abscess are all varieties of one and the same affection—namely, appendicitis.   The possibility of the inflammation of the cecum as a result of fecal accumulation is denied by Nothnagel, Sahli, and Sonnenburg and Fowler ("Treatise on Appendicitis," Philadelphia, 1894).   But according to the observations of Porter, Curschmann, Manly, Deutschmann, and Krönlein, the occurrence of primary typhlitis can not be doubted.   Osler gives a chapter to the consideration of this disease, but admits (p. 405, "Practice of Medicine") that its anatomical condition is unknown, and that it is by no means certain that these cases are really cecal.   Priebram describes it (Ebstein u. Schwalbe, "Handb. d. prak. Med.," Bd. II, S. 688) similarly to Penzoldt (Penzoldt u. Stintzing, "Handb. der. spec. Therapie innere Krankheiten," S. 486).   Judging from a critical review of the literature on the subject and from my personal experience and private practice, I do not think that we can discard the clinical conception of a simple primary typhlitis.   As I have said before, I have seen ulcers of the cecum with circumscribed catarrhal inflammation, and even a limited peritonitis over the cecum, where the appendix was to all appearances normal.   Admitting the extreme rarity of such conditions, we can, however, not entirely deny the existence of such a disease of the cecum, independent of involvement of the appendix.

Nature, Description, and Etiology.

Simple catarrhal inflammation of the vermiform process and of the cecum, either each separately or both combined, is a more frequent disease than is usually supposed.   In those cases in which the inflammation is confined to the mucosa and submucosa it may remain latent and take its course without any symptoms at all.   At most it causes but vague disease symptoms, and can be recognized only when the increasing inflammation affects the peritoneum. This may be the principal reason why the frequent occurrence of catarrhal appendicitis and typhlitis is not generally admitted.   There

PLATE 1

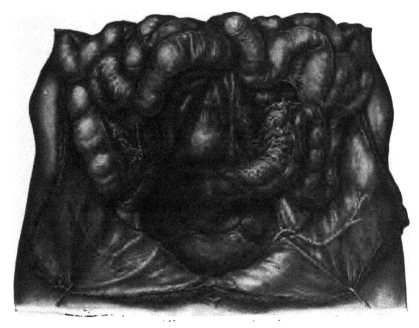

PELVIC CAVITY OF MALE (SUPERIOR VIEW).

The cecum and appendix are plainly recognizable on the left ; the sigmoid and rectum on the right. The relations of the male pelvic fossa are clearly represented. Close observance of the anatomical course of the sigmoid flexure makes the difficulty of its direct intubation and inspection intelligible.—(*From Deaver's "Surgical Anatomy."*)

can be no doubt that typhlitis often escapes detection; this is evident from Nothnagel's investigations, in which he found that in many persons who had never had any severe intestinal complaints during life the cecum alone often showed all the indications of atrophy, which is certainly to be referred to a frequently recurring and lasting inflammation of the mucous membrane; it may also be inferred from some interesting observations of Ribbert, according to which the vermiform process, with increasing age, regu-

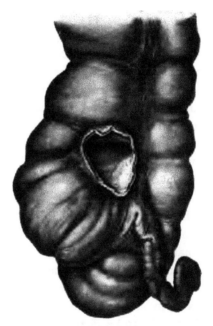

FIG. 1.—ILEOCECAL VALVE, CECUM, AND APPENDIX.
The cut edges of the ileum are separated and permit a view of the ileocecal valve.—(*From Deaver.*)

larly shows atrophic changes. These may manifest themselves in an increasing atrophy of the mucosa, which finally may be obliterated and replaced by a fine connective tissue. The muscularis, however, suffers no appreciable change. It is reasonable to assume, with A. O. J. Kelly and Sonnenburg and others, that this obliteration and atrophy are caused by a slow catarrhal inflammation of the mucous membrane of the appendix, which causes a scaling off of the epithelium, since we could hardly understand the occurrence of an oblitera-

tion in a simple atrophy of the mucous membrane.   Besides, it would
be very difficult to distinguish in its final stage an atrophy dependent
upon inflammatory processes from a simple atrophy.   Ribbert found
obliterative processes in 56 per cent. of the persons over sixty years
of age ; in persons over twenty years old he found the obliterative process was already completed in 32 per cent.   He considers that this
form of obliteration, which commences at the free end of the appendix, is a process of involution, and that it is altogether independent
of any inflammatory affections.   This would agree with the conception of the vermiform process as an organ which is degenerating.

The ancient theory that primary typhlitis was always caused by
coprostasis (hence the name, "typhlitis stercoralis"), which has
many adherents even at the present time, is certainly not correct.
It applies to only a part of the cases.   Probably the coprostasis is
more frequently the result of typhlitis, not the cause.   In those
cases in which the typhlitis does not extend to the peritoneum the
coprostasis often is its only discernible symptom for a long time.
Extraordinary accumulation of the feces may, no doubt, cause an
increase in the inflammation of the cecum if it was already catarrhally inflamed, if its mucosa be strongly irritated, mechanically and
chemically, and if its walls be excessively distended by the feces.
This inflammation may easily extend to the peritoneum and cause a
fibrinous or occasionally even a serofibrinous or a purulent peritonitis.
This explains the fact that in people who have for a long time suffered
from persistent constipation, the symptoms of perityphlitis appear
suddenly, especially if, in addition, the diet has been faulty.   The
symptoms are violent pain and a distinct resistance in the ileocecal
region.   After abundant evacuations, whether spontaneous or produced by purges, they may rapidly improve and soon cease, because
when the intestinal wall is relieved of its load, the inflammation of
the cecal mucosa and of the peritoneum may quickly subside.

Feces may easily accumulate in the cecum, because in it the
first thickening of the fluid chyme takes place, because the small
intestine opens into the cecum and makes a right angle with it as it
enters, and because the masses of feces have to move directly in an
upward direction in the ascending colon (see illustration, Fig. 1, p. 23).
Although they may occasionally be moved onward in a direction
directly opposed to the force of gravity in the small intestine, this

occurs only for short distances, and by the mechanism described in the chapter on Peristalsis. But the small intestine is often able to move in such a way as to prevent exerting its peristaltic efforts against the force of gravity (movements of the archimedian screw). The ascending colon, from the cecum upward, is, however, so bound down anatomically that the column of feces must necessarily ascend directly against gravity. In more recent times, however, Sahli has disputed the correctness of this view. He points out that the masses of solid feces which are so often found in the colon show no particular predilection for the cecum ; also that if the cecum be packed full, masses of solid feces usually are also found in the entire colon, and that the feces are softest and least harmful just in the cecum, because at this place the more fluid contents of the small intestine are constantly being added, which assist in maintaining a semi-soft state by loosening up the contents of the cecum mechanically. Besides this, as Sahli notes, the fecal tumors observed during life do not show any predilection for the cecum. Other reliable observers have frequently discovered very extensive fecal tumors in the cecum, and often when other parts of the colon were empty. When stagnation of the feces has occurred in the cecum from any cause at all and its walls are excessively distended thereby, the peristalsis of the small intestine is greatly diminished at the same time. The chyme is carried down more slowly in the small intestine, and it is thickened more than usual. Thus when it enters the cecum it is no longer liquid. The rapid passage of the chyme in the small intestine under normal conditions prevents putrefaction. Therefore if the peristalsis of the small intestine is diminished, putrefaction commences here instead of in the large intestine. Since the mucosa of the small intestine is less accustomed to the products of putrefaction, it is more susceptible to become inflamed by them, and this inflammation may extend to the cecum. The correctness of this assumption is supported by the fact that in certain rare cases of benign typhlitis and perityphlitis the symptoms of occlusion appear *early*, which is an indication of obstruction in the ileum rather than in the colon, and that the vomit or the liquid used in rinsing out the stomach may contain stercoraceous matter. After abundant evacuations, the symptoms of this variety of occlusion rapidly disappear.

The causes of catarrhal typhlitis are the same as those of a catarrh of other intestinal parts—they are bacterial, mechanical, and chemical irritations which affect the cecal mucosa. They may be the results of incorrect diet and mode of living, and occasionally the results of trauma. Thus a diet consisting principally of vegetables, of which great quantities must be ingested, may distend the intestinal walls very much, and thus favor the development of a typhlitis, from which a simple perityphlitis may then arise. Perityphlitis has been observed a short time after large quantities of hulls, skins, seeds, or kernels were swallowed. I have observed an attack of appendicitis after the ingestion of two pounds of grapes eaten with the seeds.

Fleischer (*l. c.*) observed one case recently where perityphlitis set in five or six hours after an excessive quantity of Mandarin oranges had been eaten; in another case it set in after a large quantity of gooseberries had been eaten, together with their rough skins.

In a small proportion of the cases the typhlitis is a result of a strong irritation of the mucous membrane of the cecum, caused by thickened, hardened feces, more rarely by gall-stones, genuine enteroliths, and foreign bodies.

Both typhlitis and appendicitis are caused more rarely by infectious processes combined with the formation of ulcers, such as intestinal tuberculosis, typhus, syphilis, dysentery, diphtheria, actinomycosis (Lang and Rauson), and also by cancer. The mucosa in the immediate neighborhood of these ulcers, which sometimes are confined to the cecum, is in a state of catarrhal inflammation. The conditions for the development both of a simple catarrhal, as well as of a suppurative, inflammation are more favorable in the appendix than in the cecum.

The vermiform process is a natural culture-tube for bacteria—a long, hollow appendage of varying length, which at one end opens into the cecum and is closed at the other end. In former times it was assumed that it furnished an oil which lubricated the intestinal mucosa. and rendered the peristalsis of the organ easier. Its length is about eight or nine centimeters; in some persons, however, it may be from twelve to twenty centimeters. Thus the discrepancy between length and lumen, which is considerable even under normal conditions, is considerably increased. The mouth of the appendix—that is, the beginning of its lumen—is also its narrowest point. At this place there is often a fold of mucous membrane of varying size (the valve of Gerlach). The existence of this valve has been denied by Clado, and Lefforgue found it only twice in 200 cadavers. (See "Anatomy of the Vermiform Process," by John B. Deaver, "Treatise on Appendicitis," p. 29.) This renders it more difficult for the contents of the intestine to enter, but after the entrance has been effected, it favors a retention and thickening of the feces in the appendix. The mucous

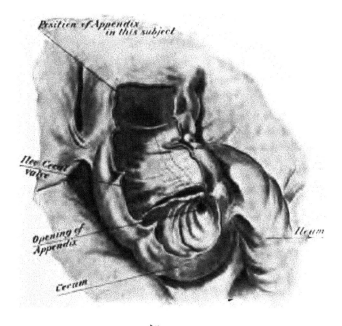

FIG. 2.—ILEOCECAL VALVE, OPENING OF APPENDIX.—(*From dissection in Anatomical Laboratory of the University of Maryland.*)

membrane of the latter has a plentiful supply of solitary glands and glands of Lieberkühn, and is a direct continuation of that of the cecum, so that catarrhal inflammations may extend in either direction very easily.

The great amount of adenoid tissue which the cecum possesses in common with the tonsils has been emphasized by American authors in more recent times (Deaver, Bland, McBurney, Lutton, A. O. J. Kelly, Ransohoff, Watney). A number of these authors associate this adenoid tissue with the very frequent diseased condition of the appendix. According to the investigations of Stöhr and Ribbert, this adenoid tissue seems to be very susceptible to infections in the direction from the mucous membrane. The physiological transmigration of the leukocytes toward the free surface of the mucous membrane is well known, and there is no reason why bacteria should not be able to pass through the tissue and the covering epithelial layers, after minute breaks have opened the way for them. Whether bacteria may pass the intestinal mucosa under perfectly normal conditions is a moot point. Bacteria participate in the development of catarrhal appendicitis and of peri-appendicitis, which starts therefrom. This is indicated by a number of observations, particularly those of Sandberg. In cross-sections of the walls of a vermiform process which was changed only catarrhally, he detected numerous bacilli in the lymph-passages (Helferich).

The appendix is for the most part covered with peritoneum. Next to this peritoneal covering it has a muscular layer which gives it a limited contractility and a capacity for emptying its contents into the cecum by means of peristaltic contractions. If the appendix is very long, these contractions may not be strong enough to expel the feces, especially if the contents are very much condensed, nor can they expel the foreign bodies which have made their way into the appendix. This explains why coproliths are so often found even in the unchanged vermiform process, playing, no doubt, a very important rôle in the etiology of the catarrhal and suppurative inflammation of the same. In 400 necropsies in which there was no evidence of perityphlitis, Ribbert found coproliths in 38 cases—about 10 per cent. It is apparent that on account of the peculiar structure of the appendix and of its inlet into the cecum the conditions are extraordinarily favorable for a stagnation and condensation of the feces, and also for the entrance of larger parasites, foreign bodies, and putrefactive bacteria from the cecum, which is ordinarily rich in parasitic fauna and flora. All these may cause great irritation of the mucous membrane. If this has caused a catarrh, a restitution to a normal estate in many cases is prevented by retention of inflammatory products and bacteria within the vermiform process, which has its explanation in the anatomical condition of the appendix. Since the mouth of the appendix is the narrowest part of its lumen, swelling of the mucous membrane and of the Gerlach valve may easily cause a stenosis, or even a complete closure, analogous to the closure of the common gall-duct in duodenal catarrh. The histological appearance of the in-fected appendix showing the interstitial exudate compression has been studied by Robert T. Morris, and pictured in his " Lectures on Appendicitis " (p. 17), and also by Herbert P. Hawkins ("Dis-eases of the Vermiform Appendix," pp. 25 and 28, "Histology of Catarrhal Appendicitis"). If there is an absolute occlusion, a

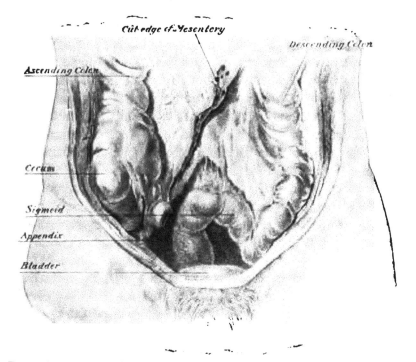

FIG. 3.—ASCENDING AND DESCENDING COLON, SIGMOID FLEXURE.—(*From dissection in Ana-tomical Laboratory of the University of Maryland.*)

very abundant secretion accumulates in the vermiform process, which is readily decomposed in the presence of numerous putrefac-tive bacteria. The walls of the appendix are excessively distended, and the mucous membrane is strongly irritated, both mechanically and chemically. Curiously enough, the very short mesenteriolum of the appendix favors a partial retention of the secretion, though the mouth of the appendix is still permeable, inasmuch as it causes a kinking when the vermiform process is distended.

The appendix occasionally contains hard fecal fragments which sometimes inclose hairs from the face or head, bristles from tooth-brushes (Edebohls, *l. c.*, Gerhardt, Eichhorst), or ascarides' eggs (Klebs), which often rapidly increase in size as a result of the deposition of mucus on the outside of the concretion (Ribbert), and thereby exert a greater pressure upon the mucous membrane and the adjacent layers. The effect of this pressure is the more injurious since the mucous membrane is already altered by inflammatory changes. If necrosis sets in and ulcers are formed, these may extend down to the serosa and cause a circumscribed fibrinous or a serofibrinous peritonitis. This may lead to the formation of various adhesions and agglutinations of the appendix with the cecum, with other portions of the intestines, and with the anterior abdominal wall. But even without this ulceration the inflammation of the mucosa may extend continuously to the serosa of the appendix and thence to the peritoneal covering of the cecum. Catarrhal ulcers located near the opening of the vermiform process into the cecum (such ulcers not accompanied by the formation of coproliths have been observed fairly often in simple appendicitis) may cause a permanent stenosis of the appendicular lumen or even an entire occlusion after healing. If the latter is the case, the secretion may be collected in such quantities that a dropsical distention of the vermiform process ensues, which may assume enormous proportions and finally present every appearance of a cyst (A. O. J. Kelly, in Deaver's "Appendicitis," second edition, p. 83, also described by Gruber, Hawkins, Shoemaker, Coats). Retention cysts of the appendix have been described by Mayland and Sonnenburg (see Edebohls, "Medical Record," November 25, 1899, p. 774). Ribbert has observed this cyst formation several times, and Guttman describes a case where the appendix attained a length of fourteen, and a circumference of twenty-one centimeters. If, therefore, from any reason an acute catarrhal inflammation of the appendix has developed, we can easily understand why it thus frequently becomes chronic, and why its final cure is, in any case, delayed considerably by acute recrudescence and relapses. Therefore we need not be surprised when simple appendicitis, just as typhlitis, causes an atrophy of the mucous membrane much more frequently than is observed in catarrhs of other sections of the intestines. If the mouth of the appendix is not permanently closed, and if the pressure within its lumen reaches a considerable degree, its contents are emptied into the cecum. If, then, the walls of the appendix lie close together, its obliteration is favored by the desquamation of the epithelial covering of the mucosa, which is extensively diseased by the inflammation. The observations of Ribbert and others as to the great frequency of obliteration in old age is explained by Sonnenburg and others as a spontaneous cure of an appendicitis. Ribbert, however, considers this to be a process of involution, just as the atrophy of the mucosa—a theory which corresponds to the conception of the vermiform appendix as a degenerated or rudimentary organ. If the infectious causes of tuberculosis, typhus, dysentery, syphilis, or actinomycosis gain entrance into the appendix when it is catarrhally changed, they often find favorable conditions there for their invasion and propagation. The anatomical and pathological characteristics of the appendix and cecum sufficiently explain why ulcers of these types are found at autopsies confined to these regions exclusively.

Simple appendicitis and typhlitis are observed much oftener in men than in women, because the intestines of the former are exposed to more injurious influences as a result of faulty diet and manner of living. There is another explanation for this—viz., the fact that females are supposed to have a greater blood supply than males, both in actual quantity and in proportion to the size of the appendices in the two sexes. Clado has described a fold of peritoneum extending from the appendix to the ovary, the appendiculo-ovarian ligament, which carries a blood-vessel to the appendix. This, together with the fact that the appendix of the female is smaller than that of the male, may account for the comparatively small percentage of attacks among women and girls (Deaver, "A Treatise on Appendicitis," p. 33).

The following table * shows the ages in the statistics of Matterstock (474), Fitz (228), Sonnenburg (130), and Nothnagel (130),† comprising altogether 962 cases of appendicitis, and showing that the disease is most frequent between the tenth and thirtieth years

---

* Quoted from Nothnagel ("Erkrank. d. Darms.," p. 622).

† In one of Nothnagel's and 7 of Sonnenburg's cases, no statement concerning the age was made.

of life. After the thirtieth the frequency of the disease rapidly
decreases, and it is rare after the fortieth year. This is a valuable
factor for differential diagnosis from intestinal carcinoma :

	MATTER-STOCK. 474	FITZ. 228	SONNEN-BURG. 130	NOTH-NAGEL. 130
0 to 10 years, ...	46	22	14	1
11 " 20 "	143	86	33	44
21 " 30 "	158	65	43	57
31 " 40 "	72	34	15	14
41 " 50 "	30	8	11	7
51 " 60 "	18	11	2	4
61 " 70 "	5	1	4	2
71 " 80 "	2		1	

This disease, according to this table, occurs in all ages, but is
found most frequently in middle age (sixteen to thirty-five). It is
not so rare in children as was formerly supposed. About 15 per
cent. of all cases occur in persons under fifteen years. The youngest
patient afflicted with typhlitis and appendicitis was a female child
of twenty-two months ; the oldest, a laborer aged sixty-eight years.
That it is so rare in advanced age is satisfactorily explained by
Ribbert's investigations, giving the evidence that the obliteration of
the vermiform appendix can be found more frequently in old age than
in youth and middle age. The obliteration naturally prevents
the entrance of disease excitants into the appendix. Catarrhal
appendicitis causes no marked disease symptoms so long as the
pathological process is confined to the mucous membrane. They
can be distinctly recognized only when the inflammatory process
spreads to the peritoneum and the characteristic symptoms of perityphlitis appear. These consist of more or less violent pains in the
right ileocecal region which are increased by pressure. A tumor
which is sensitive to pressure may often be detected in this region,
especially in those rare cases in which the typhlitis was the starting-
point of the perityphlitis. This tumor is caused by the fecal accumulation, by the inflammatory thickening of the wall of the
cecum and of the appendix, by fibrinous, and sometimes also by
a serous exudation in the neighborhood of these parts of the intestines. In simple appendicitis the tumor is much smaller or may
even be entirely wanting. In 1894 Edebohls published a method

of palpation of the vermiform appendix which placed the practitioner in a position to diagnose clearly almost every case of chronic and many cases of acute appendicitis ("Amer. Jour. of the Med. Sci.," 1894, new series, vol. cvii, p. 487). Usually both diseases result favorably if the treatment is rational and the patients conduct themselves properly. The pains soon cease, and the tumor in the right ileocecal region usually disappears rapidly, unless it is conditioned by dropsy or cyst formation in the vermiform process. The serous exudations may be absorbed very quickly, and then the cure is complete. If, as a result of perityphlitis, adhesions of the appendix to the cecum have set in, or to other sections of the intestine, or to the front abdominal wall, they may cause frequent relapses.

I am speaking here only of acute simple catarrhal appendicitis; the graver forms of the disease are considered in a separate section.

Pathological Anatomy.

The anatomical changes found in simple typhlitis and appendicitis are identical with those of catarrhs of other intestinal sections (see chapter on Enteritis). In the same way they may be accompanied by follicular and catarrhal ulcers. These extend downward, and may cause a circumscribed agglutinative peritonitis if they reach the intestinal serosa. It is only exceptionally that catarrhal ulcers extend downward in the cecum so rapidly that there is not sufficient time for the formation of firm adhesions between the base of the ulcer and the serosa of other sections of the intestine. In cases where the serosa is perforated the intestinal contents are emptied in the neighborhood of the cecum, causing a circumscribed suppurative inflammation of the peritoneum and usually also of the retrocecal extraperitoneal connective tissue. General suppurative peritonitis, which is rapidly fatal, occurs but rarely. The process may also spread to the peritoneal covering in simple typhlitis and appendicitis, even if there is no ulceration, if the disease lasts long enough. Sonnenburg, who has performed operations in a large number of cases of simple appendicitis and peri-appendicitis, and thus gained an insight into the anatomical changes which are at the basis of the nonsuppurative perityphlitis, states that the inflammation is confined to the mucous membrane alone in the less severe cases of appendicitis only. These changes vary within wide limits.

They may consist of : (1) Slight changes in the appendix itself, but numerous agglutinations of the same with the intestines and neighboring organs ; (2) changes of the appendix,—hypertrophies, kinkings, engorgements,—but at the same time hardly any symptoms of an adhesive peritonitis ; (3) very great changes both in the appendix —formation of empyemas and coprostasis—and in its surroundings.

Four varieties of the disease may be distinguished pathologically :

1. **Endo-appendicitis**, in which there is more or less inflammation of the mucous membrane and submucosa.

2. **Parietal appendicitis**, in which the inflammation attacks the interstitial or intermuscular tissue of the body of the appendix.

3. **Peri-appendicitis**, in which the inflammation attacks the serous covering of the appendix, being limited by adhesions to that portion of the peritoneum between the appendix and the serous surfaces immediately adjoining.

4. **Para-appendicitis**, in which the inflammation attacks the tissues in relation with the appendix. In the last stage we find pus-formation either localized by the limiting adhesions formed during the third stage, or general involvement of the peritoneum, etc.

The relation of the vermiform process to the cecum, Poupart's ligament, and the termination of the ileum are well illustrated in the plates accompanying this chapter, taken from Deaver's work on " Appendicitis," Plates I to IV, and by their aid the extension of the appendix inflammation becomes more intelligible.

It must be remembered that these stages are not marked by distinct lines of separation, because any one of them may be absent as a distinct stage, or, again, they may so merge into one another that it is impossible to distinguish between them (Deaver, *l. c.*, p. 45).

The last-mentioned changes are found in those cases which, according to Sonnenburg, form the transition of the severe form of the disease—the suppurative perforative appendicitis. They certainly are connected more closely with the latter than with simple appendicitis, and should, therefore, be separated from it. It is still an open question whether serofibrinous exudations (Deaver, Roux, Sonnenburg, and others) or transudations (Fowler) are present in those cases in which a serous liquid is removed by an operation or by puncture.

Dr. J. M. Van Cott, Jr., in George R. Fowler's " Treatise on

PLATE 2.

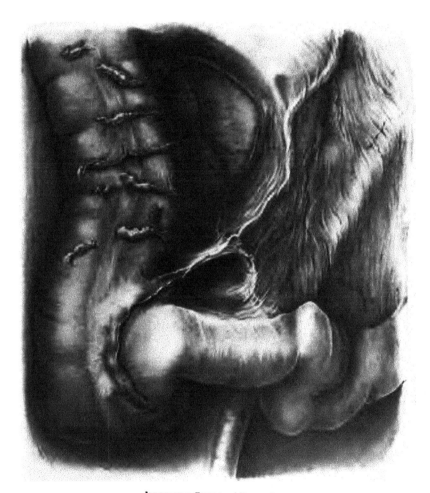

ILEOCOLIC FOSSA.—(*Deaver.*)

Appendicitis," page 92, like Clado (cited in the preceding), explains the comparative immunity of women from appendicitis by an additional blood supply which, in·the female sex, is found in the appendiculo-ovarian ligament, and which carries an artery to the appendix. The circulation of the appendix is practically a terminal one. By far the most of the blood entering it passes through a single branch of the mesenteric artery.   There is but a slight collateral circulation, derived from continuity with the structure of the head of the colon.   Van Cott, in examining thirteen specimens sent to him by Dr. Fowler, claimed to have found the presence of some form of obstruction of the blood current in the meso-appendicial vessels. There was a para-, a peri-, or an endovasculitis or organized thrombus, "conditions which must, in the nature of the case, have long preceded the intense small round-cell infiltration, coagulation necrosis, and purulent foci present in the walls of the appendices themselves." In several cases, also, a distinct chronic, interstitial neuritis supervened; in some the hyperplastic connective-tissue proliferation in the perineurium was so abundant as to have caused extensive atrophy of the nerve-fiber.   Accordingly Van Cott concludes that the real cause of the locus minoris resistentiæ which admits of bacterial infection of the appendix must be sought primarily not in a trauma of the mucosa, but rather in trophic disturbance of the appendix, resulting from : (1) Chronic vascular lesions caused by torsion of the vessels of the appendix and its mesentery, induced by great mobility of the appendix ; (2) chronic nervous lesions ; (3) both together.   According to this writer it follows that ulcerative processes in the appendix, while they may be increased by bacterial invasion, may, nevertheless, owe their origin to trophic conditions, so that it must always be difficult to prove that a given ulcerative process in the appendix is due to bacterial invasion primarily.   The source of the trophic disturbance lies in a progressive hyperplasia of the coats of the appendix, probably due to repeated or continuous hyperemia or chronic stasis, conditions which must eventually result in vascular and nervous lesions, described by Van Cott.

These investigations of Van Cott were repeated and worked over critically by Robert Breuer, on the instigation of Nothnagel (*l. c.*, p. 631). Breuer could not arrive at any definite results concerning the blood supply in the appendiculo-ovarian ligament by which Van Cott

explains the comparative immunity of females from appendicitis.
He also took exception to the description of the circulation of the
appendix as a terminal circulation, and could not find vascular
changes of that regularity and extent as were described by Van
Cott. The inflammatory alterations in the vessel, in the cases of
Breuer and Nothnagel, did not exceed those which are usually
observed in connection with acute inflammation. Above all, they
could not gain the impression that the vasculitis had long preceded
the other inflammatory phenomena. Breuer admits that the circulation of the appendix is not so abundant nor so constant as that of
other parts of the intestine, and admits also the liability to occlusion
of the appendicular artery. He also studied the changes in the nerves
in all his cases, staining them by Marchi's method, to detect the
finer alterations; but here, as well as in the vessels, he could find no
evidences which could be interpreted as causes of the appendicitis
in the sense of Van Cott. Breuer examined thirty appendices removed partially by operation and partially from the cadaver.

Nothnagel considers the two principal causes of appendicitis to be
the deleterious influence of bacteria, and coprostasis or coproliths.
The illustrations given by Van Cott certainly bear out the conclusions
he arrives at to a large extent. I have carefully studied the vermiform appendix from ten cases of appendicitis, by serial sections, and
in two of them which presented small abscesses in the terminal end
of the appendix there was comparatively little invasion of the appendicular tissues by bacteria, but there were evidences of diffuse
endarteritis and phlebitis, apparently of long standing. A number
of the nerve-fibers in the wall of the appendix presented the evidences of complete atrophy. So in the present light of the subject I am not able to decide between the investigations of Breuer
and Van Cott. Much future histological study of the diseased
appendix is required for this purpose. But Van Cott deserves much
credit for calling attention to other possible pathogenetic factors
in addition to bacteria and coproliths.

A most scholarly contribution to the pathology of appendicitis
will be found in the third edition of Deaver's " Treatise on Appendicitis." The article in question is from the pen of Dr. A. O. J.
Kelly, and enters very thoroughly into the questions I have considered in the preceding. He has studied 577 appendices removed

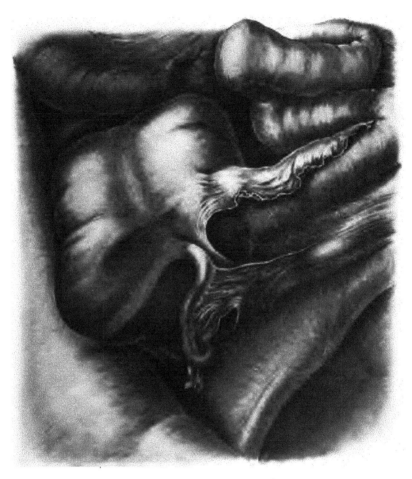

ILEOCECAL FOSSA.—(*Deaver.*)

by operation; 9 of these were removed from persons who presented no clinical symptoms of appendicitis, but who were operated upon for some other condition, the appendix being removed at the same time; 21 of these appendices were not examined microscopically; of the 547 remaining, 239 were cases of acute and 305 of chronic appendicitis; 2 were instances of primary sarcoma, and 1 of endothelioma. A. O. J. Kelly does not consider that the alterations in the nerve supply in the appendix are of such great importance as has been suggested by Van Cott. He concedes a significant place in the pathogenesis to partial or complete obstruction of the blood-vessels as a result of angulations, torsions, adhesions, etc. The increase in the virulence of the bacteria normally present in the intestine is ascribed to interference with thorough drainage of the appendix, when the lumen is constricted, compressed, or obstructed, or when the appendix is so situated that it is a physiological impossibility for it to be emptied, or the outlet has become occluded from swelling of the mucous membrane. Appendicular calculi are looked upon as a result, rather than a cause, of an attack of appendicitis. When once formed, they may act by occluding the lumen of the organ and prevent drainage, and also by inducing passive congestion in the portion of the appendix distal to their location. The efforts of peristalsis to expel the calculus may cause erosions of the mucosa and open up the way for the bacteria, thus determining a perforation. They are also an important factor in the production of chronic recurring appendicitis, provoking the acute exacerbations in this condition. The experiments of Dieulafoy, Frazier, Roger, Josué, and Roux are quoted as indicating the increase in the virulence of the colon bacillus in the appendix when its lumen is occluded. The consequent retention, stagnation, and putrefaction of the contents of the appendix favor destruction of the mucosa by the toxins formed, as well as by mechanical pressure. A. O. J. Kelly, therefore, agrees with the view which assigns to appendicitis a complex pathogenesis in which abnormalities in anatomical structure, physiological function, and bacterial activity alternate and combine in a most variable manner.

Appendicial Coproliths.—Since coproliths are often found in the appendix in peri- and para-appendicitis, an important rôle has been ascribed to them in recent times in the etiology of these condi-

tions.   I do not deny that coproliths may irritate and thus inflame
the mucous membrane by exerting a pressure upon it and the intestinal wall.   Their importance, however, should not be exaggerated,
because coproliths have often been found in an entirely unchanged
appendix by both American and European surgeons and especially
by the pathologist Ribbert.   Personally I have frequently found coproliths at autopsies in the normal appendix.   On the other hand, they
may often contribute to the aggravation of an already existing catarrhal or suppurative appendicitis, and render a perforation of the intestine easier by exerting pressure upon it and the ulcers.   Talamon
('Entérolithes ou Calculs Appendiculaires") assumed that these
coproliths were formed in the cecum and then got into the vermiform
appendix ("La colique Appendiculaire," etc., 1900, p. 45).   At present, however, most authors think that they are formed in the appendix itself. · Talamon distinguished four varieties of foreign bodies :

1. Foreign bodies properly speaking, coming from the exterior
through the diet.

2. Small concretions of fecal matter found in the appendix or
derived from the cecum.

3. Appendicular calculi or enteroliths.

4. Scybala.

There is no doubt that small foreign bodies, gall-stones, and
parasites may penetrate into the appendix from the cecum and
cause an inflammation therein.   If the specific disease excitants of
tuberculosis, dysentery, typhus, or actinomycosis get into it or into
the cecum, they may, under favorable conditions, cause an inflammation resulting in ulceration.   This inflammation sometimes is
confined to these sections alone.   The former opinion, that cherry-
and date-stones often get into the appendix and cause inflammation
(Talamon, l. c., p. 12), has not been confirmed by recent investigations.   According to Biermer's and Bossard's statements, it is entirely impossible or very difficult to force cherry-stones into the
vermiform process at autopsy.   The roundish formations found in
it usually consist of hardened feces.   If smaller foreign bodies get
into the appendix, they may facilitate the formation of coproliths,
for they constitute a nucleus for collecting the feces around themselves.   That the anatomical appearance of the simple typhlitis and
appendicitis usually is identical with that of chronic catarrh can

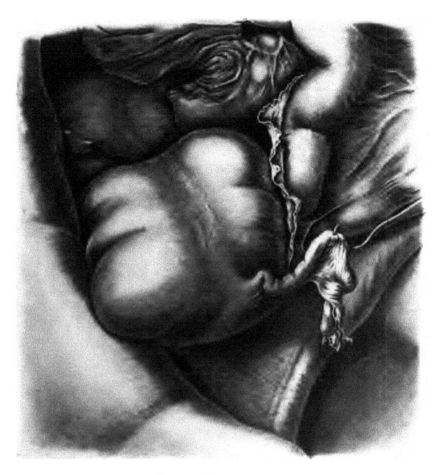

SUBCECAL FOSSA.—(*Deaver*)

easily be understood from what has already been said concerning the pathology of enteritis. We can also understand why acute aggravations of chronic appendicitis and perityphlitis may often set in. The more frequent atrophy of the mucosa resulting from these conditions is explained by the longer duration and severer character of the inflammation.

Symptomatology.

In the chapter on Intestinal Ulcers I described necropsies on cases of cecal ulcerations that had given no symptoms during life. From this we may conclude that catarrhal appendicitis and typhlitis may cause no pregnant symptoms. The constipation which is frequently observed in the former may be caused by numerous other diseased conditions. Diarrhea is not as often observed as constipation. We may suspect a typhlitis only when persistent constipation alternates with diarrhea, when a fecal accumulation may be detected by palpation in the right ileocecal region, and when the patients complain of distention, pressure, and fullness in this region. On the other hand, simple uncomplicated appendicitis usually proceeds without any symptoms. In itself it does not cause constipation. Even in those cases in which the inflammation spreads from the mucosa of the appendix or the cecum to the peritoneum its extension outward, through the layers of the intestinal wall, may be so gradual and slow that the beginning of the perityphlitis may escape detection and may not be noticed until an aggravation of the circumscribed peritonitis is caused by the action of the new pernicious agencies. As a rule, however, the spread of the inflammation to the peritoneum and the beginning of the perityphlitis cause characteristic disease symptoms. These consist more especially of more or less violent pains, which are intensified by pressure, in the right ileocecal region.

Fleischer and others have attempted to separate the clinical signs of perityphlitis developing from simple typhlitis from those of simple appendicitis or peri-appendicitis. The following is their manner of argument: If the perityphlitis is the result of a simple typhlitis, a more or less extensive resistance is usually felt in the right ileocecal region, above Poupart's ligament. The latter is often bulged out distinctly, and then one can feel a cylindrical, smooth, and nodular tumor of varying size. Sometimes, not always, it is sharply defined, and generally it is also sensitive to pressure. The skin above it is movable, but the tumor itself is immovable. The formation of the tumor is caused by accumulations of feces in the cecum, by an inflammatory thickening of the intestinal walls, by fibrinous stratifications, and sometimes also by a serous effusion in the neighborhood of the cecum and the appendix. Sometimes a large tumor is simulated by several intestinal loops if they are agglutinated, and can not escape from the palpating finger. If the tumor consists principally of feces, it may usually be indented by the finger. If, however, a serous exudation or transudation exists at the same time, and is contained within a closed space formed by agglutinations, the resistance is firmer. The percussion sound over it is often dulled or dull tympanitic. In simple appendicitis and peri-appendicitis the tumor is smaller, since these conditions cause no constipation in themselves. Under such conditions the tumor may even be entirely absent. Those cases in which a cystic dropsy of the appendix or a serous exudation in its neighborhood has developed always present a palpable tumor. In other cases where the tumor is entirely lacking, a marked circumscribed sensibility toward pressure may often be discovered at the juncture of the appendix with the cecum (McBurney's point). This is a characteristic symptom of peri-appendicitis, but the location of this point may vary considerably (McBurney, "New York Medical Journal," vol. i, pp. 676–684).

This effort at differentiating the forms of cecal and peri-appendiceal induration has more of a theoretical than a practical interest, because of the exceedingly rare occurrence of primary typhlitis as compared with appendicitis.

If there is great fecal accumulation in the cecum, there is usually a large amount of gas collected in the intestines. The latter may, therefore, force the diaphragm, the lungs, and the heart upward and cause moderate dyspnea. In association with this state there is also retention of stool. If feces pass off, they come from the lower sections of the colon. If diarrhea sets in, the pains are temporarily intensified by the rapid peristalsis.

Sometimes the symptoms of appendicitis and perityphlitis are preceded by gastric symptoms, such as eructation, nausea, vomiting, loss of appetite, and a feeling of oppression in the gastric region. Such gastric dyspepsia is actually observed if the diet has been faulty—for instance, if large amounts of indigestible vegetables have been eaten. If these symptoms occur a short time after this dietetic error and a few hours before the symptoms of appendicitis, especially if the gastric complaints continue for some time, it may safely be assumed that the objectionable diet first caused an acute gastritis and perhaps duodenitis. Thereafter, these conditions probably caused an increase in the inflammation of the cecum, which was present before, to be sure, without giving rise to symptoms. This inflammation may then have spread to the peritoneum. But it is very improbable that an acute catarrhal inflammation of the cecum caused by dietetic errors should extend in a few hours to the appendix and its peritoneal covering. If the gastric disturbances occur simultaneously with the symptoms of perityphlitis or after them, they are probably caused by the inflamed cecum reflexly. If coprostasis has caused the cecum to become entirely impermeable, symptoms of occlusion may appear, and the vomiting of fecal masses and a repulsive fetor of the breath become evident. These signs cease if the coprostasis is relieved by purges and the intestine again becomes permeable.

Fever.—In adults fever may be entirely lacking. If it does occur at the beginning of appendicitis, it rarely rises above 100° F., and usually ceases in a short time. Fever is, however, often noticed in children, since they respond more easily to an inflammation by a rise in the body-temperature. In such cases it rarely ever decreases until the inflammation of the peritoneum subsides. The pulse is correspondingly accelerated.

In suppurative appendicitis and peri-appendicitis the fever is higher and disturbances in the general health are, as a rule, very great. In simple typhlitis, however, they are very slight. The tongue has a dirty, yellowish-drab coating, and the breath is frequently offensive, even if there is no intestinal occlusion. Sometimes the patients have a persistent singultus, which always intensifies the pains for a while. Thirst is increased, and appetite is often absent. If there is a permanent coprostasis in the cecum, the urine contains large quantities of indican, due to increased putrefaction.

Simple perityphlitis, whether starting from the cecum, or, as is the case in 90 or more per cent. of the cases, from the appendix, almost always proceeds favorably if the patients conduct themselves properly and receive correct treatment. The pains in the right ileocecal region soon decrease and finally cease altogether. Then the resistance and sensibility to pressure in this region usually decrease more or less rapidly and finally disappear entirely. If the tumor consists principally of accumulated feces, it often disappears after a few copious evacuations.

The serous effusions in the neighborhood of the cecum and appendix may rapidly be absorbed again. Sometimes, however, they require a long time for their complete resorption. If a considerable dropsy has arisen in the appendix and it has developed into a cyst as a result of the closure of its opening into the cecum, the tumor resulting from this may remain for a long time. This condition is pictured interestingly in George R. Fowler's "Treatise on Appendicitis."

It is, in my experience, exceptional that the simple catarrhal inflammations of the appendix and cecum take a bad turn. This usually occurs only when the inflammation is accompanied by the formation of ulcers. One of these, contrary to the usual fashion, may extend outward through the serosa so rapidly that the perforation occurs before a sufficient agglutination has set in between the cecum and other intestinal sections or the omentum. As a result, the contents of the intestine are emptied into the neighborhood of the cecum, and this causes a suppurative, circumscribed peritonitis, as well as abscess formation in the retroperitoneal, retrocecal connective tissue (paratyphlitis), or possibly even a general peritonitis, which would soon result fatally. Such cases, however, as very minutely described by Deaver, Murphy, Fowler, and Curschmann, are rare in comparison with the great number of those resulting favorably. Perityphlitis may cause great anatomical changes, such as hypertrophies, indurations or thickenings, kinkings of the appendix, adhesions of the same with the cecum and with the omentum or other intestinal sections, or with the front abdominal wall. These may decrease the motility of the adherent intestines, render the downward passage of the feces and chyme more difficult, and thus favor the occurrence of a coprostasis in the cecum and a retention of the feces and the secretion in the appendix.

Relapses.

In this way relapses may easily be caused, and sometimes even internal incarcerations of the intestines. If large ulcers have been formed as a result of typhlitis, they may cause an intestinal stenosis after their cicatrization. Relapsing Appendicitis is described in a separate paragraph.

Prognosis.

If we except the rare cases mentioned above, the prognosis of simple appendicitis, typhlitis, and perityphlitis, as regards life, is favorable. If, however, the patient is advanced in years, the prognosis must be made cautiously, since we can not predict whether or not the perityphlitis will cause greater anatomical changes which may lead to relapses. We must also consider the fact that the catarrhal inflammation of the cecum, which often extends to the appendix, and also simple appendicitis itself, may favor the development of a severe suppurative appendicitis by penetration of septic bacteria through the intestinal walls. It is not possible to determine clinically whether suppurative appendicitis is *always* developed in the basis of a preexisting catarrhal inflammation, or whether it may not at once start up by unusual combinations of grave pathogenic factors, from a comparatively normal mucosa. In the article on " Appendicitis " in the third edition of his " Practice of Medicine," Osler says : " Recovery is the rule. Of 264 cases at St. Thomas' Hospital, 190 recovered; in one instance the appendix was removed; in 2 others attempts were made to remove it. Surgeons claim that getting well in these cases does not mean much ; this is an unduly dark view."

Diagnosis.

Simple uncomplicated catarrhal appendicitis can not always be diagnosed as such with certainty. Only when the inflammation has extended from the mucous membrane to the peritoneum, and when the pregnant symptoms of perityphlitis appear, are these conditions, as a rule, recognizable. It will always be safer to attribute any existing perityphlitis to an extension from a preexisting appendicitis, as the statistics indicate that this will be correct in from 90 to 92 per cent. of the cases. We can assume with certainty that the circumscribed inflammation of the peritoneum was caused by appendicitis, especially when the appearance of perityphlitis occurs suddenly in the midst of good health, without having been preceded or accompanied during the sickness itself by digestive disturbances; when no tumor can be detected in the right ileocecal region, and when only a circumscribed sensibility to pressure exists in the region where the appendix joins the cecum. Edebohls' method of palpating the appendix, which I have described minutely in the chapter on Chronic Appendicitis, offers the only means of instructing ourselves concerning the state of the vermiform process. W. S. Halsted, H. A. Kelly, Shrady, Deaver, Murphy, Long, C. P. Noble, Morris, Mynter, Beck, and other well-known operators have tested and approved of this method of examining the appendix. Personally I have found it useful in many cases, but there are conditions of the abdominal walls (tension, induration, obesity) where the method fails to reveal the appendix.

According to recent observations, most cases of infectious perityphlitis are the result of appendicitis. Many symptoms of the fundamental appendicular disease are observed in the secondary forms of perityphlitis, which are conditioned by the localization of tuberculous, typhoid, syphilitic, actinomycotic, and carcinomatous ulcers in the cecum and appendix. The secondary form, especially if it is caused by the infectious diseases just enumerated, is usually of longer duration than the idiopathic primary appendicitis. For the differentiation of the simple inflammation of the cecum and the appendix, and also of perityphlitis from the severer suppurative inflammation occasionally resulting therefrom, I refer to the chapter in which suppurative appendicitis is described.

Therapeutics.

A persistent constipation, occasionally alternating with a transient diarrhea, and a persistent feeling of pressure, distention in the ileocecal region, are suggestive of a catarrhal inflammation of the cecum. A thorough examination of the ileocecal region by Edebohls' method, and combined palpation with the fingers of one hand in the rectum or vagina and the other hand on the abdomen, should be executed. The first step to be undertaken is to remove the coprostasis and also to provide for regular stools. If there should be a catarrhal appendicitis, this treatment will act favorably upon it; if perityphlitis has occurred in several members of the same family, it is the duty of the family physician to warn them against a long-continuing constipation, since one apparently may inherit an abnormal situation and shape of the appendix (see chapter I, on Anatomy), such as favors the development of appendicitis and perityphlitis.

Diet.

If the characteristic symptoms of appendicitis and perityphlitis have appeared, the patient must stay in bed, even if the pains are only of moderate intensity. At the onset it is well to forbid the introduction of solid and liquid food for twenty-four hours. Later the patient should drink only albumin water, very weak tea, or lemonade. This should continue until it has been ascertained whether the symptoms are caused by a simple catarrhal or by a suppurative inflammation. This abstinence is in many ways beneficial to the patient, especially in those cases of perityphlitis where there is a coprostasis in the cecum, because it prevents the increase of the fecal accumulations and distention in the cecum, and thereby avoids increasing the peristalsis, which may heighten the inflammation. If the patients present gastric complaints, there may be an acute gastritis, and this is also favorably affected by abstinence from food. If the pains are severe, moderate doses of morphin sulphate—$\frac{1}{8}$ to $\frac{1}{6}$ of a grain—can safely be given, preferably dissolved in dilute HCl. If the paroxysms of pain are very violent, hypodermic injections of morphin may be necessary. Whether ice poultices or ice-bags, Priessnitz's, or warm poultices are to be applied in the local treatment can not be dogmatically stated for all cases. If the appendicitis is recent, acute, and associated with fever, the ice-bag is better tolerated; but if the case is of a chronic type, with a palpable tumor of long standing, the hot poultice is more rational. If we are certain, from the course of the disease, that no suppurative inflammation is present, small amounts of liquid food may be given. The early use of purges and the administration of copious enemata should be permitted only according to special indications. If the symptoms of occlusion set in, there is nothing left but to attempt to remove the coprostasis by means of enemata. If these are unsuccessful, purges must be used, even at the risk of having the increased peristalsis cause aggravation of the inflammation.   If the symptoms of inflammation are on the decline, and if a fecal accumulation may be detected in the cecum, water or oil enemata may be used to relieve the coprostasis if spontaneous evacuations have not yet occurred.   In case these enemata are not effective, mild purges may be used simultaneously.   Great caution is necessary in prescribing purges, because a typhlitis may be accompanied by the formation of ulcers, which often remain latent.   If the peristalsis is increased, rupture of slight adhesions may occur and lead to perforation of an ulcer which has extended down to the serosa.   The treatment of those cases in which eruption of pus has caused a suppurative peritonitis will be considered in a separate chapter.   If a tumor can be felt in the ileocecal region some time after the cessation of the inflammatory symptoms, the absorption of the exudation which is still present may be hastened by hot poultices (Leube). Sometimes a cautious massage has a favorable effect after all inflammatory signs have long subsided.   During convalescence, or later on, frequent relapses may occur, constituting chronic relapsing appendicitis, for which it is always advisable to consult with an experienced surgeon.

American and British surgeons have secured very good results in cases of relapsing perityphlitis where the appendix was found diseased or badly kinked as a result of adhesions.   Kroenlein, in 1884, performed the first removal of the vermiform process for acute appendicitis ("Arch. f. klin. Chir.," 1886, Bd. xxxiii); he was followed in 1886 by R. F. Weir (" Med. Record," New York, 1889, vol. xxxv, p. 449) and I. D. Bryant (" Vaillard's Medical Journal," New York, 1887, vol. xliv).   Sonnenburg also has performed resection of the diseased appendix with good results.   Thus in individual cases of simple relapsing appendicitis and perityphlitis an operation is very well justified in the intervals between the attacks.

SUPPURATIVE INFLAMMATION OF THE VERMIFORM APPENDIX (SUPPURATIVE APPENDICITIS WITH OR WITHOUT PERFORATION).

Synonyms.—Suppurative Inflammation of the Cecal Peritoneum and the Retroperitoneal Connective Tissue ; Perityphlitis and Suppurative Paratyphlitis.

For practical reasons I have described appendicitis in two sections—one which runs its course as appendicitis pure and simple, and one in which the suppurative and perforative forms are given. This necessitates the preamble that under certain conditions the simple forms may rapidly or insidiously merge into the severe forms.

Nature, Description, and Etiology.

The suppurative inflammation of the vermiform appendix almost always occurs in connection with a catarrhal appendicitis, which passes over into the severe suppurative type when the pathogenetic microbes which cause the latter find favorable conditions for their development and increase, after their invasion of the mucous membrane. This suppurative inflammation, whether accompanied by a perforation of the appendix or not, always extends to the peritoneum, causing a purulent inflammation. Frequently it also extends to and causes a suppurative inflammation of the retroperitoneal, retrocecal connective tissue (see illustration of ileocolic, ileocecal, and subcecal fossa, Plates 2, 3, and 4, this volume). In the suppurative exudations which are drawn off by puncture and operation, in suppurative appendicitis and its resultant diseases, the Bacterium coli seems always to be present.

Bacteriology.

The following is a list of the various bacteria that have been isolated from the contents and walls of the vermiform appendix, both in the stage of acute inflammation, as well as during the intervals of rest. In 20 cases examined with great regard for bacteriological detail (Tavel and Lanz, "Mittheil. aus Kliniken u. Institut d. Schweiz," Basel, 1893), Tavel and Lanz made cultures from the appendix, the fibrinous and perityphlitic deposits, pus from the perityphlitic abscesses, and exudates from the peritoneum. They found Bacillus coli communis (mobile and immobile), Bacillus fusiformis, Bacillus fœtidus liquefaciens, Bacillus pyocyaneus, Bacillus capsulatus, Staphylococcus citreus, streptococcus, pneumococcus, Coccus conglomeratus, Diplococcus intestinalis (major and minor), spirilli, diphtheria bacillus, bacillus similar to that predominating in hay infusion, organisms of glanders, tetanus, and actinomyces. Only in 3 cases of the 20 was one of these organisms found

singly in pure culture ; these were : one case each of infection with
the streptococci, with the Staphylococcus citreus, and with the colon
bacillus.   With the exception of 3 cases, the colon bacillus was
found in all.   Tavel and Lanz missed this organism absolutely in 2
cases, even in the cultures in which it usually crowds out and sub-
merges all other intestinal bacteria.   Appendicitis can, accordingly,
be considered a polyinfection in which the colon bacillus predominates.

The Bacillus coli is always present in the intestine of healthy
persons, and is found in especially large numbers in the large intestine, without causing any bad reŝults.   It can at all times get into
the appendix in company with the feces.   If it therefore is the
cause, or one of the causes, of suppurative appendicitis and its resulting diseases, we must assume that it acquires pathogenetic
qualities under definite conditions which as yet have not been ascertained.   If the assumption be confirmed that several kinds of bacteria are always concerned in the development of the suppurative
type of appendicitis, it would explain the fact that simple catarrhal
inflammation of the appendix does not, in the majority of cases, go
over into the suppurative form, even if its duration is long and relapses are frequent.   Foreign bodies, small gall-stones which penetrate into the appendix, the decomposition products of the secretion
retained in catarrhal appendicitis, coproliths—all these undoubtedly
act as auxiliary causes by causing a catarrh or an aggravation of
the same.   As to the coproliths, it has been assumed in recent times
that they played a very important rôle in the etiology of suppurative inflammation.   In themselves, however, they could hardly
cause the latter.   They may, however, facilitate the invasion of
pathogenic microbes into the peritoneum and the retrocecal connective tissue by the fact that they may cause or favor the formation and
perforation of ulcers.   In 100 autopsies Einhorn found perforation
of the appendix in 91 cases.   Matterstock found 132 perforations of
the appendix in 146 necropsies of appendicitis subjects.   In 200 cases
of appendicitis collected by MacMurtry the cecum was not affected
in a single case.   Sonnenburg operated upon 200 cases, and established that the inflammation had started from the appendix in 129.
In a more recent monograph ("Pathol. u. Therap. d. Perityphlitis,
Appendicitis Simplex, Perforativa, Gangrænosa," 4. Aufl., Leipzig,

1900), Eduard Sonnenburg reports 600 operations for suppurative appendicitis up to January, 1900, with the same proportionate origin as above stated. In by far the great majority of cases, therefore, suppurative perityphlitis and paratyphlitis are caused by a suppurative appendicitis. In an insignificantly small number of cases, however, they may be the result of a catarrhal inflammation of the cecum, accompanied by the formation of ulcers. If these ulcers, contrary to their usual behavior, quickly extend downward to the serosa before firm agglutinations with neighboring intestinal sections or the omentum have been formed, when the perforation of the serosa takes place the intestinal, or at least the bacterial, contents cause a suppurative inflammation of the peritoneum, and frequently of the retrocecal connective tissue also.

In extremely rare instances a suppurative paratyphlitis and perityphlitis, and also a suppurative appendicitis, may be caused by the fact that a suppurative paranephritis, parametritis, salpingitis, ovaritis, or inflammations of other organs or parts of organs—caries of the spine or the pelvis—may extend to the retrocecal connective tissue, and thence to the peritoneum, the vermiform appendix, or the cecum. Suppurative appendicitis sets in either very suddenly, in the midst of good health, or after stomach complaints and digestive disturbances have preceded it. It is usually accompanied by high fever and by violent pains in the abdomen, which are often intensified into paroxysms, and which soon afterward become restricted to the right ileocecal region. They are greatly intensified by pressure. A more or less sharply defined tumor of varying size may almost always be detected in the right ileocecal region, this tumor always having a suppurative nucleus (suppurative or fibrino-suppurative exudation), whether it be located in the appendix, outside of it, or outside of the cecum. It may be caused by the inflammatory thickening of the cecum and appendix; occasionally by the thickened omentum, which may place itself over the diseased intestinal sections like an open apron, and also by edematous or suppurative infiltrations of the abdominal wall and the transverse fascia, and finally by accumulated feces. The appearance of the patient is that of one gravely diseased; thirst is often increased; the appetite is gone, and the tongue is dry and covered with a thick coating. If the inflammation increases, the fever usually rises also ; the pulse is accelerated and weak. If no operation is performed, the result of the disease is decided principally by the following issues: The pus collected in the appendix may break forth outward or not ; a general septic or fibrinous suppurative peritonitis may set in, which almost always causes death, and hardly ever confines itself to one place ; the perityphlitic or paratyphlitic abscess may completely sequestrate itself; the pus may break through into the intestine, the bladder, the uterus, and the vagina, and empty itself completely or partially ; or it may make its way toward the diaphragm or toward other parts of the abdomen.   If there is no spontaneous passage of the pus outward, and no operation is undertaken, most of the patients die as a result of the loss of strength and impaired nutrition, which may be accelerrated by the formation of fecal, renal, or subphrenic abscesses, chronic pyemia, thrombosis of the portal vein, and other complications.

Suppurative appendicitis, perityphlitis, and paratyphlitis, just as the simple form of these diseases, are observed more frequently in men than in women.   They are also fairly common in youthful persons.

Pathological Anatomy.

Numerous operations and dissections have shown in recent times that the pathologic-anatomical changes caused by suppurative appendicitis, perityphlitis, and paratyphlitis are very numerous and varied, and that they may range within wide limits.   This is very easily understood, although from 91 to 95 per cent. of the cases of perityphlitis and paratyphlitis are caused by the same fundamental disease—that is, by a suppurative appendicitis.   In the few remaining cases, however, they are due to a simple catarrhal inflammation of the cecum, accompanied by the formation of ulcers, to the spread of a perinephritis, parametritis, psoitis, and suppurative inflammations about the female sexual apparatus and the biliary vessels.   The anatomical appearance of the disease varies according to the locality of the pus collection—i. e., whether the pus remains collected in the appendix or breaks outward.   Suppurative appendicitis, whether the wall of the appendix is perforated or not, often leads to a general septic or fibrinous suppurative peritonitis, which often ends · fatally.   The inflammation of the peritoneal covering of the appendix may extend intraperitoneally and extra-peritoneally to the retrocecal connective tissue and to the cecum, and may cause the formation of adhesions.   The pus of the peri-typhlitic and paratyphlitic abscesses may also break through into various sections of the intestines : oftenest into the cecum, more rarely into the ascending colon, the duodenum, the rectum, the bladder, the uterus, the vagina, or even through the abdominal wall externally.   These escapes of pus may or may not be followed by a spontaneous cure, according as the pus is emptied entirely or partially.

If the pus collected in the appendix in suppurative appendicitis does not break forth, the inflammation nevertheless always spreads from the mucous membrane to the peritoneum; sometimes it causes a general septic or fibrinous suppurative peritonitis.   The secondary peritonitis, especially if it causes a thickening of the walls of the appendix, often assists in the sequestration or in-closure of the suppurative exudation.   The longer such an em-pyema is sequestrated, the less danger it brings for its surround-ings.   If the opening of the appendix into the cecum again be-comes permeable, the pus may be emptied through it into the cecum, and a spontaneous cure set in.   In general, the nonperfor-ating, suppurative appendicitis, which is considered (Sonnenburg) a transitional form between simple appendicitis and the suppurating, perforating type, usually results more favorably than the latter.   In the majority of cases of suppurative appendicitis, perforation of the appendix results, accompanied by an eruption of the pus outward. This undoubtedly is frequently hastened by coproliths which exert a constant pressure upon the mucous membrane of the appendix and upon the deeper layers, and thus often cause necrosis and the for-mation of ulcers.   When the pus breaks through, the coprolith may pass out with it or remain in the appendix.   If no coprolith is found in the appendix or in its neighborhood, it does not exclude the possibility that the pus has softened or dissolved it.   In suppu-rative appendicitis the vermiform process often suffers extensive morbid changes.   Its walls may be thickened or it may be changed into a solid strand as a result of obliteration.   Obstructions and kinkings due to retracting adhesions are fairly common.   In many cases it is partially or completely sequestrated as a result of an annular ulceration or gangrene.   In one case mentioned by Israel, a coprolith as large as a bullet was closed up in the lumen of the appendix which had sequestrated.   Before the pus breaks out through the walls of the appendix the circumscribed peritonitis which precedes it very often causes agglutination with the neighboring organs.   When perforation, therefore, sets in and the eruption of the pus occurs into the empty abdominal cavity, general peritonitis is prevented, and the inflammation restricted to a circumscribed suppurative peritonitis (perityphlitis).   The more complete and capable of resistance the protecting wall is which separates the pus from the peritoneal cavity, the less is the danger of a general peritonitis.   If the pus is intensely infectious and if ulcers are developed, the perforation may take place before sufficient adhesions have been formed.   This also happens if the adhesions are destroyed at several places by the suppuration.   In such cases the pus gets into the free abdominal cavity, and a general septic or a fibrino-suppurative peritonitis is the result.   The former always causes death ; the latter may, in very exceptional cases, finally keep within certain limits, and after a very long time, terminate by so-called healing, in exceptional cases. Numerous adhesions between the individual intestinal loops and surrounding organs always remain as has been described in the section on External Peritoneal Constrictions.   These may, later on, cause coprostasis, obstruction, kinkings, and internal incarcerations of the intestines.   The inflammation very often extends from the peritoneum of the appendix to the retrocecal connective tissue, causing the formation of paratyphlitic abscesses.   The spread of the inflammation to the peritoneal covering of the cecum often causes agglutinations of the appendix to the cecum, to other intestinal loops, to neighboring organs, and to the front abdominal wall.   A glance at Plates 2, 3, and 4 will aid in explaining these extensions.   These agglutinations may often cause recurrences of perityphlitis and of other previously mentioned diseases. The fate of the pus of the perityphlitic and paratyphlitic abscesses is variable.   In many cases the pus is thickened by the absorption of its liquid constituents, and then sometimes it even loses its power of infection.   After the disintegration of the pus-cells, the detritus may then be gradually absorbed.   If the thickened suppuration remains infectious, a new danger arises for the patient if a part of the pus is absorbed into the blood—namely, metastatic abscess. Besides, the suppuration may break through into the intestine, the bladder, the uterus, or the vagina, and pass off, or it may take its course toward other sections of the abdomen, especially downward by gravitation and upward toward the diaphragm, causing liver abscesses, subphrenic abscesses, psoas abscesses, empyema, pyopneumothorax, and suppurative pericarditis. The subphrenic abscesses are very often caused by a suppurative perityphlitis. In one case described by Curschmann the suppurative accumulation broke through into the lungs and the bronchial tubes, and finally a cure was attained. If the suppuration has made its way into other sections of the body, it often breaks through at remote places—under Poupart's ligament, at the hollow of the knee, in the region of the spleen, or the back—after the skin has become red and sometimes edematous. Since the location and length of the appendix may vary, we can easily understand how sequestrated perityphlitic abscesses may be found in various parts of the abdomen, sometimes even in the left half.

Finally, the erosion of the blood-vessels may cause fatal hemorrhages, their compression and the spread of the inflammation to their walls may cause thrombosis and pylephlebitis, with their consequences. If the suppuration remains stagnating for some time, it may undergo ichorous decomposition, especially if it is contaminated by the intestinal contents. In such cases it sometimes contains much gas. Although such exudations may exist a long time without causing any great damage, yet there is always great danger that putrefactive matter may be absorbed and that septicemia may set in. As to the locality of the breaking through of the suppuration into the intestine, this occurs most frequently in the cecum; more rarely in the ascending colon, duodenum, or rectum. A primary perforation of the cecum, due to the formation of ulcers, also occurs in extremely rare instances. If the suppuration has passed off completely, a spontaneous cure may occur. The complete emptying of the pus is, however, usually prevented by a premature closure of the opening of the fistula. The pathologic-anatomical changes accordingly vary within wide limits. The frequent relapses occurring, especially when the resection of the appendix was impossible, have already been described.

Symptomatology.

The disease either begins very suddenly, in the midst of good health, or after having been preceded by gastric distress or digestive disturbances—constipation, alternating occasionally with diarrhea. These symptoms are often caused by catarrhal typhlitis. Sometimes the disease is directly attributed to violent bodily exertions or errors in diet. Violent pains are at first felt in the epigastrium, the left half of the abdomen, or the entire abdomen, but these soon localize themselves to the right ileocecal region. In severe cases the pains become almost unendurable, and are intensified at every bodily movement, on deep breathing, and on coughing or sneezing. They often radiate toward the back, the left side of the abdomen, or the legs, and are increased by pressure in the right ileocecal region. Usually a resistance which is very sensitive to pressure or a tumor of the size of a pigeon's or a hen's egg may be detected very early in the right ileocecal region. This is either sharply defined or is gradually lost in its surroundings. The skin over it is movable, but the tumor itself usually is fixed. The tumor may be due to various pathological factors, prominent among which are the purulent exudation of the appendix, or, in its neighborhood, the inflammatory infiltration of the diseased intestinal sections; sometimes it is due to the thickened omentum, a serous or suppurative infiltration of the abdominal wall, and a fecal accumulation in the cecum, if it existed at the beginning of the disease. When there is coprostasis of the cecum, the tumor is generally larger in size. If both a perityphlitic and a paratyphlitic abscess exist, the resistance may extend to Poupart's ligament, and backward to the region of the loins. If the tumor is small, it gives a muffled percussion sound only when deeply indented. The sound, however, is often tympanitic, because some intestinal loops filled with gas may be situated over the exudation. This is also the case if the exudation itself contains gases. On palpating such tumors by abrupt thrusting motions, a peculiar crackling sensation can sometimes be felt, according to Sahli, which is not present in fecal accumulations in the cecum. This symptom indicates a large perforation of the appendix, but I must caution against making "abrupt thrusting motions." They are very painful and dangerous. A fluctuation can be detected only when there is a copious collection of pus; its absence, therefore, does not argue against a suppuration. If the inflammation and suppuration cause considerable disturbances in the circulation, an edematous infiltration of the skin above the tumor in the right ileocecal region and in the immediate neighborhood is produced. Sometimes this edema of the skin extends beyond the middle line of the body. In the further development of the disease the resistance increases more or less slowly. It may also remain unchanged for a long time if the suppuration remains in the appendix and does not force its way out, or if the perityphlitic or paratyphlitic abscess is surrounded by a firm wall of adhesions. In many cases the resistance disappears entirely after a while, as a result of the descent of the suppurative exudation. In such cases it can be discovered in males only by an examination of the rectum; in females only by the bulging it produces in the vagina.

The general health is, as a rule, very much impaired in perityphlitis. The expression of the patient is anxious, and the eyes are sunken. The sufferer assumes a dorsal position, carefully avoiding every motion which may intensify the pain, breathing gently, and suppressing, so far as possible, all desire to cough. The legs are usually drawn up close to the abdomen, so as to relieve the tension of the abdominal walls. The temperature is greatly increased up to 103° F. or more, especially in the first few days. At this time the fever is continuous; if the patient grows worse, the fever usually increases at the same time, so that its course is a reliable indicator as to the patient's condition. For instance, the fever increases when the suppuration breaks through the walls of the appendix; when the inflammation spreads to the retrocecal connective tissue, and causes the formation of abscesses; or when the suppuration forces its way into the pleura, the pericardium, etc. If the suppurative exudation is thoroughly walled off, the fever, as a rule, diminishes or ceases entirely; even in large paratyphlitic abscesses it may be very slight or absent altogether. The pulse is accelerated. The thirst is increased, while the appetite is gone. The tongue is dry and coated. As a rule, the stools are retained, even when there are no great fecal accumulations in the cecum, because the suppurative exudation either exerts a pressure on the cecum, or the intestinal muscularis is paralyzed as a result of peritonitis. If there was a large fecal accumulation in the cecum at the beginning of the disease, so that the intestine is impermeable, the symptoms of occlusion may appear, together with vomiting of fecal matter. Meteorism may be detected in some of the cases, and often increases with the further development of the disease. The urine is scanty and contains large amounts of indican if the coprostasis is severe; sometimes it also contains albumoses, especially if the fever is very high. Suppurative appendicitis and perityphlitis, similar to simple typhlitis, may be preceded by vomiting and other dyspeptic symptoms on the part of the stomach, especially if the diet has been faulty. Sometimes, however, these gastric symptoms may occur afterward, and the pains are temporarily intensified by them. Persistent singultus has the same aggravating effect. Large perityphlitic and paratyphlitic abscesses are often accompanied by profuse sweating. If the inflammation and peritonitic irritation be very great, or if the suppuration be very copious, great pains are felt during urination soon after the first appearance of the disease. The patients, especially children, then suppress the desire to urinate, for fear of the pain, until the bladder is excessively full, and then the pains become almost unendurable, and urination is impossible because of paralysis of the bladder. It is very important to measure the daily amount of urine passed in every case of perforating appendicitis, and to use the catheter whenever inhibitory suppression manifests itself. Other symptoms, such as paresthesia and anesthesia of the legs, shivering sensations, formication, persistent erections, and elevation of the right testicle, usually indicate a large accumulation of pus, which may exert pressure upon the nerves issuing from the vertebral canal, or produce peritonitis. The prognosis of the disease will vary according to the following considerations: Whether the suppuration formed in the vermiform appendix breaks forth soon or late into the cecum, or whether a perforation of its wall takes place; whether the perityphlitic and paratyphlitic abscesses become walled off from the general peritoneum; whether a diffuse septic or a fibrinous suppurative peritonitis arises as a result of the entrance of the pus into the peritoneal cavity.*

---

* Microscopic examination of the blood yields information of value. A rising leukocytosis associated with pain, fever, and induration should be looked upon as an indication for surgical intervention, and will be considered in the chapter on Surgical Treatment (chap. VI).

According to Fitz, a general perforative peritonitis, when it occurs at all in appendicitis, usually sets in between the second and fourth days. The greater the length of time after the beginning of the sickness, the less danger there is of suppuration breaking through into the peritoneal cavity, since firmer adhesions are being formed. Many other dangers, however, threaten the patient in this case, as may be demonstrated by citing the numerous resultant conditions of suppurative perityphlitis. In some cases the most important symptoms, such as pain, fever, and disturbance in the general health, decrease in intensity a few days after the beginning of the disease; in others they continue with undiminished violence. When the improvement occurs early in the history of the case, it is seldom lasting; the pains and the fever soon increase again, because the inflammation has spread further and the amount of suppuration has increased. This alternation between growing better and growing worse may be repeated several times, until finally there is a complete cure or, if there is no operation, the patient dies from one of the numerous resultant conditions of suppurative perityphlitis. There are cases on record in which the suppurative accumulation broke through into the intestine, the bladder, the vagina, etc., and, after having been completely emptied, a cure was effected. In my experience these cases are extremely rare, however, and generally require months or years to accomplish this result. More frequently, however, the emptying is not complete; a part of the suppuration remains, and after a temporary improvement, the disease appears to start "de novo." The suppuration may be emptied into the intestine several times with the same result. If, even then, no operation is performed, a cure very rarely takes place. Usually the patients die of a gradual loss of strength, of chronic pyemia or of some other complication. There are cases in whom the improvement lasts so long that the hope seems justified that the suppuration either has been entirely discharged or has been absorbed. Later on, while the patient apparently is convalescing, the symptoms of pyopneumothorax, of pyemia, of suppurative pericarditis, etc., may often appear very suddenly, or the suppuration may break forth through the skin at a remote place, and thus prove that the suppurative exudation has continued and has made its way to other parts of the body. The conditions for a spontaneous cure are most

favorable if the suppuration does not break through the walls of
the appendix, but is encapsulated by their induration and thickening.   In such cases the suppuration may finally be emptied entirely
into the cecum through the mouth of the appendix.   The differences in the progress of suppurative perityphlitis are so manifold
that it is impossible to consider them all.   These many grave possibilities are detailed with such minuteness in order to demonstrate
that they constitute eventualities that should be avoided rather than
hoped for.   Spontaneous cures brought about by discharge of pus
through exits no one can foretell occur so extremely rarely
that I look upon them as miracles.   They must be mentioned, however, because they have really been observed.   In my own practice
I have personally seen a discharge of pus from a peri-appendicial
abscess once into the colon and once into the vagina, after operation
had been obstinately refused.   The future history of such so-called
"spontaneous cures" does not prove them to be "cures."   In my
experience such cases often suffer from enterostenoses, or new complications set up by the artificial passage burrowed by the pus.

Actinomycosis of the appendix and the cecum, which is very rare,
may take a course very like that of a suppurative perityphlitis (Lanz).
I have seen such a case at Hahn's clinic (Krankenhaus Friedrichshain) in Berlin.   It is distinguished from the latter by an extremely
chronic development, by a general, more firm infiltration, by
multiple fistulous formations, by an almost complete absence of
intestinal symptoms, and by the reaction of the peritoneum, which
remains local.   If the suppuration is removed by an operation,
actinomyces granules can be discovered in it.

Relapses are frequent, especially in the rare spontaneously cured
cases of suppurative perityphlitis.   In cases treated surgically,
relapses, in my experience, have occurred only as a result of secondary complications,—peritonitis and its consequences,—especially
when the operation was delayed.   These relapses may have the
same course as the primary disease.   It is often observed, however,
that the disease symptoms decrease in intensity in the recurring
relapses, and may finally, in extremely rare instances, cease altogether, possibly because the appendix has become completely obliterated.   The same rules hold good here as have already been stated
concerning relapsing and recurrent appendicitis.

Prognosis.

It can readily be seen, from the description of the progress of suppurative perityphlitis and of the anatomical changes found in it, that it is a very dangerous condition. The prognosis, therefore, must be stated unfavorably in all cases where it is impossible to perform laparotomy. The number of spontaneous cures in those cases of severe suppurative perityphlitis where no operation is performed is very small. Since relapses are very frequent until old age sets in, the prognosis must be guarded.

The prognosis of suppurative perityphlitis has been greatly improved by the introduction of the operative treatment, which has saved many lives. To be sure, even now patients often die after the operation. In such cases, however, the disease usually was peculiarly malignant and the infection was very great, or the operation was performed too late, often on account of the objection of the patient or of relatives. The intensity of the symptoms gives no reliable basis for a prognosis in suppurative appendicitis and perityphlitis. Experience has shown that very violent cases accompanied by high fever often result favorably if the suppuration breaks through into the intestines or other organs, while in other cases, which take a mild course soon after the beginning of the disease, the symptoms of a general septic or fibrino-suppurative peritonitis may suddenly appear. Of these two, the first always ends fatally ; the second may be cured in exceptional cases. The occurrence of general peritonitis is most to be feared on the second or the fourth day, since it is most frequently observed at this time. There is less danger of general peritonitis after the disease has lasted for some time, but other dangers are at hand. Even during apparent convalescence the symptoms of pyopneumothorax, of empyema, or of suppurative pericarditis may set in and cause the patient's death. The prognosis of perforating suppurative appendicitis is less favorable than that of simple catarrhal inflammation with slight pus-formation in the vermiform appendix. When the exudation is ichorously decomposed, we have to fear septicemia and its results. Besides this, relapses are frequent, even in those cases where an operation was performed, if the peritonitis was extensive, and more especially if it was impossible to remove the appendix.

Diagnosis.

Sometimes it is very difficult, or even impossible, to decide at the first appearance of the symptoms pointing to perforating appendicitis and perityphlitis whether it is caused by a simple fibrinous inflammation of the peritoneal covering of the cecum or appendix or by a suppurative inflammation of the same. After a brief, careful observation the former may usually, however, be distinguished from the latter with certainty. Simple perityphlitis not accompanied by suppuration is hardly ever attended with fever, and the general health usually suffers but little. In the rare instances where fever sets in at the beginning of the disease it usually ceases very soon. The pains and the tumor in the right ileocecal region also decrease after a few days if the patient conducts himself properly, and the cure is soon effected. Suppurative perityphlitis always commences with high fever. If the inflammation increases, the fever usually grows worse. The general health is greatly impaired. The tumor and the pains last for a longer time than in simple perityphlitis. The symptomatology and course may make the differential diagnosis easier. The origin of suppurative perityphlitis can not be determined with certainty : whether suppurative perityphlitis is the result of suppurative appendicitis, of typhlitis combined with the formation of ulcers, or an extension of a parametritis, salpingitis, cholecystitis, or paranephritis. Careful study of the previous history, together with a thorough examination of the rectum and vagina, may often throw light on the origin. It is a matter of indifference for the treatment whether the suppuration which is present belonged to a perityphlitic or paratyphlitic abscess. Clinically we can not ascertain, in the individual cases, whether we are dealing with an idiopathic, suppurative inflammation of the appendix or with a suppurative perityphlitis conditioned by tubercle bacilli or other specific disease excitants. It is not very easy to discover, in those cases which begin very violently, whether the suppurative perityphlitis is caused by a perforating suppurative appendicitis or by a simple purulent inflammation of the vermiform appendix without perforation. These points are critically discussed in the section on the Operative Treatment of Appendicitis.

Exploratory Puncture.—A number of German clinicians have suggested exploratory puncture for this differentiation, and also for

the demonstration of pus. If the pus which is drawn off by puncture has no fecal odor, it shows either that there has been no
perforation of the appendix or that the opening was so small
and closed so quickly that none or but little of the intestinal
contents came out. If the suppuration has a fecal odor, they
assume that there was a serious perforation of the appendix, and
that, consequently, a larger quantity of the intestinal contents
exuded. We must not, however, exclude the possibility that when
the puncture is made the pus may be drawn directly from the
appendix. The detection of suppuration is of great importance,
both for the recognition of suppurative perityphlitis and for its differentiation from other diseases which have similar symptoms. This
detection would be much facilitated by such exploratory punctures,
which Fleischer, Sahli, and Curschmann recommend if the results
could be depended upon and the methods were safe. Fleischer
claims never to have found a puncture to be followed by those
grave results which have been ascribed to them. He urges
that the puncture must be made with the proper aseptic precautions. Only a positive result, however, is of use for the diagnosis of suppurative appendicitis. I do not consider exploratory
puncture at all advisable or necessary for this purpose, even if it
were entirely free from danger. The practitioner will be right in
from ninety-one to ninety-four times out of every 100 cases if he
assumes that the perityphlitis is due to a perforating appendicitis,
and acts accordingly—namely, calls in consultation an experienced
surgeon. The presence of pus can generally be recognized by other
signs. Even if, at the operation, the inflamed appendix is not found
perforated, this does not constitute an argument against dangerous
peritoneal infection, which can take place without perforation, as I
have described elsewhere. Moreover, a small perforation may have
occurred at one time and may have healed up or closed again in
some way.

Differential Diagnosis.

Suppurative appendicitis may require differentiation from cancer
of the cecum, intussusception, psoas abscess, floating kidney,
typhoid fever, pyosalpinx, fibroid tumor, extra-uterine pregnancy,
suppurating ovarian cyst, menopause, painful menstruation, nephritic

colic, pyonephrosis, perinephritic abscess, growths of the kidney, inflammation of the ureter, perforation of some part of the intestinal tract, dysentery, splenic abscess, tubercular peritonitis, hepatic and perihepatic abscess, rupture of the gall-bladder, inguinal hernia, enlarged mesenteric glands, abscess of the abdominal wall, mesenteric hematocele, aneurysm of the iliac artery, hip-joint disease, lumbar abscess, pneumonia, pleurisy, and biliary colic. The majority of these conditions hardly require special differentiation in this chapter because they have already been considered elsewhere, or they can be distinguished by a single symptom or sign.

Cancer of the Cecum.—This occurs in advanced age, at a time when suppurative appendicitis is rare. The palpation reveals a nodular tumor or marked hardness in carcinoma; one that is not so hard, but more sensitive, in appendicitis and perityphlitis. The malignant neoplasm is of slow growth and attended by progressive loss of flesh. The extremely chronic course of the disease will argue for cancer. (See chapter on Malignant Tumors.)

Intussusception.—Those invaginations which occur most frequently have their seat in the ileocecal region. The onset is more abrupt than in appendicitis, and the pain is remissive in character. The stools contain mucus and blood, which greatly facilitate the diagnosis of intussusception. Vomiting is a prominent symptom. (See chapter on Intussusception.)

Other Forms of Intestinal Obstruction.—Onset is more abrupt, pain of severer type, remissive in character, and referred frequently, though not always, to the seat of the obstruction. There are absolute constipation and suppression of flatus, with early and persistent vomiting, soon becoming fecal, a condition rarely occurring except in the later stages of appendicitis. Intussusception is the most common form of obstruction met with in children. Shock and collapse appear early in obstruction ; not so frequently and later in appendicitis. (See chapter on Special Forms of Obstruction.)

Psoas Abscess.—The differentiation between psoas abscess and suppurative appendicitis is difficult only in exceptional cases. In the former, deep pressure over the right iliac fossa will reveal tenderness of the psoas muscles, but will fail to give evidence of either the enlarged appendix or perityphlitic abscess. One of the most important points in favor of psoas abscess is the appearance of the patient, which, as a rule, is suggestive of tuberculosis. A complete previous history, the temperature record, and a thorough examination of the lungs and spine will render the diagnosis comparatively certain.

Floating Kidney.—Appendicitis naturally presents the characteristic evidences of inflammation—fever, swelling, and pain; these are absent in floating kidney. The floating kidney should, moreover, be easily palpable and its characteristic shape detected. It should be restorable to its normal position by properly directed pressure. When the ureter has become twisted (Dietl's crisis), the resemblance to appendicitis becomes greater, but even then, there is no fever or rigidity of the abdominal wall in case of floating kidney, and there is generally a history of movable tumor previous to the attack. A careful examination of the urine may reveal the presence of blood or blood-corpuscles. I can not advise careful analysis of the urine in all cases of appendicitis too urgently. The renal irritation of appendicitis may be the result of autointoxication, reflex disturbances from the sympathetic nervous system, or the actual extension of the periappendicial or perityphlitic inflammation to some part of the urinary tract. Thus in the urine of appendicitis we may find traces of albumin, cylindroids, hyaline casts, renal epithelium, and, very rarely, pus and blood-cells.

Typhoid fever can be readily distinguished by its clinical history, its temperature curve, an examination of the abdomen, and the Widal reaction.

Pyosalpinx.—Vaginal, or combined vaginal and abdominal, or vaginal and rectal examination will reveal an inflammatory tumor in immediate relation with the uterus in pyosalpinx. When the abscess is in the right ovary, it may present all the symptoms of appendicitis: pain, tenderness on pressure in the right iliac fossa, and fever. Bimanual examination should disclose the suppurating ovary.

Fibroid Tumor.—When fibroid tumors are located in the broad ligament, the resemblance to appendicitis is confusing. The bimanual examination will detect the presence of the growth, and localize the pain and tenderness on pressure. There will also be a history of metrorrhagia.

Extra-uterine Pregnancy.—In extra-uterine pregnancy there is, as a rule, cessation of the menses for two or more periods and other symptoms of pregnancy. There will be attacks of long-continued paroxysmal pain, which may be followed by collapse. The pain is not colicky. Another symptom is an irregular sanguinolent discharge from the vagina, in which portions of the decidua are frequently found. The majority of cases of extra-uterine pregnancy present a history of sterility for five or six years previous to the abnormal conception.

Suppurating Ovarian Cyst.—See differentiation of pyosalpinx. The rigidity of the abdominal wall is not so marked as in appendicitis. The tumor is more lasting, and the characteristic ovarian pain, which differs so markedly from the colicky appendicial pains, can be brought out by pressure.

Menopause.—The localized pain in the right side and irregular gastro-intestinal symptoms of women during the menopause can be distinguished from appendicitis by the previous history, absence of rigidity of the abdominal walls, no swelling about the appendix, and the neurotic symptoms of the menopause. If necessary, bimanual local examination will be conclusive.

Painful Menstruation.—Dysmenorrhea often is accompanied by the same rigidity of the lower abdominal walls as is met with in appendicitis. The pain naturally lasts only as long as the menstrual period. If both ovaries are congested, the tenderness will be bilateral. The pain in appendicitis is at the beginning more diffuse, and becomes localized in the right iliac fossa later on. The anamnesis of dysmenorrhea will be a valuable aid in diagnosis.

Nephritic colic is usually ushered in by a chill. The excruciating pain is more perceptible posteriorly than anteriorly, and radiates along the course of the ureter down into the ovary or testicle, and is diminished by the voiding of urine. The right iliac fossa is not sensitive to pressure and contains no tender mass ; the abdominal wall is not rigid and there is no fever. Errors between these two conditions are most liable to occur in the early stages of appendicitis. I have elsewhere given the clinical history of a patient, himself a physician, who had suffered with repeated attacks of renal colic that led to the resection of what was apparently a normal appendix, thus impressing upon the clinician the necessity of a very careful examination of the patient and his excretions. In appendicitis the pain at the onset is more diffuse, is increased by pressure, and is not influenced by micturition.

Pyonephrosis.—In exceptional cases of appendicitis there may be retraction of the testicle on the right side, umbilical pain, and frequent and painful micturition. These are the cases that are liable to be confounded with pyonephrosis. In the latter disease the tenderness is more especially elicited by pressure over the kidney, and the urine contains pus and sometimes blood. In the absence of characteristic urinary signs the differentiation is still more difficult. Then the only course to pursue is a tentative one, with daily examinations of the urine and occasional catheterization of the ureters. This should especially be done in nephritic colic if there is any doubt about the diagnosis.

Perinephritic abscess does not present the characteristic symptoms of appendicitis—viz., pain, rigidity of the abdominal muscles, and tenderness. There is also absence of disturbance of the intestinal functions.

Growths of the Kidney.—Catheterization of the ureter, as well as careful palpation, absence of inflammatory symptoms, and the presence of blood and pus in the urine are the dividing-lines of diagnosis from this condition.

Inflammation of the Ureter.—This is usually an extension of inflammation of the bladder or the result of the passage of a renal calculus. The ureter may, of course, become involved in tuberculosis or carcinoma issuing from some other organ. Ureteritis is not accompanied by rigidity of the abdominal muscles, and the urine contains pus, blood, and ureteral epithelium.

Perforation of Some Part of the Intestinal Tract.—Whenever the intestinal tract has become perforated, there must be a history of previous disease, such as duodenal or gastric ulcer, typhoid fever, carcinoma, intestinal obstruction, etc. These have been described in other chapters of this work.

Dysentery.—In dysentery no localized pain or mass is palpable in the right iliac fossa (see chapter on Dysentery).

Splenic Abscess.—If pain is manifested in this rare condition, it is in the left hypochondriac region. Splenic abscess should present the previous history of trauma or septic infection, or of those constitutional diseases in which enlargement of the spleen takes place. Of course, the splenic abscess may appear as a complication of appendicitis.

Tubercular peritonitis may present great difficulty of differential diagnosis from appendicitis. The most significant symptom is the presence of ascites, which develops rather early in tubercular peritonitis. Exploratory puncture of the abdomen and sedimentation of the aspirated liquid may disclose the presence of the tubercle bacillus. Naturally, the appendix may also be the seat of tuberculous invasion, at the same time (see Deaver, *l. c.*, plate XVI). Here an exact diagnosis can not be made except by exploratory laparotomy.

Hepatic and Perihepatic Abscess.—A number of cases have occurred in my practice in which the diagnosis of appendicitis was made and the operation revealed a perihepatic abscess. This condition and **rupture of the gall-bladder** will, in the majority of cases, be preceded by a history of biliary colic. In both conditions exploratory laparotomy is needed to establish the diagnosis.

Inguinal Hernia.—A careful examination of all the hernial orifices should be made in each and every case of appendicitis, and then incipient inguinal hernia can not escape detection. It is not accompanied by fever or abdominal rigidity.

Enlarged Mesenteric Glands.—These are only exceptionally accompanied by fever, pain, and abdominal rigidity.

Abscess of the Abdominal Walls.—The swelling in abscess of the abdominal walls moves simultaneously with these walls. There are absence of intestinal symptoms and presence of local evidences of pus.

Mesenteric Hematocele.—This is a result of trauma and rupture of the mesenteric vessels. It is not accompanied by pain, rigidity, and fever. Its onset is abrupt, but it may undergo suppuration and then closely resemble chronic appendicitis.

Aneurysm of the Iliac Artery.—Circumscribed collections of pus around the iliac artery may develop in acute appendicitis, but it can be distinguished from aneurysm by the absence of the bruit.

Hip-joint Disease.—The absence of intestinal symptoms, curving of the lumbar spine when the limb is brought into a fully extended position, the characteristic deformity, inability to execute the normal movements of the joint, and pain referred to the knee are sufficient to characterize disease of the hip-joint, and distinguish it from appendicitis.

Lumbar Abscess.—This is usually preceded by history of spinal disease, presents a characteristic swelling, edema of the overlying tissue, and slow onset, but there is an absence of acute tenderness, intestinal symptoms, and rigidity of the abdominal muscles.

Pneumonia and Pleurisy.—Careful auscultation and percussion of the lungs should give the desired information concerning these conditions.

Biliary Colic.—Similarly to perihepatic abscess and perforation of the gall-bladder, biliary colic may present some confusing symptoms. It may set in with acute pain and persistent vomiting, but in biliary colic there will most likely be a history of previous attacks of less intensity, accompanied perhaps by jaundice. Fever is absent in uncomplicated biliary colic. The characteristic clay-colored stools of jaundice are an important aid to the diagnosis, as are also any gall-stones that may possibly be found by the stool-sieve. The pain of biliary colic is more continuous and intense. It radiates from the right axillary line to the umbilicus. Sometimes it is more marked posteriorly, or involves the epigastric region. The gall-bladder will be found the most acute locality upon pressure. The characteristics of pain in appendicitis have been so frequently described that they do not require repetition.

The following cases from the reports of the Pathological Institute of the Wiener Allgemeines Krankenhaus throw much light not only on the etiology and prognosis, but also upon the liability with which an erroneous diagnosis can be made in appendicitis. In the years from 1870 to 1896 inclusive there were, according to Nothnagel (*l. c.*), in 44,940 necropsies:

Cases of appendicitis and peri- and paratyphlitis, 148, or 0.3 per cent.

1 to 9 years, 2 cases	40 to 49 years, 18 cases
10 " 19 " 43 "	50 " 59 " 4 "
20 " 29 " 49 "	60 " 69 " 5 "
30 " 39 " 24 "	70 " 79 " 1 case

No statement of age, 2 cases.

Statements concerning changes in the vermiform appendix, 129 cases :

Perforation present in, ... 124 cases
Without perforation, ... 5 "
No statement concerning the appendix, ... 19 "
Coproliths, ... 42 "
Other foreign bodies, ... 2 "
Diffuse peritonitis, ... 107 "
Combination with affections of the genital tract, ... 6 "
Statement concerning genital affections alone, ... 3 "

The clinical diagnosis was stated as perityphlitis when the necropsy demonstrated the following :

Tuberculous stricture of the cecum, ... 2 cases
Pyosalpinx, ... 1 case
Metrolymphangitis, ... 1 "
Thrombosis of the portal vein, ... 1 "
Typhoid fever, ... 2 cases
Caries and abscess of the vertebræ, ... 1 case
Septicemia from abscess in the tonsil, ... 1 "

The necropsy showed perityphlitis when the diagnosis had been fixed as:

Internal incarceration, ... 3 cases
Ileus, ... 1 case
Tumor of the uterine adnexa, ... 1 "
Perforation of round gastric ulcer, ... 1 "
Tuberculosis of the peritoneum, ... 1 "

Treatment.

Referring to the classification of various forms of appendicitis given in the section on the Clinical Aspects of Intestinal Surgery, chapter VI, I am speaking in the following of groups III to VIII, not of I and II.

It can no longer be said that the question of therapeutic management of suppurative appendicitis and perityphlitis is whether it shall be purely expectant, or nonoperative, or surgical.   The views of American clinicians (Fitz, Osler, Janeway, Tyson, G. Thompson Hare, etc.) and American surgeons (Keen, Halsted, Senn, Murphy, McBurney, Weir, Bull, Finney, Edebohls, and many others) are now practically unanimous that this is a surgical condition, to be treated by operation only.   At the present time, when our knowledge of this important and common disease has been greatly increased and deepened by the numerous operations for appendicitis and perityphlitis, probably most, if not all, experienced clinicians, and especially those who have collaborated with good surgeons, admit that this demand is justified. To be sure, a spontaneous cure sets in in some cases of suppurative perityphlitis—when, for instance, the suppuration breaks through into the intestine. This, however, is dependent upon so many conditions which can not be recognized clinically that a spontaneous cure of this disease without an operation is really a stroke of good fortune. Such great dangers arise for the patient from the accumulation of pus in his abdomen that an operation is preferable to a cure by nature, even were this a more frequent event than is proved by experience. I believe that no experienced clinician will hesitate to call in the surgeon in those cases where he has detected suppuration or the formation of abscesses, or has reason to suspect them. The views of the surgeons differ only as to the choice of the time when the operation shall be performed. Some of them (Weir, Deaver, Morris, Finney, Kraft, Roux, and others) have proposed to perform it as soon as possible, for the following reasons : (1) It would be easier technically ; (2) those adhesions which would prevent recognition of the pathological territory would yet be absent ; (3) the formation of extensive abscesses and the development of diffuse peritonitis would be prevented ; (4) therefore the resection of the appendix would be easier. Others have emphasized another point of view—namely, that if the special and individual circumstances allow of waiting, in this period of time the abscess may become walled off, and that when it afterward empties itself the opening of the peritoneal cavity will have been avoided. This opening of the general peritoneal cavity is, after all, a critical matter, and can rarely be avoided in the early operation. At present we can not decide which of these opinions is the correct one. Besides, we can not formulate definite rules concerning the exact time when an operation is necessary and when not. This must be decided in each individual case. In some cases which start violently great improvement may soon set in, which may permit a delay ; in others which commence mildly the surgeon may be compelled to perform an operation very suddenly, because the symptoms of occlusion or of a threatening perforation peritonitis may appear suddenly.

The discussion of the internal treatment will precede that of the operative treatment, because in practice it always precedes the latter, and because it is the only one possible in those cases in which permission for operation is refused.

Internal Treatment.—In general this corresponds with that of simple catarrhal appendicitis : absolute rest in bed until the symptoms of the inflammation have entirely subsided ; the application of ice-bags or ice poultices on the right hypogastric region, or, if the fever is not high and the case becomes protracted, hot poultices ; for internal pains opium, and in such doses as to make the patient nearly free from pain. Excessive doses must be avoided, since they conceal the course of the disease, cause the mouth to become dry, and affect the action of the heart unfavorably. If opium does not agree with the patient, morphin must be tried. If very violent paroxysms of pain occur, subcutaneous injections of morphin render good service on account of their quick action ($\frac{1}{6}$ of a grain at first injection). Antipyretics need not be prescribed, since the behavior of the fever is a valuable indication as to improvement and aggravation. Fitz ("Practice of Medicine," Fitz and Wood) and Sahli recommend the use of leeches in the right ileocecal region, which Wood and Fitz (*l. c.*) believe to be very useful if the inflammatory action is the outcome of a typhlitis stercoralis.

In all severe cases, and especially at first, the introduction of both solid and liquid food must be strictly forbidden, because the increase in peristalsis during digestion may increase the inflammation, break tender adhesions, and facilitate the perforation of ulcers and the eruption of suppuration into the peritoneal cavity. It is only when all the symptoms of inflammation have subsided that a liquid diet may be prescribed, then a pulpy one, and eventually light, easily digested, solid food. Water, sometimes mixed with a little wine, and weak tea, may be allowed, but always in very small amounts. If there is nausea and vomiting, the stomach should remain empty and small water enemata should be prescribed. The administration of purges is of doubtful value. Great caution is also requisite in this regard, even after the suppurative appendicitis is on the wane. If the disease lasts very long, or if the general condition of the patients has suffered from former attacks of this or other disease, small nutritive enemata (milk, eggs, peptone) are to be given.

Of course, it depends upon the further development of the disease as to how long the administration of opium and the abstinence from food shall continue.

In six cases of appendicitis that all presented palpable tumors of varying sizes in the right iliac fossa, and in which I had repeatedly urged operation but was regularly refused, I met with success by large oil injections into the colon. Judging from the anamnesis, which pointed to years of persistent obstipation, they were all of the stercoral type. One pint of pure olive oil was used, in which thymol crystals were dissolved by crushing them under the oil in a mortar—a saturated solution of thymol in olive oil, in fact. This was slowly introduced at a temperature of 100° F., through a Langdon tube, as high up as possible, using from eight to ten feet of pressure. All the cases recovered from two or more recurrent attacks under this treatment, associated with diet, rest, and hot poulticing. But the danger of the method lies in procrastination—such patients should, by all means, be operated. The improvement after one attack will fortify their aversion against operation, and there is danger that they may eventually succumb to a recurrent appendicitis. I have watched these six cases since 1889, and one who was treated in June of that year died of diffuse peritonitis and intestinal paresis in 1895. Two others treated in 1890 have each had two attacks since that were serious.

Operative Treatment.—Operation should be considered when the signs and symptoms enumerated indicate a suppuration. A number of German clinicians advocate exploratory puncture if the pus which was drawn off has a fecal odor, or if it shows signs of decomposition they recommend the operation to be performed as soon as possible. Personally I do not sanction exploratory puncture and attempts at aspirating pus in appendicitis. There is a possibility of infecting the peritoneum and unnecessarily complicating the case by puncture of the bowel, and the puncture may fail to detect pus even in cases where operation proves it to be present. As to the time when the operation should be performed, the following general indications may be formulated. If the disease symptoms, such as fever, acceleration of the pulse, pains, and the condition of the abdomen in general, do not improve in two days after their beginning, but continue with undiminished intensity, or if an aggravation of symptoms follows a considerable improvement which took place in this space of time, then an operation ought to be performed at once.   The same is the case if the improvement observed at first, after the demonstrable breaking forth of the suppuration into the intestines, the vagina, the bladder, etc., is only of a very short duration, and the condition of affairs is again the same as before.   It is also the case if the resistance in the right ileocecal region disappears suddenly without being accompanied by an improvement.   Here the suspicion is present that the suppuration has forced its way into other sections of the abdomen.   An operation, also, is necessary, if the symptoms of occlusion appear ; also if the patient is seized with chills ; if the resistance in the hypogastric region rapidly increases ; and if there are signs of development of a general peritonitis.   If it has come to the development of a septic general peritonitis, the chances are bad, both with and without an operation.   In a small portion of the cases of general fibrino-suppurative peritonitis a cure has been effected by performing an operation very early.   This, however, has also been achieved in individual cases without an operation having been performed.   After the operation has been decided upon the case should not altogether be left to the surgeon to decide whether it shall be performed at once or not : the attending practitioner's experience is very valuable in forming an opinion of the general condition of the patient and any previous diseases that may have weakened it.   " The medical treatment has an important place in the management of every case of appendicitis, and should never be ignored."   (N. Senn, "Practical Surgery," p. 724.)

CHRONIC APPENDICITIS (RECURRENT AND RELAPSING APPENDICITIS).

In 230 cases of acute appendicitis which I could gather from German, French, English, and American literature, and the records of which contained a reference to the future or previous history of the case, more than one attack of appendicitis had occurred in 124 cases.   According to this complication, patients afflicted with acute appendicitis are likely to have another attack in about 54 per cent. of all cases.   In about one-half of all cases of acute appendicitis observed by Fitz there was more than one attack of the disease.

The different attacks are separated by longer or shorter intervals of apparent freedom from discomfort. The symptomatology and prognosis present the same characteristics as those of the original affection, except that the prognosis becomes graver the more numerous and smaller the intervals at which the recurrences develop. In this connection American clinicians, following the doctrines of Fitz, have come to speak of (1) recurrent and (2) relapsing chronic appendicitis.

1. If the intervals are long, perhaps months or years, each subsequent attack is regarded as a *recurrent* appendicitis. If the attacks, however, occur frequently and at shorter intervals, say of weeks or months, and the patient in the mean time is comparatively free from pain in the right iliac fossa, the condition represents a chronic appendicitis with a tendency to relapses, generally spoken of as a chronic or *relapsing* appendicitis, the difference between the recurrent and the relapsing appendicitis being that in the former we assume, on the basis of the physical examination and the general experience of the patient, that a more complete restitution to the normal condition has taken place in the appendix.

In chronic or relapsing appendicitis the histological evidences of chronic inflammation are supposed to be present as the result of a previous acute attack. The lesions characteristic of chronic appendicitis may be present, however, and may not cause the symptoms indicative of this condition. The most constant symptoms of chronic appendicitis are localized pain and tenderness, and the most important aids in determining its existence are the previous history of the patient and careful palpation. The pain is characterized by its persistence, the intervals of relief being rare. Talamon ("La Colique Appendiculaire et les formes non chirurgicales de l'appendicite," Paris, 1900) has designated this condition as " colique appendiculaire," and is of the opinion that it is an infirmity yielding to medical treatment in 72 per cent. of the cases. Personally I regard the figures of Talamon as dangerously optimistic, at least they do not agree with my personal experience with such cases.

Symptomatology.

Pain is likely to come on at any time and after the least exertion or insignificant attacks of dyspepsia. Usually these attacks compel the patient to remain in a recumbent position for several days. Careful thermometric observations have led me to believe that three-fourths of my cases of this type show a slight elevation of temperature (100° F.) during the relapses. In about one-third of the cases a resistant mass, varying from the size of a hen's egg or the index-finger to that of an orange, can be palpated in the region of the cecum. It is due either to the enlarged appendix itself or to the accumulation of fecal matter. When it consists of the latter, relief often follows evacuation of the bowel. These are the types that the older writers spoke of as "stercoral typhlitis." Just what the exact histological condition in the appendix and cecal mucosa is during these relapses it is impossible to say. The patient is, as a rule, compelled to live near his medical adviser. The constant state of uncertainty renders him irritable, timid, and neurasthenic. The enfeeblement of the patient is proportional to the frequency in the recurrence of the attacks and the shortness of the intervals of comparative freedom intervening between them.

Diagnosis.

Chronic appendicitis requires differentiation from similar symptoms caused by neurasthenia, hysteria, and hypochondriasis. Patients of this type have occasionally presented symptoms of such striking similarity to chronic relapsing appendicitis that they have been subjected to operation, and the normal appendix removed from them. On examining such patients critically the clinician will at one time or other discover that the localized tenderness in the iliac fossa is entirely absent when the attention of the patient is diverted, and that there is no palpable tumor when the iliac region is thoroughly examined and palpated.

Method of Palpating the Appendix.

Edebohls ("Amer. Jour. of the Med. Sci.," vol. CVII, 1894, p. 487) described his method of palpating the appendix in females as follows: After completion of the ordinary bimanual examination of the pelvic organs, the patient is drawn upward upon the table about a foot, her feet still remaining where they were placed for the vaginal examination. This is mainly for the purpose of unfolding the flexure of the thigh upon the abdomen, and to render the right iliac region more accessible to the palpating hand. One hand only, applied externally, is required for the practice of palpation of the vermiform appendix. No assistance can be rendered by a finger introduced into the vagina, and very little assistance, and that only occasionally, by a finger introduced into the rectum. Standing at the patient's right, the examiner begins the search for the appendix by applying two, three, or four fingers of the right hand, the palmar surface downward, almost flatly upon the abdomen, in a straight line from the umbilicus to the anterior superior spine of the right ilium. He notices successively the character of the various struc-tures as they come beneath and escape from the fingers passing over them. In doing this the pressure exerted must be sufficiently deep to recognize distinctly, along the whole route traversed by the examining fingers, the resistant surface of the posterior abdominal wall and of the pelvic brim. Only in this way can we positively feel the normal, or the slightly enlarged, appendix; pressure less than this must necessarily fail. Pressure deep enough to rec-ognize distinctly the posterior abdominal wall, the pelvic brim, and the structures lying between them and the examining finger form the whole secret of success, according to Edebohls, in the practice of palpation of the vermiform appendix. The appendix is thereby recognized as a more or less flattened, ribbon-shaped structure when normal, or as a more or less rounded and firm organ of varying diameter when its walls have been thickened by past or present inflammation. The normal appendix exhibits no special sensitive-ness on being squeezed. A good guide in searching for the appen-dix is to make out the right common and external iliac arteries first, the pulsation of which can be plainly felt. The line of these vessels corresponds to a surface line drawn from the left of the umbilicus to the middle of Poupart's ligament. The appendix is generally found almost immediately outside of these vessels. At its base it is separated from the vessels by a space of from one-half to one inch, while lower down in its course it generally crosses very obliquely the line of the arteries. In testing the method, I found that it was rarely possible to palpate the normal appendix, and in stout patients, and whenever there is much rigidity from pain or apprehension, the method has failed in my experience. Pressure sufficient to feel the appendix when there is suppuration is a dangerous procedure.

Chronic relapsing appendicitis may, under certain circumstances, have to be differentiated from all the conditions which shall be described in the differential diagnosis of suppurative appendicitis and perityphlitis. There are two conditions, however, which are especially likely to be confounded with the chronic form of appendicitis. These are cancer of the cecum and irritation of the right ureter by calculi, or even actual renal colic. An accurate anamnesis may prevent confounding cecal cancer with appendicitis; above all, the temperature is of importance. In cancer of the cecum fever is almost unknown, except where the cancer has caused perforation and peritonitis. In such cases the exact diagnosis becomes very difficult, and is often not made until an exploratory laparotomy is undertaken. Among the most interesting cases which call for differential diagnosis are those presenting pain in the right iliac fossa, due to irritation of the right ureter by the passage of crystals of calcium oxalate or uric acid. R. Cabot has called attention to the rôle of calcium oxalate in simulating the pains of chronic appendicitis. One of the most instructive cases that have come under my experience in this connection was that of a scholarly fellow-practitioner, himself a diagnostician of wide reputation. He had suffered for a long time from intense pains in the right iliac fossa, and finally was operated on by a well-known surgeon and his appendix removed. I did not see the operation, nor could my colleague give a description of it from personal observation. The statement made by the surgeon was that it presented signs of slight inflammation. There was no perityphlitis, and the cecum appeared normal. Five or six months after the removal of his appendix the doctor again suffered from pain in the same region and more intense than before, the painful attacks occurring at intervals. The same surgeon was again consulted, and suggested a second operation, but before a date could be agreed upon the patient one morning passed a ragged edged uric acid calculus in his urine, and has since then never again felt any discomfort in the iliac region. In patients who have an acquired or inherited gouty tendency repeated attacks of nephritic colic, either from the passage of calculi or of uric acid crystals, so closely resemble the relapses of chronic appendicitis that a differential diagnosis is at times impossible without examination of the urine. The presence of uric acid or calcium oxalate crystals, especially if accompanied by blood-corpuscles, should suggest a renal or ureteral nature of the attack and stimulate a very thorough examination of the ileocecal region by Edebohls' method, and catheterization of the ureters.

Prognosis.

The prognosis of chronic appendicitis is uncertain, though, as a general rule, it is favorable as to life. There is such a thing as a spontaneous cure by complete obliteration of the appendix, as a result of a severe recurrent attack.

The treatment will be considered in connection with suppurative appendicitis, but I may remark here that in a condition in which recurrences are frequent, and the relapses occur at such intervals as to keep the patient in a state of invalidism, the surgical removal of the appendix is the only treatment that gives hope of relief.

LITERATURE ON APPENDICITIS.

(In addition to that quoted in the text.)

1. Abbe, Robert, "The Problem of Appendicitis from a Medical and Surgical Point of View," "N. Y. Medical Record," Feb. 16, 1901.

2. Baldwin, J. F., "Subphrenic Abscess Following Appendicitis," "Medical News," July 14, 1900.

3. Barling, Gilbert, "Appendicitis," "Edinburgh Med. Jour.," Scotland, December, 1899.

4. Berg, A. A., "The Differentiation of Appendicitis from Other Affections in the Right Iliac and Pelvic Regions," "Phila. Med. Jour.," vol. III, p. 112.

5. Bougle, "Appendicite Chronique," "Gaz. d. Hôp. d. Paris," July 24, 1900.

6. Brown, John Y., "Pathology of Appendicitis," "Medical Review," December 9, 1899.

7. Brown, O. S., "Treatment of Appendicitis," Medical Council, Philadelphia, June, 1900.

8. Buchanan, J. J., "Treatment of Appendicitis," "Penna. Med. Jour.," July, 1900.

9. Byrne, Joseph H., "Causation and Relative Frequency of Typhlitis, Perityphlitis, and Appendicitis in Infancy and Childhood," "Jour. Amer. Med. Assoc.," September 8, 1900.

10. Carstens, J. H., "Some Facts About Appendicitis, Medical and Surgical," "Jour. Amer. Med. Assoc.," September 15, 1900.

11. Carstens, J. H., "Appendicitis,—When to Operate."

12. Carteledge, A. Morgan, "Chronic Appendicitis," "Louisville Monthly Journal of Medicine and Surgery," June, 1900.

13. Clarke, Agustus P., "Appendicitis," "Jour. Amer. Med. Assoc.," February 11, 1899, vol. XXXII, No. 6.

14. Coyne and Hobbs, "Appendicite à bacille pyocyanique," "Gaz. hebdom. d. Sci. Med. de Bordeaux," France, July 8, 1900.

15. Curryer, W. F., "Appendicitis," "Eclectic Med. Jour.," July, 1900.

16. Deaver, "Treatise on Appendicitis." Second Edition.

17. Delageniere, "De l'appendicite," "Archives Provinciales de Chirurgie," Paris, July 1, 1900.

18. Dieulafoy, G., "The Toxicology of Appendicitis," "Presse Med.," November 9, 1898, No. 92.

19. Doerfler, "Further Experience in Appendicitis," "Münch. med. Wochenschr.," April 18, 1899, 46. Jahrg., No. 16.

20. Eastman, Joseph, "Appendicitis," "Med. and Surg. Monitor," Indianapolis, February, 1900.

21. Edebohls, Geo. M., "History and Literature of Appendicitis," "Medical Record," November 25, 1899. *Containing entire literature up to the date of this publication.*

22. Ellis, R., "The Term Appendicitis," etc., "New York Medical Journal," July 15, 1899, vol. LXX, No. 3.

23. Feltz, "Some Considerations on Appendicitis," "Gaz. Hebdom.," Paris, February 8, 1900.

24. French, Pinckney, "Appendicitis—Pathology and Treatment," "Amer. Jour. of Surgery and Gynecology," June, 1900.

25. Froussard, "Appendicite et enterocolite mucomembraneuse," "Gaz. d. Hôp.," Paris, July 10, 1900.

26. Gasser, H., "Appendicitis from a Country Practitioner's Point of View," Medical Council, Philadelphia, May, 1900.

27. Gaub, O. C., "One Hundred and Twenty-four Cases of Appendicitis," "Penna. Med. Jour.," July, 1900.

28. Girard, A. C., "Early Surgical Interference in Appendicitis," "Pacific Med. Jour.," November, 1899.

29. Greer, W. Jones, "A Case of Recurrent Appendicitis; Operation; Recovery," "Lancet," May 6, 1899.

30. Hamilton, W. D., "How to Deal with the Appendix in Pus Cases," "International Journal of Surgery," November, 1899.

31. Hare, H. A., "Appendicitis and Typhoid Fever," "Medical News," July 21, 1900.

32. Hayden, A. M., "Appendicitis—Plea for Early Operation," "St. Louis Medical Era," December, 1899.

33. Hayden, A. M., "A Plea for Early Operations in Appendicitis," "Medical Review," November 11, 1899.

34. Helbing, H. H., "Appendicitis and Appendectomy," "Amer. Med. Jour.," July, 1900.

35. Hicks, R. I., "Appendicitis from a Medical Standpoint," "Charlotte (N. C.) Med. Jour.," November, 1899.

36. Homans, John, "On the Necessity of Removing the Appendix at the First Operation," "Boston Med. and Surg. Jour.," February 2, 1899.

37. Janeway, E. G., "Remarks on Some of the Conditions Simulating Appendicitis and Peri-appendicular Inflammation," "Medical Record," May 26, 1900.

38. Janeway, E. G., "Conditions Simulating Appendicitis and Peri-appendicular Inflammation," "Medical Record," May 26, 1900.

39. Jelks, J. T., "Unique Case of Appendicitis," "Jour. Amer. Med. Assoc.," May 26, 1900.

40. Keetley, C. B., "Mode of Operating for Appendicitis," "Lancet," New York, May, 1900.

41. Kellogg, C. W., "Appendicitis, Operative, in the Country," "Pacific Med. Jour.," December, 1899.

42. Kelly, A. O. J., "Pathogenesis of Appendicitis," "Phila. Med. Jour.," November 11, 18, 25, 1899.

43. Kirmisson, "Appendicitis and Gastrorrhagia," "Gaz. Hebdom.," Paris, February 1, 1900.

44. Link, W. H., "Appendicitis Far from Surgical Centers," "Amer. Jour. of Surgery and Gynecology," May, 1900.

45. Lloyd, Samuel, "Appendicitis—Results of So-called Conservative Treatment," "Medical Record," February 10, 1900.

46. Lloyd, Samuel, "Appendicitis," "Alabama Med. Jour.," May, 1900.

47. MacLaren, W. S., "Sphere of Damage in Surgery of Appendix," "Medical Record," October 28, 1899.

48. Meriwether, F. T., "Report of Sixty-one Cases of Appendicitis," "Annals of Gynecology and Pediatry," November, 1899.

49. Merriwether, Frank E., "Appendicitis," "New York Medical Times," November, 1899.

50. Middleton, W. D., "Varieties of Appendicitis," "Chicago Med. Reporter," May, 1900.

51. Morris, R. T., "When to Operate for Appendicitis," "New York Medical Journal," April 29, 1899, vol. LXIX, No. 17.

52. Morris, R. T., "Errors That I have Made in 228 Consecutive Cases Diagnosed as Appendicitis," "New York Medical Journal," April 8, 1899, vol. LXIX, No. 14.

53. Morris, R. T., "Best Methods in the Treatment of Appendicitis," "Jour. Amer. Med. Assoc.," July 15, 1899, vol. XXXIII, No. 3.

54. Moullin, C. Mansell, "Operation in Cases of Inflamed Appendix," "Amer. Jour. of Surgery and Gynecology," February, 1900.

55. Moullin, Mansell, "Preventive Operation in Acute Inflammation of the Appendix," "Edinburgh Med. Jour.," April, 1900.

56. Muehsam, Richard, "Experiments on Appendicitis," "Deutsch. Zeitschr. f. Chir.," March, 1900.

57. Murphy, John B., "Appendicitis, When to Operate and Why," "International Journal of Surgery," June, 1900.

58. Myers, E. G., "Appendicitis, Diagnosis and Treatment," "Cleveland Medical Gazette," July, 1900.

59. Nash, W. Gifford, "A Case of Suppurative Appendicitis with Secondary Liver Abscesses," "Lancet," March 24, 1900.

60. Niemack, J., "Appendicitis," "Iowa Med. Jour.," November, 1899.

61. O'Connor, J., "Appendicitis," "Phila. Med. Jour.," December 2, 1899.

62. Parker, Thos., "Appendicitis," "Medical Sentinel," February, 1900.

63. Pennebaker and Trepp, "Acute Appendicitis," "Wisconsin Medical Recorder," June, 1900.

64. Perkins, H. T., "Differential Diagnosis between Appendicitis and Inflammations of Right Ovary and Tubes."

65. Power, D'Arcy, "Prognosis and Modern Treatment of Appendicitis," "Brit. Med. Jour.," November 25, 1899.

66. Price, Mordecai, "Treatment of Appendicitis," "Therapeutic Gazette," February, 1900.

67. Quervain, "Zu welchem Zeitpunkte operiren wir bei Appendicitis?" "Wien. Med. Blätter," June 14, 1900.

68. Richardson, Maurice H., "Appendicitis," "Amer. Jour. of Med. Sci.," December, 1899.

69. Roberts, W. H., "An Atypical Case of Appendicitis," "Phila. Med. Jour.," vol. III, p. 1247.

70. Robinson, H. B., "On Some Complicated Cases of Appendicitis and Their Surgical Treatment," "Lancet," May 6, 1899.

71. Saunders, Bacon, "What is Real Conservatism in the Treatment of Appendicitis?" "Hot Springs Med. Jour.," November, 1899.

72. Senn, N., "Practical Surgery," p. 703, Aug., 1901.

73. Schmitt, A., "The Indications for Operation in Appendicitis," "Münch. med. Wochenschr.," March 20, 1900.

74. Schooler, Lewis, "What Becomes of Medicinally Treated Cases of Appendicitis," "Charlotte (N. C.) Med. Jour.," December, 1899.

75. Shnell, T. J., "Nonoperative Treatment of Appendicitis," "New England Medical Monthly," November, 1899.

76. Starr, Nathan, "Twenty-eight Cases of Appendicitis," "Clinique," Chicago, July, 1900.

77. Stewart, R. W., "Causation and Symptoms of Appendicitis," "Penna. Med. Jour.," July, 1900.

78. Sullivan, M. B., "Traumatic Appendicitis," "Medical Record," January 7, 1899.

79. Taylor, W. G., "Skin and Kidneys in Appendicitis," "Buffalo Med. Jour.," May, 1900.

80. Terrier, T., "Appendicitis," "Revue de Chirurgie," January 10, 1900.

81. Van Meter, S. D., "Two Complicated Cases of Appendicitis," "Colorado Med. Jour.," December, 1899.

82. Vineberg, Hiram N., "The Association of Chronic Appendicitis with Disease of the Right Adnexa," "Medical Record," June 2, 1900.

83. Walker, Edwin, "Appendicitis," "Amer. Jour. of Surgery and Gynecology," May, 1900.

84. Wallace, F. E., "Appendicitis," "Peoria (Ill.) Med. Jour.," November, 1899.

85. Warden, A. A., "A Note on the Safest Method of Removal of the Appendix," "Lancet," August 4, 1900.

86. Weber, Julius, "Subphrenic Abscess Following Appendicitis," "Deutsch. Zeitschr. f. Chir.," February, 1900.

87. Weir, R. T., "Improved Operation for Acute Appendicitis," "Medical News," February 17, 1900.

88. Weiss, Th., and Fevrier, Ch., "Description of Cases of Appendicitis," "Revue de Chirurgie," Decembre 10, 1898.

89. Wiener, Jos., "When Shall we Operate for Appendicitis?" "Medical Record," May 19, 1900.

90. Witherbee, O. O., "Early Radical Treatment of Appendicitis," "Southern California Practitioner," December, 1899.

91. Woolsey, Geo., "Some Points in the Treatment of Appendicitis When Pus is Present," "Medical Record," April 1, 1899, vol. LV, No. 13.

92. Wyeth, John A., "Abscess of the Appendix Discharging Through the Umbilicus," "Medical Record," January 14, 1899.

93. Zahorsky, John, "Appendicitis a Medical or a Surgical Disease," "Medical Review," February 17, 1900.

CHAPTER II.

INFECTIOUS GRANULOMATA OF THE INTESTINE. TUBERCULOSIS OF THE INTESTINE.

Prior to the views of Koch expressed at the International Congress on Tuberculosis held in London during July, 1901, the commonly accepted opinion was that infection of the human intestine with tuberculosis may occur in three ways : (1) By means of infected ingesta, particularly the milk and meat of tuberculous animals; (2) by swallowing the sputa arising from the patient's own respiratory passages that may be infected with tuberculosis ; and (3) by way of the blood and lymph channels. This latter constitutes a secondary infection of the intestinal tract, which is by far the most frequent manner of infection. In children a more frequent localization of tuberculosis in the abdominal and peritoneal lymph-glands has been found, while in adults the most frequent form of the disease is the tubercular intestinal ulcer.

The recent researches of Koch (*l. c.*) make the possibility of infection of the human intestine by ingested meat and milk of tuberculous animals, a question for future investigation.

It is important to emphasize, for the purpose of advancing our understanding of the pathogenesis and nature of intestinal tuberculosis, as well as of prophylaxis, that Koch has not asserted, as a fact proved beyond any doubt, that the human intestine *can not* be infected with tuberculosis by drinking the milk or eating the flesh of tuberculous cattle. What he stated was, that his own experiments have been carried only far enough to enable him to say positively that the bacillus of human tuberculosis can not infect cows and swine, leaving him in doubt as to the converse proposition—that is, whether the bacillus of bovine tuberculosis can infect human beings. Koch's inference is that human and animal tuberculosis are two distinct diseases, and that human beings in all probability can not be infected by the bacilli of bovine tuberculosis, any more than cattle and swine can be infected with the bacilli of human tuberculosis.   But in the absence of any experiments to prove this inference, it must for the present be considered in the light of a hypothesis.

In chapter XXI, volume I, of this work I have given a brief abstract of the views concerning primary intestinal tuberculosis (under the heading of Tubercular Ulcers).*   In answer to Klebs, Orth, and others who say that in many cases human beings and animals have been shown by postmortem examination to have been first infected in the intestinal canal, presumably by bacilli ingested in milk or meat from tuberculous cows, Koch cites the extreme rareness of primary intestinal tuberculosis, and asserts that the few cases that had been enumerated in autopsy statistics were by no means attributable with certainty to infection with bovine tuberculosis.   It was just as "likely that they were caused by widely propagated bacilli of human tuberculosis, which might have gotten into the digestive canal in some way."

In support of the rareness of primary intestinal tuberculosis he quotes the statistics of Biedert, who found but sixteen cases of primary intestinal tuberculosis in 3104 autopsies of tuberculous children; also the results of similar postmortem examinations in the "Kaiser and Kaiserin Friederich Kinder Hospital."   Among 933 cases of tuberculosis in children of this institution, only 10 cases of primary tuberculosis of the intestines occurred.   Among the great number of postmortem examinations at the "Charité" Hospital in Berlin, Koch himself remembered having seen primary tuberculosis of the intestines only twice, and he reminds us that Baginski never found tuberculosis of the intestines without a simultaneous affection of the lungs and bronchial glands.

All these references, and some others quoted by him, naturally go to show that primary intestinal tuberculosis is rare in human beings, and that therefore infection by meat and milk is also rare; for it is Koch's main argument that we can not assume with certainty that tuberculosis is caused by ingesta unless the intestine can be shown to suffer first; i. e., unless primary tuberculosis of the intestines is found.

---

* This chapter (XXI) was printed long before the report of Koch to the London Congress on Tuberculosis, and hence could not embody his recent experiments.

This argument meets with two objections that make its uncondi-
tional acceptance difficult:

I. In the first place, it has been known that the bacillus of human
tuberculosis may pass the structures of the intestinal wall (mucosa,
submucosa, muscularis) without leaving any trace of its existence
there.   After such passage without altering the intestinal tissue, it
has been known to produce tuberculosis of the mesenteric, omental,
and peritoneal lymphatic structures.

II. The positive exclusion of primary intestinal tuberculosis is a
work of enormous technical difficulty because it necessitates not
only the macroscopic, but even the microscopic, examination of the
entire digestive tract from mouth to anus (26 to 30 feet), with its
extensive mesentery, omentum, and peritoneum, and all its lymphatic structures.

The stomach and intestines give evidence of a miraculous immunity from tuberculosis infection, which is in part ascribable to
the activity of digestive ferments, to the peristalsis, and to some as
yet not understood natural provision for disinfection (see chapter
on Dystrypsia) which has been made the object of experimental
study by Schütz (*l. c.*).

Even if we accept Koch's inference that the human subject can
not be infected with the bacillus of bovine tuberculosis, we should
feel justified in assuming a more frequent occurrence of primary
intestinal tuberculosis due to the bacillus of human tuberculosis.
As this does not appear to be the case, there must be a reason for
it; either the bacillus can pass through the intestinal structures
without leaving any trace of its passage, or there is some normal
provision for disinfection, or both. These points must be the objects
for future investigation.

The relationship between human and bovine tuberculosis has
been the object of extensive experimentation by American investigators.   Dr. Theobald Smith reported his conclusions in the
"Journal of Experimental Medicine," volume III, page 451, 1898.
Whilst he agreed with Koch in the announcement that the bacillus
of human tuberculosis was incapable of infecting cattle, he differed
from Koch by asserting that the bovine bacillus may actually infect
the human subject, and attributed this to its higher pathogenic power.

The work done under the auspices of the Pennsylvania State

Live Stock Sanitary Board (Leonard Pearson, " Phila. Med. Jour.,"
Aug. 3, 1891, p. 184) showed very clearly that for experimental
animals, tubercle bacilli from cattle are in all cases as virulent,·and
usually very much more so, than tubercle bacilli from man. In view
of the fact that the bacillus of bovine tuberculosis is so constantly
more virulent than the bacillus of human tuberculosis for animals of
so widely different species as the dog, goat, rabbit, and horse (which
are classed among the more resistant animals), and the cat, guinea-
pig, swine, and cattle (which are considered vulnerable), it appears
hazardous to suggest that the bacillus of bovine tuberculosis is nonvirulent for man, on the ground that the bacillus of human tuberculosis is nonvirulent for cattle. As pointed out before, Koch by
no means asserts this ; but the idea has gone abroad, based upon
his reports, that such is the case, and therein lies a great danger.

This question could, according to Koch, only be settled by the
impossible experiment of inoculating a human being with bovine
tuberculosis. According to Pearson (*l. c.*), this inoculation has
already occurred accidentally in a number of instances. A number
of men have contracted tuberculosis and several have died from infections sustained in making postmortem examinations on tubercular
cattle. These accidents are evidence for the belief that the bacillus
of bovine tuberculosis may, under favorable conditions, become
virulent for human beings. All efforts at prophylaxis by condemn-
ing meat from tuberculous cattle, etc., must therefore continue with
unrelenting vigilance.

Orth distinguishes a specific and a nonspecific intestinal tuberculosis. By specific tuberculous changes are meant the tuberculous ulcers ; by nonspecific, the catarrhal enteritis in association
with tuberculosis. The tuberculous changes in the small intestine may be localized at any place between the ileocecal valve
and the pylorus. In the same way the colon exhibits a variable localization of the tuberculous process. Very frequently the
cecum, vermiform process, and the ascending colon are the only
parts involved. This localization often expresses itself clinically as
a tuberculous "ileocecal tumor," very much simulating the tumor
of appendicitis. This is not the only form in which intestinal
tuberculosis presents itself clinically as a tumor, for we may en-
counter enlarged tuberculous retroperitoneal and mesenteric glands

which may very much confuse the diagnostician. We will return to the consideration of this subject under a special heading, Tuberculous Ileocecal Tumor. Generally the disease, of whatever type, is preceded by a series of symptoms that correspond to those of acute or chronic enteritis or colitis. Occasionally it is even possible to arrive at a conclusion concerning the nature of this form of enteritis by the detection of tubercle bacilli in the evacuations and the positive reaction following tuberculin injections. The principal suggestive symptoms are copious diarrheas accompanied by attacks of colic and fever. If other causes can be excluded, and if they occur in individuals already afflicted with tuberculosis in another organ, or in an individual predisposed by heredity or environment, the suspicion of tuberculous disease of the intestine should be aroused. Tubercle bacilli are not found in the evacuations until the ulcerative processes have developed in the intestines and caused loss of substance. It is essential that the swallowed sputa should be excluded as a source of the tubercle bacilli found in the dejecta.

Clinically, tuberculosis of the alimentary tract may express itself in three forms : (1) The tuberculous enteritis or colitis : (2) the tuberculous ulcer ; (3) the tuberculous neoplasm or tumor. In addition to these, the possibility of peritoneal tuberculosis sometimes confuses the diagnosis.

Tuberculous Enteritis.

This at first runs its course under the symptoms of an ordinary enteritis, which are diarrhea, occasional attacks of colic, and fever reaching about 102° F. The characteristic of this diarrhea is the presence of tubercle bacilli in the dejection, but by that time we are dealing with an ulcerating enteritis which will soon express itself by discharges that contain blood and pus, and even fragments of intestinal tissue. None of these symptoms is characteristic for tuberculous enteritis. Profuse diarrhea is a more constant result of tuberculosis of the colon than of tuberculosis of the small intestine. Eventually the phenomena of tuberculous peritonitis supervene. These are meteorism, vomiting, singultus, and a free exudate in the peritoneal cavity. At first these signs are transient, but later on they become more permanent, eventuating in the formation of palpable bands in the omentum and manifold adhesions causing irreg-.

ular distribution of the exudate and distortion of the abdominal organs from their normal positions.

When constricting bands of cicatrices have developed, the lumen of the intestine may become obstructed, and we may have the clinical picture of intestinal stricture, with dilation above the constricted area. It is impossible to decide whether the stenosis in such cases is due to cicatricial stricture or peritoneal adhesions, but if intense symptoms of intestinal ulceration, with long-continued diarrhea and stools containing blood and pus, have existed, one should be inclined to attribute the obstruction to cicatrices, whereas the predominance of symptoms referring to chronic peritonitis would incline the clinician to the diagnosis of peritoneal adhesions.

Diagnosis.—The differential diagnosis between simple catarrhal and tubercular enteritis hinges upon the presence of tubercle bacilli in the evacuations under conditions where the deglutition of bacilli can be excluded. The differential diagnosis between the ordinary appendicitis and tubercular appendicitis or tubercular perityphlitis is very difficult indeed, particularly if the phthisical changes in the lungs are not very evident. These pulmonary evidences of tuberculosis are sometimes very trivial; I have had this experience in three cases of perirectal abscesses arising from tuberculosis of the lymph-glands about the rectum, and one case of tubercular tumor of the ileum just preceding and involving the ileocecal valve. In these four cases the tuberculosis of the lungs could not be definitely determined, though repeated physical examinations of the thorax were made. The patients did not bring up any expectoration. At the autopsy a small tubercular focus was found in the lungs. In all cases it is indispensable to subject the lungs to a careful examination by auscultation and percussion, and also to examine the remaining portions of the body for enlargements of lymph-glands, swollen joints, etc. A positive reaction after the hypodermic injection of 3 to 5 milligrams of Koch's tuberculin is an argument in favor of tuberculosis even in the absence of pulmonary signs.

Prognosis.—The enteritis, acute or chronic, occurring in association with pulmonary tuberculosis may cease after a varying duration and a functional restitution of the intestine take place. Even tubercular intestinal ulcers may heal. Unfortunately, the large number of secondary intestinal ulcers do not occur until the pul-

PLATE 5.

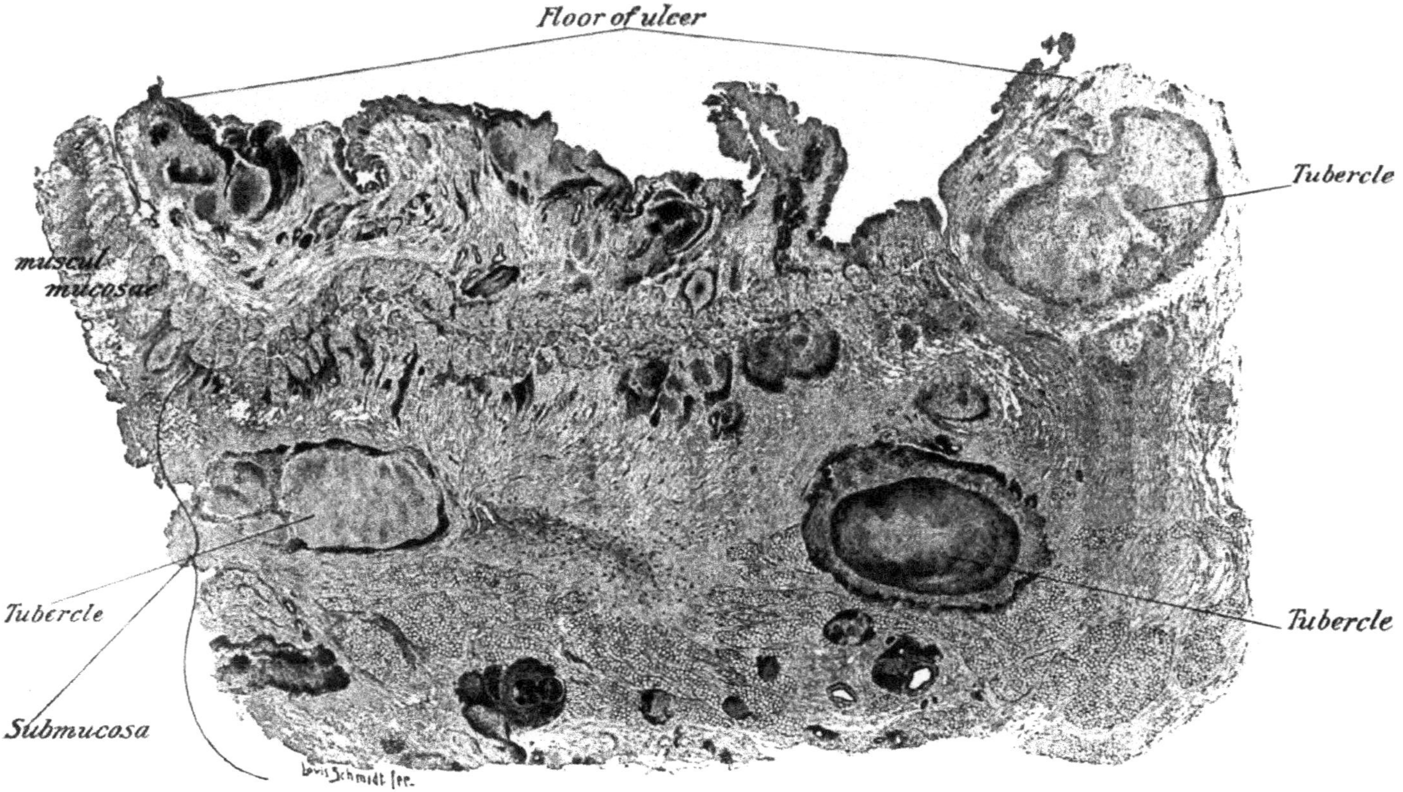

Tubercle

Tubercle

Floor of ulcer

muscosa

Tubercle

Submucosa

HISTOLOGY OF TUBERCULAR ULCER.

monary process is very advanced, so that the prognosis is grave. Such patients may continue to exist for years under alternating improvements and aggravations, so that the prognosis regarding the duration of life should not be absolutely fatal. It is a very curious experience that acute and subacute localized tuberculosis of the intestine may terminate in recovery ; even extensive peritoneal involvement may become arrested, though adhesions and functional disturbances may follow. A fatal termination by perforation or hemorrhage, while it does occur in intestinal tuberculosis, is very rare in my experience.

Mixed infections supervening upon intestinal, especially rectal, tuberculosis constitute a very serious complication. When diffuse diphtheric processes supervene upon tubercular proctitis, the evacuations become ichorous and putrescent, and a fatal result is inevitable and generally occurs under the symptoms of severe general sepsis.

Acute miliary tuberculosis also invades the intestines when it has once developed, but on account of the impossibility to determine the degree to which the intestine is involved and the hopelessness of the situation therapeutically, it has rather more of a pathological than a clinical interest.

The tubercular ulcers have already been fully considered in the chapter on Intestinal Ulcers.

Tubercular Intestinal Tumors.

Tubercular Cecal Tumor.—It has already been stated that enlarged retroperitoneal and mesenteric tubercular glands may simulate intestinal tumors. At this place, however, I wish to refer especially to the tubercular tumor of the cecum and appendix. The cecum, on account of its position, is the most favorable location for the arrest and deposit of tuberculous products which travel down the intestinal canal. The pulmonary tuberculosis which is observed together with this intestinal complication is frequently insignificant. Tubercular infection of the cecum with advanced pulmonary phthisis is a very rare occurrence. The recognition of tubercular neoplasms in this region is a modern diagnostic advance and must be largely credited to abdominal surgeons. Attention was first called to it as a disease to be differentiated from carcinoma of the cecum. Among the first to differentiate these two conditions was Durant (cited according to Conrath, *l. c.*). The fact that Durant's article was published as late as 1890 is sufficient evidence that the recognition of this condition is a very recent one. In 1891 Billroth (cited according to Conrath, *l. c.*) called attention to the tuberculous character of certain ileocecal tumors that he had encountered. Czerny (*l. c.*), König (*l. c.*), Conrath (*l. c.*), Körte (*l. c.*), Hofmeister (*l. c.*), Hartmann and Pilliet (*l. c.*), and Salzer (*l. c.*) have contributed to our knowledge of tuberculous ileocecal tumors. Tuberculous cecal tumor may originate in two ways—(*a*) from the mucosa by extensions from tubercular ulcers on the inner side of the intestinal canal, and (*b*) from the serosa by the extension of tuberculous lymph-glands. The form that originates from the mucosa represents, no doubt, an autoinfection by means of tuberculous sputa. Whether or not the tumor may arise as a primary tuberculous process from ingested tuberculous food can not be definitely stated, and Koch's recent utterances (Congress on Tuberculosis, London, 1901) cast a doubt on this question. In most cases the tumor results from three forms of changes incident to the tuberculous infection : (1) The inflammatory infiltration as a consequence of multiple tubercular ulcers which (2) may lead partly to extensive scar formation, and, by cicatricial contraction, cause stenosis of the lumen and (3) hypertrophy of the intestinal walls as a result of the stenosis.

The relation of this condition to perityphlitis of tuberculous origin has been considered in the chapters on Appendicitis, Typhlitis, and Perityphlitis. It may be stated briefly that among 120 cases of perityphlitis, Langfelt found that 20 were due to tuberculous processes. The chief stenosis occurs at the ileocecal valve, the folds of the valve being involved in the process. Professor W. P. Obrastzow, of Kiew ("Archiv f. Verdauungs-Krankheiten," Bd. IV, S. 440, "Zur Diagnose des Blinddarmcarcinoms, der Blinddarm-tuberkulose, u. s. w."), calls attention to the fact that stenosis of the ileocecal valve does not always bring about a collapse and contracted condition of the ascending colon. Theoretically one would expect to meet with this result and one ought to find that the ascending colon would be palpable, if at all, as a thin band or cord.

In some cases this is really the condition found by palpation, but the colon in other cases is found as a distended cylinder about five centimeters in diameter. Obrastzow attributes this distention to the production of gases from stagnating intestinal contents.

The Diagnosis of Tubercular Cecal Tumor.—Conrath (*l. c.*) has collected eighty-five cases, of which 65 per cent. were between the ages of twenty and forty years. In its incipiency the disease is latent; there may be constipation, or constipation alternating with diarrhea. The disease is, as a rule, not recognized as serious until the symptoms of stenosis are apparent. Then follow either localized or diffused pains of an acute, colicky character. Above all, a persistent constipation, nausea, vomiting, and frequently visible intestinal peristalsis occur. Hemorrhage from the intestine in the form of hemorrhagic admixtures in the stool are quite frequent. As the disease is a complication of pulmonary tuberculosis, elevation of temperature is frequently met with. Obrastzow, in a more recent and very scholarly contribution to the subject ("Archiv f. Verdauungs-Krankheiten," Bd. vi, S. 23), looks upon an early and rapid development of the stenosis in the cecum as carcinomatous, and a late and slow development is considered by him as characteristic of tuberculosis. In three operated cases of carcinoma of the cecum the stenosis developed in the course of from three to nine months from the beginning of the disease. In ten cases of tuberculosis of the cecum the stenotic phenomena were at no time very pronounced.

In the differential diagnosis we must consider the possibility of— (1) Cecal carcinoma; (2) dislocated kidney; (3) fibrinous appendicitis; (4) accumulated scybala in the cecum. (*a*) The differential diagnosis from cecal carcinoma is more precisely stated in the subjoined table. (*b*) From dislocated kidney, cecum tuberculosis is distinguished by the following signs: The dislocated kidney is more movable; it gives a dull sound on percussion; and is very rarely ·accompanied by signs of intestinal stenosis; a diseased kidney, when affected with carcinoma, tuberculosis, gonorrheal infection, or calculi, gives rise to nephralgia, pyuria, hematuria, etc. A dislocated kidney can usually be replaced in normal position. The differentiation from (*c*) fibrinous appendicitis is considered in the chapter on Appendicitis, and the (*d*) fecal stagnation in the cecum is considered in the chap-

ter on Obstipation.   The main supports of the diagnosis of tubercular cecal tumor are : (1) Infiltration of the walls of the cecum,
which assumes the character of a tumor; (2) the presence of
tubercle bacilli in the stools.   The presence of pulmonary tuberculosis and positive tuberculin reaction are valuable diagnostic
signs.   In the beginning the tumor is more or less movable, but
later on it may become fixed by adhesion or contracting bands in
the mesentery.   The lower edge of the cecum is located one cen-
timeter above the interspinal line in man, but when it becomes diseased by tuberculosis or carcinoma, the lower border of the cecum
rises four centimeters above the border of the linea interspinalis.
In these cases, therefore, the cecum is found in the upper part
of the iliac fossa, or even above the crest of the ilium.   Obrastzow
explains this high position of the cecum under such conditions
by a shortening of the intestinal tube caused by a sclerotic
process of a tubercular nature.   As a consequence of this high
position of the cecum the ileum is palpable for a considerably longer
distance than it would be under ordinary conditions.   Purulent
disintegration of the tumor mass may lead to the establishment of
abscesses communicating with the peritoneal cavity or adjacent
organs, or it may cause a break externally causing a preternatural
anus.   The course is protracted, particularly as the disease is generally not recognized in its incipiency ; cases have been observed that
lasted three years.

Krokiewicz ("Wien. klin. Wochenschr.," 1898, No. 29) has
made extensive investigations concerning the value of the Ehrlich
diazo-reaction in the differential diagnosis between carcinomata
and tuberculosis of the intestinal tract.   According to his results
the diazo-reaction is generally present with intestinal tuberculosis,
but is absent in carcinomata.   The diagnosis of cecal tuberculosis
thus rests upon the presence of tumor, intestinal stenosis, tubercle
bacilli in the stool, and the presence of the Ehrlich diazo-reaction.
The other rare conditions with which this disease might be confounded—for instance, actinomycosis, sarcoma, fibroma, foreign
bodies, fecal concretions, intussusception—have been considered in
their proper chapters.   Scybala, or fecal concretions, are rarely found
limited to the cecum ; if they are present there, they can be simultaneously palpated throughout the colon.   The only fecal concre-

tion that could confuse the diagnosis would be one that is strictly limited to the cecum.   If necessary, the colon could be washed out by a high irrigation, which, after several repetitions, would certainly eliminate the possibility of scybala.   The distinction from fibrinous appendicitis can frequently not be made except by observation of the course of the disease.   Improvement will follow in appendicitis of this chronic type, with a palpable induration in the right iliac fossa, on proper treatment in bed, external application of heat, counterirritation, and careful diet, but the tubercular cecal tumor will not improve under such treatment.   Fibrinous appendicitis is not a concomitant of pulmonary tuberculosis, whereas the tubercular cecal tumor is always secondary to pulmonary tuberculosis.

The following schema, which is adapted from Boas' " Verdauungs-Krankheiten," page 291, may serve to distinguish between carcinoma and tuberculosis of the cecum :

Cecum Tuberculosis.	Cecum Carcinoma.
Age : Between twenty and forty years.	Age : Rare, before the fortieth year.
Duration : From two to three years.	Duration : Eight to nine months.
Lungs : Pulmonary tuberculosis evident, more or less.	Lungs : Negative.
Tumor : Elongated ; the intestine is palpable as an infiltrated thickened cylinder.	Tumor : Sharply circumscribed, intestines not palpable.
Stenosis : Always present, develops slowly, accompanied by striking, splashing, and musical sounds.	Stenosis : Develops rapidly, acoustical signs not so pronounced.
Stool : Blood and pus rare, tubercle bacilli frequently present.	Stool : Blood and pus frequently observed ; tubercle bacilli absent.
Fever : Generally present.	Fever : Exceptional.
Urine : Ehrlich's diazo-reaction positive.	Urine : Diazo-reaction negative.

Prognosis.—This is grave under all conditions, and conditioned by the consequences of the diseases that have been described above, the principal one being stenosis, disseminated intestinal or peritoneal tuberculosis, multiple abscess formation, and amyloid degeneration of the kidneys and intestines.   The pulmonary tuberculosis in itself is one which makes the outlook hopeless.

The treatment will be considered in connection with that of the tuberculous infections of the previous types.

Prophylaxis.—The prevention of primary local infection calls for sterilization of all food, particularly of unboiled milk, avoidance of association with tuberculous patients, particularly of tuberculous nurses in the case of children, and the avoidance of autoinfection by the swallowing of sputa. Enteritis in tuberculous individuals should be treated with great care, as the mucosa which has become diseased is more liable to tubercular infection than a healthy one.

Treatment.

The treatment of tubercular enteritis or of enteritis and colitis in tuberculous patients, even where it can not be proved to be a tubercular infection localized in the intestine, demands a diet similar to that described in the chapters on Enteritis and Dysentery. Strained soups made of oatmeal, bouillon and egg, with salt, together with acorn cocoa and a little claret, should constitute the sole articles of diet for about twenty-four hours. Somatose should be avoided, because it increases the diarrhea, but eucasin and nutrose are valuable additions to the soup. The patient should be confined in bed. If an error of diet can be distinctly made out, a small dose of calomel —$\frac{1}{2}$ of a grain, repeated every three hours, and combined with $\frac{1}{6}$ of a grain of denarcotized extract of opium—will hasten the evacuation of the offending food. Concerning the specific treatment of intestinal tuberculosis by tuberculin, I may say that there is no doubt that a number of cases have been cured by a cautious administration of this substance. Elsewhere I have stated that I have personally studied the healing of a tubercular rectal ulcer under the influence of tuberculin; nevertheless I do not recommend the systematic employment of tuberculin in the treatment of tubercular intestinal ulcers, enteritis, or cecal tumor, because this form of treatment has not yet been satisfactorily tested for intestinal diseases, and also because the intestinal lesion is generally a secondary one, and the localizations in other organs also demand consideration. For the diarrhea, tannigin, tannalbin, bismuth subgallate and bismuth salicylate, as well as naphthalin, have proved useful in my experience, but I must emphasize that nothing beyond a temporary relief must be expected of these remedies. The creasote preparations have, in my experience, not proved useful. The frequent eructations which creasote causes when given in the doses recommended for these patients reduce, rather than increase, the appetite. The only partial success in the way of treatment of tubercular ileocecal tumor is to be expected from operation, wherever this is possible.*

SYPHILIS OF THE INTESTINES.

The pathological changes which syphilis may produce in the human intestine are curiously varied.   Clinically we are capable of distinguishing between three forms of intestinal syphilis : the syph-ilitic enteritis which may be both acute and chronic, syphilitic neoplasms, and syphilitic ulcerations.   The intestine may become diseased under the influence of a general diffuse syphilitic infection, and also by local inoculation and transportation of the virus.   The latter is particularly the case with syphilitic infections of the rectum. As there are no pathognomonic signs and symptoms whereby the clinician might establish the diagnosis of intestinal syphilis, the cases are rare in which this diagnosis can be positively made during life.   This will continue so, as long as the exciting cause of this disease, whatever it may be, is unknown.   Investigation of the feces furnishes no aid to diagnosis, and in this respect syphilis differs from intestinal tuberculosis and actinomycosis.   Even pathologically, when the sections of the intestine are under the microscope, it is not always possible to make the diagnosis of syphilis, particularly in such cases where the history of syphilitic infection during life is not given in the clinical reports.   Histologically syphilitic enteritis is not different from simple catarrhal enteritis in its intense type, and the syphilitic intestinal ulcer not markedly different from a tuberculous or catarrhal ulcer of severe type.   But for the possi-bility of demonstrating the tubercle bacillus in such intestines and the association of a pulmonary tuberculosis with one case, and a history of general syphilitic infection in another case, with perhaps the reported experience of the result of antisyphilitic treatment,—one could not, from the histological structure alone, decide what con-stitutes syphilitic enteritis or syphilitic ulceration, and what consti-tutes tuberculous enteritis or ulceration.   Only in the syphiloma or

---

* Literature on Tuberculosis of Intestines and Tubercular Cecal Tumor, in addition to that given in chapter XXI, vol. I, will be found in an addendum at the end of this volume.

luetic neoplasms do we possess a condition which can be pronounced characteristic. In the intestines of some syphilitics that had been subject to severe symptoms of diarrhea, with blood and pus in the evacuations, diffuse syphilomatous neoplasms have been encountered that were remarkable for their richness in spindle cells. Here and there larger nodules had seemingly, by confluence, formed a more circumscribed neoplasm. What is characteristic for syphilis in these neoplasms or gummata is a regressive metamorphosis or degeneration, which renders the substance of the gumma unstainable. I have given an illustration from a case of syphilitic gastritis of this regressive metamorphosis in a small gastric gumma in my work on "Diseases of the Stomach," second edition, Plate IX, facing page 596. Minute gummata may occur in the intestine in a miliary form, appearing like tiny tubercles, or they may develop into somewhat larger nodules, and in that case are not found so frequently. The main seat of these neoplasms is in the submucosa in my experience, though Jürgens claims to have found them prevailingly in the muscularis. They may develop from the lymph-nodules of the mucosa, though not necessarily so. Orth is of the opinion that they often develop independently of these structures; at other times they originate from isolated or agminated glands. Entire Peyer's patches may be transformed into large gummous neoplasms. As in all syphilitic neoplasms, so also in the intestine, the blood-vessels in their neighborhood are decidedly altered. Mracek asserts that the syphiloma begins around the arteries, the endothelial layer of which proliferates and eventually causes an occlusion of the lumen of the artery, to which is attributed the regressive metamorphosis of the neoplasm. Syphilitic ulcers may originate from degenerative changes in the neoplasm, but they may also develop by simple degeneration of the mucosa before a neoplasm has formed. The syphilitic ulcerations have already been fully considered in the chapter on Intestinal Ulcers.

Acute Syphilitic Enteritis.

The assumption of syphilitic enteritis as a morbid entity is based upon the observation that acute intestinal catarrh may exist contemporarily with recent lues—that is, simultaneously with the eruptive stage and the secondary manifestations in the epidermis and mouth.   It is occasionally observed in syphilitics that a slight fever, together with diarrheas and colics, accompanies the eruption of syphilis.   The assumption that this intestinal complication is due to syphilis is justifiable only when all other causes of an acute enteritis, particularly artificial production by means of drugs, can be excluded, and when the treatment directed toward the general syphilitic infection accomplishes an improvement of the remaining luetic affection simultaneously with the disappearance of the intestinal catarrh.   If, for instance, the skin eruption, with perhaps a mucous patch in the mouth, will gradually disappear and attacks of persistent diarrhea and colic cease under mercurial inunctions, the diagnosis of syphilitic enteritis is justifiable.   The enteritis may be restricted to single portions of the intestine,—for instance, only to the duodenum, where it is often associated with a catarrhal affection of the stomach, or where it may extend into the bile-passages,—or it may involve the entire small intestine.   The evacuations show the character of the ordinary intestinal catarrh, which has been described in the chapter on Enteritis.   The abdomen is distended, tympanitic, and sensitive to pressure.   In subjects that are predisposed to intestinal catarrhs, particularly in alcoholics, the acute condition may pass over into a chronic enteritis.   The anatomical changes which exist in acute syphilitic enteritis are not satisfactorily understood, because no pathological material on this subject has been reported.   Jullien ("Traité pratique des maladies vénériennes," Deuxième édit., Paris, 1885, 476 ff.) assumes that the lymph apparatus of the intestine becomes diseased by the syphilitic virus.   There can be no doubt regarding this opinion, since the intestinal lymph apparatus is affected in all intestinal catarrhs irrespective of the pathogenetic factor, especially if they assume an intense form. Acute catarrhal duodenitis may extend to the bile-passages, producing icterus.

Syphilitic enteritis may be the precursor of severe anatomical lesions of the intestine, but if diarrheas and colics disappear rapidly, it is impossible to decide clinically whether the condition had an etiological connection with the syphilitic infection or not.

Diagnosis.—If symptoms of intestinal catarrh occur shortly before or shortly after the manifestations of syphilis in the skin and other organs, the enteritis may be attributed to the specific infection.

Acute enteritis may also occur with advanced or tertiary lues. In these cases the bowel complication can be considered specific if it repeatedly occurs without any other demonstrable cause, particularly if errors in the diet can be excluded, or if the enteritis develops after a diet which the individual formerly digested without any symptoms of the intestinal distress.

Prognosis.—The prognosis of syphilitic intestinal catarrh of the acute type is not so favorable as that of enteritis in individuals that are not syphilitic, because in the majority of cases only such individuals as are disposed to bowel diseases are attacked by this complication, and also because the constitutional infection impedes convalescence.

Chronic Syphilitic Enteritis.

There are mainly two types of chronic luetic enteritis, (1) that which occurs as a concomitant of syphilitic intestinal ulcerations, and (2) that which occurs as a result of syphilis of abdominal and circulatory organs which effect a permanent stagnation in the region of the inferior vena cava, particularly of the portal vein, causing hyperemia in the intestinal canal. Occasionally an acute or subacute enteritis may pass over into the chronic type. Syphilitic enteritis, dysentery, and tormina intestinorum have been described by the older writers,—Petronius (*l. c.*), Venedictus Victorius (*l. c.*), Ambroise Paré (*l. c.*), Rondeletius (*l. c.*),—but in 1854 Cullerier ("De l'entérite syphilitique," "L'Union méd. de Paris," 1854, No. 47), in a very thorough report, called the attention of clinicians to this type of intestinal catarrh. Later descriptions, since then, are by Pillon (*l. c.*), Diettrich (*l. c.*), Müller (*l. c.*), Gallard (*l. c.*), Simon (*l. c.*), Tissier (*l. c.*), Wagner (*l. c.*), Aufrecht (*l. c.*), and Meschede (*l. c.*). Most of these cases are not simple enteritis, but a complication of the latter with syphilitic ulcerations. Microscopic investigation of the intestine in a state of chronic syphilitic enteritis shows a uniform infiltration of all layers, with proliferation of the interstitial tissue. There may be nothing more visible than the changes that are observed in simple chronic enteritis, but in some cases we may have the minute neoplasms, some of them showing the characteristic regressive degeneration. E. Müller's (*l. c.*) case is of extraordinary clinical interest : The patient was a female who showed no external signs of syphilis, and had been repeatedly treated for catarrhal affections of the larynx and bronchial tubes. At the autopsy old and recent syphilitic processes were found in the liver, larynx, and right pleura, and old cicatrices at the entrance to the vagina. The ileum was moderately distended from the ileocecal valve up to the jejunum. There were two stenoses, hardly passable by the little finger,—one near the transition of the jejunum into the ileum, and another about a foot and a half below this point. The strictures were about one and a quarter inches long, and the peritoneum was thickened by increase in connective tissue. On cutting through the constriction a hard, sinewy cicatrix with complete loss of the mucosa and even of the muscular layer became apparent. The inner surface of the cicatrix, or basis, was completely smooth. In the reports of these cases, chronic enteritis and syphilitic intestinal ulcers have been hopelessly confused, and it is necessary to separate them distinctly wherever autopsies have made this separation possible. Syphilitic enteritis, like simple enteritis, may exist without symptoms, and be recognized only at the autopsy, or it may give rise to intractable diarrheas. Whenever pus and blood are in the stool, the possibility of intestinal ulcer should suggest itself, the results and complications of which have already been described. Amyloid degeneration of the intestine may be a consequence of syphilis : it expresses itself in protracted diarrheas, pronounced albuminuria, and an enlarged liver with a thickened palpable edge. The spleen is also enlarged, and there are evidences of severe syphilis in other parts of the body, particularly in the bones and skin. Death may occur as a result of peritonitis, perforation, marasmus, exhaustion, or the consequences of intestinal strictures. Severe cases of intestinal syphilis of a chronic type may show temporary improvements under antisyphilitic treatment, but in advanced cases this improvement does not last very long.

Diagnosis of Chronic Syphilitic Enteritis.—This depends upon two factors : the presence of other phenomena of hereditary or acquired syphilis, and the exclusion of other possible causes of intestinal catarrh and ulceration. The evacuations should in all cases be examined, particularly for tubercle bacilli.

The syphilitic ulcerations of the intestine and syphilitic affections of the rectum have been described in separate chapters.

Syphilitic Tumors of the Intestine.

Syphilitic neoplasms of the small intestine, clinically representing tumors, may be brought about by the thickening of the intestinal wall in the vicinity of large specific luetic ulcers or by diffuse inflammatory infiltration and proliferation of the tissue of the intestinal layers. The accumulation of fecal masses above syphilitic stenoses, as well as the enlarged retroperitoneal and mesenteric glands in syphilitics, also demand classification under this heading. Clinically the separation as to the exact cause of the neoplasm, whether due to an ulcer, diffuse thickening, enlarged glands, etc., presents great difficulties. In this connection I will briefly report a case occurring in my own private practice.

A clerk, aged thirty-two years, had suffered with alternating constipation and diarrhea, vomiting, meteorism, and pains localized in the neighborhood of the umbilicus. His wife had gone through two miscarriages. He had two large scars over his right tibia, and three smaller scars over the left tibia. He confessed to having contracted syphilis ten years ago, and argued that he did not marry until the physician pronounced him cured. Heart and lungs were normal, urine normal, examination of stomach-contents after test-meals showed free HCl absent, combined HCl 12, total acidity 40, much mucus, and of lactic acid only a trace. There was evidence of a pronounced gastric atony. In the median line of the abdomen, extending from about an inch and a half above the umbilicus to the costal cartilages on the left side, a large tumor-mass could be palpated. On distending the stomach with CO_2, it could be distinctly palpated, and demonstrated that the tumor had no connection with this organ. On using the gastric electrodiaphane within the stomach, it was also evident that the neoplasm was not situated there. On distending the colon with 1½ liters of warm water, the tumor was slightly displaced downward, becoming much more distinct. It was not possible to pass the electrodiaphane up into the colon past the tumor: very likely a stenosis in the transverse colon prevented its passage. The diagnosis of tumor of the transverse colon was made, and the patient treated with mercurial inunctions and iodid of potassium internally beginning at once with doses of thirty grains thrice daily. Three months after this treatment had been instituted the tumor was decidedly smaller, and the symptoms of stenosis had largely disappeared. I then recommended a course of hot bathing, together with gentle massage of the transverse colon, and cessation of the mercurial treatment. After six weeks of this therapic management the mercurial inunctions were resumed. Fourteen months after the beginning of the antisyphilitic treatment it was impossible to make out any tumor or induration, even when palpation was undertaken while the patient was in a warm bath.

Riedel (*l. c.*) has reported two cases of syphilitic tumors, one of which occurred in a man fifty-nine years old who acquired syphilis in his twenty-second year. This patient presented a hard, voluminous, tightly stretched tumor in the neighborhood of the umbilicus, giving a tympanitic resonance on percussion, in the region of the cecum. At the operation the transverse colon was found distended almost unto bursting. The case ended fatally, and at the autopsy the mesentery and the entire length of the small intestine were found covered with small nodules varying from the size of a lentil seed to that of a dime, at places presenting cicatricial prolongations. The hepatic flexure of the colon and the pylorus were adherent to the gall-bladder. There was an hour-glass stomach, dilated in its cardiac portion. In the pyloric portion the mucosa was considerably thickened. The microscopic examination gave an abundant proliferation of the inflammatory tissue in the muscular layer of the intestine. The wall of the intestine was increased to ten times its normal size. The second case of Riedel was that of a woman fifty years old who had a large, painful swelling to the left of the umbilicus. Death occurred under the symptoms of collapse. The autopsy showed peritonitis due to perforation of a syphilitic ulcer. There was also a communication between two intestinal loops.

The diagnosis of syphilitic tumor can be made safely only when there are other evidences of syphilis in the skin and other organs, and when other causes of tumor formation can be excluded.

Treatment.—Intestinal syphilis of whatever kind calls for energetic antisyphilitic treatment. Inunctions should in all cases be preferred to the internal use of mercury. In inveterate cases the iodid of sodium—from thirty to forty grains in a day—should be administered at intervals. It is not wise to continue the antisyphilitic treatment without interruption, since even under the inunction treatment the stomach shows evidences of acute gastritis. One of the main objects of treatment is a highly nutritious diet, such as I have outlined in a previous chapter on Acute and Chronic Enteritis. Syphilitic infections of the rectum are treated according to the principles laid down in the chapter on Rectal Diseases by Dr. Thomas Charles Martin.

ACTINOMYCOSIS OF THE INTESTINE.

Actinomycosis is an infection of the tissues with the fungus actinomyces. The disease was first studied in animals, particularly oxen and cows, by Lebert and Davaine, about 1845. The former had discovered characteristic granules in the diseased tissue of calves, and later on found the same granules in pus from abscesses in human beings. Von Langenbeck and Israel (1845) and Laboulbene and Robin (1853) confirmed the observations of Lebert. Rivolta (1868) and Perroncito (1873) described the macroscopic structural relations of the fungus accurately and emphasized the etiological connection between it and the tissue changes with which it was found associated. But to Bollinger is due the credit of having established beyond a doubt the pathogenic significance of the fungus, based on investigations of the disease occurring on the jaws of a heifer. In 1879 Harz established the scientific position of the "Actinomyces bovis" by accurate biological methods. In 1879 Ponfick proved the pathological identity of the actinomyces of man and animals. The disease has been observed in cattle, horses, dogs, pigs, and in the elephant, but has been known under various somewhat misleading names. The most common name for the actinomycosis of the lower jaw in cattle was the German designation "Kiefer krebs," or maxillary or jaw sarcoma. In "Virchow's Archiv," volumes cxv and cxvi, O. Israel has given a classical description of the biological properties of the actinomyces fungus, and the way in which it can be cultivated, and suggested a classification which has since then been accepted in most monographs on the subject. The classification is based on the portals of entry through which the infection takes place.

First Group.—Infection through the mouth and pharyngeal cavity, generally by mechanical inoculation of the mouth and throat tissues by the actinomyces spores contained in the food.

Second Group.—Infection through the respiratory organs—pulmonary actinomycosis.

Third Group.—Infection through the digestive tract—gastric and intestinal actinomycosis.

Fourth Group.—Infection through the skin or lacrimal organs—cutaneous actinomycosis.

Fifth Group.—A number of other authenticated cases in which the portal of entry was unknown are classed under the fifth group —actinomycosis infection where the portal of entry was unknown.

The form which interests us most here is the gastro-intestinal actinomycosis. It occurs much more rarely than the cases of the first group. The diseased portions of the intestine may be only superficially invaded, or the fungus may have penetrated the entire intestinal wall, inciting them to proliferation. These forms, originating from the lower digestive tract, have become known under the names of abdominal or intestinal actinomycosis. In 1895 Grill collected 106 cases belonging to this type, including four personal observations ("Ueber Actinomycos des Magens und Darms beim Menschen," "Beitr. z. klin. Chir.," 1895). A type which has been recognized and described separately, owing to its striking resemblance to a form of appendicitis, is the actinomycosis of the ileocecal region originating from the vermiform process. Lanz has collected these cases under the name of *"perityphlitis actinomycotica"* ("Correspondenzblatt f. Schweizer Aerzte," 1892). These ileocecal types represent 50 per cent. of all intestinal affections. The remaining 50 per cent. are distributed over the small intestine, colon, rectum, and stomach. As already stated, there are a superficial and a deep form of the infection; the latter may be designated as the parenchymatous form. The only case of superficial intestinal actinomycosis has been reported by Chiari.* In this case the intestinal mucosa was covered with a thick white mycelium, not continuous, but occurring in spots, varying in size from that of a pea to the size of a ten-cent piece. The form of growth strongly resembled the aerobiotic behavior of the fungus when it is cultivated in artificial media ("Die Strahlenpilzkrankheit," by Professor Friedrich von Korányi, Nothnagel's "Spec. Pathol. u. Ther.," Bd. v). The mycelium consisted of numerous threads which partly extended into the mucosa. Between the hyphæ there were calcareous epithelia, and isolated, club-shaped formations which are so characteristic of the actinomyces fungus. There were no necrobiosis and no proliferation of connective tissue.

---

* "Ueber primäre Darmactinomycosa beim Menschen," "Prager med. Wochenschr.," 1884.

Parenchymatous Form.

In all the reports except this one by Chiari, the cases presented are of the penetrating or parenchymatous type of intestinal actinomycosis, in which the peritoneum becomes involved and reacts with an acute or chronic inflammation and the formation of exudates or pus, development of adhesions, and the consequent obstruction of the intestinal lumen, continuation of the inflammatory process to adjacent organs (ovaries, bladder, and rectum), penetration into subperitoneal connective tissue, involvement of the abdominal walls, and even of the bony pelvis. In addition to this extension by continuity and contiguity, this infectious process leads to the development of thrombi and emboli, particularly in the portal circulation.

Symptomatology.

The earlier symptoms are gastralgia and enteralgia, attacks of colic, vomiting, and constipation which in a few cases alternates with diarrhea. Occasionally severe pains occur in the thigh. The abdominal form most frequently observed is that which assumes the type of perityphlitis, the formation of tumor in the ileocecal region, pains, symptoms of descending infiltration into the interior of the pelvis, and of circumscribed peritonitis. Later on infiltrated areas develop in the abdominal wall which are very hard, extremely painful, but not sharply circumscribed. In some cases these infiltrated hard areas of the abdominal wall may soften at the anterior lower regions of the belly or about the region of Poupart's ligament; they may rupture into the region of the anus and lead to the formation of fistulæ which discharge a purulent or viscid serum containing fragments of tissue and the characteristic granules, club-shaped hyphæ, and other portions of the structure of the fungus. In a case reported by Billroth rupture of the intestinal actinomycotic invasion occurred into the bladder, and portions of the fungus were voided with the urine.

There are rare cases in which the intestinal process may progress unnoticed, without symptoms, until the peritoneum becomes involved. The course is chronic, as a rule. There are cases which seemingly run an acute course, but no doubt these are such cases in which the intestinal symptoms have remained latent for a long time.

The submucous foci of the fungus form nodules about the size of a lentil, which project slightly into the lumen of the intestine. As the disease progresses they break down at the apex and are thus converted into small ulcers very similar to the tuberculous ulcers already described, having undermined edges and a corroded base. By confluence of several such ulcerations, and also by proliferal extension, the destructive process may spread out considerably.

Diagnosis.

The diagnosis of intestinal actinomycosis is only possible if the process extends to the abdominal walls and produces the characteristic cutaneous changes, or if the characteristic fungus-granules can be found in the stools or urine; otherwise the disease will be confused with a variety of neoplasms and infiltrations of the abdominal walls, or with appendicitis, perinephritis, periproctitis, and perityphlitis.

Treatment.

The treatment of actinomycosis is almost exclusively surgical. I remember personally having observed a case in Professor Hahn's clinic at the Krankenhaus Friedrichshain, in Berlin, in which a young man, aged twenty-six, presented the typical symptoms of acute appendicitis. On opening the abdomen Hahn found the characteristic infiltration of the cecum and appendix described above, and, scooping some of the tumor-mass out with a dull curet, he exhibited to me the characteristic fungus-globules under the microscope, proving the case to be one of ileocecal actinomycosis. Whatever can not be removed surgically is injected with solution of bichlorid of mercury 1 : 1000. The injections are made at the border-line between the diseased and healthy tissue. Spontaneous cures of actinomycotic areas in the intestine are probable, since cicatrices have been observed in the same intestine together with typical actinomycotic ulcers. Whenever surgical local treatment is impossible, iodid of potash should be given internally. Thomasen-Netter has given the drug in doses of six grams, or ninety grains, for twenty-five days with varying interruptions in a case of severe pulmonary and pleuritic actinomycosis.

Rydygier has employed iodid of potash in a 1 per cent. solution for hypodermic injection into the diseased tissue. He injected from two to four syringefuls every eight days, and accomplished a cure in two months. Billroth effected a favorable result with injections of tuberculin. In the cases which I observed in the University of Maryland the iodid treatment proved useless.

LITERATURE ON SYPHILIS OF THE INTESTINES.

1. Aufrecht, "Ein Fall von Amyloidgeschwüren des Darmkanals in Folge von Syphilis," "Berlin. klin. Wochenschr.," 1869, 29.

2. Bärensprung, von, "Annalen des Charité-Krankenhauses," 1855.

3. Baumgarten, "Virchow's Archiv," Bd. CXVII, S. 39, 1884.

4. Beer, A., "Die Eingeweidesyphilis," Tübingen, 1867, 7.

5. Birch-Hirschfeld, "Lehrbuch," Bd. II, S. 589, 1885.

6. Björnström, "Fall von Darmsyphilis," "Upsala Läkareforenings Förhandlinger," 1875, XI, 72.

7. Björnström, "Arch. f. Dermatologie und Syphilis," 1876, Bd. VIII, S. 641.

8. Blackmore, A, "A Case of Syphilitic Ulceration of the Intestine," "Lancet," 1885, vol. II, p. 615.

9. Bumstead, "Bull. de la soc. d'Anat. Paris," 2 S., T. IV, 1859, p. 100, New York Acad. of Med., 1864, April.

10. Chiari, "Prager. med. Wochenschr.," 1885, No. 47.

11. Coote "On Syphilitic Constriction of the Rectum and Vagina," "Med. Times and Gazette," London, January 27, 1855.

12. Croce, cited by C. von Jullian, "Cirurgia univers.," Lib. V, tratt XII, Cap. III.

13. Cullerier, "De l'entérite syphilitique," "L'Union méd. de Paris," 1854, No. 47.

14. Dittrich, "Prager Vierteljahrsschrift," 1849, Bd. XXI, S. 20.

15. Dujardin-Beaumetz, "Observations de syph. tert. viscerale," "Gaz. d. hôpit.," 1866, 61.

16. Eberth, "Ueber eine eigenthümliche, vielleicht syphilitische, Enteritis," "Virchow's Archiv," 1867, Bd. XL. S. 326.

17. Ferrari, "De l'entero-peritonite syphil.," "Ann. de derm. et de syphil.," 1881, II, 621.

18. Fournier, "Lésions tertiaires de l'anus et du rectum," Paris, 1875.

19. Förster, "Würzburger med. Zeitschrift," 1863, Bd. IV.

20. Gosselin, "Recherches sur les rétrécissements syphil. du rectum," "Arch. gén. de Méd.," 1855, p. 666.

21. Hahn, E., "Ueber syphilitische Mastdarmerkrankungen mit ausgedehnten Geschwürsbildungen im Dünndarm," "Deutsch. med. Wochenschr.," 1892, 69.

22. Hayem et Tissier, "De la syphilis de l'intestine," "Rev. de Méd.," Paris, 1889, 281 ff.

23 Homén, "Centralbl. f. allg. Pathol. u. pathol. Anat.," 1893, 97.

24. Huët, "Ueber syphilitische Affectionen des Mastdarmes," mit Abbildungen, in Behrend, "Syphilidologie," Neue Reihe, Erlangen, 1860, 1 ff.

25. Ignatjew, Virchow, and Hirsch, "Jahresbericht für 1883," Bd. II, S. 535.

26. Israel, "Ueber eine seltene Form von Ringgeschwüren des Dünndarms (Syphilis?)," "Charité Annalen," 1884, Bd. IX, S. 707.

27. Johnson, Henry James, "Bemerkungen über Ulceration des Mastdarmes, die in Verbindung mit Kondylomen oder anderen Symptomen der secundären Syphilis vorkommt," "The London Med. and Chir. Review," 1835; and Behrend, "Syphilidologie," Leipzig, 1839, Bd. I, 388 ff.

28. Jullien, "Recherches statistiques sur l'etiologie de la Syphilis c. Mauric," cited by Neumann (*l. c.*).

29. Jürgens, "Berlin. klin. Wochenschr.," 1880, S. 667.

30. Klebs, "Handbuch I," S. 261, 1869.

31. Kleinschmidt, "Ueber Darmsyphilis mit Anschluss der Mastdarmkrankungen," Diss., Göttingen, 1895.

32. Lang, "Lehrb. d. Syphil.," S. 241.

33. Lang, V., "Vorlesungen über Pathologie und Therapie der Syphilis," Wiesbaden, 1884 bis 1886, 241.

34. Lancereaux, cited by Neumann (*l. c.*).

35. Laurenzi, "Entero-peritonite gommosa sifilitica," "Arch. di med. chir. ed igiene," Roma, p. 222-224.

36. Mason, "Venereal Stricture of the Rectum," "Amer. Jour. of the Med. Sci.," vol. LXV, p. 22, 1873.

37. Mauriac, "Leçons sue les malad. vénériennes," Paris, 1883, 729.

38. Meschede, "Virchow's Archiv," Bd. XXXVII, S. 566.

39. Mollièr, "Traité des mamal. du rect et de l'anus," Paris, 1877.

40. Monnot, "Contribute, à l'etude du syph. ano-rectal," "Thèse de Paris," 1882.

41. Mracek, "Ueber Enteritis bei Lues hered.," "Arch. f. Dermatologie und Syphilis," 1883.

42. Müller, E., "Ueber des Auftreten der constitutionellen Syphilis im Darmkanal," Erlangen, 1858.

43. Neumann, "Syphilis," Nothnagel's "Spec. Pathol. u. Therap.," Bd. XXIII, 1899.

44. Neumann, "Beitrag zur Myostitis syphilitica," "Arch. f. Dermatologie und Syphilis," 1888, 19.

45. Norman, "Path. Soc. of London," April, 1884; "Brit. Med. Jour.," 1884, vol. I, p. 668.

46. Oestreich, "Demonstration eines Dünndarms mit einer grossen Anzahl syphilit. Ulcerationen," Beilage 7 der "Deutschen med. Wochenschr.," März, 1897; und "Arch. f. Dermatologie und Syphilis," Bd. XLV, 1898, S. 312.

47. Oser, "Drei Fälle von Enteritis syphilitica," "Viertel jahrschr. f. Dermatologie und Syphilis," Prag, 1871, Bd. III, S. 23.

48. Paget, "Syphilitic Diseases of the Rectum," "Paris méd. Jour.," 1870, vol. I, p. 156.

49. Paré, "De la grosse vérole, dite malade vénérienne et des accidens qui adviennent à icelle," "Les Oeuvres d'Ambroise Paré," Lyon, 1664, 444-467.

50. Petronius, "De morbo gallico libr. Septem.," Aphrod. Luisinus, T. II, p. 1298.

51. Pillon, "De l'entérite syphilitique secondaire, ou exanthème syph. de l'intéstin," "Gaz. des hôpit.," 1857, No. 66.

52. Ponfick, "Breslauer ärztliche Zeitschrift," 1884, No. 6.

53. Riedel, "Mittheilungen aus den Grenzebieten der Medizin und Chirurgie," 1897, Bd. II, H. 3 u. 4, S. 508.

54. Rieder, "Zur Kenntnis der specifischen Darmerkrankungen bei acquirirter Syphilis," "Jahrbücher der Hamburger Staatskrankenanstalten," I. Jahrgang, 1889.

55. Rondeletius, "De morbo Italico liber unus in Methodus curandorum omnium morborum corporis humani in tres libros distincta. Lug.," 1575, Aphrod. Luisinus., T. II, p. 948.

56. Roth, "Beobachtungen über congenitale Enteritis," "Virchow's Archiv," 1867, Bd. XL, S. 326.

57. Simon, "Zur Lehre der Visceralsyphilis," "Vierteljahrsschr. f. Dermatologie und Syphilis," 1872, 533 ff.

58. Sorrentino, "Ricerche istologiche sulla sifilide intestinale," "Riforma med.," 1890, No. 147.

59. Tretat et E. Deten, "Retrecissem. du rect. Dict. encycl. des scienc. med.," 3. ser., II, 187, 726.

60. Victorius, "De morbo gallico libr.," Cap. x, Ibid., T. I, 647.

61. E. Vidat, "Ulcerat. vener. du rect.," Ibid., 687.

62. Virchow, "Ueber Mastdarmgeschwüre," Onkol. II, 415, 1865.

63. Wagner, "Arch. der Heilkunde," Bd. IV, S. 368–370, 1863.

64. Warfwinge und Blix, "Fall af Darmsyfilis," "Hygiea," Stockholm, 1877; "Arch. f. Dermatologie und Syphilis," 1879, XII, S. 452.

65. Whitehead, "Therapeutics of Syphilis of Rectum," "Amer. Jour. of the Med. Sci.," 1871.

66. Zapputa, "Observ. remarquable de retrecissem. syph. du rect.," "Ann. de derm. et de syphil.," v, 315, und Schmidt's "Jahrbücher," Bd. CXLVIII, S. 167; und "Arch. f. Dermatologie und Syphilis," 1871, 90; v. Zeissl., Ibid., 1875, 137 ff.

CHAPTER III.

INTESTINAL OCCLUSION.

INTRODUCTION TO THE STUDY OF INTESTINAL OCCLUSION.

In the clinical picture of enterostenosis and intestinal occlusion, a long series of factors merit consideration, the isolated consideration of which is of the greatest importance for a proper understanding of these conditions. When the physician is confronted with the complete case of occlusion, these individual factors are very difficult to keep apart. The pathogenesis of these conditions would never have been satisfactorily understood no matter how careful the clinical study might have been. Experimental investigation that tested the results of artificially produced stenoses in different parts of the alimentary tract, with or without simultaneous obstruction of the mesenteric vessels, was necessary. In no domain of clinical pathology is a clear understanding of the etiological factors and pathogenesis more indispensable than in the enterostenoses. A few of the more important factors in the pathogenesis I deem it necessary to consider individually, as follows :

The term intestinal obstruction is frequently considered as equivalent to stoppage of the bowels, but we shall see in the following that interruption in the permeability is not only unnecessary as a symptom of intestinal obstruction, but that it may lead to frequent errors of diagnosis :

In order to avoid misunderstanding, I feel that it will be practical to premise this chapter on the Intestinal Stenoses, Occlusions, Strictures, Constrictions, Obturations, Intussusceptions, etc., by an exact definition of these conditions.

Stenosis. In agreement with Nothnagel (*l. c.*), I designate as stenosis every narrowing of the intestinal lumen—every reduction of the diameter of its cross-section—independently of its anatomical or etiological cause. Similarly

Occlusion signifies the complete closure, blocking, or shutting up of the bowel.

Stricture designates the reduction of the lumen by circular *internal* diseases of the intestinal wall.

Constriction signifies the narrowing of the intestinal lumen from the circular binding effect of *external* causes.

Obturation—closure of the lumen by impediments *within* the intestinal canal.

Intussusception—invagination or involution (telescoping) of one part of the intestine into another.

A stenosis or narrowing is an incomplete and an occlusion a complete blocking up of the canal.

I. Stoppage of the evacuations may occur in complete intestinal occlusion without causing any detriment to the general condition. Such a state of the bowels is observed with very gradually narrowing stenoses in the lower part of the colon, where a slow accumulation of immense masses of fecal matter is possible. It is even observed without stenoses in individuals with abnormally sluggish peristalsis. Kirstein (*l. c.*) and Reichel (*l. c.*) have proved by the experimental occlusion produced in dogs that complete occlusion may exist for a long time without severe disturbances. Kirstein produced an experimental stenosis of the small intestine closely above the ileocecal valve. Every communication between the upper and the lower bowel was completely prevented, but the circulatory conditions of the intestinal wall were not injured. He closed the intestine after intersection by sewing up each end of the severed bowel separately, thereupon invaginated each end of the bowel for 1 cm., and placed a second row of stitches over the first, uniting serosa to serosa. One would expect that this animal would have succumbed in a short while, under the most tumultuous phenomena of acute occlusion. This presumption proved to be erroneous, for the dog lived six weeks without vomiting. In fact, the animal did not present a single symptom of ileus or occlusion. After he recovered from the operation, he played about good naturedly, and ate his food with apparent relish. He never had any more evacuations. At the end of the second week he showed absence of appetite, and at the end of the third he refused all food and took only water. Death occurred by starvation. At dissection the stomach was found very small, the duodenum seemed entirely absent, the jejunum and upper ileum somewhat distended with liquid and gas. Only the last 60 cm. of the ileum above the artificial closure showed a colossal dilation, filled with grayish-green pus and fecal contents. The colon was contracted and empty. In Reichel's experiments, however, vomiting occurred after several days, and all his cases had a dilation of the bowel that extended nearly up to the stomach. The point to be emphasized in these experiments is that complete occlusion may exist for some time without severe disturbances.

II. **Stagnation of feces may in itself become dangerous after a short duration**, especially if the amount of gas developed reaches great dimensions and effects an abrupt interference with the circulation and nervous system.

III. **The enormous masses of intestinal contents which are vomited do not consist exclusively of ingesta.** After the preliminary vomiting of mucus and bile has ceased, the more characteristic vomit of occlusion consists of intestinal contents resembling diarrheic passages. They are liquid and very offensive. Whatever there may be of solid material does not come from the colon, however. This character of vomit may continue for several days after all ingestion of food has ceased, and after a time when it is reasonable to suppose that all ingested food must have been evacuated. By far the largest part of this vomit consists of the immensely increased secretions of intestinal juice and the transudation which is a consequence of the circulatory disturbances. This mixture undergoes a rapid putrefaction, during which it is converted into a mass resembling thin feces.

IV. **Extreme distention can cause disturbance in the nutrition of the intestine, and bring about paralysis.** By experimental overdistention of a limited portion of the intestine in guinea-pigs, Kocher produced a passive hyperemia, tearing of the blood-vessels, and consequent extravasation of blood into the intestinal wall, accompanied by secretion of mucus and serum, which increased the distention still more. Distention of the intestinal wall, when it lasts sufficiently long, produces severer injuries than ligation of the arteries and veins supplying the corresponding portion of the intestine. Although the experiments of

Kocher are not directly transferable in their results to the clinical conditions found in man, nevertheless, although the amount of distention may be less in man, it is exerted for a longer time and the musculature must eventually become exhausted. If now a circulatory disturbance is superadded to the intestinal distention, we have a vicious circle completed. The distention injures the circulation, and the disturbed circulation favors the distention. In slight and gradual stenosis of the intestine, as we shall see later on, hypertrophy of the muscular layer develops, which may undergo fatty degeneration later on. As a consequence of this, intestinal paralysis develops gradually, the result of long-existing coprostasis.

V. When a longer or shorter portion of the intestine is paralyzed, stoppage of the downward movement of the feces is caused, even in the absence of any stenosis. The blockage of the intestine by nothing but the enormous accumulation of gas is interesting in this connection, and it will be described in the following paragraphs.

VI. Vomiting. As already stated, the fecal nature of the vomit does not mean that it comes from very deep portions of the intestine. It does not mean that the stenosis is in the colon. Even in stenoses of the jejunum we may have fecal vomiting. Constant presence of pancreatic juice and bile in the vomit is indicative of a stenosis in the duodenum above the papilla. The so-called blocking of the intestine by gas ("*Gassperre,*" of Leichtenstern) is instrumental in mechanically favoring the flow of liquid contents toward the stomach. When there is an advanced degree of meteorism, the tendency of the accumulated gases is to raise the distended loops away from the spinal column and to press them against the anterior abdominal wall. Some portions of the intestine possess a longer mesentery than others, and the duodenum is attached to the spinal column, or at least the retroperitoneal fascia, so that it can not be pushed upward. The jejunum and lower ileum have a short mesentery. It is natural, therefore, that those portions of the intestines which have the longest mesentery—viz., the middle portions of the ileum—will be raised up by the gaseous distention, and separated from the spinal column more than the other portions with a short mesentery. If, therefore, the middle ileum is immensely distended by gas and raised against the anterior abdominal wall, the jejunum, upper ileum, and duodenum, which are gravid with liquid contents, can not move away from the spinal column (owing to their shorter mesentery). As a result the intestinal contents find an easier way of exit backward toward the stomach, and not downward through the highly erected loops of the ileum. This form of meteorism occurs in consequence of paralysis of the intestine, and the effects it produces always simulate an occlusion in the upper small intestine, no matter where the location of the blocking really is.

VII. The most frequent cause of intestinal paralysis is peritonitis.   Intestinal paralysis may be caused not only by diffuse general perforated peritonitis, but by a circumscribed inflammation of the serous covering of the bowel.   The paralysis is attributable to a continuation of the inflammation into the muscular layer, or if this has not actually taken place, the muscularis is at least penetrated by a serous transudation.   Among the curious observations that have been made during autopsies, concerning this paralysis of the muscularis, are those of Ohlshausen.   This clinician reported a case in which death supervened under the phenomena of intestinal occlusion and increasing collapse.   At the autopsy neither a mechanical obstacle nor a sign of peritonitis was found.   Ohlshausen has given this disease or condition the name of "pseudo-ileus." The later investigations of Reichel (*l. c.*) made it probable that such cases can be brought about by a peritoneal infection without an exudation.   The paralysis is regarded by him as a poisoning of the musculature or its inherent nervous apparatus by the metabolic products of the bacteria.

Circumscribed Acute Peritonitis and Exudation Observed at Laparotomy, no longer Recognizable at Autopsy.—Neither Ohlshausen nor Reichel appears to be familiar with a condition of the peritoneum in which it may show intense acute inflammation in circumscribed areas during life, accompanied by diffuse saturation of the muscular layer with serum, and nevertheless no macroscopic evidence of these pathological processes may be demonstrable at the autopsy.   I have observed two such instances and made notes of them in my clinical history record.   One of these cases was a bricklayer, aged thirty-two years, who came under operation for volvulus of the sigmoid flexure. After the laparotomy it was discovered that the sigmoid had rotated about 180 degrees from the normal position. The walls of the sigmoid flexure, judging by taking them between the fingers, were about ½ inch thick, spongy, edematous, and apparently permeated by a serous transudate. The peritoneum around the enlarged area was in a state of acute congestion, and in places had even poured out a gelatinous plastic lymph between the loops of the intestine. This was washed away during the operation, which was unfortunately undertaken too late, for the case ended fatally twenty-four hours thereafter. At the autopsy there was no evidence of peritonitis nor of an obstruction of any kind, the edematous swelling had subsided, and there was no exudate. Cultures taken from the peritoneum showed the presence of the Bacillus coli communis, and no other bacteria. The second case was that of a driver who had been struck in the abdomen by the shafts of an express wagon. I will not narrate the details of this case, because they were exactly the same as in the foregoing, except that the edematous area found at the operation was in the middle portion of the ileum, where the walls of the intestine for the distance of about 8 inches were saturated with a serous transudate. Evidently the lumen had been stenosed by this edematous swelling, for immediately above the infiltrated area was an immense accumulation of fecal matter and serum. Death having occurred in collapse, the autopsy gave no evidence of acute peritonitis, which had been seen at the operation, nor of the saturation of the coats of the intestine. Cultures from the peritoneum were not taken in this case. These cases have suggested to me that there may be circumscribed peritonitis of a very acute type following very abrupt and sudden obstructions, associated with edema of the intestinal walls, which may leave no trace at the autopsy. The clinical history of direct injury to the abdominal wall just narrated brings me to speak of—

VIII. Trauma, violent compression of the abdomen. This may cause paralysis of the intestine, either by direct injury to the muscles and nerves, or by sudden overstretching of a section of the intestine. It would be very instructive to know how often abdominal sections are followed by disturbances in the motor function of the intestine. In a large number of patients who had undergone gynecologic operations, I noticed obstipation of the most persistent type. Unfortunately, I could not determine whether this had existed before the operation in a number of cases; but in a sufficiently large number of these cases there had been a clear history of normal evacuation immediately before the operation, and persistent constipation immediately following and ever since the operation, so that the epigram " Post hoc ergo propter hoc " seems justified. I have observed the same results following several operations for hernia in men, and also in extensive lateral incisions of the abdomen, necessitating intersection of the recti muscles, for appendicitis and perityphlitis, so that there seems to be good reason for believing that interference with the abdominal muscles may lead to retention of stool. In a similar way acute trauma which strikes the abdomen may produce coprostasis, by interfering with the function of the muscles that compress the abdomen. The importance of the aid of the abdominal muscles for the normal evacuation can be recognized in very adipose persons of advanced age. Here the contractility of the muscles is frustrated by the deposits of fat in the abdominal wall, and also between the intestinal loops, consequently they are frequently known to be subject to obstipation.

IX. A reflex inhibition of the muscular movements has also been described. Such arrest in the intestinal peristalsis has been observed after appendicitis, although the lumen of the intestine was free; also after incarceration of nephritic and biliary calculi. Patients who are afflicted with a painful affection of the abdomen, which, though not involving the intestine, increases its sensitiveness, seek as much as possible to prevent this augmentation of their suffering. In some way, which is not yet explained, the intestinal contents go only as far as they can be moved without causing pain. When the spot is reached where further progress causes distress, there is a coprostasis. This has been observed by myself in abscess of the ovary. No doubt the will of the patient has something to do with it, but the extent to which the will can influence this is not easy to determine. It may be an involuntary inhibitory act, a reflex.

X. Disturbances in the nutrition of the intestine. Arrest of the circulation in the intestinal walls may lead to gangrene and perforation.   Perforation and penetration of the intestinal contents into the peritoneal cavity are not absolutely necessary for the production of peritonitis ; for in acute incarcerations, for instance, the nutrition of the intestinal wall may suffer to such a degree that it can no longer resist the penetration of the intestinal bacteria.   The main resistance against the invasion of the bacteria is offered by the mucosa.   As this rapidly suffers under the severe injuries during obstructions, it soon becomes deficient in vitality and permits the transit of bacteria.   Such an occurrence has been observed in many clinical studies, where bacteria were found in the peritoneal effusion, although neither intestinal ulcers nor perforation were present. Bacteria have also been found in the serous transudates surrounding incarcerated hernias, although no loss of continuity could be discovered in the bowel.   These serous transudates in hernial sacs or into the open peritoneum are the result of circulatory disturbances in the intestine, which cause a passive hyperemia.   If both the arteries and the veins are absolutely compressed, there may be no transudate whatever, and in such cases the vitality of the intestine is most seriously threatened.   Some clinicians have attributed great diagnostic importance to the quantity and composition of this transudate.   From the absence of this liquid under the serious condition just referred to, it is evident that the amount present does not furnish any reliable diagnostic indication.   There are two practical deductions, however, that can be made from the examination of such transudates, which can often be obtained by puncture of the involved area of the abdomen by a very fine trocar or even a hypodermic needle.   If the aspirated transudate contain decided admixture of blood, the case is always a grave one, in which most probably the passive congestion has led to rupture of blood-vessels.   In such cases in which the intestinal circulation has been interrupted for some time, hemorrhagic infarctions develop, according to Conheim and Schweninger, which may end in gangrene.   The second deduction is made from the appearance and smell of the transudate. If it is not clear, but opaque and cloudy, and if it has an offensive odor, we may conclude that the transudate is at the same time infected.

XI. Effects of the intestinal occlusion on the action of the heart; incarceration shock.   Hernias may cause obstruction in two ways : (1) By incarceration ; (2) by strangulation. The incarceration is the result of sudden overfilling by fecal masses of the part of the intestine that is in the hernial sac ; the Germans call this "*Koteinklemmung.*" It is very conceivable that more fecal matter may enter a hernial sac than can get out of it in a given time, because the entrance of the feces is, as a rule, favored by gravity ; but even if not so, it is effected by the healthy intestinal muscle above the hernia. But the exit must be brought about by the intestinal muscle within the hernial sac, which is always more or less impaired in its function. Strangulation is an elastic incarceration, in consequence of mechanical constriction. It is always accompanied by interference with the circulation, and symptoms of profound nervous irritation. Incarceration is therefore from the beginning an internal process, a form of obturation of the bowel, whereas strangulation from the beginning is a process external to the intestine. Constriction of the bowel causes dangerous results which are both local and remote. The remote detriments are the reflex inhibition of the heart's action and depression of the blood pressure. The local results are injuries to the nutrition of the intestine by venous congestion. The injuries are especially pronounced if both arterial and venous circulation is arrested. In acute intestinal occlusion of these types we have first of all the sudden onset of violent pains, which is followed by a reflex inhibition of the nerves controlling the vascular tonicity. As a consequence of this, the abdominal vessels become overfilled with blood, which necessarily is accompanied by an anemia of the brain. The symptoms following these cerebral and vascular disturbances have been designated collectively as "*incarceration shock*" ; and they may often lead to death in a very short time. In a very interesting experiment Goltz has demonstrated the connection of these pathological events. When the heart of a frog is exposed, and one strikes the abdomen repeatedly with a small rod, the heart will become arrested in diastole ; but if the two vagi are cut through, the striking is no longer followed by this result. Similarly, the result is not observed if the medulla is destroyed. The same diastolic arrest of the heart's action can be observed if the stomach or intestinal canal is mechanically irritated on the serous or the mucous surface. Bernstein has demonstrated in the mammal also the existence of sympathetic nerves which transmit these reflexes.

XII. Meteorism. This is not necessarily a consequence of occlusion. We shall speak more explicitly of this symptom in the consideration of intestinal occlusion. It is well known that total impermeability of the intestines in external hernias may exist for several days without the development of meteorism. On the other hand, enormous tympanites and meteorism may develop after some acute incarceration after a few hours. According to Kader (*l. c.*), meteorism is a result of two conditions which mutually supplement each other. The first and most active and important of these is (*a*) Disturbance of the circulation in the intestinal wall, and consequent venous stagnation; (*b*) the second is stagnation and putrefaction of the intestinal contents. Disturbance in the circulation is the more important detrimental condition, because it prevents the absorption of the gases. Meteorism does not develop until the absorption is less than the formation of the intestinal gases. When that state is reached, the distention increases rapidly in intensity, because a vicious circle is established; the distention naturally injuring the circulation, and the impeded circulation paralyzing the musculature, which in turn permits of a still greater distention. This mutual supplementing and interaction of the vicious circle explains the rapidly developing meteorism which occurs in some acute incarcerations, and within a few hours causes penetrating structural changes and complete paralysis of the musculature. In the following I shall more accurately describe the condition known as "local meteorism," as distinct from "stagnation meteorism."

Local meteorism is restricted to the intestinal district that is fixed in the incarceration, and generally above the point of an intestinal occlusion, and is always necessarily associated with disturbances in the circulation in the intestinal wall.

XIII. Chronic or slowly developing meteorism due to stagnation and putrefaction of the intestinal contents, and not associated with disturbances in the circulation of the intestine, can be tolerated a long time without detriment to the nutrition of the intestinal wall. As it develops much more slowly than the previous form, and the absorption of the gases is not primarily hindered, no distention develops, but only a degree of flatus. When there is fecal obstruction the disturbances of nutrition are limited to the intestinal loop immediately above the obstacle, and then only to that portion adjoining the obstacle.

XIV. Meteorism with excessive intra-abdominal pressure may cause arrest of the heart's action and collapse. The following experiments of Jürgensen (VIII. Congr. f. innere Med., 1899) demonstrate this fact. By blowing air into the abdominal cavity of animals so that the pressure was maintained at 20 mm. mercury for a longer time, the arterial pressure became so low after several hours that the blood did not squirt out of the crural artery any longer, but simply oozed out by drops. It may be objected that this experiment is not applicable to meteorism in the human subject, because such a high degree of pressure is never reached as to make the pulse in the crural artery imperceptible. This objection to the comparison is, however, not a valid one, for although the pressure in meteorism is not so high, it is exerted for a much longer time, and simultaneously accompanied by a number of other injurious factors that depress the action of the heart.

Relative Frequency of Various Obstructions.—The following shows the relative proportion of varieties of intestinal obstruction in 500 cases collected by the author :

	CASES.	PER CENT.
Strangulation,	190	38
Intussusception,	165	33
Volvulus,	80	16
Gall-stones,	45	9
Stricture or tumor,	20	4

The situation of the obstruction in 200 of the 500 cases, in which the situation was given, was as follows :

	LARGE INTESTINE.	SMALL INTESTINE.
Strangulation,	8	70
Intussusception or invagination,	50	8
Twist (volvulus),	32	6
Gall-stones,	4	12
Stricture and tumor,	10	4

The bowel obstructed was recorded as follows in 74 per cent. of the cases reported by Fitz, *l. c.*, page 12 :

INTESTINE OBSTRUCTED.	ADHE-SIONS.	VITELLINE REMAINS.	APPENDIX.	SLITS.	POUCHES, ETC.	TOTAL.
Small, ...	39	15	6	4	2	66
Large, ...	5	. .	. .	2	1	8
	44	15	6	6	3	74

The part of the intestine obstructed in strangulation, as determined in fully three-fourths of all the cases, is the small intestine in nearly 90 per cent., and the large in 10 per cent., of the cases.

The region of the abdomen in which the strangulating object was found was as follows in 72 per cent. of the cases :

	ADHE-SIONS.	VITELLINE REMAINS.	APPENDIX.	SLITS.	POUCHES, ETC.	TOTAL.
Right iliac fossa, . .	19	21	6	1	1	48
Pelvis, ...	7	. .	. .	. .	1	8
Left iliac fossa, . .	5	. .	. .	1	. .	6
Left lumbar region,	3	. .	. .	. .	. .	3
Right lumbar region,	2	. .	. .	. .	. .	2
Umbilical region,	2	. .	. .	. .	. .	2
Right hypochon-drium, ...	1	. .	. .	. .	1	2
Left hypochondrium,	1	. .	. .	. .	. .	1
	40	21	6	2	3	72

The position of the strangulating object was thus in the right iliac fossa in 67 per cent., and in the lower abdomen in 83 per cent. of the cases in which its position was given. It was present in the lumbar and umbilical regions in 10 per cent., and in the upper abdomen in 7 per cent.

ENTEROSTENOSIS—NARROWING OF THE LUMEN AND OCCLUSION OF THE INTESTINES.

Synonyms.—Acute Intestinal Occlusion, Ileus, Miserere, Passio Iliaca.

I. ENTEROSTENOSIS.

The permeability of the intestine is capable of being injured in a variety of ways. The narrowing of the bowel demands a separate consideration from complete occlusion because of its different clinical history and prognosis, as well as widely different diagnostic indications. In studying the enterostenoses, it is above all things necessary to distinguish between processes which bring on the stenosis suddenly and those which produce this effect after a longer time. Those conditions that effect a sudden reduction of the permeability of the intestine bring the clinician at once in touch with the intestinal occlusion, or at least into that clinical field where enterostenoses and occlusions merge into each other. The sudden factors of enterostenosis are internal incarceration in hernial sacs, axial twists, clefts or gaps in the mesentery and omentum, kinking of the intestine by adhesion, coproliths, gall-stones and foreign bodies. The gradual causes of enterostenosis are neoplasms in the intestinal wall, strictures after ulceration, peritonitic agglutinations, changes in the location of neighboring organs, compression externally, and invagination. No matter what the anatomical cause of an enterostenosis may be, it is, as a rule, a slowly and gradually developing condition, requiring weeks, even months, before it is pronounced. Exceptionally a partial obturation by foreign bodies —enteroliths, gall-stones—or intussusceptions (pseudo-ligaments) may cause a sudden and rapid blocking of the passage through the bowel, or a compression may set in acutely and abruptly, but continue in a chronic course, a condition to which Leichtenstern (von Ziemssen's " Handbuch," Bd. vii, 2. Aufl., S. 416) has called attention in a masterly article on this subject. There are cases of gradually increasing bowel stenosis in which the symptoms may be entirely absent for a long time, so that no disturbance of functions is noticeable. These are the cases in which the phenomena of obstruction of the bowel seem to appear suddenly in entirely sound individuals.

Symptomatology.

The symptomatology varies according to the location of the stenosis. The stenoses between the pylorus and the jejunum are designated as *high* stenoses, while those occurring anywhere from the ileum to the rectum are spoken of as *low* stenoses. The local reduction of the intestinal lumen leads to an accumulation of intestinal contents above the compressed or stenosed locality, thus causing dilations, serving as reservoirs for the retained solid and liquid masses.   Three of the most frequent consequences of this accident are persistent obstipation, enteritis or colitis with the formation of ulcers, and in some cases formation of perforations above the stenosed portion.   It is natural that the intestinal contents which are liquid or semi-solid will pass a stenosed district with greater facility than those which are solid.   For this reason the high stenoses— those in the upper part of the small intestine—not only remain latent much longer than low stenoses,—those in the colon and sigmoid flexure,—but the higher ones will not be accompanied by such extreme suprastenotic dilations as the lower ones.   Stenoses in the large intestine require much greater exertions on the part of the muscularis to overcome them.   This is another explanation of the dilation and muscular hypertrophy found in these forms.   All forms of gradually developing stenoses are accompanied by violent tonic contractions above the stenosed area.

High Stenoses in the Small Intestine.—The stenoses of the duodenum will give a varying symptomatology, according to their location.   It is expedient, for practical and diagnostic reasons, to distinguish between stenoses that are above the papilla of Vater and those that are below it and the beginning of the jejunum.   The papilla of Vater is the slight elevation of the mucosa embracing the opening of the common bile duct, and of the pancreatic duct.   If a stenosis occurs above the papilla and completely occludes the duodenum between the pylorus and the opening of these secretory ducts, it is natural that no pancreatic juice or bile can reach the stomach under such conditions, even if antiperistaltic contractions develop. On the other hand, one of the most important signs of infrapapillary duodenal stenosis is the continuous presence of bile and often of pancreatic juice in the stomach.

When the stenosis is suprapapillary, the backward pressure of the stagnating ingesta at first causes a dilation between the stenosis and the pylorus.   This in rare instances may reach such a degree that the sphincter of the pylorus is completely effaced and the duodenal dilations become merged into one cavity with the stomach. Accordingly, the subjective signs are those of gastrectasia or permanent overfilling of the stomach, and include the same symptoms, principal among which are fullness, distention and pressure, sometimes aggravated to pain, eructation, nausea, and vomiting.   The appetite is generally lost, and thereby the general nutrition much impaired. All this will develop independently of the pathological conditions that have caused the duodenal stenosis. The meteorism, if any, is limited to the stomach. As the chyme is quite thin and liquid, it may for a long time be able to pass the obstacle; but even if this is not the case, there will be no accumulation above the obstruction, as is the case in low enterostenosis, because the chyme can readily regurgitate into the stomach. For the same reasons intense paroxysms of pain and visible intestinal peristalsis are not observed. The entire clinical picture coincides with that of pyloric stenosis; this will probably also be the nearest diagnosis that can be made. An approach to a more exact diagnosis than this might be possible by the method of duodenal intubation, which I have devised and published in the "Archiv f. Verdauungs-Krankheiten," Bd. ii, S. 85, or by Kuhn's spiral sounds, for intubating the duodenum. I have been able in one case to diagnose the complete absence of bile from the duodenum due to obstruction of the common gall-duct by this method of intubation (see Hemmeter, "Diseases of the Stomach," second edition, p. 55). If, after repeated intubation and aspiration of the duodenal contents, no bile can be found, and if the duodenal tube can be introduced beyond the normal lengths of the duodenum, the diagnosis of stenosis of the common gall-duct is logical. But if permanent absence of bile is found in the contents of the duodenum, and at the same time the tube will not pass more than a few inches beyond the pylorus, a stenosis between the papilla and the pylorus exists. The location of Kuhn's spiral duodenal tube, which contains a closely wound spiral of steel, can be made out through the x-rays. Sufficient clinical work on such cases has as yet not been done either by Kuhn or myself. The future will show whether the methods advocated will be useful for the diagnosis of duodenal stenosis.

Infrapapillary or Low Duodenal Stenoses.—The symptoms of deep infrapapillary stenoses of the duodenum are principally those of dilation of the stomach, and identical with those that have been mentioned with high stenoses. Whilst the stomach is usually dilated with high stenoses, this is not necessarily so with low duodenal stenoses; in the latter case it may be dilated, but it may also be found normal. There is no very apparent meteorism. In the

rare cases in which it does occur it is promptly relieved by eructations.   The exact location of the stenosis can only be suspected if
the previous history of the patient presents an account of diseases
of the duodenum and its surroundings, such, for instance, as have
been presented in the clinical history of duodenal ulcer; a history
of pancreatic diseases, cholangitis, cholelithiasis, and icterus will
necessarily direct the attention to duodenal complication.   The
most important clinical sign, however, of infrapapillary duodenal
stenoses is the permanent presence of large amounts of bile and
pancreatic juice in the stomach.   As a general rule, the total duodenal secretions are driven toward the stomach, including the pancreatic juice and the succus entericus.   In simple atonic dilation of
the stomach and in gastroptosis bile is also found in the stomach
before breakfast.   This is due to physical factors.   For in these
abnormalities the bile can very readily run into the stomach, which
has dragged the first portion of the duodenum out of normal location.   This backward flow of bile does not occur in the erect position, but only in the horizontal position of the patient.   In stenosis
it occurs in all positions, as it is due to obstruction.   Boas has
called attention to the fact that one is thereby enabled to exclude
a severe disease of the pancreatic duct; for instance, if the duodenal
juice and such secretions are regurgitated into the stomach and do
not give the digestive reaction of trypsin and amylopsin, disease of
the pancreas or stenosis of the duct should be suspected.   The
condition of the gastric secretions varies greatly.   In a case of
carcinoma of the descending portion of the duodenum, which occurred in my practice and which was verified at the autopsy,
the secretion of HCl was undisturbed; but it appears from the
results of Riegel and Boas that the secretion of HCl in the same
individual may at one time be abundant and at another time entirely
absent during this condition.   The presence of bile and pancreatic
juice in the stomach impedes the action of the gastric juice only so
long as the mixture is neutral (Boas).   If the gastric juice has the
preponderance, it exhibits the same digestive activity as normal
gastric juice in spite of the presence of bile and pancreatic juice.
Reversely, the pancreatic ferments are evidently destroyed if a sufficient amount of HCl is present, for they do not resume their digestive activity, although the acid may be neutralized and the medium

given an alkaline reaction. Herz has called attention to a sign which may be available when taken in conjunction with other diagnostic indications. He points out that bismuth, when administered internally, does not appear again in the stool. It is evident that this can not be a pathognomonic sign of duodenal stenosis, because the passage of the bismuth will be blocked no matter where the occlusion occurs. Frequently the stool presents the appearance of the evacuations in icterus, and the indican may be increased in the urine. Both of these signs, however, are not invariably present.

Etiology of Duodenal Stenoses.—Herz, Hochhaus, and Schüle have reported cases in which biliary concretions had caused spastic stenoses in the descending duodenum. One will have to think of this possibility whenever icterus has been mentioned in the anamnesis. The obstruction may not be caused by the stone itself, but by peritonitic adhesions emanating from a cholecystitis and compressing the duodenum. Statistics indicate that the female sex is most frequently affected with this condition. Similarly, our statistics of duodenal ulcer indicate that this condition attacks men with preference. This, then, is also a cause of duodenal stenosis. Among other factors in the etiology that occur rarely I might mention carcinoma, sarcoma, kinking, pancreatic cysts, neoplasms in the pancreas and gall-bladder, tuberculous ulcers in the duodenum, mesenteric and retroperitoneal tumors, and fat necrosis of the pancreas.

Stenoses of the Jejunum and Ileum.—The same frequent causal relation that exists between stenoses of the duodenum and inflammatory processes emanating from the biliary apparatus exists also between the genital apparatus (the ovaries, tubes, and uterus) in the female, and the appendix in the male on the one hand, and stenoses of the jejunum and ileum on the other. In enterostenoses in which it is possible for the clinician to exclude the involvement of the duodenum and the colon, and by exclusion arrive at a suspicion that the jejunum or ileum is stenosed, it is well to first think of the female genital apparatus and the appendix as the origin of the stenosis. The next most frequent cause is inflammation resulting from incarcerated hernias. Stenoses due to tuberculous neoplasms or cicatrices of partially healed tuberculous ulcers are rare in the jejunum and ileum, but that they may occur has already been mentioned in the chapter on Tuberculous Ulcers of the Intestines.

These stenoses may occur singly, but more frequently a number of them develop in the same case. Hofmeister (*l. c.*) and Fränkel (*l. c.*) have described cases in which twelve such strictures were observed. The so-called intestinal cirrhosis of English writers and the "*entérite scléreuse*" of the French must be an exceedingly rare occurrence, and in my opinion probably of syphilitic origin. Stenoses of the jejunum and ileum by carcinoma are also exceedingly rare. Küttner ("Beiträge z. klin. Chirurgie," 1899, Bd. XXIII, S. 505) has collected the literature on carcinomatous stenoses of the intestines. Among 280 cases of cancer of the intestine, only 4 were found to be located in the jejunum, and but 21 in the ileum. The symptomatology of the stenoses of the jejunum and ileum presents little that is characteristic. Therefore it will be difficult to localize narrowings of the intestinal canal belonging to this district. The observations of E. Fränkel (*l. c.*) and Litten (*l. c.*) indicate that tuberculous stenoses of the ileum which have become far advanced may run their course without symptoms. Concerning the phenomena of meteorism, diarrhea, constipation, colic, visible and palpable intestinal contractions, I will speak more explicitly in the paragraph on the general symptomatology of enterostenoses. If one has reached the diagnosis of stenosis of the jejunum or ileum in the manner indicated, the difficulties in the way of recognizing the cause are, in my experience, not insurmountable.

Stenoses of the Colon—Sigmoid Flexure.—Other things being equal, a stenosis in the large intestine will sooner lead to disturbances in function than a stenosis in the ileum, jejunum, or duodenum, though the latter lead more promptly to the manifestation of symptoms than stenoses of the jejunum or ileum, because of the proximity of the duodenum to the stomach, and the consequent very evident gastric complications which have already been described. The explanation of the prompt occurrence of disturbances in stenosis of the colon is naturally to be found in the consistency of the feces—the more condensed and firmer the intestinal contents are, the sooner will they occlude any narrow portion of the bowel lumen. In the upper portion of the digestive tract, where the chyme is of a liquid consistency, a considerable degree of stenosis may exist for a long time in a latent condition. So it may be said that enterostenoses at the beginning and at the end of the alimentary tract—the duodenum and the colon, particularly the descending colon and sigmoid flexure—give rise to symptoms most promptly, whereas those of the ileum and the jejunum are slower to react upon narrowing of their lumen.   In my experience also the course of stenoses of the colon is more often of a chronic character.   Many transient attacks precede the pronounced symptoms of stenosis, so that the patient may be treated for a long time as simply suffering from obstipation, and perhaps associated with enteralgia.   With high stenoses—those in the small intestine—when disturbances have once set in, they are at once of a grave and serious nature, the course is a stormy one, and generally without remission.   This teaches us to look with suspicion upon every case of chronic *constipation associated with paroxysms of severe pain, particularly if the abdomen has been distended and if there has been a history of vomiting*.   Such symptoms may be those of simple obstipation, but they are also generally those which precede a stenosis of the colon.   Boas has called attention to the importance of ascertaining whether the patient has been compelled to the use of more and more drastic purgatives.   The usual description which the patients themselves give of this habit is that "the purge has lost its effect," or that they "have become accustomed to it."

In stenoses of the large intestine I have observed the obstipation develop in two different ways : In one set of cases its onset is abrupt; within a few weeks the patient is compelled to use the most drastic purgatives, and sometimes enemata together with purges.   This is an especially valuable indication if this habit has developed suddenly in a patient of mature age, say after forty.   In another type of cases the constipation has existed for years, and only recently has increased in severity ; perhaps systematic treatment for constipation has been gone through, with only transient improvement, or perhaps aggravation of the disease.   This sign gains in diagnostic value if it has been associated with colic and vomiting.   I have never observed any cases of simple constipation in which vomiting has been a repeated symptom, and on the basis of a large experience with stenoses of the colon, *I am disposed to attribute to it considerable clinical diagnostic importance if it occurs in association with pain and constipation.   With those three symptoms present, one should never neglect to investigate the previous history*

and obtain an accurate anamnesis, to make a careful examination of
the abdomen, especially of the hernial orifices, of the rectum and va-
gina. Thereupon should follow a careful inspection of the rectum
and further examination by percussion and palpation, and distention
of the colon.

The **meteorism** in stenoses of the large intestine may vary considerably in degree. It is considerable when the stenosis is near
the ileocecal valve, and becomes less pronounced the nearer the
stenosis is toward the rectum. This symptom also depends upon
the amount of intestinal contents, and upon the contractile power
of the hypertrophied musculature above the point of occlusion. If
the meteorism is stationary, it may suggest to a degree where the
seat of the stenosis is located. This is, however, in my experience,
only possible in conjunction with other symptoms mentioned.
When the lumen is to a certain degree passable, the meteorism is
restricted to one or the other flank. The following signs and symptoms, should they occur in conjunction, represent the typical picture
of complete stenosis of the large intestine : (*a*) Meteorism considerable, distributed over the entire abdomen uniformly ; (*b*) voluminous
fecal contents, giving a dull sound on percussion and not changing
their volume or position by injection of water into the colon ; (*c*)
vomiting, especially if it has become offensive ; (*d*) no increase in
the amount of indican ; (*e*) secretion of urine not considerably
diminished ; (*f*) collapse not pronounced. Compare this with the
picture of a stenosis of the duodenum of the upper part of the
jejunum, where the meteorism is not prominent and is limited to the
epigastrium ; the inferior and lateral (flank) portion of the abdomen
is sunk in ; the degree of meteorism varies with the vomiting ; the
epigastrium collapses after emesis ; colon irrigation causes the
evacuation of a large amount of feces without diminishing the signs
of stenosis ; collapse is pronounced ; oliguria and, as a rule, a large
amount of indican in the urine. Between these two groups of
pictures, constituting well-defined clinical pictures, we have the
signs and symptoms of stenosis of the ileum and cecum. Here it is
claimed by some authors that the distention is limited to the middle
portions of the abdomen, whilst the colon section recedes. This,
however, in my experience, is only exceptionally the case, and is
not available as a diagnostic sign for stenoses in this section, for

when the meteorism becomes pronounced in stenoses of ileum and cecum, the upper intestinal loops are pushed over and cover the colon, producing a general and uniform meteorism. All of these groups of symptoms are unreliable in the advanced stages of stenoses. Nothnagel (*l. c.*, p. 375) has called attention to a change in the percussion resonance in the dorsal and upper lumbar region. Normally this region gives a more or less dull, high, and empty resonance on percussion, but when there is a stenosis in the sigmoid flexure or descending colon, there is a loud and deep percussion resonance of both sides of this upper lumbar region. If the stenosis, however, is in the splenic flexure or the transverse colon, this change from dull and high to low, clear, and deep resonance can be made out only on the right side. Other features of stenoses of the large intestine, as, for instance, the visible peristalsis in connection with the plasticity of intestinal loops, and the condition of the fecal evacuations, will be considered in the following paragraph on the general symptomatology.

The elucidation of the causes of stenoses of the large intestine involves a knowledge of all those conditions which can effect a narrowing of the lumen of the colon, and which have been described in previous chapters. Thus, we will have to think of the various forms of ulcers, of dysentery, tuberculosis and syphilis of the intestine, of neoplasms, of appendicitis, and inflammations emanating from the liver and gall-bladder, of inflammations of the female genital apparatus, incarcerated hernias, and any previous operations upon the abdominal cavity that the patient, may have undergone.

General Symptomatology of Enterostenoses.

The most important symptoms of enterostenoses are those: (1) Referring to the condition of the evacuations, whether there is constipation, diarrhea, or both alternating ; (2) the changes in the form of the abdomen, the plastic elevation of tetanically erect intestinal loops above the niveau of the abdomen, the increased peristaltic movement ; (3) the pain and attacks of colic dependent upon these; (4) the meteorism ; (5) the changes of the form and shape in the dejecta, whether they contain mucus, blood, pus, or bile; (6) the sounds to be elicited by auscultation, palpation, and percussion.

1. The condition of the evacuations in occlusions of the small

intestine, is, as a rule, normal ; even advanced degrees of stenoses may run their course without being associated with obstipation. From what has been said before, it is evident that obstipation should be observed, as a rule, with stenoses of the colon. The accuracy of this sign in association with such stenoses is often doubtful because the obstipation is generally promptly relieved by artificial means by the patient. I have observed a case of sarcoma of the descending colon in which the lumen was stenosed so as to barely admit of the passage of the little finger, and still the patient had daily evacuations to within ten days of the fatal termination. Nothnagel (*l. c.*, p. 190) narrates the case of a woman fifty years old who had one daily evacuation up to the 24th of February, 1886. On the 25th she had a sudden violent attack of colic, which was repeated on the next day. On March 3d, when she was presented for examination, the clinical picture of intestinal occlusion was complete. On the tenth day of her sickness she died in a state of collapse. The autopsy disclosed an ulcerated hard carcinoma, about 2 cm. broad at the transition of the sigmoid flexure and rectum. The lumen was so constricted as to be barely passable for the little finger ; nevertheless she had normal evacuations until ten days before death. The possibility of these daily evacuations was explained by the existence of an enormous muscular hypertrophy which extended through the entire colon up to the ileocecal valve. Cases of this kind and the one I have briefly referred to give evidence of the enormous difficulty which diagnosis meets in this field of clinical pathology.

It can be stated, however, that the general rule in obstruction of the colon, sigmoid, and rectum is to meet with a history of constipation. Where the patients had recourse to medication for the relief of this symptom, they found themselves compelled to use stronger and stronger purgatives. Other symptoms are gradually superadded, such as abdominal distention, loss of appetite, and nausea. Where the sufferer does not himself use laxatives, nature occasionally intervenes in the form of a diarrhea, which may last for several days, during which enormous masses of putrid feces are discharged. Immediately thereafter the patient feels considerably better. But this experience of constipation, followed by diarrhea and digestive distress, is repeated at shorter and shorter intervals.

What were considered by the patient, and very often by the physician, frequent attacks of constipation alternating with diarrhea, presently loom up as a grave intestinal disease, particularly when it is associated with attacks of colic, which will presently be described. Obstipation, therefore, is the rule, and the lower down the enterostenosis is located in the bowel, the more pronounced will it be. The most deceptive cases are those rare instances in which a chronic diarrhea has existed for weeks and months.   Here the diagnostician can scarcely avoid being misled.   These diarrheas are caused by the intense enteritis which develops above the stenosis, and also by the excitation of the peristalsis as a consequence of the stagnation of fecal matter and gas.   This intestinal catarrh causes a more abundant secretion, and hence also a liquefaction of the stagnating intestinal contents.   It is also the source of the mucus which is found in the discharges.

2. The normal peristalsis of the intestine can be occasionally observed in subjects having very thin abdominal walls, when they are able to keep them in a quiet, relaxed condition.   A careful study of the chapter on Intestinal Peristalsis (chapter IV, vol. I) will lead to a better understanding and appreciation of the pathological peristalsis met with in enterostenoses.   The peristalsis may be increased by purgatives, extremes of temperature, abnormally acid or abnormally alkaline reaction of contents, psychic affections, and acute inflammatory conditions of the bowel.   But a peristalsis as intense as can be observed through the normal abdominal wall is only observed in the enterostenoses, and particularly in those which develop slowly, because in these the muscular hypertrophy of the intestinal wall has had abundant time for development.   It is necessary to distinguish in making our clinical data, in cases of enterostenoses, between tonic contraction and the tetanic paroxysmal contractions which effect a visible erection or rigid elasticity of intestinal loops. In certain pathological conditions, particularly under the influence of certain poisons, in lead colic, and intensely acute enteritis and meningitis, tonic contractions occur in which there is a tetanus of the intestinal wall of such intensity that the lumen is actually obliterated. But such contractions are never visible.   The pathognomonic symptom of enterostenosis, however, is an increased peristalsis of such violence *that individual intestinal loops become erect, as it were, by*

tonic contractions, and are visible as plastic convolutions through the abdominal wall. The conditions for such a phenomenon are, first, an impediment or obstruction in the lumen; secondly, the accumulation of gaseous and liquid contents which can not be propagated forward by the ordinary normal intestinal contractions. The increased resistance and the irritation of the accumulated masses are a stimulus to which the muscularis responds with a tetanic reaction. Such intense peristaltic erections of the intestine are observed only in the chronic stenoses, because only in this type is sufficient time given for advanced muscular hypertrophy to develop.

The stormy peristalsis of this description is an impressive clinical spectacle. Even at the quietest moments there is a slight undulatory motion observable underneath the abdominal walls. One intestinal loop may be more distended than the others. Presently, within a few seconds it is converted into a rigid hard tube which projects upward and can actually be grasped by the fingers. In this plastic condition it may remain from thirty to sixty seconds. Thereupon it relapses into its previous condition of elasticity. Sometimes not one but several intestinal loops rise up like a huge snail shell, pushing out the abdominal integument. Alongside of these are deep grooves or ridges into which the integument appears retracted; whilst one intestinal convolution rises into a plastic hard tube, other portions of the same loop exhibit shorter vibratory peristaltic movements. All of these manifold and rapidly changing peristaltic figures are accompanied by loud borborygmi and rumbling noises. Occasionally there is a musical note. The state of plasticity rarely lasts longer than from twenty to thirty seconds. The entire paroxysm may last from thirty minutes to two hours, when there is generally an interruption from exhaustion of the musculature, or the interval of rest may perhaps also be caused by the fact that the accumulated gases and liquid contents have been moved to another point by the stormy peristalsis. There are cases in which similar attacks are caused by large gall-stones or coproliths, which can be expelled by evacuation, and are followed by perfect recovery in a short time. In others, however, the very first attack is followed within a few days by a second similar one. If we are confronted by a stenosis, the intervals between the attacks become shorter and shorter, the appetite is lost, there is evidence of embarrassed respiration and heart's action, the abdomen becomes distended permanently, and the case becomes one of pronounced intestinal occlusion. The changes in the external configuration of the abdomen, in my experience, offer very unreliable data for the localization of the occlusion. A localized meteorism will indicate the primary seat of a stenosis, but it gives no information concerning the nature of the stenosis.

3. Attacks of pain, or, as they are more frequently designated, of colic, occasionally constitute the very first symptom of enterostenosis. They occur under three conditions : (a) The ordinary intestinal contents have occluded a stenosis which is not yet absolute ; (b) the stenosis is still passable, but indigestible food substances of extraordinary volume have blocked the narrowing passages ; (c) the muscular hypertrophy which has developed in consequence of the fecal stagnation above the stenosis has become insufficient. The severity of the pain accompanying this accident baffles description. The patients act like maniacs. At. times even hypodermics of ½ grain of morphin do not relieve them, and the lamentations continue until the patient is put under narcosis. It is important to note the location of the first sensation of pain, for it will very often be in the locality of the stenosis. Soon, however, the pain becomes diffuse and spreads over the entire abdomen, and even over the thorax. Nothnagel mentions that the pain may be felt, or described as being felt, in an entirely different place from the location of the stenosis ; for instance, a cecal stenosis has been known to give pain in the left inguinal region.

4. Meteorism. The extent of this sign depends upon the amount of stagnated intestinal contents, and upon the seat of the stenosis. If the gases can escape, a possibility so long as there is any lumen whatever left through which they may be discharged, the meteorism may be very limited. Even in complete occlusion there may be but slight meteorism when the amount of absorption of gases keeps step with their formation. As a diagnostic sign meteorism, taken by itself, has only a subordinate value. Only in occlusions at the very beginning and very end of the alimentary canal do we meet with anything like circumscribed meteorism which is available as a diagnostic sign, and even then only at the onset of the stenosis.

5. **Changes in form, shape, and composition of the dejecta.**
It is natural to expect that any stenosis of the intestine will mold the
pliable fecal mass in the characteristic shape corresponding to the
size and configuration of the aperture through which it has to
pass.   That the shape imparted to the evacuation must be that
which it receives in the lower end of the intestine is also natural,
for in the small intestine the feces are liquid, and could not possibly
preserve any shape imparted to them.   Therefore we may at once
conclude that if peculiar shapes of the feces have any diagnostic
significance at all, they can only refer to stenoses of the large intestine ; but we shall presently see that even this diagnostic application of the configuration of the feces is very limited.   Concerning the various forms and configurations into which the fecal excreta
may be molded, I refer to chapter xv, on Obstipation.   Briefly to
recapitulate, there are three main types of stenotic feces: (1) The
ribbon-shaped, which are flat pieces of excrement, of varying length.
Sometimes they are shaped like a wedge ; that is, the cross-section
of the ribbon presents a triangular surface ; this is caused by one
side of the band being flat and the other having a sharp elevated
ridge.   (2) Long, thin cylinders of feces, having the shape of a
lead-pencil, which may present a ridge on the surface.   (3) Round
or oval globules, resembling the excrement of the sheep.   Whilst
such shapes may be imparted to the feces when enterostenoses are
present, they are entirely missed in stenoses of the small intestine,
cecum, and ascending colon.   I must refer here once more to the
case of stenosis of the sigmoid flexure, quoted from Nothnagel's
scholarly work, and the case reported by myself of a stenosis in
the descending colon where there were normal evacuations to within
a few days before death.   In the chapter on Obstipation I have
also described dejections which occur in that disease and are of the
exact type of those described.   It must be emphasized that they
occur in cases of obstipation in which there is no suggestion of
intestinal stenosis.   These abnormally formed dejecta are available
for the diagnosis of stenosis of the descending colon, sigmoid, and
rectum, only under the following conditions : (a) When they appear
regularly in the evacuations ; (b) when normally formed stool is
not discharged at any time ; (c) when they show evidences of blood
and pus.   This leads us to speak of these two abnormal admix-

tures in the stool.   They are, of course, not symptoms of a stenosis, but rather the result of the process which has caused the stenosis. Similarly, mucus in the stool is a product of the enteritis that has been set up above the seat of the stenosis.   Blood and pus are found as a result of tuberculous or dysenteric ulcers which sometimes accompany cicatricial strictures.   These constituents may also be present in stools of patients suffering with simple catarrhal, so-called decubital ulcers, caused by the pressure of the stagnating masses above the stenosis.   To the same class belong also the ulcers found in the rectum as a consequence of fecal stagnation. In the latter case, however, the blood most frequently originates from hemorrhoids, having the same etiology.   The most frequent sources of blood are intussusception and vascular carcinomas or adenomas.   Pus may be present in the stools as a result of the ulcers which have just been mentioned as the sources of the blood.

Prognosis.

The prognosis of enterostenosis depends upon the nature of the underlying cause.   So long as the compensatory hypertrophy of the musculature is able to overcome the increased resistance of the stenosis, the peristaltic function of the intestine will be maintained to a fairly normal degree.   Even during the period of insufficient compensation, when the patient will be compelled to resort to purgatives, the general condition will be fairly endurable.   In the clinical history of all compensatory hypertrophies a period must eventually supervene in which the musculature becomes paralyzed and can no longer overcome the obstacle.   When this point is reached in enterostenosis, the accumulation of fecal matter stretches and distends the diseased muscular fiber, thus hastening the absolute impermeability of the bowel.   At this stage there may be relief —perhaps a cure expected—from operation.   In other cases, if this can not be undertaken, death results either in consequence of perforating decubital ulcers and ensuing peritonitis, or by circumscribed fecal abscesses which develop when a previous adhesive peritonitis has prevented the rapid spread of the exuding fecal contents.   There may also be perforations into other organs and severe general septicemia.   This is the gravest form of termination of enterostenosis, and fortunately not the most frequent if the disease is treated in time.   Naturally, if enterostenosis is not recognized, or not correctly treated after recognition, it must inevitably take such a course.   There are a number of accidental complications which can scarcely be foreseen.   Among these may be mentioned axial twists, or volvulus at the transition of the sigmoid flexure into the rectum, caused by gravitation downward of the heavy and overfilled loop above the stenosis.   Prior to the descent of this gravid sigmoid, the stenosis may not have been absolute, but becomes so after the formation of the volvulus or twist.   This accident may lead to the diagnosis of an entirely acute intestinal occlusion, not preceded by a gradually stenosing process.   If an energetic peristalsis and tetanic erection of intestinal loops occurs, this may yet enable a correct diagnosis, for they cannot occur in acute occlusion, as this form of peristalsis, which can produce the projection of rigid, plastic intestinal loops through the abdominal wall, requires a preexistence of hypertrophy of the muscularis, a condition which requires a longer time for its development.   Enterostenoses which are still passable may suddenly become absolutely occluded by solid bodies in the intestinal contents, acting as obturators.   Hard fecal concretions and seeds have occasionally produced this effect.

Among the etiological factors which justify a favorable prognosis are benign neoplasms, polypi, and sometimes partial invagination. The stenosis caused by dislocated neighboring organs may also be completely removed; thus an intestinal stenosis depending upon compression by floating kidney, dislocated uterus, or a peri-intestinal exudate, may be completely cured.   Even spontaneous cures of such conditions have occurred.   In other cases the successful treatment was by means of operation.

The **diagnosis** and **treatment** will be considered in chapters devoted to these subjects after all the various forms of enterostenoses and occlusions have been separately considered.

.

II. ACUTE AND CHRONIC INTESTINAL OCCLUSIONS.

Synonyms.—Ileus, Miserere, Passio Iliaca.

The term *ileus* as a designation for intestinal occlusion is a very ancient one, and Nothnagel (*l. c.*) argues that the clinical picture which the ancients conceived under that name does not correspond to our present conception of the condition. He accordingly suggests to discard the designation entirely. Boas (*l. c.*), as well as A. Priepram (in Ebstein und Schwalbe's " Handbuch der prakt. Med.," Bd. II, p. 624), agree to the suggestion of Nothnagel, as it would be necessary in individual cases to make a special diagnosis explaining the etiology of the "ileus." This necessarily renders the distinction which Leichtenstern makes between mechanic, dynamic, and mechanico-dynamic ileus unnecessary. As these designations are all very concise and pregnant, they still force themselves into the literature of the subject for didactic reasons.

Nature and Concept, Description and Etiology.

By Occlusion or Ileus is meant the entire pathological closure of the intestine. This and the stoppage of the feces in their passage are caused either by a mechanical obstruction or by a lack of motive power. Both of these, whether acting individually or in conjunction, can cause a permanent stoppage of the fecal passage, or ileus (Leichtenstern). We therefore differentiate (1) a *mechanical* and (2) a *dynamic* (paralytic) occlusion, and in those cases where a partially closing obstruction is made complete by the fading away of the motive power, (3) a *mechanico-dynamic* occlusion. Of these three forms of occlusion the mechanical is observed most frequently, the mechanico-dynamic next in frequency, and the dynamic most rarely. The numerous abnormal conditions and diseases which cause an intestinal closure by purely mechanical means have already been considered in the preceding sections, in the discussion of these diseases. It has been repeatedly mentioned that many of them at first caused only a more or less considerable stenosis of the intestinal lumen, which after a shorter or longer time led to a complete intestinal obstruction. It has also been emphasized that slowly increasing contractions of the lumen, especially those of the small intestine, but also of the large one, may remain latent for years, if the contents of the intestine passing the contracted place are still fluid or pulpy. This is most frequently possible in stenosis of the small intestine, or also if a more permanent morbid increase of the peristalsis prevents a condensation of the feces, such as normally takes place in the large intestine; and if, in addition, a hypertrophy of the muscles of that section of the intestines lying above the contracted places completely compensates for the stenosis by causing an increase in the contractile power of the muscles (compensatory hypertrophy). As a result of improper diet, or of a decrease in the peristalsis, larger masses of undigested food or thickened feces may become heaped up at the stenosed place, so that the intestine becomes impassable. If, for any reason, the contractility of the hypertrophic muscles decreases, thus removing the previous compensation, the symptoms of obstruction may appear suddenly and unexpectedly, and lead to the assumption that a previously normal and completely permeable intestine has become closed as a result of internal strangulation, of axial twist, of intussusception, etc. If a complete compensation is prevented by a very sudden increase in the stenosing process, the symptoms of a chronic intestinal stenosis or narrowing are generally observed, and the appearance of obstruction or ileus may be observed at any time. The assumption of a dynamic (paralytic) occlusion as well as of a mechanico-dynamic occlusion, and the important part which the paralysis of the intestinal muscles above the occluded place in the intestines plays in the etiology of mechanical occlusion, are proved by the results of dissections performed on subjects who during life showed the typical symptoms of occlusion, and who died of the same. In numerous such cases no mechanical obstruction could be found, and the intestine was everywhere permeable. Further evidence is furnished by the observation, which has already been mentioned, that occlusion may occur when the intestinal lumen is stenosed, to be sure, but still permeable, and also by the observation that after the successful removal of an incarcerated hernia, or of an internal strangulation, or after the formation of an artificial anus through which the intestinal contents could be emptied from above the stenosed area, nevertheless the symptoms of occlusion continued until death. In other cases the symptoms of occlusion slowly decreased, because the previously insufficient intestinal muscles gradually recovered, a fact which is observed quite frequently in the case of chronic stenosis of the intestines.

Dynamic ileus is caused most frequently by acute or chronic diffuse or circumscribed peritonitis, by perityphlitis and permanent coprostasis, more rarely by traumas (it was observed repeatedly after laparotomy and ovariotomy), and also by the permanent strangulation or incarceration of external hernias.

In a valuable contribution to the subject of the causation of intestinal obstruction, cyst-formation and duplication, particularly with regard to the agency of persistent omphalomesenteric remains in the production of these abnormalities, Professor Reginald H. Fitz gives an interesting account of the relation of the omphalomesenteric vessels or their remains to the production of strangulation and obstruction ("Amer. Jour. of the Med. Sciences," vol. LXXXVIII, p. 30). The article is rich in pertinent abstracts from the literature of this subject, and throws much desired light on the hitherto unexplained congenital origin of bands, diverticulum, etc. According to this able investigator, the primitive intestine communicates with the umbilical vesicle by means of a tube, the vitelline or omphalomesenteric duct, toward the end of the fourth week of intra-uterine life of the human fetus. During the subsequent two weeks the abdominal plates close, shutting in a portion of this duct, which, as a delicate thread, unites to the navel the loop of intestine projecting into the depression at the origin of the umbilical cord. During the subsequent development of the intestine, that portion above the insertion of this thread becomes the greater part of the alimentary canal, while from that below this point the lowermost portion of the ileum and the large intestine are developed. The thread usually disappears. With its persistence and growth, however, there remains, more or less permanently attached to the navel from within, a tube which presents the structure of the intestine, and which may be found patent in the adult, giving rise to an intestinal fistula opening at the umbilicus. The external free surface of this fistulous tract may project as a bulging tumor, with the appearance and structure of mucous membrane. An abundant new-formation of gland-like tissue may arise from its mucous surface, possessing the characteristics of an adenoma of the intestine. There are certain well-recognized variations in the seat, size, and shape of this appendage to the ileum, to which attention may here be called.

Since the diverticulum is present, if at all, in the earliest weeks of fetal life, it is obvious that its position with reference to the ileo-cecal valve must change with the growth of the intestine. The preponderant elongation of the intestinal tube above the insertion of the duct is accompanied by a less longitudinal growth below this point, and the diverticulum is usually found in the vicinity of the valve.   In the new-born child the distance between the two is about 12 inches, while in the adult the diverticulum is found some 3 feet above the ileocecal valve.   The limits in which it may be present are thus differently stated by various authors : Rokitanski (" Lehrbuch der patholog. Anatomie," 1861, 3te Auflage, Bd. III, S. 182) finds its seat to be 1 to 2 feet above the cecum, while Förster (" Handbuch der patholog. Anatomie," 1863, 2te Auflage, Bd. II, S. 97) extends the limit to upward of 4 feet.   Klebs (" Handbuch der patholog. Anatomie," 1869, Bd. I, S. 163), among others, has attributed the origin of a large part of the esophageal diverticula to congenital anomalies.   Although other possibilities than the presence of the vitelline duct exist for irregularities of development in this region, the facts which immediately follow show that the possible presence of the duct at the upper part of the alimentary canal must be admitted as a cause of this diverticulum.   For the present this view is satisfactorily disposed of by Zenker (Ziemssen's " Handbuch der spec. Path. u. Ther.," 1877, VII ; Anhang, S. 61), but only from the lack of positive evidence.   The possibility is still recognized by him that the esophageal pulsion diverticula may proceed from congenital formations.

The following compilation, taken from the article by Fitz (*l. c.*), shows that bands and adhesions are the most frequent causes of obstruction next to intussusceptions.   Persistent vitelline vessels, either closed or open, may be found as cords or bands between the umbilical region of the anterior abdominal wall and the intestine or mesentery, or both.   They may be connected with these parts near the stomach, as well as at the lower portion of the ileum.   The band may be attached at both ends to the mesentery, and yet be of like congenital origin.   Furthermore, a band or cord of similar origin may connect a diverticulum with the intestine or with the mesentery.   An examination of the records of 4000 autopsies at Guy's Hospital, published by Fagge (" Guy's Hospital Reports," third series, 1869, vol. XIV, p. 272), gives the following results : There were 54 cases of acute and chronic intestinal obstruction ; 7 were due to intussusception, 6 due to volvulus, and 5 each due to a diverticulum and to bands.

ACUTE INTESTINAL OBSTRUCTION. APPROXIMATE RELATIVE
FREQUENCY OF THE MORE PROMINENT CAUSES.

	Number of Cases Included.	Intussusception.	Bands and Adhesions.	Twists, Knots, and Displacements.	Diverticulum.	Vermiform Appendix.	Pressure from Tumors, Abscesses, or Organs.	Diaphragmatic Hernia.	Mesenteric Hernia.	Omental Hernia.	Other Internal Herniæ.
		p. c.	p. c.	p. c.	p. c.	p. c.	p. c.	p. c.	p. c.	p. c.	p. c.
Haven, . .	163	39	24	11	6	. .	3	5	3	3	6
Duchaussoy,	347	39	19	6	6	5	6	18			
Brinton, . .	481	54	17	10	7	3	. .	. .	66	37	. .
Leichtenstern,	1134	39	9	6	6	4	4	19	. .	58	79

The following are the conclusions which R. H. Fitz reaches :

1. Bands and cords as a cause of acute intestinal obstruction are second in importance to intussusception alone.

2. Their seat, structure, and relation are such as frequently admit their origin from obliterated or patent omphalomesenteric vessels, either alone or in connection with Meckel's diverticulum, and oppose their origin from peritonitis.

3. Recorded cases of intestinal strangulation from Meckel's diverticulum, in most instances at least, belong to the above series.

4. In the region where these congenital causes are most frequently met with, an occasional cause of intestinal strangulation, viz., the vermiform appendix, is also found.

5. It would seem, therefore, that in the operation of abdominal section for the relief of acute intestinal obstruction not due to intussusception, and in the absence of local symptoms calling for the preferable exploration of other parts of the abdominal cavity, the lower right quadrant should be selected as the seat of the incision. The vicinity of the navel and the lower 3 feet of the ileum should then receive the earliest attention. If a band is discovered, it is most likely to be a persistent vitelline duct,—*i. e.*, Meckel's diverticulum, or an omphalomesenteric vessel either patent or obliterated, or both these structures in continuity. The section of the band may thus necessitate opening the intestinal canal or a blood-vessel of large size. Each of these alternatives is to be guarded against, and the removal of the entire band is to be sought, lest subsequent adherence prove a fresh source of strangulation.

The chief practical conclusion thus reached in this article is essentially the same as that of Nélaton.   This surgeon advised that the incision through the abdominal wall for the relief of intestinal obstruction should be made a little above Poupart's ligament, preferably in the right side.

Pathological Anatomy of Acute Occlusion.

The most striking alteration in the lumen of the intestines in this condition is the contrast between the size of the loops above and below the occlusion.   Those above are necessarily dilated, their walls very thin and attenuated, the color varying according to the underlying pathological conditions—sometimes very pale ; at others, particularly when the walls are thickened, they are colored a dark bloody red.

The extent to which the intestine may be expanded is limited to a certain degree by the resistance of the abdominal walls, as well as the remaining limiting boundaries of the abdomen, and the mutual hindrances which the intestinal loops themselves exert upon one another.   It is well established experimentally that the distention of the intestines during occlusion occurs by two varieties of meteorism, which are essentially different.   These have been designated as (1) *stagnation meteorism* and (2) *local meteorism.*

The distention above the point of blocking is, as a general rule, looked upon as the characteristic sign of acute occlusion or ileus. But this distention may originate in different ways.

1. **Stagnation Meteorism.**—A simple blocking of the lumen of the bowel *without causing circulatory disturbances in the intestinal wall and mesentery* brings about a kind of meteorism that is due to " stagnation " of the solid, liquid, and gaseous contents above the obstruction.   This mode of distention is observed in cases of obturation by foreign bodies, coproliths, gall-stones, and in certain forms of invagination, the indispensable conditions being the maintenance of fairly normal circulation in the bowel wall and mesentery, with simultaneous blocking of the lumen.

A further characteristic of this form of meteorism is that the narrowing process develops in a chronic manner.   The distention of the intestinal loops is brought about by a liquid mass consisting mainly of semifluid feces and gas.   If the location of the occlusion is in the small intestine, there is, as a rule, more liquid contained in the distended intestinal loops than if it is in the large intestine, because of the great resorptive power of the colon for liquids. Talma (*l. c.*) holds that the meteoristic distention is in a greater measure due to the liquids which represent an accumulation of gastric and intestinal secretions, and that it is only to a limited extent due to gas. His experiments were conducted on animals, and they are not directly applicable to the conditions in the human being, where immense distentions, due almost exclusively to gas, are also found above the location of the occlusion. Formerly every form of distention, whether it occurred during life or was found out after death, was considered due to stagnation meteorism, and ascribed to the accumulation and blocking of contents above the point of occlusion. During the last five or six years, however, attention had been called by a number of very capable clinicians and investigators to the so-called " local meteorism " in explanation of the above phenomena.

2. **Local Meteorism.**—This is a form of distention which also occurs after acute occlusion, and is conditioned by blocking of the intestinal lumen *simultaneously with grave interference with the circulation in the intestinal wall and mesentery*, thus effecting a venous congestion. The most frequent types of occlusion in which this form of meteorism occurs are those following the loop-knot formation, the internal hernia-like forms of incarceration, and the axial torsions. The first one to call attention to this differentiation was Förster (*l. c.*) in 1854, but von Wahl (*l. c.*) emphasized its great significance for the pathology and diagnosis of intestinal occlusions. These observations were confirmed by von Zoege Mannteuffel. But the most important experimental contribution to the subject, endeavoring to explain the origin of local meteorism, by experiments on animals, is by Kader (*l. c.*). The pathogenetic mechanism of local meteorism is based upon the fact that the veins are more easily compressed and obliterated than the intestinal and mesenteric arteries. If intestinal loops together with their mesentery are moderately compressed or strangulated so that the venous outflow is completely stopped, but a certain amount of arterial inflow is still possible, then the portion of the intestine involved in the strangulation rapidly assumes a dark, livid color. A primary reddish-blue

discoloration is promptly followed by venous stasis, and extravasations into the intestinal walls, producing tumefaction, so that these walls may become twice as thick as normal. At first only serum, and later on unaltered blood, are extravasated not only into the lumen of the involved loop, but also into the peritoneal cavity. Complete muscular paralysis may develop in from four to six hours in this portion. The loop becomes distended, very tight, and may reach three to four times its normal volume. This is due to the gaseous evolution which occurs no matter whether the involved section of the intestinal canal was a long or short one, whether it contained very much fecal matter or none at all, at the moment of the strangulation. The distention may become so excessive that considerable portions of the intestines leading up to and coming away from the involved area, together with their mesentery, may be drawn into the strangulation. The phenomena as they develop successively then are venous hyperemia, tumefaction of the wall, paralysis, and local meteorism. As a consequence of these, thrombosis in the mesenteric vessel and gangrene develop, leading to perforation through which the gas may escape, resulting in collapse of the involved loop. Sometimes the perforation is a capillary one, invisible to the naked eye, yet sufficient to permit of escape of the gas. The tremendous development of gas, as well as the intestinal paralysis, is attributed by Kader to the disturbances in the venous circulation. The main difference in the appearance anatomically between stagnation meteorism and local meteorism is that in the former there is a uniform distention reaching upward toward the stomach from the uppermost location of the intestinal loop involved in the occlusion, to a greater or less extent. In local meteorism this may (in rare cases) occur also, but not necessarily so. As a rule, the intestine above and below the occluded area is completely empty, and only the loops caught between both points of occlusion are distended, of a blood-red color, and filled with gas and liquid contents. In local meteorism, therefore, we have a distended balloon between the two points that are blocked ; the intestinal loops above and below are usually empty. In stagnation meteorism there is distention upward toward the stomach from the point of occlusion. If the phenomena of local meteorism are absent, in typical cases in which the conditions are given,—viz., occlusion of the intestine, together with interference with the circulation in the mesentery and intestinal wall,—there are generally good reasons which can be found in explanation of this absence; either the exit of the intestinal contents downward is found incompletely blocked, or, as Kader has shown, there are minute capillary perforations which permit of the escape of gas. Local meteorism, therefore, may be said to occur regularly after the conditions indicated, and is conformable to certain pathological and physiological laws, as it is capable of being reproduced experimentally. An essential factor to bear in mind is that the gaseous distention can not be attributed so much to fermentation of the intestinal contents as to the circulatory disturbances in the veins of the involved intestinal loop, for it occurs even when there are no intestinal contents contained in the loops. Nothnagel has called attention to the following experimental observation, which proves the same point. If the intestine is experimentally stenosed in one place by ligation that *does not involve* the mesentery, and the mesentery is ligated at a place somewhat below the locality at which the intestine is ligated, we may have *stagnation* meteorism above the intestinal ligature, but also *local* meteorism in the loops below this point, although access to this loop from above is blocked and the exit of the contents downward is not interfered with, thus proving that local meteorism can occur in the absence of intestinal contents in the involved loop.

In occlusions due to axial twists, torsions, strangulation, and loop-knot formations, it is the loop that is involved in the obstruction itself that is the main seat of the meteorism. The diagnostic importance of this phenomenon may be estimated by the fact that this distended, resistant portion of the intestine, which is immovably fixed in the abdomen, can not fail to be recognizable by inspection of the form of the abdomen and a distinct resistance to palpation." The technic of this clinical investigation is described by von Zoege Mannteuffel ("Verhandl. d. VIII. Congress. f. innere Med.," 1889, S. 93). "After the preliminary history of the patient, and his general condition is noted, a careful ocular inspection of the abdomen is next made. The slightest asymmetries must be considered. One observes whether the asymmetries are constant, whether they change their form as a result of increased peristalsis, whether intestinal movements are observable, or whether a dismal rest predominates in the tense, greatly distended abdominal walls. Then follows the palpation, which seeks to determine differences in the resistance; a strangulated distended loop must feel entirely different from a normal intestine filled with liquid stool. A distended loop, which demands the greatest possible amount of space, pushes up against the receding abdominal walls, thus facilitating this investigation. If vomiting occurs, one can distinctly grasp the more resisting section of the intestine during the interval when the abdominal tension relaxes. This is especially facilitated under chloroform narcosis."

The palpable, prominent, and resistant intestinal loop described in the preceding has been designated by the term "von Wahl's sign." In rare cases it may be wanting, particularly where other distended intestinal loops, situated above the obstruction, overlap and cover the fixed loop. It may also be difficult of recognition when a very large section of the intestinal loop is strangulated. Nevertheless, it is a valuable sign, and the diagnosis of intestinal obstruction has been made repeatedly, based upon the presence of this sign alone, and successful operations have followed its recognition.

Pathological Anatomy of Chronic Occlusion.

The principal pathological changes that develop in the course of chronic occlusion are: (1) distention of the intestine above the stenosis, firm contraction below the stenosis; (2) genuine muscular hypertrophy; (3) enteritis and colitis followed by ulceration, which, again, may be followed by peritonitis; (4) elongation of the intestinal district above the stenosis. To speak of these changes in detail, I might emphasize that the distention above the stenosis in chronic occlusion does not attain the enormous degree of meteoristic dilation which one observes in acute occlusion. In rare instances, where complete blocking is superadded immediately before death, so that the passage of the gases was made absolutely impossible, one may exceptionally observe considerable meteoristic expansion. The hypertrophy of the muscularis is observable on the fourth or fifth day after the first development of a stenosis. The connective tissue is not increased, but only the individual muscle-fibers themselves. It is a genuine hypertrophy due to overwork. The ulcerations which are observed in association with the inflammation of the mucosa and submucosa belong to the type of stercoral or decubital ulcerations. They may lead to perforation and fecal abscesses.

This leads us to speak of the pathological changes in the peritoneum. Every intestinal occlusion is, in my experience, accompanied with more or less extensive peritonitis, which is due to the invasion of bacteria. Occasionally one single bacterium is found in pure culture, but more frequently the peritonitis is a mixed infection. The organisms which are most frequently found as the cause of this complication are, above all, the Streptococcus pyogenes and the Bacillus coli communis. The recent investigations lend support to the view that the intestinal walls in the paralyzed districts involved in the meteorism rapidly become permeable for the microbic inhabitants of the bowel, which thereafter induce either a peritonitis or a general infection. In very acute occlusion the peritonitis is localized to the area involved, but the longer the occlusion has existed, the more extensive will be the peritonitis.

Symptomatology.

The symptoms of obstruction often occur suddenly, and without any apparent cause; usually unnoticed messengers precede it, such as diarrhea, constipation, and a discomfort which may increase to moderately strong colic-like pains. Sometimes the anamnesis indicates that a short time before a severe trauma acted upon the abdomen as the primary cause, or that there was a cold, or excessive bodily exertion, or that a large meal was ingested, or that a strong purge had been administered. The patients suddenly experience extremely violent pains, which are described by them as tearing, pulling pains, occasionally also as cramp-like and resembling the pains of parturition. These pains are felt in some cases at the seat of the closure, but more frequently in the neighborhood of the navel, and in some cases they are from the beginning spread over the entire abdomen. Even if the pain is at first circumscribed, it soon extends over the entire abdomen. The pains either continue with undiminished intensity (provided they are not lessened by large doses of opium) or they diminish somewhat after a while, without, however, ceasing entirely, only to grow more severe and to increase almost beyond endurance. If the abdominal walls are thin, very quick peristaltic

movements may often be observed through them.   These are due
to the forcible contractions of the muscles in the intestinal loops
lying above the closure, and are the chief cause of the paroxysms
of pain.   As the periodically recurring pains in intestinal occlusion are caused by periodic, spasmodic contractions of the intestinal muscles, it can easily be understood why the pains become
still more severe after the administration of aperients.   In case
of complete closure, the stool is generally suppressed for long ·
periods.   Aperients or enemata may cause the evacuation of small
quantities of feces.   If the occlusion is in the small intestine, and if
at its beginning the large intestine contains a great amount of fecal
matter, in the cecum or ascending colon for instance, then very
abundant evacuations may take place for a time at least.   Evidently, therefore, these stools always come from that section of the
intestine which is situated below the occluded place.   These evacuations often give support to the false hope that the pains were
caused by coprostasis alone, and that the intestine is again permeable.   The long-continued retention of stool causes a nervous excitement in many of the patients, because they suppose that this is
the principal cause of their pains and other complaints.   Under
such a state of affairs it is a test of good judgment to resist the
solicitations for purges and enemata to remedy this stoppage of the
evacuations ; it must be borne in mind that aperients can do no
good, but may do great harm.   The statement of the patient that
no more flatus at all passes off, whereas the abdomen is becoming
more and more inflated (meteorically), is of very great importance
for the positive proof that the intestine is completely closed.   If
flatus again passes off after a time, it is a favorable sign, because it
proves that the mechanical occlusion of the intestine has been
removed, or that the previously insufficient intestinal muscles have
recovered, and that the intestine is once more permeable to a certain degree at least.

Soon after the beginning of the pains,—soonest, indeed, in occlusion of the small intestine,—other important symptoms of ileus
occur—namely, eructation, persistent vomiting, and frequently also
a torturing singultus.   First the particles of food remaining in the
stomach are vomited ; soon afterward abundant yellowish, bilious
masses.   These are followed by discolored, dirty green, later on

brownish, crumbling masses, which at first have only a faint fecal odor; later on, however, the odor of feces grows stronger and more distinct with each vomiting. Finally, only liquid, feculent masses are vomited, which have the appearance of diarrheic evacuations, but they are only seldom of a pulpy consistency. By this *stercoraceous vomiting*, which represents one of the most nauseating, unendurable consequences of occlusion, the patients and also their relatives are naturally put in the greatest consternation. After the fecal vomiting, and not infrequently before it, the eructations and the breath of the patient sometimes have a fecal odor (*fœtor ex ore*), and the air in the room, especially in the immediate neighborhood of the patient, may become unbearably offensive. The vomiting, which is rarely lacking, may last a long time; occasionally it ceases for a few hours and then returns. Permanent cessation of it occurs when paralysis of the intestines has set in, or after a perforation of the intestines has let out the collected gases into the peritoneal cavity, these gases being the main cause of the antiperistalsis—the cause of the vomiting. Brignet, Jaccoud, Rosenstein, and Dr. Quintard (Am. Gastro-Enterologic Assoc., Washington, May, 1901) report the vomiting of firm scybalæ. Leichtenstern, Boas, and Nothnagel emphasize that they have never observed this. Personally I may add that this phenomenon has never occurred in any of my cases. The abdomen often, but by no means always, appears asymmetrical or meteorically inflated *in toto* (barrel-shaped) soon after the beginning of the intestinal occlusion. If the diaphragm is then pushed upward by the excessively inflated intestinal loops, thus exerting a strong pressure upon the lungs, heart, and blood-vessels, other symptoms occur, prominent among which are a torturing oppression and dyspnea. The very shallow breathing is owing to the difficulty with which the diaphragm makes its excursions. This respiratory embarrassment may grow in intensity, so that at times suffocation threatens. The very rapid and compressible pulse increases in frequency. The great loss of water by vomiting, profuse perspiration, and the greatly disturbed absorption in the intestines causes a marked diminution in the amount of urine excreted (oliguria). Occasionally this secretion even ceases entirely (anuria). The patient has an unquenchable thirst, and at the same time a dry tongue and mucous membrane, but as soon as water is taken, it is

promptly vomited.   Sooner or later the symptoms of a very severe
collapse appear.   The eyes lie deep in their sockets, surrounded by
dark rings, the nose is pointed, the color of the face is pale, and a
cold sweat is upon the forehead.   The voice becomes hoarse, un-
melodious, whispering, shrill (just as in Asiatic cholera).   The
pulse is weak, soft, rapid, rarely retarded.   The temperature of the
body is below the normal.   The extremities are cold,—the hands
and feet are sometimes as cold as ice,—livid, and covered with a
cold, clammy sweat.   The tongue usually has a dirty brown coating.   The patients toss about restlessly.   In the sharply drawn
features the greatest fear, helplessness, and desperation are expressed, and this can readily be understood, because the psychic
functions of the miserable sufferers usually remain undisturbed up
to death or just before it, and they are usually aware of their terrible
condition.

Individual Symptoms.

Pain.—The extremely violent pain which always sets in as one
of the first symptoms of occlusion immediately after an acute internal strangulation, intussusception, or axial twist, is largely due
to the great stretching which the peritoneal covering of the intestine
undergoes at the point of occlusion under these diseased conditions.
The secondary inflammatory changes at and above the point of
closure, and also the mechanical and chemical irritation of the
nerves of the mucosa, which are exposed by ulcerations, tend to
increase and continue the pains which are felt in the various stages
and forms of occlusion.   The excessive distention of the intestinal
walls and of the peritoneal covering above the occluded loop (peritonitic irritation), and finally the occurrence of general peritonitis,
which is a very frequent result of occlusion (see paragraph on
Pathological Anatomy), also tend to increase the pain.   Those
pains which recur at greater or less intervals, and then diminish, are,
on the other hand, probably attributable to the periodical and very
energetic contractions of the muscles of that section of the intestine which lies above the occlusion.   These contractions cause
quick peristaltic movements of the individual intestinal loops.   In
mechanical occlusion this periodical increase of the intestinal peristalsis is not caused by the obstruction as such, but by the enor-

mous accumulation of gases, acting as a direct irritant on the plexuses of Auerbach and Meissner.

Under normal conditions the peristalsis of the small intestine is much greater than that of the large intestine ; the contractions of the circular and longitudinal muscles of the former succeed each other more rapidly, and the irritability of the sensory and motor nerves is probably greater in the jejunum and ileum than in the colon. We can therefore easily understand why, in occlusion of the small intestine, the paroxysms of pain occur not only sooner, but are also distinguished by a greater intensity and occur at more rapid intervals than in occlusion of the large intestine. If, as is often seen just before the death of the patients, both the paroxyms of pain and the vomiting cease, while the meteorism—the indirect cause of both of these—and the collapse increase, we may assume that either a complete paralysis of the muscles of the intestinal section above the obstruction has set in, or that perforation has taken place. The initial pains are occasionally somewhat diminished by a moderate pressure on the abdominal walls, rarely increased ; in the further course of the disease, especially if there is a peritonitic irritation, or if general peritonitis has set in, even the slightest pressure, such as that of the bed-cover, often causes an increase in the pains. In occlusion of the small intestine the pains are usually felt in the neighborhood of the navel ; if the occlusion is in the large intestine, the pains are often felt along its anatomical course. Since the positive determination of the place of the initial pains is of great importance for the localization of the intestinal occlusion, it is extremely advisable for the physician to ask the patient, immediately after their appearance, where he or she first experienced a circumscribed pain. On the other hand, the localization of the pains felt in the abdomen some time after the beginning of the occlusion gives no reliable data for the determination of the seat of the occlusion.

Vomiting.—*Stercoraceous Vomiting.*—The first vomiting, which in acute internal strangulation of the intestine may occur contemporaneously with the initial pain, is caused by peritoneal reflexes, because great traction is exerted upon the peritoneum at the point of strangulation. If it does not occur contemporaneously with the onset of the pains, but some time after, it is either the result of a mechanical irritation of the peritoneum of the suprastenotic section of the intestines, the walls of which (and therefore also the serosa) are excessively distended by gases, and by the stagnating contents of the intestines, or it is due to an actual peritonitis.   Both of these may cause an increase in the peristalsis of the intestines.   The abnormally powerful and quickly succeeding contractions of the intestines always play the most important rôle in the causing of the stercoraceous vomiting.   These antiperistaltic contractions are caused soon after the occlusion by the collection of gases, which constitute an irritant to the intestinal nerves.

According to Nothnagel, the obstruction as such (the intestinal occlusion) does not cause this increase in the peristalsis, since the intestine remains perfectly quiet for some time after it has been experimentally ligated at one place.   Besides the gases, the toxins arising from the decomposition of the albuminates, to the action of which the nerves of the small intestine are not accustomed, probably irritate the nerves more strongly in the case of occlusion. Thus, Bokai observed that skatol, when injected into the intestines of rabbits, even in very small doses (2 mg.), caused energetic contractions of the intestines, and even tonic cramps.

The beginning of the fecal vomiting may be determined with certainty by means of the sense of smell.   The former opinion that stercoraceous vomiting occurred only in occlusion of the large intestine, and at the same time proved the insufficiency of the ileocecal valve, has long since been disproved both by numerous reliable clinical observations and by the results of autopsies, so that at present we know that stercoraceous vomiting may occur in occlusions of the small intestine as well as of the colon and sigmoid, and thus has no diagnostic value for the localization of the occlusion.   The transformation of the intestinal contents into feces, under normal conditions, takes place in the colon.   The lowest portions of the ileum however, at times contain ingesta of a fecal character, and therefore it is intelligible that in occlusions of the jejunum and ileum, stercoraceous vomiting may occasionally take place.   Naturally, the occlusion must not be absolute,—i. e., it must still permit the passage, antiperistaltically, of some fecal matter,—if it occurs above the district where feces normally are formed.   Or the occlusion is absolute, but is situated below the intestinal section that transforms the contents into feces.

It has been repeatedly emphasized that under normal conditions the rapid passage of the chyme in the small intestine prevents the beginning of decomposition in the same, and that putrefaction therefore usually begins in the large intestine, the contents of which, as a result of much slower peristalsis, move more slowly and often stagnate completely.   Since the rapid passage of the chyme in the small intestine is the main reason why the chyme does not decompose, it is intelligible that, if the chyme is considerably retarded, as a result of muscular paresis of the small intestine, its contents may become decomposed.   After the occlusion of the ileum, when a complete stoppage in the passing of the chyme sets in, the conditions in this state are still more favorable for the beginning and increase of the decomposition, and consequently also for the transformation of the chyme into feces, than in the large intestine ; because the contents of the small intestine are liquid or pulpy and rich in albuminates, which decompose much more easily and quickly than the other food elements, and the decomposition products of which give to the feces their characteristic odor.   The important fact, demonstrated by Jaffé, in his experiments on animals, and confirmed by observations made during disease, that in occlusion of the ileum the urine contains more indican (indoxyl-sulphuric acid), which comes from the indol arising from the decomposition of the albuminates in the large intestine, while in occlusion of the large intestine this amount is not increased, is a positive proof for the correctness of the previously mentioned opinion, aside from its great importance for the differential diagnosis of occlusions of the large and the small intestine.   Under normal circumstances the indol, the parent substance of indican as it occurs in the urine, is formed only in the large intestine and by the decomposition of albuminates.   The chyme which passes out of the small intestine into the colon at a normal rate of intestinal peristalsis contains but little albumin, and the amount of indol formed in the large intestine of healthy persons (and consequently also the amount of indican in the urine) is slight. Since after the beginning of an uncomplicated occlusion of the colon (as, for instance, the result of a simple fecal obturation) the decomposition of the albuminates in the large intestine, and consequently also the formation of indol in the same, suffers no change, the amount of indican in the urine of the patients remains the same.

The circumstances are entirely different, however, in occlusion of the ileum, because considerable amounts of indol, skatol, and phenol may be formed by the greater decomposition of the chyme, which stagnates in the small intestine and contains larger amounts of albumin. These substances (indol, etc.), after their absorption in the blood, are secreted as indol-, skatol-, and phenol-sulphuric acid. The amount of indican can also be increased in occlusion of the large intestine, especially when a general peritonitis accompanies it, and when this, as is usually the case, leads to paresis of the intestinal muscularis with its consequences (decomposition of the stagnating contents of the small intestine). According to Leichtenstern's observations, the same holds true for those cases of intestinal occlusion which are caused by strangulation or compression (incarceration), since in these cases the passage of the chyme is usually delayed quite early, and the decomposition in the ileum thus favored. If the amount of indican is not increased, it can be interpreted as an indication of an occlusion of the large intestine.

If the patient has received abundant nutritive enemata, rich in albumin, an increased amount of indican in the urine is of no diagnostic value for the localization of an occlusion of the small intestine, since the albumin soon decomposes in the rectum and gives rise to the formation of indol.

Mechanism of Stercoraceous Vomiting.—The idea originally represented by Galen was that stercoraceous vomiting was caused by a reversal of the peristalsis, by antiperistaltic movements, which caused a retrograde passage of the feces from the lower to the upper sections of the intestines, and finally to the stomach, and has very few adherents at the present day. It is displaced by the theory which Haguenot (of Montpelier) advanced in 1713, based on many experiments on animals. This theory of Haguenot, which is now almost universally accepted, was called by his contemporaries the " hydraulic theory," because it traced stercoraceous vomiting back to mechanical laws. The theory is perfectly simple and convincing. Up to recent times it has been ascribed to van Swieten, although this clinician denied emphatically that he had originated the theory, and it is one of Leichtenstern's services that he corrected this literary error and proved Haguenot's priority of discovery. According to the latter's explanation, the stercoraceous vomiting arises as follows : If the intestinal lumen is completely occluded at any place, the liquid or pulpy contents of the intestine are collected before the place of occlusion in great quantities.   As a result of a contemporaneous collection or development of gases in the intestine, a considerable pressure is exerted upon these collected masses, which is still further increased with every inspiration during the muscular efforts of emesis, especially during the energetic contractions of the intestinal muscles.   Under the influence of this pressure the liquid contents of the intestines, which are stagnating above the point of occlusion, are readily displaced, and yield in the direction of the least resistance,—that is, upward,—and thus get into the upper intestinal loops next to the stomach.   If these are completely filled with the decomposed, feculent masses, a regurgitation, or, as Henle has fitly characterized it, an overflow, of a part of this fluid takes place into the stomach ; the gastric mucosa is strongly irritated by the contents of the intestines, and vomiting sets in.   For physical reasons either liquid or pulpy, easily moved intestinal contents can be transferred from the lower sections of the intestines to the higher ones ; but thick contents or already formed hard feces can not progress upward antiperistaltically.   In occlusion of the large intestine, just as in that of the small intestine, solid particles of feces are never vomited, but only fluid contents, or, at most, thin pulpy masses.

There are clinical observers (quoted in the preceding) who have often had the opportunity to treat patients suffering with occlusion, and who assert that they have not observed one case where formed fecal balls were vomited.   In the extremely rare cases in which the latter phenomenon is described, it is suggested that they probably had to do with patients in whom a fistula of the stomach and the colon had resulted from a cancer or from ulcerations.

The shorter the distance between the seat of the intestinal occlusion and the beginning of the intestine or the stomach, the quicker the uppermost intestinal loops are filled with the fluid intestinal contents, and the sooner the regurgitation or overflow into the stomach takes place.   Thus the theory of Haguenot explains why stercoraceous vomiting sets in sooner in occlusion of the small intestine than in that of the large.   Since a much larger quantity of a feculent liquid is often vomited by persons suffering from occlusion of the small intestine than had been introduced previously with the food and drink, we are justified in assuming that in occlusion of the small intestine—probably as a result of the great increase in the peristalsis—considerable amounts of intestinal juice, and possibly also of pancreatic juice, are secreted into it, and that as a result the upper loops are filled still more rapidly. In occlusion of the large intestine the vomited feculent masses might also consist partly of the digestive juices of the intestines. In this condition, just as in Asiatic cholera, a very abundant transudation out of the blood-vessels into the intestines probably takes place. If the fluid collects above the place of occlusion, a part of the thickened feces is dissolved in it and is later carried outward by vomiting. The mechanism by which those loops of small intestine which have the shortest mesentery are most readily filled with intestinal contents (upper ileum and duodenum) has already been described.

Meteorism.—It was formerly held that the intestinal gases for the most part (if not entirely) passed off with the flatus, and that a greater collection of gases in the intestines (meteorism, tympanites) was the result of an abnormally increased gas generation, and especially of a restricted discharge of the flatus. This has been disproved in more recent times by the beautiful experimental observations of Zuntz, which completely explained the pathogenesis of meteorism. Zuntz has determined by experiments on animals that the *intestinal gases for the most part are absorbed by the intestinal blood-vessels, and carried out of the body by the lungs together with the expired air, and that only in a limited degree do they leave the body with the flatus.*

The absorption of the gases is dependent upon the integrity of the blood circulation of the intestinal walls, and so long as this is undisturbed, even if the gas generation is increased and its discharge per anum hindered, meteorism may not set in. On the other hand, the gases often accumulate in the intestines when the resorption does not keep pace with the formation, and this accumulation will increase all the more rapidly, the more the production of the gases is augmented, and the more the passage of the flatus is hindered, if at the same time the absorption has completely ceased. The clinical observations, which could not be reconciled with the old view concerning meteorism,—indeed, even contradicted parts of it,—completely agree with the newer view.   For instance, in former times one could not explain why, after persistent constipation lasting several weeks, during which no feces and flatus were passed, as a result of a stenosis of the colon, meteorism was often wanting or but slight in spite of the increased gas formation, while in other cases, only a few hours or days after the beginning of an acute occlusion of the intestine, caused by incarceration, or after a peritonitis, an advanced tympanites of the intestine usually sets in. At the present time the explanation meets no difficulties, because it is known that, on the one hand, in those diseases which cause constipation, if the blood circulation in the intestinal walls, and consequently the absorption of gases, remains. undisturbed, a considerable amount of the intestinal gases can be absorbed, and their accumulation in the intestines prevented.   On the other hand, when the intestinal closure results from incarcerations, axial twists, intussusceptions, etc., and also in advanced peritonitis, the blood circulation in the intestinal walls may be greatly disturbed, and the gas absorption consequently considerably lessened or even stopped entirely.   If these disturbances are lacking in obstruction, as it occasionally happens, the meteorism may be entirely wanting, as is proved by an observation of Touchard.

Acute intestinal occlusion almost invariably causes meteorism. The further down the occlusion is situated in the intestinal canal, the more pronounced the meteorism.   Both when general peritonitis sets in and when the muscles of the intestine are paralyzed, the meteorism is increased.   Although the meteorism is at first circumscribed (the characteristic barrel-shaped abdomen does not appear until paralysis of the muscularis has reached its most advanced stage), it later goes over into the diffuse form.

If one has the opportunity to examine the patient just after the beginning of the occlusion and before the beginning of the diffuse meteorism, one can often, by means of careful palpation and percussion of the abdomen, discover a local, circumscribed meteorism in the immediate neighborhood of the seat of the occlusion ; this is easiest and most distinct in volvulus of the sigmoid flexure, but is also true of other forms of occlusion due to strangulation.

The intestinal loop which borders on the occlusion becomes excessively distended by gases as a result of paralysis of its muscularis.   Inflammatory changes, great stretching of the peritoneum, interference with the blood supply, are some of the main causes of this muscular paresis.   The loop is crowded against the anterior abdominal wall, thus bulging it out asymmetrically.   If the abdominal walls are yielding, the dilated intestinal loop may easily be grasped in palpation.   It has an entirely different feeling from a loop filled with a fluid.   On account of the excessive distention of its walls, it does not give a tympanitic or metallic sound on percussion, like other loops that contain air and the walls of which are less distended, but it gives a deep, non-tympanitic tone similar to that of the lungs.   So long as its muscles stay paralyzed, this tone does not change, and the inflated loop also remains at the same spot.   As von Wahl first emphasized, this is an important indication as to the location of the occlusion, which gains still more in importance if the initial pain was also felt at this point.   Since this valuable symptom evades discovery when the meteorism has become diffuse, one must look for it at the very first examination.   In occlusion of the colon, a local circumscribed meteorism may also appear in the lower portions of the abdomen, and this is then a sign that the ileocecal valve is still capable of closing.   If the latter is the case, the section of the intestines lying between the valve and the point of occlusion is very much distended by gases, and the abdominal walls at the point in question bulge out asymmetrically. If the obstruction is at the right or hepatic flexure, the right side of the abdomen will bulge out.   If it is in the rectum, the left side of the abdominal wall above Poupart's ligament is first to become inflated, and soon afterward the abdominal wall above the navel is also bulged outward by the greatly inflated transverse colon.   It is well to note, however, that in occlusion of the colon also—just as in occlusions of the small intestine—the abdomen may appear distended by uniformly diffuse meteorism at the same time when the inflation by gases is yet confined to the colon, and this is especially so when the colon is displaced into the epigastric region.   One can also observe diffuse general meteorism in occlusion of the colon when the ileocecal valve has become insufficient as a result of excessive distention.   In occlusion of the duodenum, and also of the upper part of the jejunum, the meteorism is entirely lacking or is confined to the epigastrium, which sinks in after every evacuation of the stomach by means of vomiting, whilst the lower parts of the abdomen are retracted. If the intestinal lumen is occluded in the lower section of the ileum, the abdomen may be symmetrically bulged out in the umbilical region. If this diffuse symmetrical dis-tention is restricted to the umbilical and subumbilical region, there is, as a rule, no distention of the transverse colon. Deductions from the localization of the most pronounced meteorism must be made soon after the initial symptoms to be of any diagnostic value.

Appearance of Collapse.—The symptoms of great collapse, appearing soon after an acute intestinal occlusion, are the result of the strong mechanical irritation which acts upon the roots of the splanchnic nerve during the incarceration (strangulation shock). The strong irritation of the splanchnic, which is not only the sen-sory, but also the vasomotor nerve of the intestines (its stimulation causes anemia, its paralysis an advanced state of hyperemia), often leads to its paralysis and consequently to an overfilling of the intes-tines and other hypogastric organs with blood. Since the blood-vessel area of the intestines is the greatest in the entire body, its overfilling with blood causes an anemia of other organs and parts of organs, and this is the cause of the most important symptoms of collapse : fainting spells, roaring noises in the ears, flashes be-fore the eyes,—sometimes coma and delirium occur,—which often precede the collapse, and are usually ascribed to anemia of the brain. It is presumed that the tonus of the vagus is decreased in this cerebral anemia, and as the vagus is the inhibitory nerve of the heart, the pulse in collapse is therefore more rapid when this nervous control is lost, and very soft and of low tension, besides, as a result of the incomplete filling of the arterial system. The skin, to which less blood flows than usual, is anemic, cool, especially in the pendent parts of the extremities ; the body temperature is usually subnormal. The decrease in the arterial pressure, making itself felt in the blood-vessels of the kidneys, causes oliguria.

Water Impoverishment of the Blood.—It has already been mentioned that many symptoms of occlusion—such as the torturing thirst, the dryness of the tongue and mouth, the oliguria and an-uria, the decrease in the amount of blood in the skin, muscular cramps—are to be explained by the great loss of water which the blood sustains as a result of vomiting, sweating, supersecretion of the

intestinal juices, and transudation of liquids out of the intestinal
vessels.   In spite of the loss of water, uremic symptoms do not at
all, or extremely rarely, occur.   This is ascribable to the usually
very rapid progress of the occlusion and to the decreased formation
of excretory products in this condition.

Sweat.—The profuse cold sweats which so often occur with
occlusion cannot be explained by changed conditions in the circulation ; they may possibly be the result of the paralysis of a nerve-
center which inhibits the sweat secretion, just as hyperhidrosis
during a faint, and also the death-sweat.

Behavior of the Urine.—It has already been stated that in an
occlusion of the large intestine the amounts of indican and conjugate
ethereal sulphates in the urine are increased, but not in uncomplicated occlusion of the small intestine.   The albuminuria often
observed in occlusion is either the result of decreased blood-pres-
sure, of disturbances of nutrition in the kidneys, or of an irritation
of the kidneys by toxins.   Hematuria has also been occasionally
observed.

Tetanus, coma, cramps, delirium, fever, which are observed more
rarely, and the symptoms similar to those of typhoid fever resulting
from an incarceration, and also the symptoms of severe nephritis,
are perhaps the results of an autointoxication by means of products
formed in the intestines during the putrefaction of proteids (pto-
mains), which are formed in great quantities in obstruction, especially if it is caused by an occlusion of the ileum.   It was recently
emphasized by Mollière and Lépine that many of the symptoms
found in occlusion remind one of poisoning by atropin.

Results of Examination of the Abdomen in Intestinal Occlu-sion.

Inspection.—The abdomen in intestinal occlusion appears either
uniformly inflated, like a barrel, or the protrusion of the abdominal
wall is confined to a restricted portion, varying according to the
time which has elapsed since the beginning of the intestinal occlusion, and according to its seat.   Thus, for instance, in occlusion
of the duodenum, it is restricted to the epigastric region ; in occlusion of the colon, so long as the ileocecal valve can be closed,
sometimes only to the left, or the right hypogastric region.   When

the abdomen is distended uniformly,—*i. e.*, barrel-shaped,—one can not note any quick peristaltic movements of the intestinal loops lying above the occlusion, nor can the contours of strongly inflated sections of the intestine be made out, because by this time an intestinal paralysis has usually set in.   In acute intestinal occlusion, caused by strangulation or axial twisting, the visible motions of the intestines usually cease quite early for the same reason.   In chronic strictures of the intestines the stenosing process itself, whatever it may be, does not go on to complete obliteration of the lumen as a rule, but the complete occlusion is effected by accumulating fecal masses.   It is, as it were, an acute obstruction then, supervening upon a chronic stenosis, and the intestinal paralysis sets in after a while, as described above with regard to the acute form.

Palpation.—In some of the cases of acute intestinal occlusion, at the very first a circumscribed sensibility to pressure may be detected at the seat of the occlusion; in the remaining cases either the umbilical region or the entire abdomen is sensitive to pressure from the start.   In cases of intussusception a resistance in the depths of the abdomen may be felt; in cases of tumors of organs lying close to and exerting pressure upon the intestines, and finally compressing the lumen, as in fecal tumors and also incarcerations, strangulations, or axial twists of the intestines, this resistance is felt but rarely, in my experience.   When it is felt, it is dependent upon the inflation of that intestinal loop which is next above the point of occlusion.   After the external palpation of the abdominal walls, a careful digital examination starting with the rectum and with the vagina, and also a thorough examination of the external hernial orifices or of any hernial sac or protrusion, must be made. The necessity of this mode of examination can not be emphasized enough, because, as experience has shown, many a human life has been lost in consequence of its omission.

Auscultation.—Loud, dry, rattling, clashing, hissing, or moist rustling noises (borborygmi), which are considerably increased by a change in the patient's position or by a light pressure upon the abdominal walls, indicate that the muscularis is still capable of contracting, and that intestinal paralysis has not yet set in.   The passage of gases in the intestine may also proceed noiselessly, and sometimes even ceases entirely when the intestines are quieted by larger doses of opium ; therefore a negative result of an auscultation of the abdomen does not prove that the intestinal paralysis has already set in.

Percussion.—Among the useful signs that can be made out by percussion is the elevation of the diaphragm, which occurs in diffuse meteorism (barrel-shaped abdomen). In diffuse uniform meteorism the percussion-sound is deep and not tympanitic, when the intestinal wall is exceedingly distended by the accumulated gases ; but if the tension of the intestinal wall is only moderate, the sound is tympanitic or even metallic. When the movements of the gases in the various intestinal loops have ceased, as a result of the paralysis of the intestinal muscles, the tone emitted from the various loops under repeated percussion changes but little, if at all. If, on the contrary, the sound over an intestinal loop under long-continued percussion changes rapidly or slowly from a deep, untympanitic sound to a higher tympanitic or metallic sound (or reversed), or if it suddenly changes from a high ringing sound to a deep one, from a clear sound to a muffled one, because the percussed intestinal loop was displaced by another, these results go to show that the motility of the intestine has not yet been destroyed. According to the observations of Leichtenstern, the pleximeter percussion, simultaneously with auscultation, is especially suited for detecting the changes in the sounds which accompany the alterations in the tension of the gas in the various intestinal loops. After an intestinal perforation large quantities of gas pass over into the peritoneal cavity ; then the liver dullness, and occasionally also the splenic dullness, usually cease. Where general peritonitis has set in, as well as when serous, bloody transudations are secreted into the peritoneal cavity (as a result of axial twisting, the formation of knots, intussusceptions, etc., which have caused a compression of the mesenteric vessels, or peritonitic infection in the method described in the introduction to this chapter), the symptoms of freely moving or circumscribed exudations or transudations may often be detected in the lateral lower parts of the abdomen. The amount and weight of contents of excessively distended loops are sometimes sufficient to drag them down toward both sides of the abdominal cavity, in the horizontal position. This may simulate a moderate ascites or free exudate within the peritoneum, for the lateral abdominal regions then give a marked dullness on percussion ; when the position of the patient is altered, the tone becomes resonant and clearer, because the heavy intestinal loop has been made to change its position.   This occurs with stenosis of the sigmoid flexure and ileum, for loops of the small as well as the large intestine may sink toward the sides in this manner.   Nothnagel suggests a very simple method of arriving at a differentiation between localized exudate or ascites outside of the intestine on the one hand, and liquid inside the dislocated loops on the other.   He advises the examiner to direct rapid but short blows and pushes perpendicularly against the questionable area of dullness ; if a splashing sound is elicited, one is dealing with fluid *inside* of the intestinal lumen.   Considerable amounts of liquids may escape detection entirely, when they are situated between or behind intestinal loops that are agglutinated at various points, and thus to some extent float in the liquids.

Course, Duration, and Termination of Occlusion.

In some cases the patients succumb to this condition in a few hours, or in others on the second day after the beginning of the occlusion, from heart failure resulting from shock ; in other cases the disease continues for a number of days up to a week ; in occlusion resulting from intussusception it may even last several weeks or a month, with alternating aggravation and diminution in the pain. If the patients survive the initial collapse, and the intestine, as a result of the spontaneous resolution of an intussusception or of an internal strangulation, or as the result of the return of an axial twist to its normal position, etc., again becomes permeable, the passage of very offensive flatus is usually the first sign that the occlusion has ceased to exist.   Some time afterward there is also a stool, which likewise has a putrefactive odor, and this is quickly followed by other evacuations.   The first evacuation after the resolution of the intussusception (often also before) almost always contains blood ; after that of an axial twist it contains blood occasionally.   Blood has also been detected in the evacuation in a case of an incarcerated hernia which was replaced by Schnitzler, and in two cases after herniotomy (Henoch, Wilms).   The stercoraceous vomiting ceases, the meteorism decreases, and the patients, if there is no relapse, gradually recover from their great exhaustion. If the acute intestinal occlusion has caused advanced anatomical changes in the intestinal wall at the point of occlusion or above it (such as the formation of ulcers, gangrene, or adhesions), after a time the symptoms of a chronic contraction of the intestine may be observed. This chronic constriction may remain latent for reasons given in the preceding, then suddenly give rise to the symptoms of an acute intestinal occlusion, coming on a considerable time after the first attack. If this apparently acute or subacute attack soon ceases, only to be followed after a short time by another, and if the rapidly succeeding attacks of occlusion grow more and more severe, it is an almost certain indication that there is a chronic intestinal stricture.

In those cases in which the intestine remains impermeable,—and this includes most of the cases,—the life of the patient is often ended by a general peritonitis with or without perforation (ulcer, gangrene, and rupture of the intestines).

Even without a perforation of the intestinal wall, general peritonitis may easily set in when a paralysis of the intestines has taken place. According to the experimental observations of Bönnecken, Nepoen, and Reichel, the intestinal wall can not be penetrated normally by the intestinal bacteria, but it soon becomes permeable for them after paralysis. The invasion of the peritoneum by bacteria sometimes causes a severe general infection, with a severe collapse, even before it has led to peritonitis, just as strangulation of the intestinal wall with its peritoneal covering may do at the beginning of an intestinal occlusion. In occlusion due to strangulation, the disturbance in the circulation of the intestine at the point of occlusion, and above it, is usually much severer than in occlusion due to obturation, and is all the more grave the tighter the intestine is constricted. Since the gaseous inflation and also the paralysis of the intestine are caused more especially by disturbances in the circulation, it can not appear strange that general peritonitis and also the appearance of a severe collapse, which are traceable to sepsis, are observed more frequently and sooner in occlusion due to strangulation than in obturation.

At the beginning of the peritonitis the temperature quickly rises to 102° to 104° F. or more, having usually been subnormal previously. Severe general peritonitis, and even the suppurating (ichorous) form, may run its course from beginning to end at the collapse temperature. As the frequency of the pulse increases, the tension decreases still more. The dyspnea reaches a very advanced degree, especially in very diffuse meteorism. If the diaphragm is forced up to a considerable height, and considerable pressure is thus exerted upon the lungs and the heart, death by suffocation may take place unexpectedly. General peritonitis also causes persistent vomiting, and often a torturing singultus, which may continue until death. The patients complain of very severe pains over the entire abdomen, which are considerably increased by the slightest pressure. In cases where active peristaltic undulations of the intestine were previously visible through the abdominal walls, or if the intestinal contortions and individual loops were distinctly marked in rigid plastic relief through the abdominal wall, this is no longer recognizable after the beginning of the general peritonitis. A partial or local meteorism soon changes into the diffuse universal form, and the abdomen is bulged out like a globe. In the lower parts of the abdomen in some cases a peritonitic exudation, which is usually of a serosanguinolent composition, may be detected. The severe collapse which sometimes precedes the general peritonitis caused the same symptoms as the initial strangulation's shock.

Perforation.

If a perforation of the intestinal wall should take place during the existence of a general peritonitis, this is often introduced by the symptoms of severe collapse or unconsciousness, that may continue until the fatal termination, which usually occurs very soon in this state of shock. I have observed instances where patients that were comatose regained consciousness from the effect of the pains, which are especially violent if the peritoneum was previously inflamed. Paroxysms of pain which are caused by the increased movements of the inflated intestines often cease entirely because the intestines, which have been partially relieved by the escape of the gases into the peritoneal cavity, come to rest. The escape of gases into the peritoneal cavity after perforation causes a degree of meteoristic inflation of the abdomen rarely observed under any other conditions; the liver-dullness, if it indeed was still present, disappears. Whilst any possible peritonitic exudates forming dur-

ing peritonitis without perforation may escape detection, for reasons
already mentioned, in perforation peritonitis the discovery of a
freely moving, usually quickly suppurating exudation is not difficult.

Among the rarer consequences and complications of occlusion
which may hasten or cause death the following may be mentioned :
traumatic (aspiration) pneumonia,—which is usually caused by the
aspiration of the contents of the stomach into the lungs during
the stercoraceous vomiting,—septicemia together with embolic
processes in the lungs, and metastatic abscesses in the liver and in
other organs.   This process is a result usually of intestinal perforation and the emptying of the intestinal contents into a peritonitic
exudation or into the retroperitoneal connective tissue (fecal abscess formation).   After the agglutination of an intestinal loop lying
above an occlusion with the front abdominal wall, gangrenous
destruction of a part of the intestinal and abdominal wall may in
exceptional cases lead to the formation of a preternatural anus.   In
rare cases a fistula is formed between intestinal loops above and
below the occlusion.   Even though, in the latter case, the channel
has again become free, healing does not set in, because the gangrenous destruction of the intestinal wall continues.   In some cases
fistulas are formed between the intestine, the bladder, the uterus,
and the vagina.

Diagnosis.

The diagnosis of occlusion alone is generally made without
difficulty, but it does not represent the limit of the duty and object
of clinical examination ; we must seek to discover the seat of the
occlusion, and the nature of the disease which is the cause of it.
Although the recognition of the intestinal occlusion is usually safe
and rapid, especially when the most important and pregnant
symptoms of occlusion—the complete retention of the stools and
flatus, appearances of collapse, meteorism, pains, stercoraceous
vomiting—can be discovered, it is very much more difficult, and
in many cases of acute intestinal occlusion entirely impossible to
determine its location and causes in time.   Difficulties, as well
as failures and wrong diagnoses in previously treated cases of occlusion, should not deter the conscientious clinician ; he should

rather, in every new case, try to determine the seat and cause of the occlusion, by means of a thorough anamnesis and examination, in which, besides inspection, palpation, percussion, and auscultation of the abdomen, he should make a careful digital examination of the various hernial orifices, a combined exploration through the vagina and rectum (the latter also during chloroform narcosis), an examination of the urine (for indican), of the feces (for blood), and also of the vomit, since the success of an operation depends chiefly upon the timely discovery of the exact location and cause, and the chances of operation are the more favorable, the sooner it is performed and the more rapidly it is completed.

Differentiation of Occlusion from Other Diseases.

The symptoms of occlusion are very characteristic, yet they may be confused with other disease symptoms, especially with general peritonitis, acute typhlitis, perityphlitis, and appendicitis, less easily with Asiatic cholera, bilious colic, nephrolithic colic, lead colic, incarceration of a floating kidney, of the uterus, of the testes in the inguinal canal. It is not very likely that intestinal occlusion could be confused with twisting of the pedicle of ovarian tumors, or with acute arsenical poisoning. There are cases on record, however, where a primary peritonitis was discovered during laparotomies which were made for occlusion. On the other hand, the opposite case, where an experienced diagnostician made a diagnosis of primary peritonitis, and afterward an undoubted primary intestinal occlusion was found, has probably never occurred. If it has, the clinician in control did not have the courage to report it.

Differential Diagnosis between General Peritonitis and Occlusion.—*Distinguishing Marks: (a) Behavior of the Body Temperature.*—General peritonitis, as a rule, causes high fever, rising rapidly from the onset, whereas in occlusion or ileus the body temperature usually is subnormal. The absence or presence of fever does not furnish any reliable data for a differential diagnosis, because severe general peritonitis, even of the suppurative type, may be accompanied by the low temperature, as is usual in collapses, and also because occlusion occasionally causes fever (up to 102° F.) at the beginning (Naunyn).

(*b*) *Pain.*—In general peritonitis the patients complain of violent pains in the entire abdomen, which are greatly increased even by slight pressure upon the abdominal walls.   In occlusion the pain is at first circumscribed, in some cases at least, and is located, in these cases, either at the seat of occlusion or in the umbilical region. At the onset it is not increased by pressure, but on the contrary is sometimes alleviated by it.   In the further course of occlusion, the pains, which at first were circumscribed, spread out over the entire abdomen, and then they are increased by external pressure, as soon as the local meteorism has passed into the diffuse form.   Pains which occur in paroxysms, and which are the result of an increase in the movements of the intestines, peristalsis visible through the abdominal walls, and also recognition of intestinal contortions which appear in plastic relief, or of intestinal loops contracted in tenesmus, all these signs speak for occlusion and against general peritonitis, because in this disease the intestinal peristalsis is soon paralyzed. Abdominal pains felt during micturition speak for general peritonitis.

(*c*) *Meteorism.*—In general peritonitis the meteorism is diffuse from the very start, the abdomen is inflated symmetrically, and the abdominal walls are under great tension.   In occlusion the meteorism in most cases is at first slight and circumscribed.   According to the seat of the occlusion, in one case the lower parts of the abdomen are curved out, in another the upper, or the upper and the middle together, as the walls of the abdomen have only a moderate tension.   In the further development of the occlusion the meteorism likewise passes from the local into the diffuse form.

(*d*) *Vomiting.*—This symptom is common to both general peritonitis and occlusion.   In the former, however, it often continues for some time without any interruption, but in occlusions it often ceases after a while, only to recommence later on.   Stercoraceous vomiting, which is a characteristic of occlusion, does not occur in general peritonitis ; if it occurs, a secondary or paralytic occlusion has developed.

(*e*) *State of the Urine.*—A great increase in the amount of indican contained in the urine occurs both in general peritonitis and in occlusion of the small intestine.   If this increase is lacking, it argues for an occlusion of the large intestine.   Albuminuria occurs as well in peritonitis as in occlusion.

. The discovery of an exudation of liquid into the lower parts of the abdomen can not be utilized with any degree of certainty for the diagnosis of a general peritonitis, because large amounts of a serous, bloody liquid are also secreted into the peritoneal cavity in axial twists, intussusceptions, and volvulus, when the mesenteric vessels are strongly compressed.

The diagnosis of general peritonitis is rendered considerably easier if one can succeed in demonstrating that those diseases which can eventuate in peritonitis—for instance, diseases of the stomach (gastric ulcer), of the intestines (appendicitis, perityphlitis, typhoid, tuberculous and other kinds of intestinal ulcers), of the liver and gall-bladder, and of the female sexual organs—have preceded or still exist. We must finally consider, in the differential diagnosis of the two diseases, that general peritonitis may cause occlusion and occlusion may cause general peritonitis.

Appendicitis and Perityphlitis.—Since perityphlitis and appendicitis may cause vomiting, the symptoms of collapse, meteorism, pain, and stool retention, a confusion of the same with occlusion is possible at the very onset, but only then. Fortunately these symptoms are extremely rare in appendicitis. After a longer thorough examination the diagnosis of perityphlitis may be made with certainty, especially if, besides the previously described characteristic symptoms of the disease, an edema of the abdominal walls, disturbances in the sensibility of the right leg, and pain during urination can be observed. · The diagnosis is facilitated by the fact that perityphlitis and appendicitis often cause fever, and that in spite of complete stool retention the passage of flatus rarely ceases. It has already been emphasized that perityphlitis may sometimes cause an occlusion.

Discovery of the Location of the Intestinal Occlusion.— *Where is the site of the occluded loop?* This is the burning question that will be asked of the diagnostician. In the small or in the large intestine? If in the former, is it located in the duodenum, jejunum, or ileum? If in the latter, is it located in the cecum, ascending, transverse, descending, or sigmoid colon?

The discovery of the location of the occlusion is of the greatest importance, in view of the operation which may have to be undertaken; the surgeon must know at what portion of the abdomen he must make an incision (it will not be the same incision for occlusion of the cecum as it would be for occlusion of the sigmoid, etc.). If the patient can state exactly where the initial pain was felt in his abdomen, or is still felt, and also if this pain does not increase under pressure, but rather decreases, the discovery of the seat of the occlusion has been furthered by one essential factor. Circumscribed pains which are felt later on can not be utilized at all, or but little, in the determination of the occlusion. Unfortunately, in only a portion of the cases—namely, in the strangulations—is the pain felt at the seat of the occlusion. In the cases due to chronic intestinal stenosis this is hardly ever the case, and in the others the pain is either transferred to the umbilical region or is diffuse from the very start.

Another important guide to the location of the intestinal occlusion is the inflated intestinal loop, which extends to the place of occlusion, and by which the abdominal wall is moderately bulged out asymmetrically. This is von Wahl's symptom. And I must not omit to emphasize again that this loop is motionless; there is no peristaltic contraction in it (*the so-called fixed, motionless, inflated loop of von Wahl*). The percussion sound over this loop is not the ordinary intestinal tympanitic resonance, but a deep, non-tympanitic sound. According to Schlange, a suppressed slight peristalsis can be observed in the suprastenotic loop before it comes to complete rest (*the so-called distended fixed loop with peristalsis of Schlange*). This clinician, and also Naunyn, regards this sign as valuable for the diagnosis of acute occlusion and the locality of it. The slight peristalsis referred to must not be confounded with the stormy contractions that always run in a direction toward the occlusion, and which are found only after chronic stenosis when hypertrophy of the muscular walls has developed. In the acute occlusions that have come under my observation, I was unable to detect Schlange's peristalsis; and I am disposed to believe that even if it occurs, it must be of such short duration that it has ceased before the physician sees the case. By the time cases of acute occlusion are seen by the physician, the pre- or suprastenotic loop, if distinguishable, is in a state of quiescence.

If the peristaltic movements, which are usually combined with more or less severe pains, also proceed in a definite direction, one may assume with certainty that the occlusion is in the neighborhood of that place in the abdomen whither they go (Naunyn). In acute intestinal occlusion, energetic (tetanic) contractions of the intestinal muscles (above the point of occlusion) are not observed, in my experience. These contractions are perceived most frequently and distinctly in chronic intestinal stenosis, and are often felt by the patient himself a considerable time before the complete occlusion of the intestine. There are also peristaltic contractions observable in the suprastenotic loop of acute obstruction, but they never reach such a degree of intensity as to deserve the name *tetanic*, nor do they ever effect a plastic erection of the loop in question. During the palpation of the abdomen one must also be on the lookout for a tumor or a deep-seated resistance. These, however, are frequently lacking in acute intestinal occlusion, and in only a portion of the cases of intussusception can a cylindrical tumor be felt. In carcinomatous stenosis of the intestines an irregular knotty tumor, which is sensitive to pressure, may sometimes be felt. The accumulation of thickened, hardened feces above the stenosis may, however, often simulate the appearance of a malignant tumor.

If the examination of the abdomen has given no definite result, a careful digital examination of the various hernial orifices must be made. Besides the more common forms, all the rarer hernias——lumbar, umbilical, ischiorectal (rupture through the perineum), ischiadic, obturator hernias, etc.—must also be considered. The omission of the examination of the hernial orifices is a great neglect, which may bitterly avenge itself upon the physician. If the orifices of the hernial sacs have been found to be open, a thorough simple and combined exploration by vagina and rectum is imperatively necessary. In the former, one must search for those changes in the position of the uterus which may exert a pressure upon the lower parts of the intestine. One must also look for tumors of the ovaries and of the other pelvic organs which may also act in this manner. Prostatic hypertrophy must be looked for by rectal palpation. Fecal accumulations, strictures, and tumors of the lower section of the rectum may be discovered by such digital examination. If the suspicion is present that the obstruction to the course of the feces is situated in the lower section of the intestines, and if the digital investigation has given normal results, palpation through the rectum with the entire hand during chloroform narcosis may be executed in such cases where the rectum is found sufficiently large to permit of this way of palpating.   If during this examination the lower part of an intussusception is felt in the upper section of the rectum, both the location and the kind of the occlusion are made apparent.   The advance of the intussusception into the sigmoid flexure and the rectum is often manifested by a relaxation or gaping of the anus (paralysis of the sphincter) and by the involuntary rectal discharges of an ichorous bloody fluid.

The first step to be undertaken is to determine whether the occlusion is in the large or in the small intestine.

Occlusion of the Small Intestine.—It has been repeatedly emphasized that in occlusion of the small intestine, especially if it is caused by internal strangulation, incarcerations and flexures, the symptoms of intestinal occlusion, such as vomiting, pains, and the symptoms of collapse, are more intense, and the course more rapid than in occlusion of the large intestine.   A violent and very copious vomiting spell sets in immediately after the occlusion, and stercoraceous vomiting occurs very soon afterward.   The meteorism is at first confined to the epigastric, hypogastric, and mesogastric regions, while the lateral and lower portions of the abdomen are flattened or even retracted.   It is only in the further course of the disease that the lateral portions of the abdomen, which correspond to the situation of the ascending and descending colon, and also the lower parts of the abdomen, are bulged out.   Rapid peristaltic movements and contractions of the loops of the smaller intestine, which can be distinctly seen and felt through the abdominal walls, also indicate an occlusion of the small intestine.   The higher up the occlusion is situated in the small intestine, the earlier and more frequently does the anuria set in.   The shock of strangulation is very severe, and likewise the septic collapse, which occurs later.   The latter is observed so regularly that its absence argues against the location of the occlusion in the small intestine. The amount of indican contained in the scanty urine is soon considerably increased.   As early as the second day one often finds a bluish-black color of the urine, or of the chloroform in the Jaffé test, and indigo blue is precipitated in heavy flakes.   After the use of enemata, feces which have already been formed may pass off abundantly, and then large quantities of air and water may be introduced into the unobstructed colon by the rectum.

Occlusion of the Large Intestine.—In this case the symptoms of intestinal occlusion are less pronounced than in occlusion of the small intestine, and usually also occur later. Stercoraceous vomiting especially may not set in till some time after the beginning of the occlusion. It may even fail entirely to put in its appearance in an occlusion of the descending colon or the sigmoid flexure—for instance, in volvulus of the latter—and of the rectum. The septic collapse is also much less severe in incarcerated occlusion of the large intestine. This is probably due to the fact that the walls of the large intestine are much thicker than those of the small, and that consequently the blood-vessels of the former are much less severely compressed by a strangulation than the vessels of the jejunum and ileum. So long as the ileocecal valve can be closed, the meteorism in most cases, but not in all, is confined to the lower portions of the abdomen. In occlusion of the colon one sometimes notices in the lowest portion (of the abdomen) that the left iliac region is first distended meteorically, and then only the transverse colon, and finally the ascending colon. The diagnosis of an occlusion is made still easier if one can perceive peristaltic motions of single sections of the colon, if these motions are always in the same direction. It is also aided if the contours of these intestinal sections are plainly visible in relief through the abdominal walls as plastic rigid cylinders. The amount of indican in the urine is not at first increased. According to the observations of Naunyn, however, the urine, in occlusion of the large intestine, may show a deep blue color under the Jaffé test, as early as the fourth day.

A more exact localization of the intestinal obstruction usually succeeds in those cases in which it is situated in the duodenum, or the upper part of the jejunum, in the lower part of the large intestine (descending colon and sigmoid flexure), or in the rectum. Thus the beginning and end sections offer more ready signs for this recognition than the middle ileum.

Occlusion of the Duodenum.—In this case pure bile (undecomposed bile pigment) is vomited in very great amounts (Cahn). The substance vomited often has an acid reaction, and is never feculent. The amount of indican in the urine is not increased. Usually the region of the stomach is very much inflated; after severe vomiting it sinks in for a while. See clinical history of supra- and infra-papillary duodenal stenosis for full account of symptoms.

Occlusion of the Jejunum.—In this case the vomiting, which at first is green, is followed by yellow decomposed bile pigment. This in turn, if the occlusion is situated but a few inches below the pylorus, may occasionally become fecal (Naunyn). At intervals the substances vomited or brought forth by means of a stomach-tube may again become purely bilious. Indicanuria is usually absent.

Occlusion of the Descending Colon and the Sigmoid Flexure.—Diagnosis by Distention.—It has been mentioned that only in the first days an increase in the amount of indican is regularly absent (Naunyn). Determining the capacity of the colon by pouring water into this section gives variable data for the more exact localization of the intestinal occlusion. If the occlusion is situated far down, the patient can retain but little water, seldom more than ⅓ to ¾ liter, even when the intestines have become accustomed to its irritation. If more than 1 to 1 ½ liters are retained, it is very probable that the occlusion is not located in the rectum nor in the sigmoid flexure nor descending colon (Naunyn, Schraum). It is very essential that this water distention should not be undertaken until the patient has become quiet. If there is much suffering and consequent nervous tension, the results are unreliable for judging the capacity of the sigmoid, as it is impossible for the patient to retain any water under those conditions.

According to the investigations of Brinton, which were made almost fifty years ago, if only ½ liter can be poured in, the occlusion is located no further down than the upper part of the rectum. If 1 to 2 liters pass in, the sigmoid flexure is free, without a doubt, and the occlusion is situated no further down than the descending colon, and usually higher. If the ascending colon is occluded, large amounts (4 ½ liters) may be retained. In those rare cases in which several liters of water may be poured in, although the occlusion is situated far down in the rectum, we probably have to do with abnormal dilations of the rectum.

Can the colon be sounded or intubated? For the exclusion of stenoses of the rectum, sigmoid, and colon, no method has proved itself more useful in my experience than direct exploration of the rectum and sigmoid flexure, as described by Dr. Thomas Charles Martin, in the scholarly article he has contributed on "Diseases of the Rectum," and sounding the colon by means of the Langdon or Kuhn tube. As I have stated in my work on "Diseases of the Stomach" (second edition, p. 105), I have been able to illuminate the entire human colon by the method of Heryng and Reichmann ("Therap. Monatshefte," 1892). Rosenheim ("Darmkrankheiten," Leipzig, 1893, S. 26) states that it is impossible to pass a tube beyond the sigmoid flexure. E. Graser (in Penzoldt and Stintzing's "Handbuch d. spec. Therapie innere Krankheiten," Bd. IV, S. 560) expresses himself similarly. His words are: "*Some have dreamt that they had advanced as far as the cecal region with their tube; this is doubtless a deception; the tube or sound never passes beyond the sigmoid flexure. Frequently it is bent around backward in the ampulla, or it pushes the distended flexure upward to a certain degree,*" etc.

By means of the electrodiaphane and also by a Kuhn spiral sound—a Langdon tube containing a steel spiral—it is possible to demonstrate conclusively that a tube can be passed into the cecum from the rectum; namely, the metallic spiral sound can be recognized by the fluoroscope and the Röntgen rays. By alternately insufflating air and irrigating with water one may auscultate the gurgling noises over the cecum produced by these procedures. In patients with very thin and relaxed abdominal walls I have been able to palpate the Langdon tube within the cecum. If there is any doubt about the location of an occlusion, whether in the large or small intestine, direct inspection, distention of the colon with air or warm water, and sounding of the colon with the Langdon tube, are methods available for excluding stenoses of the colon. The technics of these procedures have been described elsewhere. With the permeability of the colon clearly made out in this manner, the clinician has advanced an important step. By no means is it necessary in all cases to execute these mechanical methods of colon exploration. In many cases the diagnosis becomes evident by other physical methods already described.

Determination of the Character of the Intestinal Occlusion and its Cause.—The determination of the character of the intestinal occlusion and of its cause, which are so exceedingly important for the correct judgment and treatment of occlusions in individual cases, often offers greater difficulties than the determination of its location.

Causes of Acute Intestinal Occlusion.—This may be caused, as is well known, by internal incarcerations of the intestine in holes and slits of the omentum and mesentery, by abnormal ligaments, compressions, constrictions, sudden bendings, axial twistings, intussusceptions, and also by intestinal obturations (gall-stones, foreign bodies, enteroliths, and fecal tumors).

Internal incarcerations, which are observed most frequently in persons under forty years of age, concern the small intestine in the great majority of cases. The more the peritoneal covering is distorted or irritated by this incarceration or strangulation, the more severe and sudden are the symptoms of the initial collapse, as well as of other consequences of acute occlusion of the small intestine (meteorism, vomiting, etc.). This is of great importance for the differentiation of obstruction due to incarceration and that due to obturation, because in the latter the initial collapse is wanting. Since the symptoms are about the same, one can not decide with certainty whether the occlusion of the small intestine is due to an internal incarceration in a break in the omentum or mesentery, whether it is caused by pseudo-ligaments or diverticula, or due to sudden bendings caused by adhesions, or to a compression, or to an axial twist. We may, however, suspect an intestinal bending or kinking, caused by peritonitic bands and adhesions, if a general peritonitis has preceded. We may also suspect it in ruptured patients in whom a hernia was reposited by a hernial operation or by taxis, or in whom a hernia still exists, because, if an intestinal occlusion sets in, adhesions and bands are often found in the neighborhood of the orifice of the hernial sac when an operation is performed. These adhesions and ligaments frequently pull upon or compress the intestines. Torsions occur more rarely. In internal incarceration we find neither tenesmus nor tumor; at the start the circumscribed sensibility to pressure is also absent. After the excrement which may have been in the intestine previously is excreted, the stool retention is complete. Large quantities of air and water may be introduced into the colon.

Axial Twistings (Volvulus).—Although we can not prove with certainty the existence of axial twists of the small intestine, the determination of the fairly frequent volvulus of the sigmoid flexure is usually easy and certain.   Volvulus of the sigmoid, which often recurs, is especially frequent in persons over fifty years of age. The axial twist of the intestine makes either an entire revolution (about 360°), or a partial one (about 180°).   Only in the first case is the occlusion complete.   In the latter the intestinal lumen is considerably contracted, but it still remains permeable.   In this manner Naunyn explains the great variations observed in the course of volvulus of the sigmoid.   If the axial twist made only a half revolution, intestinal occlusion will set in only when the stenosed intestinal lumen is occluded by feces.   The symptoms of occlusion caused by this partial twist, just as the symptoms of an intestinal occlusion caused by coprostasis in cicatricial enterostenosis, are not pronounced, and the development is comparatively benign.   The collapse and the meteorism are slight, and flatus passes off from time to time.   If the obstructing fecal mass is forced out, the intestinal occlusion ceases.   If the partially revolved intestine does not make a retrograde revolution to its former state, the symptoms of a chronic intestinal stenosis continue, and the intestinal occlusion may occur again after some time.   Stool retention and diarrhea alternate.   If the axial twist is an entire revolution (360°), the suddenly commencing symptoms are much more severe.   Constipation usually precedes them.   The sigmoid flexure generally remains permanently impermeable, because it very rarely returns to its normal situation spontaneously.   The patients feel a severe and very often intermittent pain, which is usually located in the umbilical region.   A sensibility to pressure can be detected quite early in the left inguinal region.   When the intestinal loops situated above the flexure are inflated very much, this sensibility to pressure may later on be felt over them also. The meteorism increases at a varying rate, sometimes rapid, sometimes slowly.   It may become so great that the entire front abdominal wall up to the epigastrium is bulged out and greatly distended.   If the inflation of the intestine is not yet excessive, the immovable distended intestinal loop in the immediate neighborhood of the sigmoid flexure (prestenotic, distended, immovable loop) may distinctly be recognized (von Wahl, von Zoege Mannteuffel).   The vomiting is moderate, and usually decreases after a time. It rarely becomes feculent, and sometimes is altogether wanting. After the resolution of the volvulus, blood is often found in the diarrheic evacuations. Whether it may be found in the stools before this is not evident from any clinical reports. Tenesmus frequently sets in quite early. The amount of indican in the urine does not increase for the first few days. It is impossible to pour more than one liter of water into the rectum, and also to inflate the descending colon with air. Loop knot formations between the sigmoid flexure and the ileum cause the same symptoms as the axial twists. It is said, however, that in this case bloody diarrheas are much more frequent than in axial twists.

Intussusception.—The diagnosis of acute and chronic intussusception has been thoroughly discussed in a separate chapter.

Acute Intestinal Obturations.—(*a*) *Obturation Caused by Gall-stones.*—Obturation due to gall-stones is not at all rare. It usually occurs in elderly persons, principally women. It is sometimes observed as a direct consequence of biliary colic; at other times this colic has preceded it a long time. Occasionally a gall-stone, or a fragment of one, is found in the last stool previous to the obturation. An obturation by means of gall-stones may occur, however, without being preceded by the symptoms of cholelithiasis. The only way in which large stones can get into the colon or the small intestine is by the formation of a fistula between the gall-bladder and the intestine, or the gall-duct and the intestine. The formation of gall-bladder fistulas causes either the symptoms of a violent cholelithiasis or cholecystitis, but it also may remain completely latent. If, however, a stone is present in the common gall-duct, and a fistula of the latter is formed, the symptoms of cholelithiasis are hardly ever absent. If the gall-stone ulcerates directly through into the large intestine, it usually passes off without causing any disease symptoms, even if it is of considerable size. It may even remain for a considerable length of time in the large intestine without causing any complaints. But if, in its downward passage, it sticks fast in the rectum, it may become an obstruction to defecation, and then must be removed artificially. If stones of any considerable size get into the small intestine, they stick fast in it; the most frequent location of blocking being immediately in front of the ileocecal valve.   Then the symptoms of an acute occlusion of the small intestine set in (gall-stone occlusion)—abundant bilious vomiting, which may later become feculent when the ileum is occluded, and a quick stormy peristalsis associated with pains.   Usually the stone can be felt distinctly.   Even if stercoraceous vomiting has set in, the meteorism as a rule is slight, and the passage of flatus does not cease entirely.   This is probably due to the fact that the stone does not obstruct the intestine entirely, and that its complete closure is brought about only by the accumulation of condensed feces before and around the stone.   In many cases the symptoms of a slight occlusion alternate for a long time with diarrhea.   Since larger gall-stones may cause the formation of ulcerations at various places in the intestinal wall, the diarrheic dejections often contain blood (sometimes in considerable quantities).   If the gall-stone gradually passes downward, the previously mentioned disease symptoms change their location, but usually remain for quite awhile in the ileocecal region.   After the stone has passed the ileocecal valve, the intestinal occlusion usually ceases.   If ulcers of the mucous membrane have been formed in the intestine, the pains, increased peristalsis, and diarrhea continue for some time, until the ulcers have healed.   Indeed, if a perforation of the ulcer and an agglutinative peritonitis had developed, the symptoms of intestinal occlusion may even continue, due largely to the secondary peritonitis.

(b) *Obturation by Means of Foreign Bodies and Enteroliths.—* Bodies of considerable size can not pass the pylorus; still the largest ones that are capable of being passed may cause the symptoms of a severe intestinal stenosis, if they get into the normal intestine, but not the symptoms of a complete occlusion. The latter can only occur when the feces or chyme are accumulated between the foreign body and the intestinal wall, or in front of it.   If, however, the intestinal lumen is considerably stenosed at any place, foreign bodies of a very small size may cause complete occlusion of the intestine.   It has repeatedly been observed that plum- or cherry-stones, which had been wedged in at a stenosed part of the intestinal wall, and which had obturated it, caused intestinal occlusion.   The symptoms of an obturation caused by foreign bodies are identical with those of an obturation caused by gall-stones.   The foreign bodies, especially if they are angular or sharp, may also cause ulcers of the mucous membrane. The danger of intestinal perforation, however, is much greater in ulcers caused by gall-stones. The diagnosis, then, of an obturation due to foreign bodies is naturally only possible when it is known that such an object has been swallowed.

Enteroliths.—Enteroliths occur very rarely. They also usually stenose the intestinal lumen, but only exceptionally do they occlude it entirely. The enteroliths usually are lodged in the cecum or rectum.

Coprostasis.—The symptoms and detection of coprostasis have been fully discussed in the chapter on Obstipation. In coprostasis the amount of indican in the urine is rarely increased. It seldom causes intestinal occlusion. Even if the coprostasis lasts a long while, the meteorism may be but slight, if there is no great circulatory disturbance; the passage of the flatus never ceases entirely. Coprostasis itself causes intestinal occlusion only in weakened persons, or those suffering from some disease of the spinal cord. In such cases the colon and the rectum up to the anus are stuffed with balls of excrement, which occasionally are as hard as stone. Illoway describes a number of such cases in his interesting book on "Constipation."

Finally, we must note that a diseased condition greatly resembling intestinal occlusion is occasionally observed in hysterical patients. It is caused by paresis or paralysis of the intestinal muscularis. It is accompanied by great meteorism and complete stool retention, rarely by violent vomiting, and only in isolated cases by stercoraceous vomiting (Briquet, Jaccoutt). The abdomen is very much distended, and the abdominal walls are under great tension, and sometimes sensitive to pressure. The passage of flatus ceases. If the diaphragm is forced up very much by the great meteorism, severe apnea sets in and collapse may occur. Besides these symptoms other nervous appearances can be detected. The general health is but little disturbed. The meteorism usually ceases quite soon, and the collapse likewise is of short duration.

Diagnosis of Chronic Intestinal Stenosis.

It has been repeatedly emphasized that stenoses of the large and small intestines, if they are not very severe, may escape detection for a considerable time. Indeed, the classic description of Cruveilhier proves that it may continue for years undetected. If, therefore, in such cases, the symptoms of intestinal occlusion appear very suddenly, we are justified in assuming that a previously normal intestine has suddenly become occluded as a result of internal incarcerations, sharp bendings, volvulus, axial twists, etc. Since the contents of the small intestine have a pulpy consistency, we can easily understand that even severe stenoses may remain latent for a considerable time. This is more rarely the case in stenoses of the colon and of the rectum, the contents of which have a firmer consistency. The symptoms of a stenosis of the large intestine have been discussed in a special section devoted to this subject, and also in the chapter on Carcinoma of the Intestines. Besides disturbances in the evacuations and changes in the form of the feces, quick peristaltic movements of one fixed loop or of several intestinal loops form an important symptom of intestinal stenosis. If it can be demonstrated that the portions which are in motion belong to the colon, it is a sign of a stenosis of the large intestine. The peristaltic movements are very active; they can be plainly seen and felt through the abdominal walls, and always proceed in the same direction. I have stated previously that if an intestinal occlusion appears suddenly without having been preceded by the symptoms of a stenosis, we may assume in the first place that it is the result of an internal incarceration, axial twist, etc. We can not, however, exclude the possibility that the occlusion was due to a chronic enterostenosis which has acutely become occluded (see definitions). If the intestinal occlusion recurs at long intervals, there is no proof of the existence of an enterostenosis, since this is also observed in the case of incarcerations, volvulus, intussusceptions, etc. If, however, the recurrences quickly succeed each other, and the attacks grow more severe, and if the circumstances are favorable for cancer (advanced age, cachexia, a deep location of the impermeability), the existence of enterostenosis is probable (Naunyn). The location of the stenosis may usually be determined with some degree of certainty by means of the results obtained by inflation with air and distention with water, and sounding of the colon as previously described.

Stenosis of the Small Intestine.—The diagnosis of a stenosis of the small intestine is made much easier if we can determine by means of the anamnesis that peritonitis, tuberculous affections, peptic ulcers, perityphlitis, lesions, trauma, or hernial strangulations have preceded or still exist, or that operations for hernia have been performed. If the lumen of the small intestine is considerably stenosed at any place, pains, meteorism, and also violent vomiting set in. · The pains occur in paroxysms, at first at long intervals, later on more frequently. So long as the small intestine is still permeable, the vomiting does not become feculent. Tenesmus and indicanuria are absent. The condition of the evacuations varies. Often constipation exists, or it alternates with diarrhea. If we have to deal with elderly persons who were formerly healthy but have suddenly become cachectic, and in whom a tumor can be discovered, we are dealing in all probability with a carcinomatous stenosis, especially if the stool occasionally contains blood. It must not be overlooked, however, that even benign stenoses of the small intestine may very early cause great disturbances in the general nutrition.

Prognosis.

According to recent statistics (collected by Curschmann, Für-bringer, Senator, and others), out of 100 patients suffering from obstruction, only 30, or at the most 35, recovered. Since relapses often occur even in those cases which turn out favorably, and the formation or increase of an enterostenosis is to be feared, therefore the prognosis is always bad. In those cases in which the intestine again becomes permeable without any operation having been performed, we have usually to do with coprostasis, either alone or combined with enterostenosis. Other favorable cases are obturations caused by gall-stones or foreign bodies, with intussusception or with *partial* axial twists. On the other hand, a spontaneous healing is extremely rare in cases of internal incarcerations, sudden kinkings, and *complete* axial twists. The prognosis in the former class of cases is therefore relatively more favorable. If in enterostenosis the recurrences of occlusion rapidly succeed each other, each new attack growing severer, the prognosis is also bad, unless an operation is performed. If, in addition, a cancer is present, the prognosis is absolutely fatal. If singultus, pneumonia, pyemia, general peritonitis, and even perforation peritonitis set in during the intestinal occlusion, there is no hope of saving the patient. The same is generally true also if fistulas are formed between the intestine, the bladder, the vagina, and the uterus; because the fistulas are usually formed only by severe (usually cancerous) intestinal stenosis, and because soon after a rupture of the intestine takes place. The prognosis is often considerably improved by an operation, and more especially in those cases in which the seat and the kind of the intestinal occlusion can be determined. If this is not the case, the chances of an operation are not much better than those of internal treatment in this class of cases.

Therapeutics.

The Use and Abuse of Opium and Morphin.—The main reliance of internal treatment is based on avoidance of purges, quieting the intestine by means of small doses of opium or morphin, not taking food or drink by the mouth. Just as in perityphlitis the administration of purges is absolutely forbidden, so at the present day there can be no reasonable doubt that the purgation is not only useless, but positively harmful. The only exceptions are those cases of intestinal occlusion which are caused by coprostasis. It has been repeatedly shown that soon after the beginning of an acute intestinal occlusion there is an abundant accumulation of gases, with considerable distention in the section of the intestines lying above the occlusion. This condition causes abnormally severe muscular contractions, quickly following one upon the other, in the distended loop, and to these contractions the quick peristaltic movements are due. The latter are the chief cause of the paroxysmal pains and of the stercoraceous vomiting. The more energetic the contractions of the muscles are, the greater is the exhaustion of the muscularis and the sooner muscular paresis may be expected. If the distention of the intestinal walls on account of the gases is long continued, temporary paresis often goes over into complete paresis, which is one of the worst results of intestinal occlusion, since it favors the appearance of a severe general collapse, as well as of peritonitis.

The increase in the movements of the intestines aggravates an already existing intussusception, at the same time rendering its resolution more difficult. In a similar manner axial twists are aggravated and their return to normal position rendered more difficult. It may even happen that by these movements new intestinal loops are telescoped into the already formed intussusception or incarceration. Therefore it is wrong to increase the peristalsis artificially in the first stage of acute intestinal occlusion, by giving purges, because it is already abnormally increased. On the contrary, it is the duty of the physician to reduce the peristalsis or to bring it back to a normal condition. For this purpose opium and morphin are best suited. They exert a quieting influence on the peristalsis, which is probably due to the fact that they act upon the inhibitory fibers in the splanchnic nerves of the intestine (Nothnagel). Opium may be administered internally by the mouth, or in in the form of strong suppositories. Morphin gives its best and safest results when injected subcutaneously. This method, which in recent times has been advocated by Bāumler in intestinal occlusions, has the disadvantage that the effect is more transient than that of opium. On the other hand, hypodermic injections have this advantage, that the effect sets in more promptly, and is often at first attained by means of slight amounts. Thus an exact calculation of the doses is possible. If the opium introduced by the mouth is vomited, or if a distinct result is absent because of the general depression of the intestinal absorption, opium suppositories must be used, or morphin injections. The opium suppositories might also have been used in the beginning. I must warn against a frequent introduction of opium by the mouth, because if the absorption is decreased in the stomach, a great amount of it may stay there. Later on, when the normal absorption is resumed by an improved circulation in the mucosa, great amounts of opium will enter the blood at one time (Frerichs, Curschmann). Even if the patients suffering from intestinal occlusion seem to have a certain indifference or tolerance toward opium or morphin, nevertheless large doses must not be given, on account of their doubtful effect on the heart. Since in some cases even very moderate amounts of opium and morphin suffice to decrease the peristalsis, to alleviate the pain, and to stop the stercoraceous vomiting, whereas in others the same result is attained only by the use of much larger doses (as much as 7 to 15 grains of pure opium in twenty-four hours have been given), the proper amount must be ascertained in each individual case. It is advisable for the physician himself to

administer the opium and carefully watch for its results.   How long
the narcotics are to be given depends upon the further development
of the disease in each individual case.   This may vary within a
wide range, according to the seat of the occlusion, its causes, and
also according to the presence or absence of certain complications
due to intestinal occlusion.   If paralysis is imminent or has already
set in, the drug must either be decreased or omitted altogether.

The use of opiates in intestinal occlusions (as well as in suppurative appendicitis) has been criticized by several American surgeons,
who say that by it the appearance of the disease is obscured, that the
patient does not decide to allow an operation because of the apparent
improvement, and that consequently the physician is deceived in his
prognosis, and loses the most favorable opportunity for an operation.   This claim, however, is not sufficiently logical to justify the
physician in omitting the administration of opiates, for, as Naunyn
says ("Ueber Ileus, Mittheilungen a. d. Grenzgebirt der Med. u.
Chir.," Bd. x, No. 1, 1896), "*it is not the privilege of the physician
to withhold the benefits of his science from his patient in order to
coerce him to a more correct view.*"   On the contrary, it is his duty
to ameliorate as far as possible all of his sufferings.   If the means
in question at the same time conduce to his cure, even if only in
individual cases, this duty is made more attractive.   Besides this,
the possibility is by no means excluded that the normal intestinal
movements which set in after the quieting of the intestines by means
of opiates may cause a removal of the obstruction to the fecal passage in intussusception, axial twists, and intestinal incarceration.
For it is conceivable that intestinal loops that are caught in bands,
slits, or ligaments are still further distended by the previous violent
peristaltic movements ; such pulling and tugging as must occur in
the stormy peristalsis must inevitably place the inclosing bands,
etc., as well as the caught loops in the greatest possible tension.
This occurs in abrupt kinking of the bowel, internal incarcerations,
invaginations, axial twists, and volvulus.   There is no doubt that
an abnormal peristalsis is pre-eminently active in the production of
these conditions.

Opium should not be withheld during the first symptoms of
reaction ; then there can be no better treatment for the intensified
peristalsis and the excruciating pains.   If the symptoms of primary

irritation cease after 20 drops of the tincture of opium have been given every three hours (or 0.03 gram denarcotized extract of opium) for a day, the remedy should be discontinued. Should the peristaltic storm and pains continue after the first day, the dose must be reduced to 10 drops of the tincture of opium. Wherever the first stage has already passed by unutilized, and there are indications of frequent and very compressible pulse,—the precursor of collapse,—especially if the sufferer presents a dejected, exhausted expression, opium must not be administered. There are rare cases in which opium has no effect when given internally; here a subcutaneous injection of ¼ grain sulphate of morphin should be given under the conditions stated above. Desperate indeed are those cases of occlusion to which even this form of administration brings no relief. If the symptoms of primary reaction are over, or if they have existed for three days, I advise to keep away from opium or morphin.

The objection of certain authors, particularly surgical authors, that opium and even gastric lavage should not be employed in the treatment of occlusion because they effect a condition of pseudo-euphoria, under the disguise of which the pathological alterations may clandestinely become aggravated and the most favorable period for operation may be lost, has no doubt some logical foundation. For such danger as they describe does to a degree exist, but it can be avoided by the observance of rules laid down above, and by the most strenuous attention to the action of the heart.

In many of my cases the effect of opium was very favorable, sometimes even magical, and although I have transferred numerous cases to the surgeon, I have not yet had occasion to regret the legitimate use of opium. The general health is improved, the pulse grows stronger, the appearances of collapse disappear, the terrible strangling and stercoraceous vomiting and also the pains cease or are greatly diminished. The sleep is quiet and refreshing. This improvement, however, will not deceive the experienced physician, or indeed the beginner, except possibly in his first case of intestinal occlusion. The mortal peril in which the patient is continues to exist so long as the intestine remains impermeable; indeed, it becomes greater the longer the occlusion lasts. The physician will therefore use this period of betterment in deciding whether an operation is to be performed or not, before the severe resultant effects of intestinal occlusion set in and thus make the prognosis worse.

Murphy has made the demand upon physicians that they should give no opiates until the diagnosis is certain, as the sedatives suppress the peristalsis, which is of great importance for the diagnosis. This statement goes beyond the mark, however. To be sure, moderate doses of opium quiet the irritated peristalsis, but do not suppress it entirely (Naunyn). It is only by means of excessive doses of opium and morphin that a complete arrest of the peristalsis can be effected. If the violent pains, the stercoraceous vomiting, and sensibility of the entire abdomen toward pressure, which is partially due to the increased peristalsis, have ceased after the administration of opium or morphin, a thorough examination of the abdomen can be made much more readily than before. If the use of narcotics is then stopped, the peristaltic movements of the fixed intestinal loop or of several loops (above the occlusion) usually occur again after a while. These are of great importance for the detection of the location and kind of the intestinal occlusion, and their localization and direction can be discovered all the more easily if the other sections of the intestines are quiet (under the influence of the narcotics, if need be) or not in evidence.

Purgatives.—These are to be avoided in intestinal occlusion combined with stercoraceous vomiting. They are to be allowed only in those rare cases in which intestinal occlusion is manifestly caused by coprostasis. They may also be used for a time in chronic enterostenosis which has led to persistent constipation as a result of the fatigue of the muscularis adjoining the stenosis, and also of the fecal accumulation. In the latter case the use of strong purges is at first to be avoided, since a paralysis of the muscularis may thus be hastened (Nothnagel). Milder remedies are to be prescribed (castor oil, magnesia, rhubarb, etc.), and their action is to be assisted by water or oil enemata. If these have no result, it is advisable to prescribe opium at first, rather than a strong purge, because it is often observed in such cases that evacuations occur a short time after the administration of the sedative, the opium acting both as a tonic and purge. This is due to the fact that the muscularis of that section of the intestines lying above the stenosis, which previously exhausted itself in vain attempts to force the feces through the stenosed place is made to rest a while, and as a consequence is once more able to conquer the hindrance by means of powerful contractions. If we can demonstrate the existence of a slowly increasing enterostenosis, we may often delay the appearance of an intestinal occlusion by means of a rational diet—the avoidance of such foods as leave a great amount of residue, or tend to cause an abundant formation of gas in the intestines, by a regulation of the evacuations by dietetic (somatose) and medicinal purges, by enemata and electricity. If the attacks of intestinal occlusion recur in rapid succession and with increasing severity, an operation should be performed if possible. This is best done when the intestine is empty ; therefore if possible after an attack of occlusion has passed over.

Enemata and Colon Irrigations.—An abundant introduction of water into the rectum and colon is frequently of great service in fecal accumulations of the large intestine. It is useless in an occlusion of the small intestine, because in this case the water gets into the small intestine only when the ileocecal valve is insufficient—a very rare occurrence. The mechanical irritation which the water exercises on the mucous membrane causes contractions in the muscularis ; and what is still more important, the condensed, hard, stagnating feces are also softened and to a certain extent dissolved in the water. If, in a stenosis of the large intestine, one succeeds in forcing the water introduced per anum through the stenosed place, and if this softens the feces accumulated above the stenosis, it materially assists the muscularis in its function of forcing the feces downward. For the purpose of pouring the water into the rectum, a fairly stiff, yet elastic, tube of considerable caliber is used, or a thick-walled rubber tube (Langdon or Kuhn tube). This is introduced about 15 cm. into the rectum. The irrigator must be connected with the intestinal tube by a long rubber hose. Since the water has to overcome great obstacles in the fecal accumulations and stenoses of the larger intestine, it has to be under considerable pressure. Thus it can also get into the higher portions of the large intestine. To get this pressure I generally place the irrigator several meters above the body of the patient. Sometimes the patients at first (even if the occlusion is situated high up in the intestine) can retain the water but a short time ; it must therefore be poured in repeatedly, three or four times a day. Cold enemata (ice-water) cause greater contractions of the muscularis than warm ones. The effect of the enemata may be increased by the addition of spirits of turpentine (1 tablespoonful), soap (6 to 10 grains), and table salt (1 to 1½ teaspoonfuls) to the quart.

In an interesting series of experiments Grützner demonstrated that under certain conditions particles of charcoal, finely cut horse-hair, or sawdust, when injected into the rectum of rabbits, guinea-pigs, and rats, were found six hours later all along the small intes-tine, even in the stomach, while the rectum was empty. This anti-peristaltic progress of fine particles only occurs, however, if they are impregnated with normal salt (0.6%) solution. When the sus-pensions of these particles were made in distilled water, HCl or KCl solution, instead of physiological NaCl solution, the particles did not ascend in the digestive tract (Grützner, "Deutsche med. Wochenschr.," 1894, No. 48). He also injected starch suspen-sions in normal NaCl solution into the rectum of human beings, and after a number of hours demonstrated starch grains in the gastric contents microscopically.

Nothnagel first showed that NaCl placed on the serous surface of the intestine is capable of starting antiperistaltic movements ("Beitr. z. Phys. u. Path. d. Darms, 1884), and Grützner interprets this observation as explaining the antiperistaltic progress of minute particles saturated with normal NaCl solution. He also cites Nothnagel's studies as explaining the digestion of egg enemata con-taining salt by assuming that the food mass, after being injected into the rectum, is moved upward through the entire small intestine and there becomes digested and absorbed. Even Riegel ("Krankh. d. Magens," S. 245) seems satisfied with this interpretation, and adds that it explains the negative results of Voit and Bauer without salt being added, and the positive results of Huber's experiments, in which salt was added.

In a large number of carefully conducted experiments on men and animals I was able to confirm the main conclusions of Grütz-ner, viz., that under normal conditions minute particles do move antiperistaltically from the rectum to the stomach when injected in normal NaCl solution, and this antiperistaltic progress does not take place when the particles are injected in HCl or KCl (Hemmeter, "*Études expérimentales sur l'Action motrice et digestive des Intes-*

tins," "Trans. XIII International Congress of Medicine," Paris, August, 1900). But I do not consider that the antiperistalsis as described by Grützner is capable of moving ingesta in bulk. The name antiperistalsis is not correctly applied in this case, as the movement is invisible, and can only be judged by the progress of minute particles; the intestine itself appears at rest whilst this antiperistaltic movement of particles goes on. Nothnagel's antiperistalsis is quite a different phenomenon; it is a strong, visible antiperistaltic wave, but occurs only under abnormal conditions, whilst the antiperistalsis of Grützner is only a marginal movement, probably physiological, and present at all times (Hemmeter, "Diseases of the Stomach," second edition, p. 212).

In four cases of complete intestinal occlusion I made tests with subnitrate of bismuth and lycopodium, to see whether these substances would find their way from the rectum to the stomach. The results of repeated lavage of the stomach were negative; not even in the stercoraceous vomit which set in could any trace of the bismuth or lycopodium be discovered microscopically. My experiments with normal human subjects show that ordinarily the particles injected into the rectum should be found in traces in the stomach in from eight to ten hours. It occurred to me, therefore, that this antiperistaltic progress of minute particles might be used as a test of the permeability of the intestines. As the procedure is a painless and harmless one, I hope it may be taken up by clinicians, particularly in suspected cases of developing enterostenosis, where purgatives have already been resorted to for the relief of the coprostasis.

A teaspoonful of lycopodium, starch, or bismuth subnitrate is mixed with half a pint of warm normal salt solution, and slowly injected into the rectum. After twelve hours of fasting (overnight) the stomach is washed out and the wash-water examined under the microscope after centrifugalizing. Normally these substances should be found in traces in the stomach. Personally I have not had opportunity to test this phenomenon in more than four cases of obstruction, in all of which no evidence of the particles was found in the stomach. The utility of the method would be greatest in those cases of gradually developing enterostenosis due to strictures or neoplasms. Such cases may run their course, extending through

months or even years, without giving any evidence of absolute occlusion, but only at intervals the signs of more or less complete
enterostenosis.

Fleischer recommends large enemata of normal salt solution for the
resolution of recent intussusceptions, upon the ground that the solution is worked upward through the telescoped loops of bowel according to Grützner's explanation; large normal salt enemata undoubtedly
favor the resolution of such a condition at times, but the explanation of this action by Fleischer in attributing the ascent to antiperistalsis of Grützner is not well founded.   Enemata can find their
way up to the stenosed area, and in rare and favorable cases gradually penetrate through it, but this occurs under the antiperistalsis
as described by Nothnagel.   This author specifies as one of the
causes of this reverse movement, "Entrance of food by an unphys-
iological entry, the rectum"; accordingly, enemata may be gradually moved up into the transverse and descending colon.*

While the water is being introduced in large quantities, the pulse
and the respiration of the patient are to be watched.   If the symptoms of collapse appear, as sometimes occurs in extremely weakened
persons, this introduction must be stopped at once.   A very
unpleasant complication results in rare cases, when the water is
completely retained during an already developed extensive meteorism, and this may cause great complaints and increase in the tension already existing.   This accident is a rare one in my experience,
and occurs when the intestinal wall is already paralytic.   In such
case I use a double or recurrent colon tube with a wide lumen for
the outflow, and first proceed to wash out the rectum and those
portions of the sigmoid that are accessible, assuring myself by
inspection that these parts are really clean.   Retention of an enema
has never occurred in my experience if a recurrent colon tube was

---

* Whilst I am at the consideration of this subject, I might add my own views regarding the cause of the digestion of nutritive enemata.   It is by no means necessary to
assume an antiperistaltic movement of food injected into the rectum in order to account
for its digestion, for an abundance of proteolytic and amylolytic ferment occurs in the
contents of the human colon to effect proteolysis and amylolysis of any food injected into
the lower bowel.   It is probable that these ferments are trypsin and amylopsin which
have survived the passage through the intestinal canal.   (See Hemmeter, "Das Vor-
kómmen proteolyt. u. Amylolyt. Fermente," etc.   "Pflüger's Archiv f. d. gesammte
Physiologie," Juli, 1900.)

used.   Unfortunately it can not always be used if we wish to bring water beyond a stenosis, for the simple reason that it is impossible to pass a tube of so large a caliber through the obstructed area. If peritonitis or intestinal ulcers exist, or if the suspicion of a rupture in the intestinal wall or of gangrene is present, no water at all should be introduced.

Enemata of olive oil, linseed oil, cotton-seed oil, or poppy oil of the first pressing, one-half to one pint (200 to 500 cubic centimeters or more), which were first recommended by Kussmaul and Fleainer, have rendered valuable service, in my experience.   Since the oil does not irritate the mucous membrane, even the first oil enemata are retained quite well.   The oil easily ascends in the large intestine, softens the hardened feces, and makes the intestinal mucous membrane slippery, so that the balls of excrement may glide downward more easily.

Air inflation of the rectum has been recommended by von Ziemssen, Runeberg, and others, and in favorable cases it actually renders good service in stenoses of the large intestine, especially if the intestine has kinked, and also in recent intussusceptions.

Air is introduced into the rectum by the following simple means : A thick-walled rubber tube (stomach-tube) is deeply inserted into the rectum.   The nates are pressed together and air is slowly forced in by means of a double bulb attachment.   Between the blower and the intestinal tube there should be a forked glass tube. One branch of this tube should be connected with the blower, and the other one with a rubber tube supplied with a pinch-cock.   If severe complaints or discomforts are caused by the introduction of the air, they may easily be relieved by opening the pinch-cock. Instead of the double bulbs one may also use a large syringe of a known capacity, and having a double valve.   If neither of these is at hand, Fürbringer suggests that the physician, may use his own lungs as blowing power.   As soon as he ceases blowing into the intestinal tube, however, he must firmly compress the rubber hose, since the air may easily come out from the intestinal tube and into his mouth—a danger which should suffice to prevent cautious men from using this method.   Air inflation is of no use whatever in occlusion of the small intestine so long as the ileocecal valve is in working order, except indeed under great pressure, which in time may have a bad effect on the occlusion. Air inflation, just as introduction of water, is also contraindicated if there is a suspicion of the possible existence of peritonitis, intestinal ulcers, perforation, or gangrene. Jürgensen reported a case of intestinal rupture during inflation with air, no doubt due to one of these complications.

Air inflation and the copious introduction of water are to be recommended in quite recent intussusceptions, since they may cause a resolution of this condition, or at least impede the progress of the intussusception. They are not advisable in volvulus, however. Of course, a resolution of the intussusception is only possible when no adhesions have occurred. Before the air inflation, the feces which have accumulated below the intussusception should be removed by an enema. When water is introduced, the patients should try to retain it as long as possible (at least one-quarter of an hour). If this is impossible the lower part of the rectum is to be closed with a tampon (Rosenheim).

If the lower part of the intussusception can be felt in the rectum, it should be reposited to its normal situation by means of the finger, if possible, or by a long forceps guarded by as large a bunch of sterile cotton as can be introduced. After reposition, the sigmoid should be held in place by a tampon such as is described by Dr. T. C. Martin in the chapter on Rectal Diseases. If relapses occur, the tampon must be left there for a longer period of time. If, in spite of all this, relapses do occur, or if the reposition is not successful, an operation becomes necessary.

Intestinal Puncture.—In a previous paragraph I have described the danger of great accumulation of gases in intestinal occlusion. Curschmann has in more recent times recommended a direct puncture of the intestine for this condition. This method was formerly practised, but later on it was neglected again. Curschmann, however, emphasizes especially that it is to be used only with great caution and discrimination. If intestinal paralysis is present, or if we suspect a peritonitic irritation, or changes in the intestinal walls which may lead to gangrene, it must not be used. Not only Curschmann, but also many other experienced clinicians,—von Ziemssen, Jürgensen, Fräntzel, Fürbringer, Rosenbach, and others,—have achieved admirable results by the direct puncture of the intestine at various places. This is easily understood, since the partial removal of the gases relieves the intestinal wall above the occlusion and decreases its tension very much. Considerable improvement and amelioration in the condition of the patient and sometimes even an indisputable direct cure are claimed for this procedure. Under the aforesaid conditions Curschmann has not observed any evil results at all due to puncture, and more especially peritonitis and perforation were absent.

According to Curschmann, the puncture should be made in the following way : A long, very thin and carefully disinfected hollow needle belonging to a Pravaz syringe is used. It must have a stop-cock, which is to be closed before the puncture. This needle is thrust through the carefully cleaned and disinfected abdominal walls into one of the most distended intestinal loops. This loop must be carefully chosen in each individual case. After the needle is thrust in, it must be connected with a rubber tube, which is led into a bottle filled with a weak solution of salicylic acid, the bottle inverted in a basin containing the same fluid. When the cock of the needle is opened, the intestinal gases enter the flask, first in a continuous stream, then in great globules, and finally in intermittent bubbles. In this way the amount of the escaping gases can easily be deter-mined. If a mercury manometer is connected with the hose, the tension of the gases may also be ascertained. Curschmann's method has this advantage, that the rubber hose (if long enough) permits the needle to move freely in obedience to an active peristalsis. If the needle is firmly held in any one place, it may easily cause a tear in the intestinal wall (Fürbringer). If the meteorism is very great, the puncture may have to be repeated at various regions of the abdomen. In some cases, where the gas pressure in the punc-tured intestine is slight, and the muscularis is paretic, the intestine gives off its gas only after a time, even under massage of the ab-domen, and then only in small quantities (Rosenbach). In other cases liters of the gas may come forth from the intestinal loop, im-mediately after the first puncture. If the liquid contents of the intestine get into the needle, it must be drawn out and inserted at another place (von Ziemssen). In this case, however, it is advis-able to force a little air or salicylic acid solution into the intestine, in order to avoid a contamination of the peritoneum by the intes-tinal contents.

Although Curschmann and other clinicians have never observed any bad results following an intestinal puncture, reports by T. A. Hoffman, of Leipzig, on the contrary, indicate that under certain conditions the procedure may result in dangerous complications. He relates a case in which, in spite of the greatest care, fecal masses exuded from the intestine after it was punctured with a very thin Pravaz needle. Frāntzel described one in which a large amount of gas passed from the intestine into the abdominal cavity. The autopsy also showed that the intestine had been torn at the point of puncture. Fürbringer and also Naunyn, in more recent times, stated that in some cases they could demonstate at autopsy the evidence of peritonitis located at the point of puncture. A very striking case indicating the possible danger of intestinal puncture is reported by Körte ("Berlin. Klinik," No. 36). In these cases the harmful results of the intestinal puncture were possibly caused by the fact that the muscularis of the loop in question was already paralyzed, and that the channels caused by the puncture consequently remained open for a longer period of time. So long as the muscular coat of the intestinal walls has not lost its contractility, these channels probably close immediately after the puncture. This is proved by two facts : (1) If the intestine of a person suffering from ascites is punctured, no pathological changes in the intestinal wall can later on be discovered at the autopsy (Naunyn); (2) by the fact that no evil results were observed in the numerous intestinal punctures performed by Curschmann and other clinicians.

My first experience with intestinal puncture occurred in connection with severe volvulus of the sigmoid flexure in a negro, aged forty-two, and living in the mountains of western Maryland. The usual nonsurgical means of replacing failed. I had used ¼ grain of morphin subcutaneously with but transient relief; the meteorism was enormous. The only instrument I had with me was a hypodermic syringe, with the needle of which I punctured the most distended loop, after washing the patient's skin with soap and hot water. Gases escaped in large quantities ; at the end of five minutes the intestine had not yet completely emptied itself. On the following day, when I arrived to give a large enema of warm salt water, every symptom of obstruction had disappeared, and the negro asserted himself to be well. Since then I have been compelled to

employ the method on four other cases, partly because other therapeutic measures had been exhausted, operation refused, or because
no other instrument but a hypodermic needle was at hand.   Three
of these four cases were types of sigmoid volvulus, the fourth an
ileocecal intussusception.   I had every reason to believe that the
puncture aided in restoring the bowel to its normal state.   Whilst
I am fully aware of the dangers of the procedure, and far from
advising its application to every case, I can see no reasonable
objection to it when performed by experienced hands in the first
stage of intestinal occlusion, before intestinal paralysis has set in,
and when peristaltic movements of the intestine may be plainly
seen and felt through the abdominal walls, after the use of opium
has been stopped for some time.   The nonsurgical methods of replacement should be tried first and the prospects of the puncture
as well as of the operation made plain to the relatives of the patient.
It should require no emphasis to impress that where the surgeon is
at hand, the operation should be given the preference.

Gastric Lavage.—The washing out of the stomach, which was
introduced in the treatment of occlusion by Kussmaul and Cahn,
has given good results in many cases.   Its beneficial effect is due to
the fact that the intestine above the occlusion is relieved, the tension
is diminished, and the terrible choking and stercoraceous vomiting
are prevented.   That the artificial emptying of the stomach may
cause the intestinal loop above the occlusion to be relieved of its
load is proved by the following observations.   Frequently a large
quantity of fecal matter is found in the stomach a few hours after
washing out.   This can be removed by means of lavage.   In
the suprastenotic intestinal loop there is considerable pressure,
forcing the feculent contents in the direction of least resistance
—that is, toward the empty stomach and through the insufficient
pylorus.   It is intelligible that many patients are greatly relieved by
these washings, that the violent peristaltic intestinal movements and
the accompanying paroxysmal pains decrease.   Many times I have
observed that the disagreeable singultus and the repulsive stercoraceous vomiting ceased altogether, the meteorism decreased, the
previously tense abdomen became soft, and the feeling of oppression disappeared.   Although stomach washing usually has only a
palliative effect, yet the possibility is not excluded that gastric

lavage may occasionally cause a cure or a removal of the obstruction.

After the burden of the suprastenotic intestinal loops and the tension of their walls and of the abdominal integument have decreased as a result of the outflowing of the contents of the loops above the occlusion, it is conceivable that the normal intestinal movements incited reflexly from the stomach may cause the liberation of an incarcerated section of the intestine, the resolution of a fresh intussusception, or the return of an intestinal loop twisted around its axis. So long as they are weighed down by fermenting excrement and overdistended, the restitution of the occlusion to normal permeability is not only impossible, but the conditions causing the occlusion are even further aggravated. Experiments carried out for the study of the mechanism of hernial incarceration argue for the correctness of this assumption. Schede's experiment illustrating this mechanism was conducted as follows: An intestinal loop with its mesentery still attached is drawn through a moderately large ring so as to cause the two halves or pendants (limbs) of the loop to hang down from the ring suspending them. If now a syringe is fastened into one of the two limbs and water injected into it, it will project further and further into and through the ring as it becomes filled until so much mesentery has been drawn along that a wedge-like occlusion is formed. Both pendants, afferent and efferent, will now be firmly compressed and reposition is impossible. If the afferent pendant is relieved of its burden, however, by letting out the water, reposition follows without difficulty, especially if slight lateral pressure or traction is exerted upon it.

Necessity of Gastric Lavage Prior to Operations for Occlution.—It is highly advisable to thoroughly rinse out the stomach before every operation. If this is not done, stercoraceous vomiting may set in during the narcosis. In a case reported by von Ziemssen, the vomited stomach contents entered the lungs by aspiration, causing sudden death.

When gastric lavage is undertaken immediately after the beginning of the occlusion, one often finds that the stomach is already at this time filled with fecal matter. The rinsing out is especially desirable because the esophageal foramen may be closed by a slight displacement of the stomach, according to Aufrecht, and thus prevent stercoraceous vomiting. For the same reason the washing out ought also to be repeated, even if the stercoraceous vomiting has ceased for a long while. In the lavage, I advise using the largest sized stomach-tube obtainable. It is a false impression that practitioners have when they assume that a small tube will irritate the patient less than a large one. The small tube is just as annoying in the beginning, and will have to be tolerated with the same initiating discomfort as a large one. But on account of its small caliber it can not discharge the thick gastric contents, and will frequently become clogged. First the stomach's contents must be removed by means of the tube; to start with, a small quantity of water, not more than a pint, may be poured in. Secondly, the stomach is to be thoroughly washed with large quantities of lukewarm water. If the contents are feculent, disinfectants may be put into the water, such as salicylic acid, boric acid, thymol, etc.

Duodenal Intubation for Determining the Permeability.—By a method originally devised and published by myself ("Versuche über Intubation des Duodenum," "Arch. f. Verdauungs-Krankheiten," Bd. II, S. 85) it is possible to pass a hollow rubber tube into the small intestine. In eight cases of intestinal obstruction I have assured myself of the permeability of the duodenum and ileum in this manner. F. Kuhn has suggested another method directed to the same purpose ("Sondirumgen am Magen, Pylorus, und Dünndarm des Menschen," "Arch. f. Verdauungs-Krankheiten," Bd. III, S. 19). Neither of these procedures can be unreservedly advised in all cases. In suspected neoplasms, for instance, with their well-known tendency to ulcerate in the intestine, I would be loath to make use of them. In the cases in which I did make use of them, however, it was a great comfort to find out and rest assured that there was no stenosis and only a severe coprostasis in six out of the eight cases. The greater the extent of the large and small intestine which we can exclude from the condition of stenosis by colon and duodenal intubation, the more favorable the prognosis. Above all things, the limit of doubtful regions in the intestine which might be occluded is narrowed. If, for instance, the physician is able to pass a flexible tube through the entire colon to the ileocecal valve, and thus convince himself that the large intestine is open throughout, and at another occasion pass a tube of 2 meters' length through the duodenum and jejunum into the ileum, any possible stenosis must be in the lower ileum. In the presence of a number of physicians I have repeatedly passed tubes of 3 to 4 meters' length through the coils of the small intestine, so that the metal spiral (which is so constructed in the Kuhn tube as to be as flexible as rubber) could be felt in the inguinal region. The ileum is too long to intubate it entirely with a tube only 3 meters long, but I find that it is possible to get past even the ileocecal valve and enter the ileum from below. For this work thick-walled Langdon tubes are to be preferred to the tubes of Kuhn, which contain a metallic spiral, because the Langdon tubes are more elastic and yielding, and not so heavy. In my work on "Diseases of the Stomach" I have given evidence that it is quite practicable to wash out the duodenum by this method. Professor Fleischer (*l. c.*, "Krankheiten des Darms") expressed the hope that a method of intubation might be invented and utilized for relieving the suprastenotic loops of fermenting semifluid fecal masses, and for removing the gases and disinfecting these intestinal loops by harmless antiseptic solutions—weak solutions of boric acid or thymol, for example. In three cases of obstruction I attempted to carry out this suggestion. Whilst it is trying on the patient, it is not nearly so exhausting as the terrible vomiting and singultus that call peremptorily for gastric lavage. The internal lavage is justifiable only when the heart action is normal and the blood count shows a normal number of leukocytes. It is executed by steps; first, gastric lavage, then ten minutes' rest, then duodenal lavage, thereupon jejunal lavage; when the tube is in the intestine only one pint of water can be allowed to flow in at a time, and must be immediately siphoned back. This is repeated several times until the water comes back quite clear. Then the tube is pushed in 10 inches further, and the same procedure gone through. By careful studies on cadavers I have learned that it is rarely possible to wash out more than 10 inches of the bowel at one time. The effects on the vomiting and symptoms of autointoxication have been very gratifying in the three cases in which I executed this method. Still, it must not be understood that I recommend it in all cases of occlusion as a method that can be relied upon as safely as gastric lavage. In the original article ("Arch. f. Verdaunngs-

Krankheiten," Bd. ii, *l. c.*) I have given the criticism of my own method, for like all new means of treatment, it must not be recommended for general practice until thoroughly tried in the hospital by other clinicians.

Massage and electricity have a very limited application in the treatment of occlusion even when used in paralytic intestinal occlusion due to coprostasis; and in obturations of the small intestine caused by gall-stones and foreign bodies, these means have proved of little utility in my experience. If the obturating body should be pointed, angular, or sharp edged, and there is no means of telling whether it is or not, great harm may be done in massage. Electricity and massage are also excluded if it can be proved that lesions, ulcers, malignant neoplasm, intestinal hernia, hemorrhages, peritonitic irritation, and peritonitis itself exist. Martin, it is true, has reported a case in which an obturating gall-stone was carried from the small intestine into the large one by means of massage, thus removing the occlusion. But that was a rare bit of good fortune, and it may become dangerous unless very delicately carried out.

The electrical treatment, which requires fairly strong faradic or galvanic currents, is best carried on if one electrode is inserted in the rectum. The faradic current is given as strong as can be comfortably tolerated, the galvanic current in the strength of 25 to 35 milliamperes. If it is to be of any use in paralytic intestinal occlusion, it must be repeated several times daily, and must continue for fifteen to twenty minutes.

Abstinence from Food and Drink.—If an intestinal occlusion really exists, the introduction of food and drink must be absolutely prohibited, especially at the onset of the case (Curschmann, Ewald, Gottdammer, Nothnagel). At most, only small amounts (teaspoonfuls) of iced milk and cold tea may be given in order to alleviate the annoying dryness of the mouth and throat. If the patient is weak, small amounts of champagne and a mixture of crushed ice and brandy may be allowed.

Personally I favor total abstinence from food in occlusion of the small intestine only, because any ingestion of food in these cases means a new burdening of the muscularis. But in occlusions of the large intestine vomiting occurs more rarely, and when it does occur it is not as severe as in occlusions higher up. Boas does not consider it proved that the motor paralysis and loss of resorptive power above the occlusion occur in the colon, but only in the small intestine. He calls this assumption "a hypothesis proved by no sure experiment" (*l. c.*, p. 453). Whilst I agree with him in the "rationale" of allowing amounts of food to sufferers afflicted with stenoses of the colon, such as milk, beef jellies, somatose, and nutrose,—as every calorie absorbed must be considered a valuable gain,—I do not consider the loss of motor and absorptive power in the suprastenotic loops of the colon a hypothesis, for I have become convinced of the existence of muscular paralysis of the suprastenotic portion in occlusions of the colon, and with the development of intestinal paresis the resorptive power is lost also.

If food or drink be given in larger amounts during the first few days, it is either vomited or the intestine is further burdened with the (solid) food, which is usually not digested nor absorbed in the stomach, and which thus furnishes the material for generating more gas in the intestines. The thirst is best relieved by enemata of lukewarm normal salt solution (100 to 200 c.c.). These enemata are usually completely retained and quickly absorbed, especially if opium suppositories have been used. If the blood has suffered great water impoverishment (anuria, crural cramps), and if enemata are not retained, subcutaneous infusions of a physiological solution of salt (0.6 per cent.) are recommended. Since the general nutrition usually suffers very soon in high intestinal occlusion, nutritive enemata—milk and eggs (Ewald), meat extracts with bouillon, albumoses or peptones—are to be administered. In case of a weak heart or collapse, strong wine or cognac may be added.

The patients, naturally, must lie in bed on their backs during the entire course of the disease. Great bodily exertions are to be avoided, and fecal as well as urinary evacuations must also take place in this dorsal position. If pains occur during urination, the urine is to be removed by means of a catheter, if this is possible.

The Use of Metallic Mercury in Intestinal Occlusions.— The internal administration of metallic mercury was formerly the last resort of the older physicians, and was used when all other means had failed. If the observations of these clinicians are reliable, it sometimes seems to have had a good effect. The assumption in former times was that its effect was due to its weight, by which it might, for instance, liberate an incarcerated intestinal loop. At present we know that this idea is wrong, and that mercury may do more harm than good when it arrives at an occluded place in acute intestinal occlusion, such as acute incarcerations, kinkings, and intussusceptions. When it was given in cases where the occlusion was the result of a coprostasis combined with a paralysis of the muscularis, after all other means had been tried in vain, it was assumed that it thoroughly penetrated the accumulated feces, and thus loosened them sufficiently to permit of their onward progress. This is hypothetical, and there are no well-founded reasons to justify the therapic use of metallic mercury for obstruction.

After this more general consideration of the occlusions we will proceed to a special consideration of each individual type.

STRANGULATION AND INTERNAL HERNIAFORM INCARCERATION OF THE INTESTINE.

Not so very long ago, during the first half of the nineteenth century, all forms of impermeability of the intestine were classed under the collective name of "ileus." This designation comprised diseases of the most varied anatomical character. Even peritonitis, appendicitis, and perityphlitis were included under it. We owe our modern insight and more scientific knowledge of the various forms of intestinal occlusion to the development in two medical sciences. First the rise of pathological anatomy, and secondly, the perfection of abdominal surgery, particularly to the improvement of surgical technic, since and during the era of antisepsis and asepsis. The first step was the exclusion of diseases of an inflammatory nature, such as appendicitis, peritonitis, and perityphlitis ; then pathologists and clinicians began to make distinctions between coprostasis and impermeability. The latter was separated into a number of conditions based upon the anatomical changes found to be the underlying causes. Thus authors began to distinguish between a strangulation by peritoneal bands and an axial twist or volvulus, and between occlusions due to a neoplasm and those due to a cicatricial stricture. Even at the present day, I regret to say, Wahl's requirements that an anatomical diagnosis of the kind, nature, and seat of the occlusion should be made, above all things, before the knife is taken in hand, is not always fulfilled. Unfortunately, the surgeons must frequently operate with no other diagnosis than that of intestinal obstruction, with no intimation whatever of the anatomical foundation of this impermeability. The development of clinical diagnosis has not kept pace with the progress in pathological anatomy and surgical technic with regard to intestinal occlusions. In this connection I must confess, much to my regret, that it has been my experience that unsuccessful operations for occlusion are only exceptionally attributable to the surgeon (defective technic, infection, long duration of the operation, inexperienced assistants, etc.). In the greater majority of cases of fatal results which I have had opportunity to study they were due to error in diagnosis by the clinician who had charge of the case before the surgeon, or, what is more often the case, to unjustifiable delay before the patient was transferred to the surgeon for operation. I shall return to a consideration of this subject under the heading of treatment.

In this chapter I shall consider the pathology, clinical history, and diagnosis of

1. Strangulation and incarceration by peritonitic bands or adhesions.

2. Strangulation and incarceration by omphalomesenteric (vitelline) remains (Meckel's diverticula).

3. Strangulation and incarceration by mesenteric and omental slits.

4. Strangulation and incarceration by internal hernias into peritoneal pouches and openings.

There is no essential difference in the character of the symptoms which arise from these causes of obstruction. The mechanism which produces the intestinal occlusion in all of these cases corresponds exactly to that which produces the incarceration of so-called external hernia. These occlusions almost always involve the small intestine and only extremely rarely the colon. The pathogenesis, symptomatology, prognosis, and treatment are practically the same for all these anatomical types. The classification which I have given is original with Leichtenstern (von Ziemssen's "Handb. der spec. Pathol. u. Ther.," 1876, Bd. VII, 2, S. 528), and has been adopted by Treves ("Intestinal Obstruction, Pathology, Diagnosis, and Treatment"), Nothnagel (*l. c.*), and more especially in a very clear-cut monograph by R. H. Fitz ("Trans. Congress Amer. Physicians and Surgeons," vol. I, 1888). The statistics given in the paper by Professor Fitz merit especial appreciation because they have been submitted to the severest criticism, with the result of the exclusion of a large number of doubtful cases. They were collected from English, French, and German literature, between 1880 and 1888. The comparative frequency of strangulations in contrast to other forms of obstruction is given in his first table as follows; the entire number is 295 cases of acute intestinal obstruction :

	CASES.	PER CENT.
Strangulation,	101	34
Intussusception,	93	32
Abnormal contents,	41	15
Twists and knots,	42	14
Strictures and tumors,	15	5
	295	100

A comparison of these figures with a larger number in the collection of Duchaussoy, Brinton, and Leichtenstern follows :

PERCENTAGE OF RELATIVE FREQUENCY OF THE MORE PROMINENT CAUSES OF ACUTE INTESTINAL OBSTRUCTION.

	NUMBER OF CASES INCLUDED.	STRANGULATION.	INTUSSUSCEPTION.	TWISTS AND KNOTS.
Duchaussoy,	347	54	39	6
Brinton,	481	33	54	10
Leichtenstern,	1134	35	39	6

The immediate anatomical causes of the 101 cases of strangulation are as follows, the numbers being regarded as equivalent to percentages :

	CASES.
Adhesions,	63
Vitelline remains,	21
Adherent appendix,	6
Mesenteric and omental slits,	6
Peritoneal pouches and openings,	3
Adherent tube,	1
Pedunculate tumor,	1
	101

Thus 84 per cent. were due to bands and cords in the restricted sense.

Age.

Strangulation in early youth, according to the table of Fitz, was

comparatively rare.   At least 40 per cent. of his cases occurred
between the ages of fifteen and thirty; and adhesions were the
cause more than twice as frequently as vitelline remains.   After the
age of thirty, adhesive bands were found to be the usual cause.

Sex.

According to the figures of this clinician, 70 per cent. of the cases
of obstruction from strangulation occurred among males.   Further,
nearly all the cases of obstruction from vitelline remains, adherent
appendices, and mesenteric and omental slits were found among
men.   The percentage of bands of intestinal origin and those of
pelvic origin was about equal in both sexes.

I. Strangulation and Incarceration by Peritonitic Bands or Adhesions.

Bands and cords resulting from pre-existing peritonitis are first
in numerical importance as a cause of strangulation and incarceration.   These bands are chiefly of two varieties:

First, isolated peritonitic adhesions of a round or ribbon-like shape,
varying from the size of a string to that of the index-finger (I have
seen them 2 inches broad between the colon and stomach).   In length
they are also very variable.   They may be so short that they bring
two different parts of the intestine, or two different organs, in juxtaposition; then, again, I have observed them 18 inches (46 cm.)
long, extending from the pylorus to the left inguinal canal.   They
may occur singly or a number of them at the same time.   Treves
(*l. c.*) has stated that there is no conceivable combination of various
localities in the abdomen, but that the actual anatomical demonstration of such adhesions had really occurred.   In the accompanying
illustration (Plate 6, p. 213) I present a case which occurred at my
own clinic.   The small intestine is dissected away; only the mesentery remains.   It was impossible to demonstrate the adhesion
between the colon and the abdominal wall and between the colon
and the sigmoid flexure with the small intestine remaining *in situ*.
There were several adhesions between the individual loops of the
small intestine, and between the small intestine and omentum.   Those
plainly visible in the illustration are adhesions of the stomach to the
liver and gall-bladder (a^3), of the stomach to the transverse colon

(a^4), of the hepatic flexure to the abdominal wall (a^1), of the transverse colon to the descending colon (a^5), of the descending colon to the abdominal wall (a^6), and of the hepatic flexure to the liver (a^2). The other possible adhesions that have been observed are as follows : Adhesion of the cecum with a loop of the small intestine in the right hypochondriac region, of the cecum with the sigmoid flexure, of the cecum with the abdominal wall, adhesions between the intestine and mesentery, between mesentery and mesentery, between individual loops of the small intestine, between the intestine and the uterus, ovaries, bladder; adhesions between any of the female generative organs and the parietal peritoneum of the pelvis ; adhesions between the limbs or ring of an external hernia on the one hand, and the mesentery, intestine, and parietal peritoneum on the other hand.

Secondly, omental or mesenteric bands. These owe their origin to peritonitis, issuing either from the uterus and its adnexa, the appendix, or the biliary apparatus. They are most frequently the result of tuberculous peritonitis, however. The entire mesentery may retract, drawing some of the intestinal loops posteriorly as far as the vertebral column. Mesenteric bands are usually thicker and longer than the isolated peritonitic bands. They are more frequently of a round shape, and may occur singly or in multiples. The entire omentum may be adherent and form one solid conglomeration, attached to the abdominal wall, intestine, or a pelvic organ ; the base of this conglomerate spreads out toward the transverse colon. Mesenteric as well as isolated peritonitic adhesions may give rise to two different incarcerations or strangulations in different parts of the abdominal cavity.

There are in the peritoneal cavity a number of freely movable structures—for instance, the vermiform process, the Fallopian tubes, Meckles' diverticula or omphalomesenteric remains, and epiploic growths which are pouch-like fatty projections of the peritoneum of the large intestine, usually spoken of as *appendices epiploicæ*. Any of these structures may be so fixed that its free end becomes adherent to the mesentery, intestine, or abdominal wall. It has been observed that the vermiform appendix was attached to the mesentery of the ileum or cecum in such a way as to form a tight string with two firm points of insertion. The diverticula of Meckel are frequently found attached to the inner side of the navel by persistent

PLATE 6.

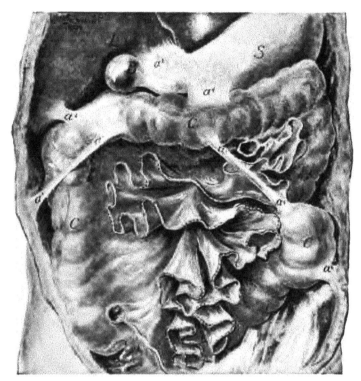

ADHESIONS OF ASCENDING, TRANSVERSE, AND DESCENDING COLON TO ABDOMINAL
WALL AND OTHER ORGANS.

S. Stomach. *L*. Liver. *B*. Gall-bladder. *C, C, C.* Colon. Adhesions of stomach to liver and
gall-bladder (a^3) and transverse colon (a^4). Adhesions of hepatic flexure of colon to abdominal wall (a^1, a^1). Adhesions of transverse colon to descending colon (a^5, a^5) and of descending colon to abdominal wall (a^6). Adhesion of hepatic flexure to liver (a^2). The small
intestine has been dissected away, only the mesentery remaining. The end of the ileum is
visible in the lower left-hand corner.—(*From Author's Clinic.*)

omphalomesenteric vessels, thus forming another arch under which the intestine may become incarcerated. Whenever a band or an arch of new-formed tissue is developed by the fixation of one of these free structures in the method described, it constitutes a ridge under or over which a strangulation or incarceration may occur.

There are four different ways in which incarcerations and strangulations may develop: (1) Under a band; (2) over a band; (3) by loop or knot development of the band or string itself, catching the intestine, as it were, in a noose or lasso; (4) kinking or sharp bend produced by traction.

1. *Incarceration under a band, bridge, or arch or a peritonitic adhesion.* This occurs usually when the band is short and very tight, and is capable of grasping the caught intestine in such a manner as to compress it against a relatively hard basis. The band in such cases rarely exceeds two inches in length, and the width of the arch incarcerating the intestine is rarely greater than to admit the passage of three fingers. The basis against which the strangulated bowel is pressed is formed by the wall of the pelvis, the right iliac fossa, hard masses of conglomerates and adhesions formed in the mesentery, enlarged tuberculous glands or other neoplasms, or the uterus.

2. *Incarceration over a band* is compared by Treves to the obturation produced in a thin rubber tube filled with water when it is laid over a tightly drawn string. Naturally, at the point where the rubber tube rests on the string, its lumen will be completely obliterated. It is conceivable that an analogous condition occurs when a long filled intestinal loop lies over a tightly drawn adhesion.

3. In contrast to the short and tough nature of the bands just described, those which strangulate the bowel by the *formation of loops or knots in the bands themselves* are very long, loose, and relaxed. Accordingly they are naturally found to be developed from the omentum, and known as omental pseudo-ligaments. Leichtenstern (*l. c.*) has pointed out that the intestinal loops which are caught in these nooses frequently present certain preformed peculiarities. The two basic or fulcrate points of the intestinal loop, corresponding to the free ends of a horseshoe, are very closely approximated, so that it separates and projects from adjacent loops like a pedunculated neoplasm. It is this projection beyond the other intestine that brings the eccentric loop into trouble. The noose in

the relaxed omental pseudo-ligament, when once accidentally pushed over it during the course of the manifold intestinal peristalsis, lassoes it and the strangulation becomes complete.   The strangulation may be a simple constriction, or a genuine knot may develop. Leichtenstern and Treves both describe the strangulation under a band as being much more frequent than the knot or loop formation in the band.   According to Treves, the proportion is 6 of the former to 1 of the latter.   According to Leichtenstern, who had a larger number of cases, there are 62 of the former to 27 of the latter.   This loop or knot formation in the constricting band itself must not be confounded with axial twists and knot formation occurring in the intestine.   Loops or knots in the bands themselves, inasmuch as they require a great length of the string, occur almost exclusively in the greater peritoneal cavity, and they may strangulate entire convolutions of the intestine ; whilst on the other hand incarceration under the arch of a short band, whilst it does occur in the greater peritoneal cavity, is much more frequent in the pelvis, and because of the shortness of the band it can only incarcerate short intestinal loops.

4. *Sharp bends or kinks produced by tractions upon adhesions.* Incarceration of the intestine of this type occurs when one end of the adhesion is attached to an organ which undergoes sudden change of position or form.   It is claimed to have been observed after evacuation of an ovarian cyst by puncture, and after evacuation of the uterus.

II. Strangulation and Incarceration by Omphalomesenteric (Vitelline) Remains (Meckel's Diverticula).

The diverticula of Meckel may occur in two forms : first, those with a freely floating end, only attached at the intestine ; secondly, those with a double insertion, one from the intestine, with which it communicates, and the other attached to the umbilicus, or to the abdominal wall above the umbilicus.   When it is attached to the umbilicus, incarcerations underneath it can not readily occur ; but there is another type of insertion of the free end,—that by peritonitic adhesions,—which may attach it at a variety of points, most frequently on the mesentery.   According to Fitz, the possibility of the presence of the vitelline duct at the upper part of the alimentary canal must be admitted as a cause of diverticula.   Meckel states that Lobstein and Wrisberg observed a connection of the vitelline duct with the duodenum ("Beitr. z. vergleich. Anat.," 1808, 1, S. 92). In his comprehensive paper on persistent omphalomesenteric remains, Fitz refers to other similar cases ("Amer. Jour. of the Med. Sci.," vol. LXXXVIII, p. 32), so that one may expect such abnormalities almost at any part of the intestine. These diverticular strings may lead to incarcerations similar to the peritoneal pseudo-ligaments, which have been described in the preceding. The strangulation may occur either under the arch of the tightened diverticulum, over the strings by traction or kinking, or by the formation of loops and knots in the diverticulum. The accompanying illustration represents a very long diverticulum which has at its

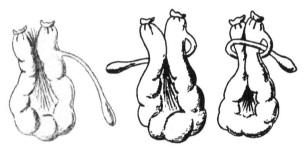

FIG. 4.—STRANGULATION OF INTESTINE BY MECKEL'S DIVERTICULUM.—(*Regnault*.)

free end a bulb-like swelling or ampulla. When this ampulla is filled, it may (by aid of gravity and the peristaltic movements of the intestine) form a ring into which an intestinal loop may happen to push itself. In its efforts to push further or to retract, the noose formed by the elongated diverticulum tightens. A very much elongated appendix has in very rare cases been known to act in the same way.

III. Strangulation and Incarceration by Mesenteric and Omental Slits.

This is a very rare cause of strangulation and incarceration. In Fitz's table of 101 cases, only 6 of this type are recorded. They are therefore more of a pathologic-anatomical than of a clinical interest. The slits may be congenital or acquired by trauma, and are usually found in the omentum of the lower portion of the ileum. Sometimes slits occur in broad peritonitic pseudo-ligaments, or crevices are formed between the pseudo-ligament and a normal fold of the peritoneum,—as, for instance, the broad ligament of the uterus, —and into these slits and crevices intestinal loops may be taken up and incarcerated.

Incarceration in Holes, Rings, or Crevices Caused by Adhesion of Abdominal or Pelvic Organs.—These are pathological curiosities; similarly the incarcerations which occur into tears or ruptures in the bladder or uterus, into a slit of the suspensory ligament of the liver, etc. To diagnose the nature of such strangulations and incarcerations as described in this paragraph is manifestly impossible, except perhaps that protruding through the uterus.

IV. Strangulation and Incarceration of Internal Hernias into Peritoneal Pouches and Openings.

Internal hernias are those which are entirely located in the peritoneal or thoracic cavity. They extend subperitoneally or retroperitoneally into the abdominal cavity, without even tending to protrude outwardly. These hernias extend into preformed folds and recesses of the peritoneum, into crevices of the omentum, and rarely through the diaphragm. It is a well-known fact that external hernias—for instance, an inguinal or a crural hernia—may become incarcerated without showing any swelling or tumor externally; that is, the condition runs its course like an incarceration of an internal hernia. This has occurred in my experience with a hernia of the linea alba. In special works on this subject cases of this kind have been described where obturator, ischiatic, vaginal, rectal, lumbar, perineal, abdominal, or intercostal hernias have become incarcerated, showing no external manifestation of tumor. Hernias have developed between the muscles and fascia of the abdominal wall, either independently or together with a manifest inguinal or femoral hernia, the one in the interstitial hernial sac remaining hidden. It has occurred that operations have been undertaken for evident symptoms of incarceration; an inguinal hernia, for instance, was operated and replaced; nevertheless the symptoms of incarceration continued, and later on an interstitial hernial pocket was found in the abdominal wall, either at the second operation or at the necropsy. The better known internal hernias are the following:

1. *Duodenojejunal or Treitz hernia.* About 70 of this type have been reported, several of which were incarcerated.   It is the most frequent type of internal hernia.   Treves found the duodenojejunal fossa 48 times in 100 cadavers.   If this fossa is deepened and the bowel enters, the upper jejunum is admitted first and may drag the entire ileum after it.   In extensive cases only the stomach and colon remained outside.   Strange to say, many cases presented no symptoms, and were only discovered accidentally at the autopsy. Where incarceration occurs a cyst-like tumor can be palpated to the left of the umbilicus, and the region of the ascending colon is sunken in.   In my opinion a Treitz hernia can not be diagnosed, as such, by clinical methods, not even if it is incarcerated.

2. *Omental hernia.*   Six incarcerations of the small intestine and two incarcerations of the large intestine have occurred through the foramen of Winslow.   When the hernia is not incarcerated it may run its course without symptoms.   In a case operated on by Treves, the cecum, ascending colon, and a part of the ileum were incarcerated in this form of hernial sac.   They could not be reduced at the laparotomy, and even at the necropsy the reduction was only possible after severing the hepatic artery, portal vein, and common gall-duct.

3. *Retrocecal hernia, or Rieux hernia.*   Under this type various forms have been described, the best known of which is the ileo-appendicular hernia.   About twelve cases are known, four of which ran a latent course.   The others, becoming incarcerated, proved fatal in a few days.   The sub- or retrocecal fossa is represented on Plate 4, opposite page 42, this volume.

4. *Intersigmoid hernia.*   Whilst the pericecal or retrocecal hernias are very small, the intersigmoid hernias, which occur in a recess of the mesocolon, may reach the size of a child's head. Usually, however, they are small.   The cases that have been reported all terminated fatally.

5. *Diaphragmatic hernia.* Whilst the diagnosis can not, in my opinion, be made in any of the preceding types of internal hernias, it is actually possible to make the diagnosis of diaphragmatic hernia in individual cases.   Though a very rare form, it occurs more frequently than the previous forms, with the exception perhaps of the Treitz hernia. Diaphragmatic hernias may be congenital or acquired.   The

latter are, as a rule, traumatic. Leichtenstern distinguishes true and false diaphragmatic hernias, and, curiously enough, the false are more frequent than the true. The true diaphragmatic hernias are characterized by a hernial sac consisting either of peritoneum or pleura, or both. The false hernias of this type are those in which an open communication exists between the abdominal and thoracic cavity; a hernial sac composed of serosa appears to be absent. The most frequent locality of the penetration of the diaphragm is the esophageal foramen; other localities are a place immediately behind the sternum, through which the colon and small intestine may enter the anterior mediastinum, or either of the two pleural cavities; then a space between the lumbar and costal part of the diaphragm, and finally the spot where the sympathetic nerve passes through the diaphragm. These hernias occur much more frequently on the left side, because the right side is protected by the liver. The organs that enter the thorax are the stomach, spleen, transverse colon, part of the duodenum, pancreas, and liver. When the stomach enters, it may be completely turned around, so that the greater curvature comes above, and the posterior surface toward the anterior thoracic wall (axial twist of the stomach). The symptoms of this condition strongly resemble pneumothorax,— that is, when it gives symptoms at all,—for it is possible that it may run its course in a latent manner. The corresponding half of the thorax is dilated; there is a full resonance with a tympanitic after-sound on percussion. On auscultating whilst pleximeter percussion is executed, a metallic sound is perceived. The respiratory murmur is absent over the invaded area. The differentiation from pneumothorax is made by the auscultation of metallic borborygmi and the rapid change in the percussion and auscultation sounds as the stomach and intestines are filled or emptied. Filling of the stomach with water causes disappearance of the full tympanitic resonance on percussion, but it is a procedure attended with considerable risk, because of the possibility of the presence of a genuine pneumothorax. If occlusion should result as a consequence of this condition, the only hope of relief is from operation, and that is a very small one.

Pathological Physiology and Etiology.

Internal hernias are more frequent among men than among women. According to Leichtenstern, both sexes are affected with incarcerations by peritoneal pseudo-ligaments with the same frequency. One would presume that the female sex, being more liable to pelvic peritonitis, would also present a greater frequency of incarceration by pseudo-ligaments. The greater frequency of pelvic peritonitis in females is counterbalanced, however, by a far greater frequency of peritonitis starting as appendicitis, or from the various hernial gates, in men. All incarcerations due to Meckel's diverticula, the appendix, and the omentum, are by far more frequent in men than in women. Men are more frequently subject to peritonitis starting from the biliary apparatus, the appendix, and the hernial sacs; and as the omentum in men, on account of its anatomical length, may come in contact with these structures much more easily than in women, it follows that men are much more subject to these forms of incarceration than women. The etiology of all forms of congenital abdominal abnormalities,—for instance, the congenital slits and crevices, the intra-abdominal hernias, omphalo- mesenteric remains,—is unknown. In rare instances the diagnosis can be aided by etiological factors if the clinician is capable of eliciting a history of chronic peritonitis resulting from the gall-bladder, the cecum or appendix, the female generative organs, the rectum, or trauma of the abdomen. When such dangerous structures, slits, and abnormalities exist in the abdomen, the intestines make their way into it by means of the peristalsis. The question has been raised, "What prevents the intestinal loops from escaping from their dangerous position, from a crevice, or from under an arch of pseudo-ligament, by means of this same peristalsis?" Older views held that the intestine was retained in its dangerous position by spasmodic contraction of the pseudo-ligament or slit. This is manifestly impossible, for peritonitic bands and slits in the omentum contain no muscular tissue, and therefore can not contract suddenly. The strangulation may occur very suddenly or gradually. It is not absolutely necessary that the intestine should be functionally destroyed the moment it enters such a dangerous position. Although there are such sudden incarcerations which present the symptomatology of an abruptly developing absolute intestinal occlusion, they are rather exceptional. As a rule, the development of the symptoms of strangulation is gradual. Many theories have been propounded attempting an explanation of the direct causative factors of an incarceration or strangulation. They can be found in text-books on intestinal surgery—for instance, Treves (*l. c.*), Bardaleben ("The International Encyclopedia of Surgery," Wm. Wood & Co., New York, vol. VII), König, B. Schmidt, and Nicholas Senn ("Practical Surgery," Phila., 1901). They are mostly based on experimental investigation, aiming at an explanation of the mechanical and physical conditions which are responsible for the development of incarcerations. Suffice it to say that mainly three factors or pathological changes are active in retaining an intestine once caught in one of the manners described above. First of all, the effects of the disturbances in the circulation of the intestine and mesentery ; these consist of serous transudation and bloody extravasation, associated with enormous development of gas that accumulates in the lumen of the incarcerated intestine. The walls of the intestine themselves begin to swell, and the lumen itself expands owing to the distention. This has already been more fully described under the heading of local and stagnation meteorism, and in the chapter on Meteorism. Secondly, in most cases of incarcerated or strangulated intestine a subsequent axial twist occurs which fixes the loop in its abnormal position. Thirdly, the entrance of intestinal contents into the incarcerated loop increases the distention by their own bulk as well as by adding to the fermentation.

Symptomatology.

The clinical picture is the same as that given in the chapter on Intestinal Occlusion. In this place I simply wish to repeat the most characteristic symptoms of strangulation and incarceration. From a practical and surgical standpoint all forms of impermeability of the intestine may be divided into two great groups : First, impermeability in consequence of strangulation or incarceration, in which both the intestine and its mesentery are constricted, and the serious changes are dependent on the circulatory disturbances, especially the impediment to the venous outflow. Secondly, impermeability due to obturation, in which only the lumen of the intestine is blocked, but the mesentery is not included in the obstruction or constriction.   Here the changes are principally dependent on the stagnation of intestinal contents.

The first and fundamental question to decide in each case will be, *" Is it a case of strangulation or obturation ? "*   In all strangulations and incarcerations, the forms which we are considering now, the nutrition of the intestine soon suffers as a result of the circulatory disturbance.   The incarcerated loop becomes distended and ultimately paralyzed.   The distention may acquire colossal dimensions ; a single loop of the large intestine, for instance, when distended, apparently fills the entire abdominal cavity and extends up into the dome of the diaphragm.

In all strangulations we always have a fixed, distended, and paralyzed intestinal loop.   The parts lying above the strangulated portion, the suprastenotic loops, show no distention, or very little, in the first stage.   We have already given the causes of strangulation, and those of obturation are given in another chapter, yet to follow.   It is necessary to repeat here that as there are no circulatory disturbances in the mesentery in obturations, the nutrition of the intestine suffers comparatively little.   We do not observe any distended paralyzed loop, and the portions of the intestine above the obstruction are not only free from paralysis, but the peristalsis is distinctly increased.

Invaginations occupy an intermediate position ; sometimes they involve the mesentery, and sometimes they do not.   Therefore we may have in one case the phenomena of strangulation, and in another those of obturation.

The most important symptoms may be arranged in the order of their frequency, as follows : (1) Gas and stool retention, (2) pain, (3) vomiting, (4) meteorism, and (5) incarceration shock.   There are other symptoms of minor importance ; for instance, tumor, fever, singultus, anuria, or diminished excretion of urine, exudations into the abdominal cavity.

Retention of Feces and Gas.—This is, in my opinion, the first important symptom in all cases that can be noticed from an early date.   It occurred in 84 per cent. of the 500 cases in literature in which any statement concerning this symptom was made at all, as the first deviation from the normal condition.   The reason why it has not been more frequently put down in the literature as the first symptom is in my opinion due to the fact that the retention of stool and flatus is often considered as an attack of simple constipation and treated as such by the patient, as well as by the physician. In all cases of strangulation the mechanical closure of the intestinal lumen causes a complete stoppage to any gaseous, liquid, or solid discharges from the bowels. There are very rare cases where fecal masses have been discharged from sections of the intestine lying below the obstacle, and there has also been described an extremely rare form of acute impermeability accompanied by diarrhea,—the so-called "*cholēra herniaire*" of Malgaigne,—which is probably due to a hypersecretion of the intestinal juices. These clinical curiosities can not invalidate the importance of the fundamental symptom of suppression of stool and flatus. In contradistinction to volvulus, and especially invagination, *blood* is never present in the stools of strangulations or incarcerations.

Pain.—This is the next most important symptom in frequency. It was found to appear on the first day in 70 per cent. of those of the 500 cases referred to in which it was possible to determine the date with any degree of accuracy. The pain is more or less constant, very severe, and most pronounced in the acute herniaform incarcerations of the small intestine. It is less intense in strangulations of the large intestine, where it may under rare conditions be absent altogether. External pressure on the abdominal wall does not increase the pain. Fitz (*l. c.*), in accord with Treves and Nothnagel, is not inclined to attribute any diagnostic importance to the seat of the pain as an evidence of strangulation, or of its special cause. He found it to be associated early with nausea and vomiting, either alone or together, in 69 per cent. of the cases compiled by him. It took place on the first day in at least one-third of the cases of adhesion, and in more than one-half of those of vitelline remains, and in five-sixth of those of peritoneal slits. The proportion is much greater when the numbers of cases are considered in which the date of occurrence could be definitely ascertained. The relative frequency of pain on the first day, according to Fitz, then comes to more than one-half in cases of adhesions, two-thirds in those of vitelline remains, five-sixths in adherent appendix, and one-half in strangulation by a slit.

Vomiting.—The initial nausea and vomiting noticed at the beginning of the attack, and sometimes actually ushering it in, must be carefully distinguished from the stercoraceous vomiting, which occurs only in the later stages of the disease.   Stercoraceous vomiting is the classic symptom of all kinds of impermeability ; it is caused by the overfilling of the intestinal sections above the obstacle—as I have designated them, the *suprastenotic loops*—with decomposed offensive secretions and ingesta.   I have already spoken of Huguenot's explanation of stercoraceous vomiting in which he attributes it to a retrograde movement of the contents of these loops, caused by abdominal and diaphragmatic pressure, and not due to antiperistalsis.   The initial vomiting occurs at a time when there can be no idea of overfilling of the suprastenotic loops ; it is a result of the sudden and intense irritation of the peritoneal and intestinal nerves at the moment of the incarceration.   Therefore it is of a purely reflex character.   For this reason I consider that the initial vomiting has an important diagnostic significance, because in my experience it has occurred almost exclusively in the strangulations.   The first vomit is composed of the last food that was taken.   It next becomes yellow from the admixture of bile, and finally fecal.   But the stage at which the vomit becomes fecal is in my experience not reached until the third day.   A sufficient length of intervening time therefore elapses to separate the initial from the fecal vomiting.   A number of cases of strangulation have been reported in which entire absence of nausea and vomiting was mentioned.   These were two cases of strangulation by adhesions, one of which recovered after laparotomy, and the other terminated fatally.   From a therapeutic standpoint it is of importance to notice the report frequently made in the literature of the subject, that the vomiting only became constant when material was persistently taken into the stomach.   The term fecal vomit is indiscriminately applied in the literature of the subject.   Of course no hard-and-fast line is to be drawn between vomit that is fecal and that which is not fecal.   The odor of the vomit is usually the only criterion ; but as was the case in my experience, many times I have observed that the physician was not overanxious to get near to the vomited masses with his nose, and the diagnosis " fecal vomit " was simply made from the appearance ; and thus the term applied to the ejection of yellow, almost odorless, duodenal secretions. If the term were applied more strictly to the offensive ejections that are distinctly fetid and which come from the loops directly above the obstruction, we should have fewer cases in the literature of so-called fecal vomit.

Meteorism and Visible Peristalsis.—In the general chapter on Intestinal Obstruction I have already considered this symptom, and given a description of its varieties—the "local" and "stagnation meteorism." Suffice it to call attention here once more to the signs of von Wahl and Schlange. Von Wahl's sign is a distended immovable loop, usually representing the very loop itself which is strangulated. It is forced up against the abdominal wall, causing an asymmetric projection of the same, and on account of its excessive tension it does not yield the ordinary intestinal sound on percussion, but a deep, non-tympanitic resonance. The thick, distended loop of von Wahl shows no peristalsis. Schlange has described a peristalsis in the distended loop above the obstacle which occurs before complete arrest of peristalsis has developed—a fixed intestinal prestenotic loop with peristalsis. According to Naunyn, it is not a sure sign of strangulation, as it occurs in any acute obstruction, even those without strangulation. Personally I have never observed the sign of Schlange, although I have carefully watched and searched for it, and even the sign of von Wahl is not always easy to recognize. I have personally never seen it in the classical volvulus of the sigmoid flexure, where the distended loop may fill the entire abdomen. Von Wahl and his pupils Zoege von Mannteuffel and Kader emphasize the necessity of examining the abdomen during deep narcosis, and that examination by the vagina and rectum should never be omitted. Should the slight peristalsis to which Schlange calls attention be observed, however, it should not be confounded with the powerful and stormy peristalsis as it is observed in chronic stenoses, in which it always runs in the direction toward the obstruction. Such a peristalsis means the chronic process, and can only be caused by hypertrophied intestinal muscularis. In strangulations, peristalsis is either entirely wanting, or if it occurs at all, it is not pronounced. This absence of peristalsis in the presence of all the previously mentioned symptoms of strangulation offers a possibility for the differentiation of obstruction due to strangulation from that due to obturation in the majority of cases. If we find on examination no single immovable loop, we must consider the fact that in strangulations the incarcerated loop may be paralyzed or that the intestinal sections lying above the obstruction are not at all or very slightly distended; for there are rare cases in which meteorism was wholly absent as late as the eighth day. Fitz (*l. c.*) records its presence in 56 per cent. of the cases compiled by himself.

Incarceration Shock.—The intensity of this condition runs parallel with that of the pains and of the initial vomiting. It is more pronounced with strangulation of the small intestine, and in my experience is an almost invariable accompaniment of this type. Incarceration shock is chiefly a grave depression of the cardiac and respiratory functions and nervous system. This form of collapse is generally regarded as a reflex phenomenon produced by intense irritation of the sensory nerves of the intestine and diaphragm; also as a reflex paralysis of the vagi and splanchnic nerves. A second theory explains incarceration shock as a septic collapse, dependent upon the rapid infection of the peritoneal cavity in consequence of the permeability for bacteria of the altered intestinal wall. A third theory is based on the autointoxication hypothesis, which attributes the shock to the absorption of the products of bacterial proteid putrefaction in the intestine. Whilst both of these latter theories are plausible, and no doubt the conditions described play an important rôle in the later stages of strangulation, they cannot explain the gravity of the primary incarceration shock, which usually appears in the first hour after the strangulation, when we could hardly assume the presence of an intoxication or infection.

General Appearance and Condition.—The disease befalls the individual as a rule during a state of complete health, without any prodromal pathological symptoms. Occasionally a very sudden bodily movement, a jump, fall, or blow against the abdomen, lifting of a heavy weight, or pressure at stool is assigned as the direct cause. Sometimes the outward progress of an old hernia, the ingestion of voluminous food, or the administration of a purgative is assigned as cause. After this the patient is suddenly taken with a violent pain in the abdomen. In an hour or a few hours we have the initial vomiting. The face has the expression of intense suffering. The eyes are sunken in their sockets. The skin is deprived of its normal flesh color, cold sweat stands upon it, the lips are cyanosed, and also the fingers and toes. The voice is without resonance, later on hoarse; the pulse is scarcely perceptible. It is a grave clinical picture, all the more depressing because the consciousness of the patient is generally clear.

Prognosis and Course.

Internal strangulation and incarceration are fatal if left to themselves. In more than one-half the cases compiled by Fitz (the table included thirty cases of strangulation treated by purely medicinal means) death occurred from the second to the fourth day. Le Moyn observed two cases of sudden strangulation in young soldiers; one died after ten and the other after eighteen hours. As a general rule, the fatal termination is more rapid after very intense and severe initial symptoms, and the course is more protracted when the symptoms begin more gradually. The severity of the symptoms depends upon two factors: the length of the incarcerated section of the intestine and mesentery, and the force of the incarcerating agency. A number of cases (I shall speak of them in the section on surgery of the intestines) may be saved by operation. Operative interference took place in 76 per cent. of Fitz's cases. The percentage of recoveries after surgical interference, in these cases of strangulation, was 39 per cent., a mortality of 61 per cent. The total mortality in the 1000 operations reported by Chas. L. Gibson ("Annals of Surgery," November, 1900, p. 704) was 47 per cent. A still smaller number of cases are reported to have been saved by so-called internal or nonoperative treatment.

The question has been raised whether spontaneous cure of strangulations can occur. As the incarceration may not be complete, and the involved loop may have undergone a simultaneous partial axial twist, keeping the incarcerated portion in its perilous trap, it is conceivable that the axial twist which has occurred secondarily may become resolved, thus making possible the escape of the incarcerated bowel. Another condition making plausible the possibility of spontaneous cure is the gangrenous condition of the incarcerating bands which has been found at the time of operation and autopsies. The nutrition of the pseudo-ligament must necessarily suffer by compression, just as well as that of the incarcerated intestine. The gangrenous condition found at the operation makes it conceivable that the band may tear and thus release the bowel. It is also conceivable that the partial incarcerations and strangulations may become released by reduction of the intra-abdominal pressure, after lavage of the stomach and colon, and the substitution of a more favorable peristalsis for the abnormal one. Death occurs by shock, exhaustion from pain and profuse vomiting, and in rare cases from peritonitis. Death from perforation and gangrene is very rare in strangulations, because the fatal termination follows long before these conditions have time for development.

Diagnosis.

There is no single sign or symptom that has pathognomonic significance. What is required of the clinician is not simply the diagnosis of the condition, but also of the seat of the strangulation. From the reports of the cases in the literature of the subject, it is evident that an exact diagnosis of obstruction from strangulation is only possible by exploratory laparotomy. To determine the seat and kind of the incarceration with exactness is simply impossible in the present state of our knowledge. Concerning this point, however, I may refer to the statistics of Fitz once more. In fully three-fourths of all cases collected by him, it was the small intestine that was strangulated in 90 per cent. of the cases, and the large intestine in 10 per cent. It will not be far from wrong if we assume that the lower ileum is the most frequent location of the incarceration. By a process of logical exclusion of the other acute intestinal occlusions,—(a) incarceration of external hernia, (b) invaginations, (c) obturations by foreign bodies, (d) partial intestinal paralysis and diffuse peritonitis, (e) axial twists, (f) sudden absolute occlusion in chronic stenoses,—we may in extremely rare cases also reach a conclusion regarding the diagnosis of strangulation. The differential diagnostic points concerning these possibilities will be considered in a separate chapter after all the various types of intestinal obstruction have been especially described.

Synoptic Diagnostic Résumé.—Here I wish simply to emphasize the cardinal points upon which the meager possibility of the diagnosis is based. The chief symptoms are gas and stool retention, abdominal pain, nausea or vomiting, meteorism, incarceration shock, and abdominal tumor.   In strangulation these symptoms develop rapidly; onset with violent pain, followed rapidly by vomiting, absolute obstipation, and early development of shock.   No reliable indication on examination of the abdomen.   Pronounced meteorism as a rule absent; in some cases a distended loop is palpable ; absence of bloody stool ; a history of internal incarcerations, old hernias, perityphlitis, gall-stones, appendicitis, or inflammations about the female generative organs.

In many cases every support for a definite anatomical conception of the case is absent.   Whether we are confronted with a constriction by pseudo-ligament, by elongated appendix, by a diverticulum, by a band of the mesentery, by adhesion, by slits in the omentum, by a loop knot formation or axial twist, will in most cases not be possible to determine when the cases are presented for treatment. Nevertheless nothing should be left undone to arrive at a diagnosis ; it is of the greatest importance that the previous history and the present status should be taken down in writing.   I therefore supplement this chapter with a synopsis for determining such a clinical history of the past and present state.   It has been of great value to me, inasmuch as it compelled me to regard critically the important clinical points, and therefore has made possible a later comparison of the facts recorded for diagnosis.   I regard it as impracticable to present actual clinical histories for each of the above possible conditions, for there is no such thing as a stereotyped clinical picture to answer for all emergencies, and in a concrete case, as presented, such clinical histories generally leave the practitioner in the lurch.

The **treatment** will be considered with that of the remaining forms of intestinal obstruction, and in the chapter on Surgery of the Intestines.

OBTURATIONS.

When the lumen of the intestine is obstructed by abnormal contents, such as biliary or intestinal calculi, hardened feces, or foreign bodies, we speak of it as an obturation.   It is then a plugging up of the lumen by a body which is movable within it.   Mostly the conditions result in an occlusion, though partial stenosis occurs in rare instances. There are principally five varieties of obturating bodies of clinical interest: (1) Gall-stones; (2) intestinal calculi (enteroliths); (3) foreign bodies; (4) fecal masses; (5) entozoa.

1. Obturation by Gall-stones.

Gall-stones which are sufficiently large to obstruct the lumen of the intestine by themselves can only get into the bowel as a result of a pathological communication between the gall-bladder and the intestine. The most frequent communication is that between the duodenum and the gall-bladder; the next most frequent, that between the ileum and the gall-bladder; and the communication between the colon and the gall-bladder is the rarest of all. The visceral changes which occur as a result of inflammatory processes originating from the gall-bladder have been pictured in a scholarly article by Geo. E. Brewer ("Contributions to the Science of Medicine," dedicated to Wm. Henry Welch, p. 344). In 7 of 9 cases of irregularities, Brewer describes the gall-bladder as adherent to the first and second portions of the duodenum, the transverse colon, and the omentum; in two instances the gall-bladder was firmly bound down by adhesions to the duodenum only; in one to the first, and in the other to the first and second portions of the duodenum.

The penetration of the stone must be preceded by adhesive inflammation and the formation of a fistula. Stones that pass through the common gall-duct are not of sufficient size to obstruct the intestine. But a fistula may also develop between the cystic end of the common gall-duct and the duodenum. According to Leichtenstern, the obturation may occur at different locations in the intestine. Of 42 cases collected by him, the obturation was 10 times in the duodenum and jejunum, 15 times in the middle ileum, and 17 times in the lower part of the ileum. There are other varieties of obturation of the intestine by gall-stones. Mikulicz found the gall-stones that caused the obturation not in the intestine, but in diverticula of the cystic duct, which had become superimposed upon the duodenum and compressed it ("Arch. f. klin. Chir.," 1895, Bd. LI). There is no doubt that even smaller gall-stones may, under rare, unfortunate conditions, by the apposition of fecal masses, cause impermeability, whilst relatively large stones may pass without doing any damage. Přibram describes the uneventful passage through the entire intestine of two large gall-stones as "thick as the thumb," which had passed from the gall-bladder into the intestine under severe chills ("Handb. d. prakt. Med.," von Ebstein u. Schwalbe, Bd. II, S. 637). On the other hand, Israel described a case of obturation of the ileum by a gall-stone the greatest diameter of which did not exceed 2 cm. (about ¾ inch). He expressed the opinion that the effect must have been caused by a dynamic stricture, a reflex contraction of the intestine, set up by the stone, the relatively small circumference of which could not have caused the obturation. Nothnagel and Naunyn agree with him in this view. Obturation of the colon by gall-stones is an extremely rare occurrence. In a compilation of 200 cases from the literature in which I could find a statement concerning the location of the gall-stones, the obturation was present 12 times in the small intestine, and only 4 times in the large intestine. Females are more frequently subject to obturations by gall-stones than males, the proportion being 127 females to 34 males, according to Naunyn. In Fitz's statistics the proportion is 18 females to 5 males (*l. c.*). I have investigated critically the literature on gall-stone obstruction, and admitted only those cases into my statistics in which there was no doubt as regards the diagnosis, judging from the reports of the various authors. In quite a number of these publications the presence of a gall-stone, found during operation or at autopsy, obstructing the bowel was considered sufficient evidence to make the diagnosis of gall-stone obstruction. In a surprisingly large number of the same cases the reporters give an account of peritonitis which naturally must have been present, set up by the destructive processes of adhesion and formation of fistulæ which preceded the entrance of the stone into the intestine. As I have stated in the introduction to the chapter on Intestinal Obstruction, peritonitis itself may cause intestinal paralysis by the infiltration of the muscular coats with a serous transudation. If now the bowel becomes immovable, a fecal stagnation results, and a gall-stone may even be caught in it. This, however, is by no means a condition which we can designate as gall-stone obstruction ; it is an obstruction due to peritonitis and coprostasis, in which the gall-stone has accidentally been caught. An analogous condition prevails with regard to the reported cases of obstruction from inspissated feces, of which I shall treat in one of the following paragraphs. Very large gall-stones, particularly if they possess sharp edges, may cause gangrene, peritonitis, and perforation.

Age.—It is apparent, from the tables of Fitz, that obstruction from gall-stones occurs only in adults. Eighteen of his 22 cases, or about 82 per cent., occurred after the fiftieth year. Of 40 cases compiled by Chas. L. Gibson (*l. c.*), 33 occurred after the fiftieth year. Of 120 cases observed by Naunyn ("Mittheilungen aus den Grenzgeb. d. Med. u. Chir.," Bd. 1), only 5 were under thirty years, 7 occurred at from thirty-one to forty, but 96 between forty-one and sixty.

Symptomatology.—In about one-fifth of the cases the anamnesis gives a distinct history of cholelithiasis, and in some of the cases, of icterus. In about four-fifths of the cases there is no history of biliary colic, which becomes intelligible on reflecting that the stone does not pass through the common gall-duct, but enters the intestine by a fistula communicating with the gall-bladder and the intestine. If the stone is not very large, it may give rise to but very slight symptoms, indicating a partial and transient obstruction of the bowel. When the symptoms of severe obstruction occur, they begin gradually with severe pain and followed by intense, even fecal, vomiting. This occurred in 77 of 120 cases collected by Schüller. Then, as in the typical cases of severe obstruction, constipation, meteorism, and collapse follow. The meteorism is rarely extensive, although there may be fecal vomiting. Naunyn emphasizes that flatus may be discharged at the same time that the patients are suffering from fecal vomit. The obstruction, therefore, is not necessarily absolute. Even evacuation of stools has been observed during the fecal vomiting. The stone can only very rarely be felt. I have observed two cases, and Naunyn also described cases in which the passage of the intestine became free again transiently, only to become absolutely impermeable after days and weeks. Gall-stone obstruction has been observed twice in the same individual. Death may occur under the phenomena of severe collapse between the fifth and the tenth day. Very rarely the symptoms of obstruction may be drawn out to the fifteenth day. The mortality of inoperative cases is stated variously at from 44 to 56 per cent. Chas. L. Gibson gives the mortality of operated cases among females as 53 per cent., and 33 per cent.

among males.   When a fistula exists between the gall-bladder and
colon, naturally very large stones can be passed without any of the
phenomena of obstruction, but when the gall-stone becomes impacted in the duodenum, we may have all the symptoms of duodenal or pyloric stenoses, which have been described in the chapter
on Enterostenoses.   There are rare cases of spontaneous recovery,
the gall-stone having passed the narrow portions of the intestine
and entered the colon.   Such recoveries have been observed even
after three weeks of symptoms of occlusion by gall-stones.   Sands
reports a case in which there was fecal vomiting on the third day,
which continued for three weeks.   The absolute retention of stool
was present even in the fourth week.   At the expiration of this
time evacuations were again resumed after the patient, a woman,
had been treated with purgatives and enematas.   On the seventh day
thereafter a gall-stone was passed 7½ cm. (3 inches) in circumference, and the patient recovered entirely.   The stone does not
always appear in the passages immediately after the cessation of the
phenomena of obstruction, which are continued only as long as the
stone is in the small intestine, and cease as soon as it has entered
the large intestine.   It is possible that the stone may remain a long
time in the large intestine before it is evacuated.   Kölliker reports
a case of incarcerated gall-stone which was mistaken for appendicitis, because phenomena of both gall-stone colic and appendicitis
had been recorded in the anamnesis.   The operation confirmed the
diagnosis and led to a cure.

Bradbury reported two cases of gall-stone occlusion of the small
intestine without previous phenomena of cholelithiasis.   The vagaries
and wanderings of gall-stones have been interestingly described by
Henry L. Elsner ("Medical News," February 5, 1898).   He reports
six extraordinary cases, only the first one of which seems to have
caused symptoms of intestinal obturation.   The patient was a woman
fifty-seven years of age, who had a tumor in the right hypochondriac
region for fifteen months.   There was gastrectasia with retention of
the contents, and absence of free HCl during this time.   This, together with the presence of an enlargement of the pylorus, certainly ·
very much resembled gastric carcinoma.   The symptoms of intestinal obturation followed upon a violent attack of pain in the upper
part of the abdomen.   The obstruction was incomplete, and there-

fore operation was delayed. Sixteen days later she passed an enormous gall-stone 13 cm. (about 5 ¼ inches) in circumference, and weighing 368 grains. Eleven months later a second gall-stone weighing 240 grains was discharged. The patient recovered completely. Elsner supposes that there was ulceration with the formation of a fistula between the gall-bladder and the duodenum, through which the stone was originally discharged into the intestine. According to his report, perforation occurred in 19 of 421 cases of cholelithiasis which came to autopsy at Basle. Rehn has reported the case of a woman who had symptoms of intestinal obstruction for which no reason could be found. At the operation two gall-stones larger than walnuts were found in the deep loops of the ileum ("Arch. f. klin. Chir.," Bd. LX, H. 2). In the case of stone smaller than the lumen of the bowel, Rehn attributes the obstruction not to mechanical blockage, but to inflammation, the result of the irritation of the foreign body. Wilkinson observed the spontaneous discharge of a gall-stone as large as a chicken egg in a patient who had suffered from the symptoms of incarceration for eleven weeks. In some of the cases in literature there were several attacks of intestinal obturation that were broken by long intervals of comparative well-being.

Diagnosis.—If the gall-stone becomes impacted in the duodenum below the papilla (see Geo. E. Brewer, *l. c.*) there will be profuse bilious vomiting, which should awaken the suspicion of gall-stone obturation if there has been a history of cholelithiasis, or signs of perforation of the gall-passages into the intestine. Increase of the hepatic dullness, painfulness of the gall-bladder on moderate pressure, pain and great sensitiveness over the anterior and posterior hepatic regions, should awaken the suspicion of cholelithiasis even in the absence of a history of this disease or of jaundice. The palpable tumor is rare. Whenever such a tumor was discovered, its position was variable, owing to the downward progress of the calculus by peristalsis. Fitz reports that in 11 cases, or nearly one-half of his compilation of obturations from gall-stone, there was a previous attack of biliary calculi. Jaundice was present in only 2 cases. He reports the presence of tumor in 5 cases, once in the right iliac fossa, which proved to be a calculus; twice the tumor was in evidence at the umbilicus on the third day. In one of these cases it is

reported to have been as large as a child's head.   In a fourth case
tumor was present in the left inguinal region, and in a fifth it was
found on rectal examination.   Of 23 cases of gall-stone obstruction
by this author, there were 13 deaths and 10 recoveries.   Twelve
cases were treated medically and 11 surgically.   Of the former, 8
recovered and 4 died.   The passage of the gall-stone, in those
cases which recovered, occurred on the fourth, fifth (2 cases), tenth,
fourteenth, fifteenth, seventeenth, and twentieth days.   Of the 11
cases treated surgically, 2 recovered and 9 died.   Since all the
operative methods after the seventh day terminated fatally, and as 5
cases under medical treatment after this date recovered, Fitz is of
the opinion that the condition of the patient must determine the
treatment to be followed ; that is, it should not always be treated
surgically.

2. Obturation by Intestinal Calculi (Enteroliths).

The so-called enteroliths are rarely composed of the same material throughout ; they are rarely of exclusively mineral composition.   As a rule the nucleus is formed of some organic substance,
or some chemical substance taken as a medicine.   Leichtenstern (*l. c.*)
describes three kinds of such stones : (1) Intestinal calculi of a very
hard consistency and quite heavy, on cross-section showing a uniform, homogeneous structure ; on the surface they are dark brown,
and internally of a dirty gray color.   They are round, oval, or
when several of them are present they may be faceted.   Their size
varies from 2 cm. to 3 cm. in diameter, to enormous dimensions.
Some have been described 23 cm. in diameter and weighing four
pounds.   Very often the mineral parts of such stones have been
deposited around a distinct nucleus, such as foreign bodies, particles
of bone, seeds of fruits, and indigestible plant residue.   They are
composed generally of the phosphates of ammonium, calcium,
magnesium, and ammonio-magnesium.   In rare cases they contain calcium sulphate.   (2) Enteroliths due to the continuous
ingestion of medicinal preparations.   Kiaer reported the case of an
enterolith weighing 9 grams and composed mainly of bismuth.   It
was found in a hernial sac within the intestine. Baumberger
describes an enterolith composed of 80 per cent. of carbonate of
calcium in a patient who had eaten chalk for years.   Hutchinson

published a case of an enterolith composed of magnesia and iron. (3) The third group of enteroliths are those which are composed of intertwined masses of indigestible vegetable residues of the food. They are found in persons who live largely upon a diet which leaves an enormous indigestible residue—for instance, the coarse oatmeal which is abundantly used in Scotland. Such stones are usually very light, and occasionally float on top of water. Avenoliths, or oat-stones, the origin of which is due to the diet described above, are found among the inhabitants of certain regions in Scotland, who use a great deal of oats in their diet. The stone of iron and magnesium described by Hutchinson was found in the rectum, and could only be removed after crushing. The nucleus consisted of thousands of gooseberry seeds. Dowen described a fatal case of obturation of the lower ileum by an enterolith composed of cocoanut fibers. Quain reported a case of enterolith weighing four pounds and composed of cocoanut fibers. Among the forty-four cases of obstruction from abnormal contents reported by R. H. Fitz (*l. c.*, p. 24), there were two of enteroliths which offered grave symptoms. One was composed of date seeds and gritty material, and the other was a shellac calculus present in a cabinet-maker who was accustomed to drinking alcoholic solution of shellac.

A most interesting condition of gouty enterolithiasis is described by Dieulafoy. I have referred to this opinion in the chapter on Membranous Enteritis, as well as on that on Gouty Intestinal Ulcers. This versatile French clinician holds that there is an intestinal uric-acid diathesis, giving rise to the formation of grit or calculi, similarly as we have a urinary or biliary diathesis with tendency to form calculi.

3. Obturation by Foreign Bodies.

Foreign bodies that occur in the intestines are, above all, such as are naturally taken in with the food, but can not be dissolved by the digestive juices. These are the stones and seeds of fruits, the indigestible shells of fruits, leguminous plants, etc., fishbones, shells of mollusks, and bones.

A tumor of the sigmoid colon in a boy aged fourteen who came under my observation puzzled me for three weeks. By large colon enemata I gradually succeeded in washing off pieces of it, which consisted of grape skins and seeds. By the combined effect of large doses of castor oil and colon enemata the whole mass was finally evacuated, containing thousands of grape seeds and weighing 8 ounces. The boy made an uneventful recovery. Another class of foreign bodies are those that are taken into the stomach or rectum by the insane and hysterical, by children, from mischief, or in the performances of charlatans. The most wonderful objects have been found in the intestinal canal as the result of such performances. Spoons, knives and forks, coins, needles, glass balls, dagger blades, pieces of wood, iron, a small flute, pieces of porcelain, false teeth, nails, screws, hair and wool, fishbones, pieces of oyster shell, etc. In a patient who had complained of pain in the left iliac region for four or five weeks and a rapidly developing tumor of the right iliac fossa, H. A. Beach and F. B. Mallory found an inflammatory mass at operation containing a small abscess cavity, the origin of which was traced to a fishbone that had perforated the intestinal wall ("Boston Med. and Surg. Jour.," November 17, 1898). In one case an artificial set of teeth with six teeth was passed six months after it was swallowed. Among things that were put into the rectum from the anus, are a bottle of cologne, a pair of shoemakers' pliers, a pestle, pig tail, a beer glass, and other almost incredible things. Those who are interested in these curiosities will find a full record of them in Gould and Pyle's "Anomalies and Curiosities of Medicine," page 645. Concerning the foreign bodies that may enter through the stomach, see "Diseases of the Stomach," by the author, pages 492 and 610, second edition ; also the contribution by W. S. Halsted to the surgery of foreign bodies in the stomach ("Contributions to the Science of Medicine," dedicated to Wm. Henry Welch), page 1047.

Symptoms.—Larger foreign bodies sometimes cause transient obturation with colic and vomiting ; others cause ulceration and perforation, and acute chronic peritonitis. The ulceration, if it occurs, may even lead to the formation of a fistula through which the foreign bodies may be expelled. The fistula may communicate between the ileum and colon, or between the colon and rectum ; it may also open into the bladder and vagina. Sewing needles may penetrate the intestinal wall, and migrate to the remotest portions of the body. If the foreign bodies are not of excessively large size, they pass the intestinal tract without accident. In fact, the large majority of foreign bodies are expelled from the digestive canal in this way.

Diagnosis.—The diagnosis can be made by the anamnesis, and also by the presence of the foreign body in the stool or in the gastric wash-water. They can not be palpated in the intestine even if they are large enough to cause obturation; but if they are of a metallic nature, they sometimes can be recognized by the skiagraph and the Röntgen rays.

Treatment.—Many times the patients will present themselves with a history of active purgation for the purpose of removing the foreign body, a practice by no means to be encouraged. When a foreign body has been swallowed, the best thing to do is to avoid purgatives, and to encourage the patient to eat a great deal of food in gruel form—for instance, mashed potatoes, purée of peas and beans, etc. But if symptoms of obturation occur, one should not wait too long with the operation.

The repeated finding of foreign bodies in the stools, provided they are not fruit seeds or substances derived from the diet, should excite the suspicion of a psychosis, and such patients should be watched. Articles that have been stolen—for instance, watches and chains and jewelry—have been hidden in the rectum for a long time without causing any distress to the criminal. But in Gould and Pyle's remarkable work numerous instances are cited of the introduction of foreign bodies provided with bristles and hooks, such things as were introduced with malign intentions upon other individuals, and gave rise to severe proctitis and periproctitis. Strange to say, very sharp objects, such as bones of poultry, have passed the entire intestine and did not become arrested until the rectum was reached, where they caused considerable distress, either by directly producing ulceration, or by setting up a reflex spasm of this organ. Such accidents occur in persons who bolt their food, and in old toothless persons, in whom proper mastication is difficult. In hysterical persons, and especially the insane, swallowed foreign bodies often exist only in the imagination of the patient. Boas (*l. c.,* p. 436) reports having freed a hysterical patient from a swallowed needle by showing her a needle surreptitiously thrown in the wash-water of a rectal enema.

4. Obturation by Fecal Masses.

In the chapter on Constipation I have already described the accumulation and condensation of fecal masses in the colon which occur in habitual obstipation. This condition is more frequently the result of defective innervation of the intestine, and in rare instances of congenital or acquired debility of the muscular peristalsis. The formation of fecal concretions or coproliths, under such conditions, occurs preferably in such localities of the colon in which the progress of the feces is to a certain extent impeded by natural difficulties of the lumen. We therefore find them preferably in the cecum, the flexures, and the sigmoid colon. The longer they remain, the harder they become. At first they are simply condensed stagnating masses, which do not obstruct the bowel entirely; gradually they become hardened by the loss of water by absorption, and larger by the further deposition of solid material. In such cases the clinical picture of a slowly progressing stenosis may develop, occasionally becoming suddenly aggravated to an absolute occlusion. If the loops that are made gravid by this accumulation are dislocated, they give rise to kinking or the development of a volvulus of the sigmoid flexure. The lethargy of the colon may be still more aggravated by the distention or the weight of the stagnating material and the gases formed therefrom. Paralysis of the musculature, including all the symptoms of intestinal occlusion, may follow. If a stenosis has previously existed,—for instance, one depending on an ulcer or a carcinoma,—a fecal concretion may become lodged in front of it and render it an absolute obstruction.

Symptomatology.—The symptoms of coproliths will be those of chronic enterostenosis or of intestinal occlusion, with the features that are characteristic of these conditions. When the fecal accumulation is in the sigmoid or rectum, tenesmus will be a prominent symptom, which will not be present if the mass is in the ascending or transverse colon.

Diagnosis.—The diagnosis is not always easy, and the fecal tumor has been mistaken for neoplasms, abscess, and floating kidney. The statistics of H. Illoway, in his scholarly monograph on "Constipation," give numerous cases of this sort. There are cases of this kind in which there may be an enormous accumulation of hard and dry feces in the rectum, and still a spurious kind of diarrhea exists at the same time (Morris Price, "Brit. Med. Jour.," 1886, vol. II, 1211). One should never omit to examine by the vagina and rectum. If the fecal tumor is in the lower section of the large intestine, it can as a rule be palpated. A previous history of chronic constipation is always suggestive, particularly when associated with repeated attacks of transient occlusion. Naturally such transient occlusions can also be due to one or the other form of intestinal obstruction described in other chapters. If meteorism exists, it is impossible to palpate the fecal tumor. If a tumor can really be felt, the question may arise whether it is really a fecal tumor or a neoplasm. Under such conditions the best course to take is to give the patient several oil or soap enemata. If the tumor does not move from its position, as it often will, these injections will at least render it soft, so that it can be indented by the pressure of the fingers. Repeated enemata and examinations are sometimes necessary. Gersuny ("Wien. klin. Wochenschr.," 1896) describes a so-called "*adhesive sign*," which consists in adhesion of the intestinal mucosa to the fecal tumor after it has been pressed against it for some time by the examining finger. When the pressure is interrupted, the intestinal mucosa releases itself from the fecal mass. According to Gersuny, this releasing movement is perceptible and characteristic for fecal tumor. Hofmokl ("Wien. med. Wochenschr.," 1896, S. 43) investigated this sign of Gersuny, but failed to confirm it as a reliable diagnostic means. Although I have personally attempted to discover the sign in a number of fecal tumors, I have also failed to recognize it. In forty-four cases of obstruction from abnormal contents, Fitz (*l. c.*) collected nineteen as due to fecal concretions. A critical consideration led him to exclude many cases as doubtful. Many of the symptoms of the obstruction which are attributed to the fecal accumulation, or coproliths, are due to an associated peritonitis or an inflamed appendix. Fitz emphasizes that if fecal tumors are found, and the symptoms of intestinal obstruction are present, it by no means follows that they are due immediately to the feces. An associated inflamed appendix is of so frequent occurrence that it alone suffices to suggest the diagnosis of obstruction. Enormous fecal accumulations may exist, in other cases, and very few symptoms arise to suggest an attack of acute internal obstruction. It is obvious from the considerations of Fitz that obstruction from feces may be excluded from the series of acute internal mechanical obstructions, because abdominal pain, meteorism, and stercoraceous vomiting were very rare and late symptoms, while nausea and vomiting were also of late occurrence. A tumor was present in half the cases, but by rectal injections, etc., positive evidence was obtained that it was not a neoplasm, but characteristically fecal. Fever was absent. As the seat of the obstruction from fecal accumulation was the large intestine, and the lower part was more often involved than the upper, this may be interpreted in favor of the view that the accumulation of feces in so-called stercoral typhlitis is not the cause of an inflamed cecum and appendix, but rather the result.

5. Obturation by Entozoa.

Although Leichtenstern (von Ziemssen's "Handbuch," Bd. VII, 2, 2. Aufl., 1878, S. 491), Davaine ("Traité de Enterzoaires et de Maladies vermineuses," second edition, Paris, 1871), and Heller ("Darmschmarotzer," S. 586) doubt the possibility of intestinal obturation by parasites and worms, yet Mosler and Peiffer (Nothnagel's "Spec. Pathol. u. Ther.," Bd. VI, S. 197) are inclined to accept this condition as a clinical fact. The obturation occurs mostly by ascarides lumbricoides, and the location of the obturation is mostly near the ileocecal valve, and in children. The authors last quoted affirm the occurrence of obstruction, incarceration, and volvulus by enormous accumulation of spool worms. Simon reported the following interesting observation ("Revue médicale, de l'Eto," 1892, No. 8), also cited by Mosler and Peiffer (l. c.): A child eleven years old became unconscious as a result of violent pains in the umbilical region. After three days symptoms of peritonitis set in. In the subumbilical region there was a distinct resistance with localized pain. On the following days bloody evacuations. Nothing abnormal on rectal examination. Operation for artificial anus was performed; and thereafter an evacuation of a stream of liquid feces, and collapse of the distended abdomen occurred. On the following day a conglomeration of seven live ascarides lumbricoides was expelled from the artificial anus. After this the stools were evacuated by the normal anus, and later on five more similar worms were expelled. The artificial anus healed completely, and recovery was perfect. Heidenreich ("Semaine médicale," 1891, No. 42) performed an enterostomy for similar indications, resulting in recovery. In recent American literature I have found the following case bearing on this condition: E. H. Bartley ("Archives of Pediatrics," April, 1898) reports a case of intestinal obstruction due to lumbricoid worms, simulating appendicitis. On opening the abdomen a ball of intertwined lumbricoids was found in the ileum, resting against the ileocecal valve, and completely occluding the opening. An attempt to force the worms through was without success. As the appendix was swollen, edematous, and intensely congested, it was thought best to remove it. The ileum was then opened by a small incision and about forty worms removed with forceps. The incision was sutured and the abdominal cavity cleansed and completely closed. All went well for forty-eight hours, then sharp pain was complained of in the left leg, which became very cold; gangrene set in, and seven days after the first operation an imperfect line of demarcation was formed about 4 inches above the malleoli. Amputation was performed at the knee-joint and the child made a slow but perfect recovery. Přibram reports the case of ileus verminosis of the small intestine, which was also cured by operation (Ebstein and Schwalbe, " Handbuch der prakt. Med.," Bd. II).

Characteristic Subjective and Objective Signs of Obturation, as Distinct from Other Forms of Obstruction.

The signs I shall consider are (1) meteorism, (2) gas and stool retention, (3) nausea and vomiting, (4) pain, (5) incarceration shock, and (6) the condition of the peristalsis.

1. **Meteorism.**—While it is always present in obturations, it is restricted to moderate limits, and it never acquires the colossal degree (at least not in the early stages) which is observed in strangulation. All the signs of which I shall speak as valuable in the diagnosis are of use only in the *early* stages. In order to determine the nature of the various impermeabilities, only the *early* stages of the disease can be utilized. In the later stages, when paralysis has involved entire districts of the intestine, the dead quietude of the distended abdomen does not even permit of a differential diagnosis between strangulation and diffuse peritonitis, or

between any of the various forms of obstruction. According to Kader's experiments, which have been repeatedly cited, the main cause of meteorism is the disturbance of the circulation in the intestinal walls, which impedes the absorption of gases from the intestinal lumen into the blood, and therefore a local distention with gases develops. Such circulatory disturbances occur only in strangulation of an intestinal loop. In obturation, which represents the simple blocking of the lumen, without circulatory disturbance of the intestinal wall, the absorption of gases from the intestine into the blood is not disturbed (Zuntz). Therefore the development of meteorism of considerable dimensions is prevented. In the later stages of obturation a disproportion ensues between gas formation and gas resorption, as a result of which meteorism develops. At first it takes place in the loops immediately above the obturation, then it extends to other loops in advance of the obstacle. In the beginning of each case the prestenotic loop, which is distended more than the rest, may serve as an indication of the seat of the obturation.

2. Gas and Stool Retention.—Whilst gas and stool retention is absolute in strangulation, it is only relative in obturation. Gases frequently pass in the latter condition. This is intelligible from the mechanism of the impermeability, which may suffice for the retention of firmer particles whilst gases can still make their escape.

3. Nausea and Vomiting.—Whilst these signs are present from the very beginning in strangulation, they may be wanting for a long time in obturation. The so-called initial vomiting of reflex origin, which I have described in the strangulations, is very rarely observed in obturation. In later stages, however, of the latter condition, vomiting as a rule sets in and may assume the character of fecal vomiting, as a result of overaccumulation in the prestenotic loops. If the question were asked, "In which condition does stercoraceous vomiting occur most often as a constant symptom—obturation or strangulation?" I think it would have to be answered that it occurs most constantly in obturation, for in the strangulations the violent vomiting from the very beginning of the disease prevents the overfilling of the prestenotic loops and the decomposition of their contents. Frequently death occurs even before the offensive putrefying masses can accumulate.

4. Pain.—The pain in strangulation is very intense, but constant and uninterrupted. In obturations the pain, while it also may be severe, is periodic, occurring at intervals, for it accompanies the peristaltic contractions of the prestenotic loops. During obturation these contractions may occasionally become tetanic, and the pain which is dependent upon these is described as being of a colicky nature.

5. Incarceration Shock.—The general condition suffers surprisingly little during obturations; whilst the painful colics are very torturing, they are not accompanied by the rapid decrease of strength, nor the cardiac debility, which occur in strangulations. When collapse occurs eventually in obturations of long standing, it is produced by the pains, the exhaustion and insomnia, perhaps from autointoxication, and is unlike the incarceration shock of strangulation, which occurs much sooner, and is not dependent upon these conditions, but is of reflex origin. Incarceration shock, therefore, which is a characteristic accompaniment of strangulation, may be said to be wanting entirely in obturation.

6. Peristalsis.—The peristaltic contractions in the intestinal loops above the obstacle are so pronounced in obturation that they may be said to be characteristic of it. This sign is most pronounced in acute obturation occurring on the basis of an already existing enterostenosis. Here the already developed hypertrophy of the muscularis enables the intestinal wall to give rise to peristaltic contractions of exceptional intensity. Intestinal loops may actually become so tetanically contracted that they become rigid, and are raised above the niveau of the abdomen, as plastic, hard cylinders. This sign has been called by Nothnagel "Darmsteifung" (bowel stiffening, or erection), and is characteristic of a chronic stenosis; but also in the other forms of obturation which attack an intestine that has been hitherto entirely permeable, increased peristaltic movements are most always discernible. The "Darmsteifung" may not be visible, it is true, but we can almost always detect and follow a peristaltic wave, generally running in one direction, and terminating at a certain point, which corresponds to the seat of the obstruction.

The tetanic contractions which occur in impermeabilities on the basis of chronic stenoses are maintained a long time, whereas in obturation where a muscular hypertrophy of the intestinal wall has not developed the peristalsis weakens and relaxes much sooner, and is gradually replaced by muscular paralysis, in consequence of over-distention. Like the pains, the increased peristalsis in the supra-stenotic loops presents a periodic character, occurring in paroxysms and accompanied by more or less colic. The periodicity of the attack in obturations is explained by the temporary exhaustion of the intestinal musculature, and perhaps also by the change in position of the intestinal contents, which exert an irritation upon the intestinal nerves and evoke the contraction.

The following is a comparative statement of subjective and objective signs of strangulation and obturation :

STRANGULATION.	OBTURATION.
Meteorism : Acquires colossal dimensions.	*Meteorism :* Present, but limited.
Gas and Stool Retention : Absolute.	*Gas and Stool Retention :* Only relative. Gases frequently pass.
Nausea and Vomiting : Present from the beginning. Initial or reflex vomiting.	*Nausea and Vomiting :* Absent for a long time. Initial or reflex vomiting rarely observed.
Pain : Very intense, constant, uninterrupted.	*Pain :* Periodic, occurring at intervals.
Incarceration Shock : Characteristic. Cardiac debility. Rapid decrease of strength.	*Incarceration Shock :* Shock wanting. Exhaustion may supervene after some time.
Peristalsis : No peristalsis in the supra-stenotic loops.	*Peristalsis :* Peristaltic contractions in suprastenotic loops pronounced and characteristic.

INVAGINATION OR INTUSSUSCEPTION.

Invagination or intussusception is a term designating a condition in which one section of the intestine is telescoped into the lumen of another, one section surrounding the other like a sheath. It is one of the most frequent abnormalities that give rise to intestinal occlusion. In 295 cases of obstruction compiled by Fitz (*l. c.*), 93, or 32 per cent., were intussusceptions. In 1000 operations for intestinal obstructions, compiled by Chas. L. Gibson ("Annals of Surgery," October, 1900), 187 were intussusceptions. Of all the various forms of acute intestinal obstruction this type presents the most definite and clear-cut symptomatology.

An invagination consists of three cylinders pushed into one another in the following way :

The outer cylinder, which embraces the other two, is called the vagina, sheath, or "intussuscipiens"; the two other layers contained within it are called the "intussusceptum." It consists of the middle and inner cylinders. The innermost of these, that which is nearest to the central lumen, is called the "entering," and the middle tube is called the outwardly receding or "returning cylinder." The lower part where the innermost or entering cylinder curves over into the receding or returning cylinder is called the head or

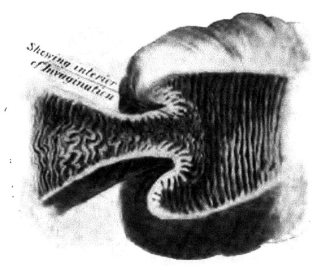

FIG. 5.—SHOWING INTERIOR OF INVAGINATION.—(*From preparation in Anatomical Laboratory, University of Maryland.*)

apex. It is always directed toward the anus. The upper part of the invagination, where the sheath or vagina curves over into the middle or returning cylinder, is designated as the neck. The external cylinder or sheath and the middle or returning cylinder are in contact with each other by the mucosa. The middle and internal cylinders are in contact by the peritoneum or serosa. Leichtenstern describes double invaginations consisting of five cylinders, and triple invaginations consisting of seven cylinders. There are also total or complete, and partial, lateral, or incomplete invaginations. In the latter only a circumscribed area of the intestinal wall is arched forward into the lumen, just the reverse of

what has taken place in diverticular expansions.   Partial invagination occurs in association with benign and malignant neoplasms,
which draw the intestinal wall into its lumen by their own weight.
Leichtenstern distinguishes between an "agonal" invagination on
the one hand, and a "vital" persisting or inflammatory invagination on the other.   Nothnagel designated these two conditions
as the "physiological" and "pathological" forms of invagination.
Invaginations most always occur in such a manner that a superior
portion of the intestine is telescoped into an inferior one, toward
the anus (descending form).   In extremely rare cases an inferior
section of the intestine is sheathed into a superior one (toward the
mouth (ascending form).   The portion called the apex or head
is always formed by the same part of the intestine.   The advance of the invagination occurs at the expense of the external
sheath, vagina, or intussuscipiens, which continually rolls itself
over the intussusceptum.   Only in the ileocolic invagination does
the neck or head itself advance, and in this type alone is the apex
composed of different portions of the intestine as the invagination
advances.

Physiological (Nothnagel) or Agonal Form (Leichtenstern) of Invagination.

This very probably always occurs after death, during the agony,
its origin depending on the fact that one part of the intestine dies
sooner than other parts, thereby making it possible that a portion
of the bowel which is still contractile may become invaginated into
one which is already paralyzed.   At autopsies they may be found
at three to five different places in the same subject.   They occur in
the small intestine almost without exception, and rarely exceed 2
inches (about 5 cm. in length).   They are most frequently found in
the bodies of children, and are rare in adults.   They may be either
ascending or descending, and are distinguished from the pathological or inflammatory forms by non-inclusion of the mesentery
and by absence of anatomical changes in the intestinal wall and
peritoneum.   Very slight traction suffices to draw them out.

Figure 5, page 247, represents this form of invagination.

Pathological Invagination (Nothnagel). Vital, Persistent, or Inflammatory Form (Leichtenstern). Obstructive Form (Treves).

This is the type that concerns us most, clinically. As a rule, it occurs singly, and in any part of the intestine. This form may reach considerable length of invaginated portion, and is, as a rule, always a descending invagination. Leichtenstern found but eight ascending pathological invaginations among 593 cases. Even these eight cases are not free from objection, since Leichtenstern remarks that they had developed at a time when the normal peristalsis was arrested and antiperistalsis had developed as a result of peritonitis and paralysis of a considerable district of the intestine. Besnier, Hektoen, Jones, and d'Arcy Power have described ascending pathological invaginations. Invaginations occur with greatest facility in the movable portions of the bowel, those which possess a mesentery. This mesentery is drawn into the invagination, and, being compressed, grave circulatory disturbances develop as a result of the obliteration, first of the veins, and later on of the arteries, by compression. Serous transudation soon invades the walls of the intussusceptum, and hemorrhages into the lumen occur. If the compression of the arteries is advanced, gangrene may develop, and if a well-defined line of demarcation has formed, a kind of spontaneous cure has been known to occur by sequestration of the invaginated portion. A large number of terms have been invented to designate the different forms of invaginations as they occur in various parts of the intestine.

Terminology.

If a portion of the intestine is invaginated into another portion of the same section of the bowel, bearing the same name, the whole invagination is designated by the name of that particular district of the intestine. For instance, an invagination of the duodenum into itself is called a "*duodenalis.*" One of the jejunum into itself is termed a "*jejunalis.*" If, however, one section of the bowel is invaginated into another section, the abnormality is designated by the conjoint name of the two sections ; for example, an invagination of the duodenum into the jejunum is called a "*duodeno-jejunalis.*" An invagination of the jejunum into the ileum is termed a "*jejuno-*

iliaca.'' Sometimes a portion of the bowel which is invaginated into another portion of its own section may again become ensheathed into a still lower adjoining section. This is what occurs, for example, when the ileum, after it is invaginated upon itself, is telescoped into the colon, through the ileocecal valve. This intussusception is called the *"iliaca-ileocolica."* The latter is the most complicated of all invaginations. All types in which the ileum and cecum are simultaneously involved are grouped under the name of "ileocecalis." The typical form of this is that in which the ileum and cecum are invaginated into the colon in such a manner that the ileocecal valve precedes as the apex of the intusssusceptum. The innermost cylinder is formed by the ileum, and the vagina or sheath is formed by the colon. The apex of the whole invagination is the ileocecal opening, including the valve. This form (the ileocecalis) is divided into two subtypes—(*a*) the "ileocolica" and (*b*) "iliaca-ileocolica." The ordinary ileocecalis has just been described. The ileocolica differs from it in that the valve does not form the apex of the intussusceptum, but the lower end of the ileum projects through the valve into the colon. The valve itself and the cecum remain at first in their normal position. If this invagination advances still further, the colon and the cecum are inverted, and become the middle cylinder. In this form, the apex is always formed by the prolapsed ileum. The first step of this type of invagination, where the ileum simply prolapses through the ileocecal valve into the colon, leads to an adhesive inflammation between these two cylinders, which is a necessary condition to the subsequent inversion of the cecum and colon, and their becoming the middle cylinder. The ileocecalis is the type which may develop into the largest dimensions. It may extend through the entire colon as well as sigmoid and rectum, and appear through the sphincter at the anus, the ileocecal valve all the time forming the apex.

All these forms may be arranged in the following three great groups :

I. *Enteric invagination*, in which small intestine is invaginated by small intestine.

II. *Colic invagination*, in which large intestine is invaginated by large intestine.

III. *Ileocecal invagination*, in which small intestine is invaginated by the colon.

Age.

The years of early childhood are those in which invaginations occur most frequently. Thirty-four per cent. of the cases collected by Fitz were under the age of one year, and 56 per cent. under the age of ten years. His statistics (*l. c.*, p. 15) include 91 cases, 51 of which occurred prior to the tenth year. This agrees fairly well with the statistics of Leichtenstern, who collected 593 cases, 134 of which occurred in the first year of life. Of these, 80 occurred from the fourth to the sixth month of life. The second to the fifth year included 49 cases of invagination. Pilz ("Jahrbuch f. Kinder-heilkunde," N. F., Bd. III, H. 1) collected 163 cases in children. Of these, 91 occurred in the first year of life. From the second to the fourteenth year there were 71 cases. Those that occurred in the first year of life were distributed as follows : Under two months, 3 cases; three months, 10 cases ; from the fourth to the sixth month, 55 cases ; from the seventh to the twelfth month, 23 cases. All the cases of intestinal obstruction that occurred in children under one year, in Chas. L. Gibson's table (*l. c.*, p. 490), were intus-susceptions. Widerhofer collected 58 cases, of which 32 occurred in the first year of life, and 11 from the second to the tenth year.

Sex.

At all ages the male sex exceeds the female as far as the relative occurrence of this abnormality is concerned. In 79 cases collected by Fitz, 52 were among males and 27 among females. Raffinesque, however, among 71 cases of the chronic form, had 38 men and 33 women. Chas. L. Gibson's statistics (*l. c.*) show that 72 per cent. of the cases of intussusception occurred in males, and 28 per cent. in females.

Pathogenesis.

It is probable that almost every experimenter in physiology who has worked on the abdomen of living rabbits and guinea-pigs has observed the formation and resolution of invaginations. The first physiologists to make note of this observation was Albrecht von Haller. Nothnagel also mentions having observed the formation and resolution of invaginations in the intestines of rabbits when the entire abdomen was submerged in warm physiological salt solution.

Some of them lasted for ten minutes. They originate by the telescoping of a strongly contracted part of the intestine into one that has remained quiescent and relaxed. Nothnagel ("Zeitschr. f. klin. Med.," 1882) and Senn ("Annals of Surgery," 1888, VII, 4) have conducted exact experiments throwing light upon the method of production of invagination. The formation of this condition in guinea-pigs seems to have a physiological character, and Nothnagel has suggested that also in the normal human intestine such small invaginations may form and become resolved spontaneously, without giving rise to disturbances. Cruveilhier, Raffinesque, and Treves also favor the view of momentary (transient) invaginations in the human being. Cruveilhier explains the transient but very sharp attacks of colic which occur after the ingestion of especially indigestible food by assuming a momentary formation of invaginations. Joseph Bell (cited from Nothnagel, *l. c.*), on performing a laparotomy for internal incarceration, found an invagination 10 cm. (about 4 inches) long on opening the abdomen. It was easily replaced. The question arises, "How is a severe pathological form of invagination developed from a physiological one?" There are two principal views which conflict in explanation of this question. They may be called the theory of invagination by paralysis, and that of invagination by spasm of the intestine. The former is held by Leichtenstern. He assumes a paresis of a limited portion of the intestine, and during this relaxed and helpless state, any accidental, intense peristalsis may supply the force for telescoping a normally contractile portion of the intestine into the paralytic portion. Nothnagel (*l. c.*) favors the view of production of invagination by a spasmodic contraction of the intestine. Whenever a tetanic contraction of a limited portion of the bowel was produced by the application of the faradic current, a small invagination developed at the boundary between the powerfully contracted and the normal intestine. This invagination is not formed, as some observers state, by the pushing of the contracted portion into the passive portion, but by the arching over of the normal intestine onto and around the end of the contracted district. The further development of the invagination occurs exclusively at the expense of those parts of the bowel from the sheath toward the anus. The contracted portion which develops below the point of irritation becomes the entering cylinder of the intussusceptum. The returning cylinder and the intussuscipiens are formed by the passive intestine lower down, which is drawn over the contracted part of the longitudinal muscular fibers. The intestine lying above the tetanic contracture does not take any part in the formation of the invagination. The growth of invagination at the expense of intestinal districts lying always toward the anus of the contracture—that is, at the expense of the sheath—makes it possible that the intestinal segments which have formed the original starting-point always remain at the apex or point. This is the explanation of the fact observed in the ileocecalis, namely, that the ileocecal valve may appear at the anus, and the

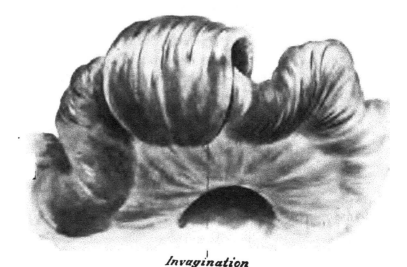

Invagination

FIG. 6.—EXTERIOR OF INVAGINATION.—(*From preparation in Anatomical Laboratory, University of Maryland.*)

entire large intestine be telescoped upon itself. But the ileum, excepting the lower portion, which is primarily contracted, is entirely outside of the invagination. The stimulus or irritant for the further pathological contractions which draw the lower segments of the intestine over the intussusceptum is, according to Nothnagel, furnished by the incarcerated head of the invagination. This head, which constitutes a thickening formed by the entering and returning layers of the invagination, constitutes the foreign body, which is treated like any other of the intestinal contents—that is, the peristalsis tends to propagate it downward. But it is necessary to emphasize once more that the originally contracted portion is not shot into the lower intestine from above downward by the peristalsis; on the contrary, the intestinal segment below the point of spastic constriction is drawn upward over this tetanic portion by the contraction of the longitudinal muscular fibers. Cruveilhier, Brinton, Bristow, Dance, Raffinesque, and Treves have accepted these interpretations of Nothnagel, and even Leichtenstern, while still adhering to his hypothesis of a primary paresis as an inciting factor in the production of certain invaginations, accepts a kind of tenesmic spasm of the sphincter of the ileocecal orifice as explanation of the most frequent form of invagination (44 per cent. of the cases)—the ileocecalis. The type known as ileocolica, where the large portion of the ileum is wedged through the ileocecal valve into the colon, is in its incipiency a genuine prolapse of the ileum into the colon, according to Leichtenstern. A similar condition exists at the end of the digestive tract, where the rectum has been found prolapsed through the anus. Whilst Nothnagel does not deny the possibility of origin of invagination from paralysis of a limited intestinal district, he could never produce an invagination experimentally by causing a circumscribed intestinal paralysis.

A third hypothesis attempting an explanation of the origin of invagination does not recognize either spasm or paresis as a necessary etiological factor, but conceives invagination to be a purely mechanical process. This is the theory of Besnier ("Des étranglements internes de l'intestin," Paris, 1860), who conceives invagination to come about in the following way: If a certain district of the intestine undergoes a moderately strong contraction whilst gravid ingesta accidentally make the district immediately above the contracted portion heavier than usual, the latter may slip or be pushed into the intestine immediately below it.

Etiology.

D'Arcy Power has studied the mechanism of the most frequent of all invaginations—the ileocecal type—experimentally, in animals, by causing violent intestinal paralysis with turpeth mineral. The peristaltic wave coming from the ileum becomes arrested at the ileocecal valve and a new active peristalsis begins at this place. This ending of the ileac peristalsis and beginning of the colon peristalsis does not occur simultaneously, and according to the conception of D'Arcy Power ("Virchow-Kirsch Jahresberichte," 1886), the invagination is brought about in such a manner that the cecum actually swallows or gulps up the ileum. The ileocolic invagination, where the ileum passes through the ileocecal valve into the colon without involving the valve, is extremely rare. The intussusceptum here is formed by the ileum, and the valve and cecum are not taken along until the invagination reaches extremely advanced degrees.

The direct causes of invagination may be any of the following conditions : neoplasms of the intestinal wall, both benign and malignant, polypi, as well as carcinomas and sarcomas, foreign bodies, ulcers, strictures, chronic enteritis, dysentery, which run their course with stormy peristalsis, traumas and violent agitation or concussion of the body. Weak, emaciated individuals are predisposed to this pathological condition. As it occurs sometimes in a number of individuals of the same family, similar to hernias, it is supposed that there is a hereditary factor which is active in the production of this condition. H. Zeidler ("Mittheil. a. d. Grenzgebieten und Chir.," Bd. v, S. 593) has reported two cases in which the invagination was caused by a polypoid form of neoplasm. N. Petroff ("Arbeit d. Gesellschaft Russischer Aerzte," January, 1896) has reported a case of multiple gastric and intestinal polypi which seemed to involve the entire gastro-intestinal tract. Benign tumors or polypi, when they cause an invagination, usually have their seat in the lower ileum, and the invagination resulting is generally. an ileocecalis. Strange to say, the carcinomas rarely cause invaginations, but fibromas, lipomas, adenomas, and myomas do so more frequently. Nothnagel looks upon the causation of an invagination by a polypus as confirming his view of an etiological spastic contraction. He believes that the presence of a polypus may evoke a vehement peristalsis with intestinal constriction, leading to formation of an invagination, according to his conception. He explains the rarity of invaginations in association with enterostenosis and carcinoma by the changes which are caused in the intestinal tube in these processes. The stenosis dilates and hypertrophies the intestinal wall,—frequently it is adherent in addition,—and for these reasons can not be embraced and converted into an intussusceptum by the lower lying districts. The carcinoma, especially the scirrhus, changes the entire region it involves into a rigid cylinder, which can not become an intussusceptum for the same reasons.   Carcinomas give rise to invaginations only under rare conditions, especially when they have their seat at the ileocecal valve (one case operated by Czerny).   The immediate causes in 593 cases published by Leichtenstern (" Prager Vierteljahresschr., Bd. CXVIII) were assigned as follows :

1. Absence of every statement of anamnesis, ...	267 cases.
2. Sudden development in healthy individuals, ...	111 "
3. Intestinal polypi, ...	30 "
4. Carcinomas and strictures of the intestine, ...	6 "
5. Preceding diarrheas, ...	21 "
6. Other symptoms of abnormal intestinal functions, ...	25 "
7. Ingesta, ...	28 "
8. Contusions of the abdomen, ...	14 "
9. Concussion of the body, ...	12 "
10. Invagination during pregnancy or child-bearing, ...	7 "
11. Catching cold, ...	6 "
12. Invagination after various acute and chronic diseases or after different and etiologically doubtful factors, . . .	66 "
Total, ...	593 cases.

Fitz (*l. c.*) states that the exciting causes were absent in 42 cases, and the following were the possible causes in 45 cases :

Diarrhea, ...	13 cases.
Habitual constipation, ...	12 "
Protracted abdominal pain, ...	7 "
Indigestible diet, ...	6 "
Violent exertion, ...	4 "
Injury, ...	3 "
Total, ...	45 cases.

Individual cases occurred in the course of typhoid fever, pregnancy, variola, and gastro-enteritis after the use of cathartics and after an operation for incarcerated hernia ; in all, six cases.

Symptomatology.

The principal symptoms of intussusception, ranged in the order of their importance and frequency of occurrence, are the following : (1) Abdominal pain, (2) nausea and vomiting, (3) tumor, (4) hemorrhagic evacuations, (5) meteorism, (6) tenesmus.   The relative frequency of these symptoms in 180 cases of invagination and intussusception, of which I found a record in literature, was as follows :

Abdominal pain, ...	84 per cent.
Nausea and vomiting, ...	72 "
Tumor, ...	70 "
Hemorrhagic evacuations, ...	65 --
Meteorism, ...	36 --
Tenesmus, ...	34 --

The date of the appearance of these principal symptoms of intussusception is represented in the following table (Fitz, *l. c.*, p. 16) :

DATE.	PAIN.	NAUSEA OR VOMITING.	METEORISM.	TUMOR. ABDOMEN.	TUMOR. RECTUM.	BLOODY STOOLS.	TENESMUS.
First day, ...	61	51	1	9	10	32	15
Second day, ...	2	4	2	12	8	7	4
Third day, ...	1	3	8	8	7	6	5
Fourth day, ...	1	3	8	2	3	3	. .
Fifth day, ...	. .	1	4	. .	2	1	2
Sixth day, ...	. .	. .	3	3	4	3	3
Later or not given, . . .	. .	4	5	5	6	4	4
Total number of cases, . .	65	66	31	39	40	56	33

These symptoms are largely due to the circulatory disturbances as a consequence of the incarceration and compression of the mesentery. In the so-called physiological invagination the mesentery is not incarcerated, but in the pathological invagination we are confronted with the same processes as in strangulations. According to the degree in which the mesentery participates in the invagination, this may present either the phenomena of strangulation or those of simple obturation. The mesentery is usually caught between the entering and returning cylinders of the intussusceptum; the further the invagination progresses, the greater will be the traction upon the mesentery, which forms an extended wedge, the apex of which is at the point of the intussusceptum, and the basis at the neck of the invagination. In the so-called ileocecal invagination, in which the ileocecal valve occasionally projects from the anus, the intestine, according to Treves, describes an arc in its invagination from the cecum to the anus. The center of this circle or arc

is the root or attachment of the mesentery, and the radius is the
mesentery itself.   The traction which is exerted upon the intussusceptum by the mesentery naturally produces a curve in the invaginated portion of the intestine, which is directed with its concavity
toward the attachment of the mesentery.   The sheath is not curved
as much as the intussusceptum.   This difference in the degree of
traction made upon the intussusceptum and the intussuscipiens,
being stronger upon the former, causes a divergence of the axes of
these two cylinders.   The mouth of the cylinders composing the
intussusceptum can not open straight in the direction of the intestinal lumen, but it is drawn against the wall of the vagina or sheath.
This evidently must make the intestinal impermeability complete.

The veins being more compressible than the arteries, a bluish-red
venous hyperemia of the mesentery and intussusceptum results, with
progressive stagnation and edema; hemorrhages and serous transudations occur into the parenchyma of the intestinal wall, as well as upon
the surface.   The swelling and induration are more pronounced along
the convexity than along the concavity of the invagination, and the
apex of the intussusceptum becomes transformed into a thickened
tumor with a central opening of the lumen, which has been compared
to the os uteri.   A certain degree of this passive hyperemia and
edematous swelling may be recovered from, and the permeability
of the intestine may be restored for liquid foods at least; but if
they exceed a certain limit, absolute interruption of arterial and
venous circulation and gangrene ensue.   According to Leichtenstern and Nothnagel, gangrene occurs most often in the acute
cases which run a rapid course.   According to Leichtenstern, it
occurred 94 times before the fourth week in 125 cases; after the
sixth month it only occurred 3 times.

It happens, sometimes, in the ileocecal invagination, that the
internal ileum cylinder sequestrates before the middle or colon
cylinder, after a previous peritonitic adhesion at the neck of the
invagination.   When this occurs, the mucosa of the sequestrated
ileum is directed toward the mucosa of the vagina or sheath, and
in this inverted position, the inner side turned toward the exterior,
the ileum is discharged, after the middle cylinder has also been
loosened by gangrene.

The section of the intestine above the invagination is altered only in the chronic forms, when it develops the hypertrophy and dilation, and sometimes decubital ulceration, that are consequent upon chronic intestinal stenosis. The place at which the sequestration has taken place, at the neck of the invagination, naturally continues in a state of ulceration, which may continue, in fortunate cases, to heal and form a circular cicatrix. In this way invagination which has healed spontaneously may give rise to an enterostenosis; for not only does the cicatrix form an internal stricture, but there is, as a rule, an adhesive peritonitis established around the neck.

The following compilation from Gould and Pyle's "Anomalies and Curiosities of Medicine" will give an idea of the various lengths of intestine that may be sequestrated:

Lobstein ("Traité d'anatomie pathologique," Paris, 1829) mentions a peasant woman of about thirty who was suddenly seized with an attack of intussusception of the bowel, and was apparently in a moribund condition when she had a copious stool, in which she evacuated three feet of the bowel with the mesentery attached. The woman recovered, but died five months later from a second attack of intussusception, the ileum rupturing and peritonitis ensuing. There is a record in this country ("Amer. Jour. of the Med. Sci.," Philadelphia, 1846) of a woman of forty-five who discharged 44 inches of intestine, and who survived for forty-two days. The autopsy showed the sigmoid flexure gone, and from the head of the cecum to the termination the colon measured only 14 inches. Vater ("Philosophical Transactions of the Royal Society of London," 1719–33) gives a history of a penetrating abdominal wound in which a portion of the colon hung from the wound during fourteen years, forming an artificial anus.

Among others mentioning considerable sloughing of intestine following intussusception, and usually with complete subsequent recovery, are Bare ("Amer. Jour. of the Med. Sci.," Philadelphia, 1863), 13 inches of the ileum; Blackton ("Med. Times and Gaz.," London, 1853), 9 inches; Bower ("Annals of Medicine," Edinburgh, 1803), 14 inches; Dawson ("Western Jour. of Med. and Surg.," Louisville, Kentucky, 1840), 29 inches; Sheldon ("Med. Times," London, 1850), 4½ feet; Stanley (Gould and Pyle's "Anomalies and Curiosities of Medicine"), 3 feet; Tremaine ("Canada Med. and Surg. Jour.," Montreal, 1879), 17 inches; Grossoli

("Spallanzani (Lo)," Modena, 1875), 40 cm.; and Cruveilhier (cited by Nothnagel, *l. c.*), 3 meters. Osler ("Practice of Medicine") refers to a specimen of sequestrated invagination 17 inches long in the Museum of McGill University.

The onset of the symptoms enumerated is, as a rule, very sudden, and the attack strikes the individual in the midst of perfect health, as a rule. Only in rare instances have disturbances of the intestinal functions been reported as preceding it. Isolated cases are on record where a trauma striking the abdomen was accused as the direct cause. The onset is described in some cases as striking the sufferer during sleep and as befalling nursing children whilst they were being suckled. After the first severe pain, which is of a colicky character, nausea and vomiting set in; thereupon there are one or more offensive evacuations. Following upon these we are confronted with diarrheic stools which may consist of mucus, blood and mucus, or pure blood, or any of these three forms of stool with an admixture of ingesta. In connection with these evacuations there may or may not be tenesmus. The pulse is rapid and compressible. On the third day, as a rule, phenomena of collapse are evident; vomiting, which may have ceased, may return and even become stercoraceous. The stools contain only blood and mucus by this time. In grave cases, especially in children, death occurs in this state of collapse. The abdomen presents in many cases the characteristic tumor, but meteorism is observed in only about one-third of all cases. Other clinical types present a stormy onset, after which the violent symptoms abate, and the practitioner is confronted with the signs and symptoms of chronic enterostenosis. Invaginations which involve the small intestine, the ileac and the ileocecal form, as a rule set in vehemently and abruptly, whilst those in which the colon or rectum alone is involved exhibit a more gradual development. The more acute cases may terminate in temporary spontaneous cure by sequestration of the intussusceptum or in death from strangulation. The slower types terminate fatally also by gradual emaciation and exhaustion, in consequence of pain, loss of sleep, and malnutrition.

Individual Symptoms.

Abdominal Pain.—This is the first symptom of acute invagination. It attacks the sufferer without the slightest premonition. The character of the pain is colicky ; it may be continuous or intermittent. As a rule it is uninterrupted at the onset, and becomes slightly intermittent later on. It is located in various abdominal regions, according to the character of the intussusception. It may be located at the navel, in the right or the left iliac fossa, or in the epigastrium. When it is located in the right iliac fossa it may lead to a diagnosis of appendicitis, perityphlitis, typhlitis, or enteric fever. The seat of the pain in rectal and colicorectal varieties was referred to the left iliac fossa. Its position at the umbilicus usually suggests the small intestine as the seat of the invagination. If the invagination becomes chronic, pains of a spasmodic character torment the unfortunate sufferers for months, with remission at intervals lasting from one to three days. Sometimes there are continuous periods of pain lasting for a week, which are interrupted by one or two days of rest. In children it is impossible to ascertain any definite abdominal region as the seat of the distress, but in adults it is occasionally possible to limit the affected region with accuracy. They generally define the right iliac region as the one most intensely painful, which corresponds to the seat of the ileocecal invagination. In chronic invagination visible peristalsis increasing to intestinal stiffening or plastic rigidity may be observed, caused by the hypertrophied intestinal walls above the invagination.

Nausea and Vomiting.—Nausea and vomiting set in either simultaneously with the pain or immediately after it. Distinction must be made between the ordinary vomiting of ingesta and characteristic fecal vomiting. The latter only very exceptionally occurs on the first day in this form of obstruction. Ordinary vomiting occurred on the first day of the attack in nearly nine-tenths of the cases in which any definite date could be fixed by Fitz. It is more of a constant symptom in children, and may at times be absent in adults. Among 93 cases of intussusception collected by Fitz, fecal vomit was noted in only 12 cases, and it appeared on or after the fourth day in all but two of these. The vomiting of ingesta and intestinal secretions, as it occurs on the first day in the great majority of cases, may be regarded as a reflex phenomenon, analogous to the reflex vomiting which has been described as marking the onset of other acute intestinal diseases, especially the strangulations. It may be continuous or occur at intervals. The higher up in the intestinal canal the invagination has occurred, the more prompt and constant will be the onset of emesis. The lower down in the intestinal canal the invagination takes its origin, the more likely is this vomiting to be absent as an initial symptom. Not only does it depend upon the seat of the invagination, but also upon the degree of completeness of obstruction, the extent to which the mesentery is incarcerated and compressed. Invaginations involving the colon alone are, as a rule, characterized by a relatively mild course. Those involving the ileum, ileum and cecum, or ileum and colon present the severest vomiting and the most unfavorable prognosis. When the invagination involves only the colon, it does not cause vomiting on the first day, as a rule. This symptom may, under that condition, be delayed to the third or fourth day, and cases are on record where it did not show itself until the fourteenth day. The variable intensity of the vomit, or its cessation for a day or two, does not justify the prediction of a favorable termination. There are records of fatal cases with a history of cessation of vomiting for two or three days. Occasionally this form of emesis is accompanied by a torturing singultus. In acute cases which later become chronic it shows itself as an initial symptom, but later on becomes less and less constant, or does not return at all, until the recovery or fatal termination. If, however, these chronic types become complicated by an absolute occlusion or a secondary peritonitis, the vomiting returns.

Nature of the Vomit.—The substances vomited consist of mucus, gastric and duodenal contents, and bile. It becomes fecal in one-eighth of all the acute cases in the reports of which I could find a record of this symptom. According to the statistics of Raffinesque (*l. c.*), fecal vomit occurred in only 3 of 40 chronic cases.

Tumor.—The tumor of invaginations is the most important physical sign from the diagnostic standpoint. It differs in important features from all other varieties of tumors that are observed in the abdominal cavity. In 610 reports of cases of invaginations of all kinds in which I found a statement concerning this sign, it was present in 308. In 84 chronic invaginations recorded in American and foreign literature, the tumor was present in 40 cases. In 433 invaginations of all kinds, collected by Leichtenstern, tumor was

present in 222.   Raffinesque found it in 24 of 53 chronic invaginations.   In very small invaginations, involving but a short distance
of the intestine, and not much of the mesentery, no tumor can be
palpated, because none is formed.   But there are other cases in
which a tumor does actually exist, but it can not be palpated, this
being prevented by great thickness or tension in the abdominal wall,
or because the tumor is covered by the liver, ribs, or tympanitic intestinal loops.   It is a more constant sign in children.   The size varies
from that of a hen's egg to that of the forearm of an adult.   Treves
(*l. c.*) gives warning that the absence of tumor should never be positively stated until the abdomen has been palpated and thoroughly examined during a paroxysm of pain, for the tumor of invagination may
occasionally disappear during the relaxation.   But during the colicky
pains, if it is present at all, it can be discerned with the greatest dis-
tinctness.   During palpation it may appear smaller than it really is,
because it may be partly hidden under the right or left hypochondrium.   But occasionally it appears larger than it really is, because
the volume of the fecal accumulation above it is added to the bulk
of the tumor during palpation.   In Treves' statistics of 61 cases of
invagination tumor, it was found only in the abdomen in 23 cases,
only in the rectum in 21 cases.   In no case should it be omitted to
palpate through the rectum, and in females through the vagina and
abdomen bimanually.   One of the most characteristic features of an
invagination tumor is that its resistance changes within a short period
of time in one and the same case.   Whilst it never feels as hard as
a carcinoma, yet it presents a considerable feeling of density.   In
two of the cases which I could observe in private practice, during
1901, I detected the tumor during a paroxysm of pain, and keeping my fingers upon it, I could feel how it relaxed and almost
vanished from touch, so that I imagined it had slipped from my
grasp, and began to palpate for it elsewhere with the right hand,
keeping the left on the spot where I had first perceived the tumor,
when another paroxysm of pain reproduced it in the identical position in which I had last felt it.

The location of the tumor is variable.   According to the table of
Leichtenstern, the most frequent seat is the region of the sigmoid
flexure ; the locations next in frequency may be arranged in the following order : (2) tumor projecting from the anus, (3) in the rectum,

(4) in the region of the cecum, (5) in the descending colon, (6) in the transverse colon, (7) in the ascending colon, and (8) in the hypogastrium. This latter is the rarest location of all, and is only noticed in invaginations of the ileum. When a tumor is prolapsed from the anus—ileocecal or colic invagination—the apex presents the opening of the ileocecal valve, and frequently a second opening, that of the appendix, can be made out adjacent to it. In cases where the tumor is palpable in the rectum by the finger, it gives an impression similar to the uterine cervix. Invagination tumors are relatively very movable, though in rare cases with a chronic course they may become fixed and immovable by adhesions. Unless bound down in this manner, the invagination tumor is capable of being moved around by the hand to a considerable extent, or it may even apparently migrate of its own accord. That is, a tumor which has been localized in the cecum may in twenty-four hours be palpated in the transverse colon or sigmoid flexure. It may even appear at the anus. This outward progress of tumors has been observed in acute as well as chronic invaginations, and in the ileocecal invagination of children the progress may be so rapid that a cecal tumor may be palpable in the rectum after twenty-four hours. This movability of invagination tumors, both the locomotion caused by the progress of the intussusception, as well as the movability which can be imparted to it by the hand, is sufficient proof that the location of the tumor can not be made use of diagnostically for the determination of the anatomical situation of the section of the intestine that is involved. A so-called retrogressive or backward locomotion of the tumor is also observed, either under the influence of therapeutic measures (large enemata) or because of spontaneous resolution of the intussusception. In connection with invagination tumors that have become stationary and chronic, a kind of chronic enterostenosis develops in the suprastenotic loops, and augmented peristalsis, as well as occasional plastic erection of intestinal loops, is observed as a result of this condition.

Evacuations.—The evacuations from the rectum in invaginations are of the greatest importance for the diagnosis. It is also very important that we should distinguish between acute and chronic cases in a description of the rectal discharges. Whilst we have persistent obstipation in acute cases, the condition of the evacuations may be most variable in the chronic type. In the acute forms the evacuations do not cease at once ; one or two fecal movements which evacuate the intestinal contents below the point of obstruction occur before the complete suppression of the stool. In acute invaginations we have stool suppression or obstipation, and nevertheless we have evacuation ; that is, there is no discharge of feces after the section of the bowel below the intussusception has been emptied, but there are frequent discharges of blood and mucus. The normal intestinal contents and the intestinal flatus are no longer discharged ; the passage from above is completely blocked ; but the various layers of the intussusceptum, altered by the passive hyperemia and transudations, which I have described in previous paragraphs, furnish pathological intestinal contents, consisting almost exclusively of blood, serum, and mucus. Hemorrhagic evacuations represent one of the most constant symptoms of invagination. They occur in 80 per cent. of all acute cases, and in invaginations of all descriptions and locations. They are most constant in the ileocolic and rarest in the rectal type. The amount of blood lost is variable ; sometimes the stools are largely mucus and only streaked with blood. At other times the hemorrhages are so profuse as to be the direct cause of death. There are, however, rare cases in which there is no absolute blockage for the passage of feces. In such cases we may have the typical appearances of dysentery, stools consisting of feces, blood, and mucus. The typical evacuations of intussusceptions, however, should contain no feces, but only blood, serum, and mucus. In those rare cases in which the stenosis caused by the intussusception is not absolute, small amounts of fecal matter may constitute an admixture of the stools, which may number ten to twenty in twenty-four hours. When the process assumes a subacute type, the hemorrhagic evacuations may cease, transiently or permanently. But when the expulsion of sequestrated gangrenous intussusception takes place, bloody evacuations will begin again and be characterized by an indescribably offensive odor (the odor of carrion).

Character of Evacuations in Chronic Invaginations.—The only characteristic (if it may be so called) of the stools of chronic invagination is their exceeding variability (Treves). In 140 cases of chronic invagination in which I could find any reference to the character of the stools, the following results could be tabulated: Normal stool, 20; diarrhea predominating, 49; constipation predominating, 36; diarrhea and constipation alternating, 35. In chronic forms there may also be blood in the evacuations; at least hemorrhagic stools are found much more often in this form than in any other form of chronic enterostenoses. It should be emphasized, however, that the stenosis is not absolute in chronic invaginations. Laxatives are, as a rule, capable of producing bowel movements.

Meteorism.—The tympanitic distention of the abdomen depends upon the degree of obstruction of the intestinal lumen, upon the seat of the invagination, and upon the presence or absence of diarrhea. It occurred in about 36 per cent. of the cases I have collected from literature.

Tenesmus.—Tenesmus was present in about one-third of the cases collected by the author. It was severer in children, often leading to paralysis of the sphincters, and can be stated to be generally severer the lower down in the intestinal canal the invagination has taken place.

The Condition of the Abdomen.—Aside from the comparatively rare tympanitic distention already spoken of, there are no characteristic symptoms or signs recognizable on the abdomen superficially. In the older literature of the subject one meets with the description of a depression in the right iliac fossa, which was called the "signe de Dance." Raffinesque mentions it only twice in 53 chronic invaginations. It therefore can have little diagnostic significance.

Fever.—Fever occurs in about one-third of all the cases of invagination in which this symptom is referred to. In many of the reports on this subject no mention is made of this symptom. It is natural that we should expect fever when peritonitic inflammation, rupture of the intestine, etc., have developed.

Clinical History.

Experience teaches that the fatal termination is the most frequent, and therefore the prognosis, generally speaking, is grave. Notwithstanding, there are undoubted resolutions and recoveries of invagination. These occur mainly in adults, and are occasionally entirely independent of treatment. There are cases of complete restitution to integrity, actual spontaneous cures, where no firmer peritonitic adhesions had developed. Nothnagel (*l. c.*, p. 316) cites the case of a man fifty years old who had a typical acute attack of invagination in April, 1892, from which he recovered in June of the same year without operation. He then enjoyed one and one-fourth years of excellent health. In November, 1893, his former complaints returned. On examination he presented the classical picture of invagination tumor in the transverse colon—intensified peristalsis, plastic rigidity of the loops of small intestine, and attacks of colic and vomiting. He was eventually operated, and a typical ileocecal invagination, at the apex of which there was an intestinal polypus, was discovered. Every trace of peritonitis was absent; the two serous surfaces were not agglutinated, and the invagination could be drawn asunder readily. This case is remarkable because of its long duration and the spontaneous resolution of the invagination of the first period,—April to June, 1892,—for Nothnagel believes that the identical condition was present during the first period that was found at the operation. The course of the disease is different in the two forms, the acute and chronic. Raffinesque distinguishes three groups of acute cases: (1) The peracute, or intensely acute, in which a fatal termination occurs in the first twenty-four hours; (2) the acute cases with a duration of one week; (3) the subacute cases, running a course of about four weeks. In 51 cases tabulated by Fitz, 16 recovered and 35 died. Of those that terminated fatally, death occurred before the sixth day or within the first week in 19 cases. The peracute type is the rarest. In 269 cases of Leichtenstern's table there are only 5 of this form, 4 of which occurred during the first year of life, and 1 in an adult. The cases of the acute type—those lasting about a week—are also predominantly made up of children during the first year of life. The mortality was 80 per cent. The subacute cases, lasting from two to four weeks, include prevailingly persons over ten years of age. Most of the so-called spontaneous recoveries are found in this group. The chronic cases are, again, very unfavorable in their prognosis.

Cause of Death.

In the peracute and acute cases death is due to shock and collapse, caused by the same factors which I have described in the chapter on Strangulations and Internal Incarcerations. The terrible effect of the overwhelming pain can be more readily understood when we reflect that these cases are mostly children. The next most frequent cause of death is conditioned by the results of the intestinal occlusion, which have already been described; viz., traction upon the point or apex of the intussusceptum, pulling it against the sheath or vagina, angular kinking of the intussusceptum by traction upon the mesentery, congestion and tumefaction of the intussusceptum. Naturally, these conditions occur mostly in the acute and subacute types; they are rare in the protracted cases. A third fatal complication causing death is produced by gangrene and the discharge of the sequestrated intussusceptum. Naturally, if the sequestration occurs before adequate adhesive agglutination has occurred around the neck of the intussusceptum, a tear will occur and open the peritoneum, when the intussusceptum is expelled; the result is a fatal peritonitis. The sequestration occurs in the first week in children, and in the second week in the majority of cases of adults. Peritonitis may occur without perforation; it is then caused by an extension of the gangrenous process before the expulsion of the intussusceptum. Sometimes a septic process starts (phlebitis in the mesenteric veins, thrombosis, encapsulated peritonitic abscesses) after the intussusceptum has been discharged. In one of my cases death occurred two months after the spontaneous discharge of an intussusceptum, and at the autopsy an ulcerating surface was found in the intestine, which had led to a minute perforation and septic peritonitis. After the sequestration profuse diarrhea, which could not be controlled by our dietetic and medicinal methods, was continuous up to the day of death. Even if such ulcerated surfaces heal, they may result in a cicatricial enterostenosis, or they may continue to destroy the intestinal tissue, and in rare cases penetrate into an artery, causing death by hemorrhage. We unfortunately have no statistics concerning the duration of so-called recoveries after the sequestration of the intussusceptum. One of the necessary conditions to the successful termination of this process is an extensive peritonitic adhesion around the seat of separation. Although the possibility of recovery during this spontaneous discharge of the invaginated portion of the intestine is conceded, it involves such great danger, during the actual process of gangrenous separation and in the complications which may follow, that we are by no means justified in depending upon the occurrence of this phenomenon as a means of cure. My experience has taught me to prefer operation wherever this is permitted. Spontaneous expulsions of invaginations are rare prior to the fifth year, because children of this age have not the strength to endure the suffering for a sufficient length of time to permit of the gangrenous elimination of their invaginated intestine. As regards the occurrence of sequestration in the various locations of invaginations, Leichtenstern's tables give the following information : The ileac invaginations present 61 per cent., the colon invaginations 28 per cent., and the ileocecal invaginations 20 per cent. of sequestrations.

Course of the Chronic Forms.

Chronic forms of invagination develop in two ways : (a) The process begins like an acute type, and, gradually abating, is transformed into a chronic invagination. (b) The invagination begins very slowly ; there are no acute onsets, but a very gradual clandestine development. We have in these conditions only a moderate degree of mesenteric incarceration, which does not lead to the development of gangrene, and which makes it possible that the various parts of the intussusceptum can recover a certain degree of blood supply. All the symptoms and signs that have been mentioned in acute invagination may be present in the chronic form, but they may also be absent or alternate in the most varied manner. The duration may extend for years. Cases are on record of eleven years' standing. The most frequent picture of the chronic type is that of a chronic enterostenosis.

Diagnosis.

Although the subjective and objective signs and symptoms of invagination are more characteristic than those of any other form of intestinal impermeability, the diagnosis is not exactly easy in the majority of cases. The following are the most valuable factors upon which to base a recognition of this abnormality : (1) Sudden onset of intense pains during perfect health. (2) Pains may be continuous or intermittent. (3) Nausea and vomiting, which is fecal in only one-eighth of all acute cases. (4) Tenesmus. Boas (l. c., p. 422) attributes considerable diagnostic importance to this symptom, as the only other form of obstruction in which it occurs is volvulus of the sigmoid flexure, and even there but rarely. (5) Hemorrhagic evacuations consisting of blood and mucus, very rarely diarrhea evacuations containing traces of actual feces. (6) Tumor presenting the characteristics already described. Examination per rectum and vagina. If the tumor can be palpated in the rectum the diagnosis is at once conclusive. (7) Suppression of fecal evacuation and flatus. In exceptional cases slight fecal admixture, even after the first or second fecal stool, which occurs in all cases. (8) Discharge of purulent or gangrenous shreds of tissue. Whilst bloody evacuations may occur in the incarcerations and strangulations, fragments of intestinal tissue are typical for acute invaginations.

Diagnosis of the Chronic Form.—Whilst the diagnosis of the acute form in the majority of cases should be possible, it becomes a matter of great difficulty when we are confronted with chronic forms. According to the statistics of Raffinesque (*l. c.*), a wrong diagnosis was made in 27 of 55 chronic cases. If the tumor of the invagination can be palpated the diagnosis is facilitated. Outside of this the only other factors to which we can attach diagnostic importance are the pain and the visible intestinal contractions which are sometimes intensified to plastic rigidity of the intestinal loops. One-half of all chronic cases present intestinal hemorrhages, which might be available as a diagnostic sign. Taken as a whole, the chronic cases of invagination in the absence of any palpable tumor can be diagnosed if they are seen often, very thoroughly examined, and other abnormal possibilities excluded by logical diagnostic argument.

The **treatment** of invagination will be considered in conjunction with that of other intestinal occlusions.

VOLVULUS AND AXIAL TWISTS OF THE INTESTINE.

The word volvulus comes from the Latin "*volvere*," to roll, and is used to designate a twisting of the intestine either upon itself or upon its mesenteric axis, so as to occlude its lumen. In modern literature on the subject two kinds of intestinal occlusions are included under the term of volvulus : first, that which I have already mentioned—the axial twists ; and, secondly, the intestinal knot formations. These knots should be carefully distinguished from the loop-knot formations caused by the strangulation of an intestinal loop by a pseudo-ligament or peritoneal band. The latter have already been described in the chapter on Strangulation and Incarceration. By knot formation in the present sense is meant the entangling of one intestinal loop by another. The most important forms are the volvulus of the sigmoid flexure, that of the ascending colon, and that of the small intestine. The twist of the sigmoid flexure around its mesenteric axis is by far the most frequent of all forms composing two-thirds of all cases of volvulus,

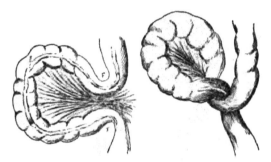

FIG. 7.—VOLVULUS OF SIGMOID FLEXURE.
F, F indicate the fulcrate points, between which the mesocolon is very narrow, thus facilitating the rotation of the abnormally elongated sigmoid flexure.—(*According to Potain.*)

so that it represents the only actual and typical form of this abnormality. The anatomical condition necessary for the development of a volvulus of the sigmoid is an excessive elongation of the sigmoid flexure and its mesentery, which may be either inherited or acquired. More frequently it is an acquired condition. If we have, in addition to this elongation, a very narrow mesentery, there will be two fulcrate points of the elongated sigmoid loop, which will become very closely approximated, and the portion of the mesocolon between them will be reduced to a kind of stem around which the twist of the two limbs of the sigmoid can easily take place. This tendency is pictured in the accompanying illustration. The causes of volvulus are direct and indirect. We have no accurate knowledge concerning the causes that may produce a narrowing of the mesocolon. Of course it is possible that this condition may be congenital, but the most frequent causative factor seems to be habitual constipation. The elongation of the sigmoid and its mesentery is produced by the weight of the accumulated fecal masses. It is conceivable that the persistent irritation of this traction may cause a peritonitis of the mesocolon, eventually resulting in secondary contraction which narrows the so-called mesenteric stem, thereby approximating the beginning and the end of the sigmoid flexure. (See *F*, *F*, in Fig. 7.) The frequency of volvulus in the rural population of Russia is explained by the predominating vegetable diet upon which the inhabitants live (Lingen and Küttner). After these anatomical conditions for the development of volvulus have been brought about, the perfection of the abnormality is caused by any opportune etiological intervention, such as violent bodily exertion, falls, or leaps. It may also be brought about by the burdening of one limb of the extended flexure with feces, as a consequence of which it falls over the other limb. This may also occur as a result of any unusual forcible peristalsis. The following predisposing etiological moments may be enumerated : Accelerated intestinal peristalsis or acute intestinal paralysis, neoplasms, foreign bodies, gall-stones, cicatrices, traumas, laparotomy. The increased intestinal peristalsis is very often caused by powerful drastic purges ; then the two limbs having been thrown upon each other, a rotation occurs of 180°,—in rare instances of 360°,—thus bringing the colon end and the rectal end of the sigmoid in contact. Generally the colon end is brought to lie upon the rectal end. The rotation around the mesenteric axis necessarily brings about a partial rotation of the sigmoid around its own axis, *i. e.*, around the axis of the intestinal loop itself.

In the chapter on Invaginations I referred to certain physiological intussusceptions which might undergo spontaneous resolution. A similar condition of volvulus has been described by Leichtenstern. At a necropsy on a boy eleven years old who had never had constipation, he discovered a chronic axial twist of the sigmoid flexure, with very close approximation of the fulcrate points. When air was injected into the colon limb, the twisted loop unturned itself immediately, but returned into its abnormal position when the blowing in of air was discontinued. This process must have occurred during life every time flatus and fecal masses passed through the sigmoid. This case makes it conceivable that axial twists may become resolved spontaneously. They are probably prevented from doing so by the great weight of the loops in consequence of fecal accumulation or the congestion caused by hyperemia, the formation of transudates, and the distention by gas in the portion that has been twisted off. Whenever a stenosis has occurred by such an axial twist the distention in the higher sections of the colon will prevent a resolution of the volvulus, because it mechanically encroaches upon the intra-abdominal space. Finally, we must assume that the sigmoid, as a result of long-standing constipation and distention, has been reduced to a state of atony. Other rare conditions which prevent an untwisting of a volvulus are compression by convolutions of the ileum, pseudo-ligaments, and peritoneal adhesions. In 1836 Rokitanski devised a scheme of the various forms of intestinal axial twists based on observations made at necropsies ("Oesterreichische med. Jahrbücher," Bd. x, 1836). He distinguished mainly three types of torsions: (1) A section of the intestine undergoes a half or a complete turn around its own longitudinal axis, whereby the opposite walls are approximated and the lumen is obstructed. (2) In this type there is a rotation around the mesenteric axis. The entire mesentery, or a section of it, and also the intestinal loops belonging to it, makes either a semi-rotation, a complete rotation, or several complete rotations around its axis. (3) This includes the intestinal knot formation, where one portion of intestine, together with its mesentery, serves as the axis, and another portion of the intestine, with its mesentery, is looped around it.

Sex.

Of 38 cases of volvulus collected by Fitz (*l. c.*), 26 occurred in males and 12 in females. I have collected 208 cases from literature in which the sex was stated; still, the percentages as stated by Fitz were maintained even in this large number; that is, 68 per cent. for males and 32 per cent. for females.

Age.

The greatest number of cases in Fitz's table—that is, about one-third of all—were found between the ages of thirty and forty, and indeed volvulus is a rare occurrence before the fortieth year. This is explainable by the fact that chronic constipation, the most frequent cause of volvulus, is also a disease of maturer age. In 1888, when Fitz read his memorable paper on the acute intestinal obstructions, he had collected only 40 cases which had occurred since 1880; i. e., there were only 40 cases collected from the literature in eight years. In the last ten years I have been able to collect 168 cases of undoubted volvulus, but I do not believe that I have by any means exhausted the literature. I therefore believe either that there are more cases published than formerly, or that volvulus has become a more frequent disease.

Hitherto I have spoken chiefly of volvulus of the sigmoid flexure, which is the most frequent form, and generally serves as the clinical type for other and rarer forms. I do not wish to deny that other parts of the colon can undergo rotation about their mesenteric axes, but in other sections of the colon this abnormality is very rare. In a case reported by E. Schreiber (" Zeitschr. f. klin. Med.," Bd. xxxviii, H. 4, 5, 6), a boy nine years old had repeated attacks of intestinal obstruction, which were accompanied by fecal vomiting. The postmortem examination showed a volvulus formed by the jejunum and ascending colon, which had been produced through the fact that the cecum and ascending colon were not fixed to the posterior walls of the abdomen, but were free, excepting for the attachment to the mesentery, which was similar to that of the small intestines. Schreiber insists that when one has a case of severe constipation with vomiting, even though the latter be not feculent, and if severe prostration ensues within a short time, one should consider the possibility of obstruction, and if this cannot be absolutely excluded, the patient should be operated upon as soon as possible. I repeat these indications from this writer because they agree exactly with my own experience in three cases. Axial twists in the transverse or ascending colon are conditioned by the same anatomical abnormalities that were mentioned in connection with volvulus of the sigmoid. These conditions are mainly three : (1) Congenital abnormalities of position ; (2) malformations of the intestine ; (3) abnormally long mesocolon.

Torsions of the Mesenteric Axis of the Small Intestine.

These types are among the rarest, and when they do occur they occasionally complicate incarceration of the ileum by bands and pseudo-ligaments. Such volvulæ of the small intestine may take in only small sections of the ileum, or larger convolutions or the entire small intestine from duodenum to the ileocecal valve. The cases in which the entire small intestine is involved are, according to Leichtenstern, such abnormalities in which the colon, cecum, and ileum have a common mesentery. The peculiarly elongated mesentery presenting a narrowing at its attachment may be either congenital or acquired by a contracting mesenteric peritonitis—a condition sometimes spoken of as "*chronic mesenteritis.*" Such a condition is most often observed in intestinal loops that have been inclosed for a considerable time in external hernias. The occurrence of volvulus in association with hernia has been the subject of an interesting study by R. Lawford Knaggs ("Annals of Surgery," April, 1900). He recognizes four groups: (1) Volvulus of the hernial contents, the neck of the volvulus being either within the hernial sac or close to the hernial aperture; (2) cases in which the hernial contents are implicated,

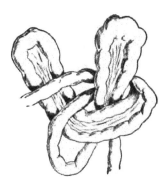

FIG. 8.—VOLVULUS OF SMALL INTES-
TINE.—(*Leichtenstern.*)

but the neck and some of the affected coils lie within the abdomen; (3) cases in which volvulus is produced in the abdomen by reduction of the hernia; and (4) those occurring in the abdomen from some predisposing condition more or less directly connected with a hernia. He reports two cases which have come under his care. A woman of sixty-two years had a strangulated umbilical hernia as large as a Rugby football (?). Under anesthesia the sac was opened. It was occupied by several feet of small intestine; the bowel was distended and black with blood; the whole of the affected intestine, about 4 to 6 feet in length, had been twisted, constituting a volvulus; the constriction was released and the operation concluded. Death followed forty hours later. In a second case a man aged fifty-six years, who for some years had had an irreducible left inguinal hernia, was taken with severe pain and vomiting.   On examination the sac was found flaccid; there was impulse on coughing, and the contents could be easily moved about.   The sac was opened, and a small quantity of dark fluid escaped.   A coil of small intestine about 3 feet long occupied the sac; it was not strangulated and its appearance varied; on one side it was of nearly a healthy color, on the other it was congested and covered with bloody fluid.   On pulling down the herniated coil a broad line of constriction was reached and the diagnosis of volvulus was certain.   The patient's condition was such as to contraindicate further intervention.   Death occurred twenty-seven hours after the operation.   At the necropsy it was found that the lowest 4 feet of the ileum had undergone a single half-twist from right to left, so that at the neck of the volvulus the termination of the ileum lay over and directly against the gut at a point some feet above the valve.

Rotations of the Intestine Around its Own Vertical Axis.

In the description of the various twists around the mesenteric axis, I have already indicated that the fulcrate points of the intestinal loops which are caught in the volvulus undergo a certain degree of twist around their own axis in addition to that around the mesenteric axis.   Whoever has seen a volvulus at operation or autopsy, or whoever has attempted to reproduce one experimentally upon the cadaver, will recognize that this secondary rotation around the axis proper of the intestine must of necessity occur in any volvulus. There are, however, rare cases in which the intestine experiences a twist or rotation only around its vertical axis proper.   It occurs exclusively in the cecum and ascending colon.   Leichtenstern regards these abnormalities mostly as a sign of kinking in consequence of dislocation.   They do not always lead to absolute obstruction unless other complicating factors are associated with it. For example, it may happen that an entire convolution of the small intestine with its mesentery may fall upon the locality of the kink, closing it completely by compression of its mesentery.

Knot Formations Between Two or More Intestinal Loops.

The symptoms of these very rare forms of volvulus are essentially the same as those from strangulation.   They present little importance from the clinical standpoint, and in my opinion will, as a rule, be diagnosed as strangulations. A very clear explication of these conditions is given by Leichtenstern (von Ziemssen's " Handbuch," Bd. VII, 2. Aufl., p. 73) and also by Küttner ("Virchow's Archiv," Bd. XLIII, 1868). In all these knot formations a rotation of the intestinal loops around their mesenteric, as well as to a certain extent around their own axis, is unavoidable. They most frequently occur between the ileum and the sigmoid flexure, in rare cases between different portions of the ileum and jejunum, and in still rarer instances between the ascending colon and cecum on the one hand, and a loop of the ileum on the other. It will not serve for the elucidation of the clinical recognition of these extremely rare forms to give elaborate descriptions of the miraculous serpentine contortions which the various portions of the intestine can undergo when their mesentery is abnormally long and narrow.

Etiology.

The principal etiological factors that are active in the development of actual rotations and loop-knot formations are the following : (1) Abnormal length of the mesentery or of the intestine. W. Gruber and Küttner have called attention to the fact that the Russian intestines exceed in length the German, English, and French intestines. Gruber describes a Russian small intestine 56 feet long, which he attributes to the fact that the diet of the poor and middle classes of Russian inhabitants consists predominantly of vegetables. Very often this is necessitated by the rigorous observance of religious fast days, and explains the frequency of volvulus among this nationality. This is an acquired form of elongation of the intestine. There must be a normal relation between the breadth of the insertion of the mesentery and the length of the intestine. When a disturbance of the proper proportion ensues there is danger of axial twists. (2) Chronic retracting mesenteritis. (3) Habitual constipation. (4) Various causes, such as acute diarrhea, trauma, violent muscular exertion. Israel has reported a case (" Berlin. klin. Wochenschr.," 1897, No. 1) in which a sigmoid volvulus occurred immediately after a copious rectal enema. (5) Predisposing causes are mature age, emaciation causing a relatively increased intra-abdominal space, and loss of fat in the omentum and mesentery.

Pathological Anatomy.

The loops comprised in the volvulus may be so excessively distended as to cover the entire remaining intestine. Its walls become hyperplastic, rigid, and thickened by a transudate. The enlarged sigmoid may extend to the right hypochondrium, pass over the liver and stomach, and even force up the diaphragm. The lumen of this portion of the bowel is filled with a mixture of blood, mucus, and liquid feces. Tears may develop in the muscular layer and peritoneum. The remaining portions of the small and large intestines are usually collapsed, pale, and empty, though there are exceptions to this rule. I have seen two cases of sigmoid volvulus in which the transverse colon was also considerably distended by gases. The peritonitis which generally results from gangrenous destruction of the twisted limbs of the volvulus may be local or diffuse. Perforations are rare, generally because the cases terminate fatally before they have time to develop.

Individual Symptoms.

In many cases of volvulus the symptoms which usher in the development of the abnormality are persistent constipation, vomiting, and rapidly developing collapse. The principal symptoms are pain, tenesmus, vomiting, constipation, and disturbed general conditions.

Pain.—Pain is present in all cases from the first stage ; whilst it is very intense, it is not as unbearable as that which is described in the acute internal incarcerations. It is always risky to speak of the pain in one condition being severer than that of another abnormality, especially when the pains in both are violent. In most cases of volvulus the pain is continuous, but in my experience it subsides to smaller doses of morphin or opium than are necessary for the relief of incarcerations. It is as often localized around the navel as in the left hypochondriac region.

Tenesmus.—Whilst tenesmus is a frequent symptom, I do not consider that it is available for a differential diagnosis from other forms of obstruction, for this symptom is a frequent occurrence in acute invaginations.

Vomiting.—Vomiting usually occurs simultaneously with the paroxysms of pain. It need not always be present. Fitz (*l. c.*, p. 21) reports two cases in which it was very light, and in 3 instances of twists of the small intestine there was no fecal vomit at least. In some cases nausea, eructation, and singultus seem to take the place of the vomiting. Fecal vomiting may occur, and is reported in 6 cases of the 34 studied by Fitz. In a larger number of cases which I have collected (64) it occurred in only 10. As Treves correctly remarked, fecal vomiting is of sufficient rarity in volvulus to serve as a distinctive factor in the differentiation from internal incarceration.

Constipation.—Whilst other forms of intestinal impermeability are, as a rule, not preceded for any length of time by a definite intestinal disease, volvulus in by far the great majority of cases is preceded by chronic habitual constipation. In fact, repeated colics, in association with chronic constipation, may be regarded as the prodromal stage of this abnormality.

Disturbed General Conditions.—The general condition is disturbed in a manner identical with that described under the chapter on Strangulations and Incarcerations. The collapse is similar to that occurring in these conditions.

Sensitiveness to Pressure.—The abdomen is always sensitive to pressure over the seat of the volvulus. It becomes intensely sensitive to pressure when peritonitis has developed.

Intestinal Symptoms.—The principal intestinal symptoms to which attention should be paid are the local meteorism and the cessation of evacuation of intestinal contents and flatus. The local meteorism, which I have already described in the general chapter on Intestinal Obstruction, is more pronounced in volvulus than in any other form of intestinal impermeability. The so-called sign of von Wahl—*i. e.*, meteorism in the loop involved in the volvulus— may be developed after twenty-four hours. Local meteorism, to be of diagnostic value, must be hunted for on the first or second day of the disease. It is true that the meteorism may in some cases not be restricted to the region of the sigmoid flexure, but may extend upward and toward the right. Sometimes there is no meteorism at all in the sigmoid flexure, whereas the entire abdomen may seem filled with tympanitically distended intestinal loops. This is, in my experience, not the case during the first and second days. During this period the distended loops of the sigmoid flexure can almost regularly be made out in the left lower abdominal region. Later on the distention increases and the sigmoid volvulus rises toward the right upper abdomen, and in addition to this there may be a stagnation meteorism in the colon, or a general tympanitic distention resulting from peritonitis.

Symptoms of Axial Twists in Other Sections of the Intestine.—These are not essentially different from the typical symptomatology of the sigmoid volvulus. Naturally, the seat of the pain and of the greatest distention of the local meteorism may vary considerably, according to the portion of the small intestine that is twisted. The tenesmus and admixture of blood in the stool, which are quite constant in sigmoid volvulus, are wanting in volvulus of the small intestine, or of the transverse and ascending colons. Naunyn (*l. c.*), however, describes a case of torsion of the small intestine in which almost one liter of pure blood was passed in one day per anum. It is also natural that there need not be absolute suppression of stool and feces when the volvulus is high up in the small intestine. The seat of the twist in 39 of the cases collected by Fitz (*l. c.*) was as follows :

SEAT.	NUMBER OF CASES.	PER CENT.
Sigmoid flexure,	19	49
Ileocecal region,	6	16
Cecum,	5	13
Small intestine,	5	13
Ascending colon,	2	5
Colon,	1	2
Descending colon,	1	2
	39	100

It is thus evident that about one-half of the cases of twist took place at the sigmoid flexure, and that nearly one-third of them were present in the ileocecal region. It is further evident that, for all practical purposes, eighty-seven per cent. of the cases occurred in the large intestine.

Recurrent and Consecutive Attacks.

In my experience the forms of sigmoid volvulus that are amenable to purely medical treatment are liable to recur. In September, 1888, I had occasion to treat a physician for the first time for this type of volvulus. In January, 1890, he had a return of the accident, and in June, 1890, it recurred for the third time. Since then I have observed four similar cases. But recurrences may take place after the volvulus has been replaced surgically. Ed. M. Foote describes a case of sigmoid volvulus ("Boston Med. and Surg. Jour.," March 9, 1899) in which a deaf-mute, aged twenty-two years, was three times relieved of the abnormality by operation. The second attack occurred six months after the first, and the third attack seven months after the second. The third operation consisted of stitching the sigmoid to the abdominal wall, and the patient recovered. Ellsworth Elliott, Jr., has reported three interesting cases of sigmoid volvulus, in one of which there were three consecutive attacks within three years, the patient being operated upon each time and eventually recovering ("Annals of Surgery," July, 1899).

Course.

All forms of sigmoid volvulus, unless they can be treated by bloodless mechanical means or by timely operation, must end in death. The administration of purgatives aggravates the danger. Sometimes, in very acute cases, death may occur in twelve hours, under symptoms of collapse. But in the uncomplicated cases of sigmoid volvulus the duration is about eight days. The longest was three weeks, and the shortest three days, on the average.

Course of Chronic Forms.—Whether the volvulus affects the small or the large intestine, there is practically no possibility of spontaneous return to the normal condition. Cases of so-called spontaneous cures reported in literature can not, in my opinion, stand the test of critical judgment.

Diagnosis.

An absolutely reliable diagnosis can only be made by abdominal section. The sudden abdominal pain, the vomiting, the tenesmus, constipation, and collapse do not, in my opinion, permit of the establishment of a logical diagnosis. In rare cases the local meteorism or partial axial twists of the sigmoid flexure are so well localized and restricted over this portion of the bowel that the clinician is justified in establishing a diagnosis, especially when the local meteorism is associated with blood in the discharges from the rectum and tenesmus.

The **treatment** will be considered in connection with the other forms of intestinal impermeability.

INTERNAL STRICTURES OF THE INTESTINE.

Intestinal strictures may be external or internal. The internal are the result of pathological changes in the layers of the intestinal wall itself. The external intestinal strictures are caused by chronic circumscribed peritonitis. Internal strictures may be congenital or acquired. The congenital strictures of the intestine manifest themselves during the first stage of life. Up to the third month of fetal life the intestinal canal is a closed tube at its lower end, possessing a narrow communication with the urogenital apparatus and terminating in a common cloaca. The blind end of the intestine is opened into by an invagination of the skin from the anal region, which, extending upward, eventually communicates with the intestine, being separated from the bladder in males and from the vagina in females by a partition, the perineum. Abnormalities in the formation of this fetal development of the invagination from the anal region may cause an atresia of the anus in which the blind end of the bowel has no communication with the exterior, and no skin invagination has been formed from the outside. There is also an atresia of the rectum, in which an invagination has been formed, but has not extended upward sufficiently to meet the blind end of the intestine. These conditions are abnormalities rather than strictures (see Mathews, "Diseases of Rectum," and Penzoldt and Stintzing's "Handbuch d. spec. Therapie," Bd. iv, S. 656, for illustrations). Genuine congenital strictures result, however, in consequence of the imperfect communication between the external skin invagination and the blind end of the bowel. They consist sometimes simply of a tough membrane, presenting a smaller or larger opening in the center, like a perforated diaphragm stretched across the lumen of the rectum. E. Graser (Penzoldt and Stintzing, *l. c.*, p. 658) describes such a diaphragm in a girl fifteen years old. She was so badly nourished that she gave the impression of a child but five years old.   She had been compelled to use purgatives since her youth, and even with the aid of these only narrow bands of offensive, tough feces could be evacuated.   An examination by rectum had never been made.   On introducing the finger Graser found a circular diaphragm 5 cm. above the anus.   He could not penetrate it with his finger, but during narcosis the obstruction was removed by operation.   V. A. Robertson ("Amer. Gynecolog. and Obstet. Jour.," May, 1899) reports three cases of imperforate anus, for which he advises immediate operation.

There are congenital atresias of the colon and small intestine. They have been most commonly observed in the duodenum and the ileocecal communication.   The most frequent congenital occlusions, however, are those of the rectum.   The great rarity of this condition can be judged from the fact that in 66,654 newborn children, atresia of the anus was found only three times.   The congenital strictures of the rectum, colon, and small intestine are still rarer than those of the anus.   Of 375 collected cases, 10 occurred in the colon, and 74 in the small intestine.   Nothnagel distinguishes three groups of internal intestinal strictures : (1) Those due to carcinoma ; (2) those due to cicatrices ; and (3) those due to chronic inflammatory infiltration of the intestinal wall.

In 1884 Treves gave the synopsis of 78 cases of intestinal strictures which he was able to collect from the literature of the subject up to that year (" Intestinal Obstruction," American edition). Of these, 26 were strictures of the small intestine, 8 strictures of the ileocecal region, and 44 of the colon.   Of the 26 cases of stricture in the small intestine, 10 were due to cicatrices following ulcer, 2 to cicatrices after trauma, 4 followed strangulated hernia, and 10 were caused by carcinoma.   The subject of carcinomatous strictures I have already considered in a separate chapter.   I will therefore not consider them in this connection again, but limit the chapter to the discussion of strictures due to ulcerations and those due to chronic inflammatory infiltration of the intestinal mucosa.   The latter condition is so extremely rare that the etiology of intestinal strictures may be, for practical purposes, limited to a consideration of cicatricial stenoses.   The so-called chronic inflammatory infiltrations of the intestinal wall, the nature of which is not thoroughly understood, are extremely rare.

For the accompanying illustration of the application of the Röntgen rays in determining the location of obstructions and strictures in the intestinal canal, and also for determining the distance to which the rectum is not perforated in cases of imperforate rectum, I am indebted to Dr. Mihran K. Kassabian, who is in charge of the Röntgen ray laboratory of the Medico-Chirurgical Hospital of Philadelphia. The case described by Dr. Kassabian occurred in the practice of Dr. William V. Laws, assistant surgeon in this same institution.

The value of the X-rays application for the detection of metallic foreign bodies, such as a penny, button, needle, pin, etc., in the alimentary tract, can not be doubted, and for the most part is of great service to the general practitioner and surgeon. The presence of any foreign body in the alimentary tract can easily be determined ; and, what is of still greater importance, we can with certainty discover whether or not that body is movable or stationary. Should it be determined that a particular foreign body in the above stated tract is immovable, for any length of time, we are thus justified in resorting to operative procedure if it gives rise to symptoms.

It is not possible for us to discover, or rather locate, the exact seat of intestinal obstruction or stricture, but we can diagnose an obstruction by the following procedure : The patient should be requested to swallow a hard-rubber capsule containing a small bullet, or, preferably, a keratin-coated capsule filled with bismuth subnitrate. This foreign body will travel that portion of the alimentary tract between the mouth and the seat of the obstruction, and upon meeting the latter will remain there ; and upon examination by the X-rays the obstructed area of the intestinal tract will be shown by the stationary location of the bullet at the seat of the obstruction. But as the intestinal loops are superimposed upon one another, it is not possible to state just where that seat is. (See " Value of X-rays in Diagnosis of Dis. Intest.," Prof. J. C. Hemmeter, London " Lancet," Sept. 28, 1901, p. 829.)

Congenital imperforate rectum can also be diagnosed by the use of the X-rays, as is plainly evident in the following case, which I have the pleasure of reporting through the courtesy of Dr. William V. Laws.

Case : Master W., age twelve, was brought to the Hospital by his parents, asking whether or not surgical skill could do anything to relieve him of a colostomy, which latter had been performed when the child was three days old. The sphincter ani was normal and the lower portion of the rectum was open for about 1½ inches. The feasibility of an operation was settled by the use of the Röntgen rays.

Röntgen ray examination : Bowels purged, followed by the introduction of a hard-rubber tube through the artificial anus, and an emulsion of bismuth subnitrate injected. While the patient was lying on his back, the skiagraph taken, the latter (Plate 7, B) showing a dark area, indicating the pouch above the seat of obstruction. Plate 7, A, shows the introduction of a steel sound through the sphincter ani. This was skiagraphed also, and thus we determine the distance or length of obstruction between the pouch above and the open portion of the rectum below. This gave the surgeon a clean-cut idea of the *exact location* of the pouch, and, secondly, the *length* of the imperforate portion of the rectum. An operation was performed, the obstruction and a small portion of the coccyx being removed, and the pouch anastomosed with the upper open portion of the rectum. A few days after the operation had been performed the patient passed his feces through the newly made channel.

PLATE 7.

SOUND

BISMUTH EMULSION

RUBBER TUBE

This illustration shows the steel sound introduced through the sphincter ani; the distance between the end of the sound and the bismuth emulsion represents the imperforate part of the rectum.

rea above center of illustration is the bismuth emulsion accumulated in the dilatation or pouch above the obstruction.

Hypertrophies and Chronic Inflammatory Thickenings of the Intestinal Wall.

These conditions are, as a rule, hypertrophy of the musculature or of the mucosa, or of both. All chronic inflammations of the intestine may be associated with circumscribed hypertrophy. In the neighborhood of neoplasms they may occur also. The muscular hypertrophies are not due to simple increase in the muscle substance exclusively, but also to increase in the connective tissue. Local hypertrophies of the muscle substance have already been described in the chapter on Benign Tumors, under the heading of Myomas. The compensating muscular hypertrophy occurring above stenoses has already been considered in the chapter on Enterostenoses.

Hypertrophies of the mucosa develop as a consequence of chronic enteritis, dysentery, or tuberculosis. They usually take the form of polypoid neoplasms, in which the glandular elements of the mucosa are in excess of the other histological elements. Chronic inflammatory infiltration of the intestinal wall is not confirmedly due to simple chronic enteritis. Some specific factor must be super-added to the chronic inflammation in order to cause an inflammatory hypertrophy of the intestine sufficient to bring about a stricture. Nothnagel (*l. c.*, p. 264) describes a case in a physician forty years of age, who for many years had had intestinal disturbances. About eighteen months before his death he suffered from constipation, which he had to regulate artificially. During this period, when he had constipation he suffered from three or four attacks of colic analogous to those which occur with enterostenoses. In spite of very careful examination, no objective proof of neoplasm could be found until two months before his death, when a round tumor, the size of a walnut, and hard as cartilage, was palpated in the ileocecal region. Most of his colleagues considered it a probable carcinoma. It was painless and very easily movable. An operation was performed, and the unfortunate patient died three weeks thereafter. The part of the bowel which was removed presented a very hard tumor as large as a hen's egg, somewhat larger above, and tapering off funnel-shaped downward, and involving the ileocecal valve. The lumen was narrowed down to the diameter of a lead pencil, and there was no trace of ulceration. At first sight the pathological anatomists also considered it a carcinoma, but on histological examination all characters of malignant neoplasm were wanting. It presented the appearances of a chronic inflammatory infiltration containing giant cells, and after long searching a few tubercle bacilli. The difficulty of diagnosing such cases is not only evident from this example, but Nothnagel has presented us with another instructive case (*l. c.*, p. 236), in which a tumor of the ileocecal region, which was very hard, uneven, and movable, in the absence of preliminary disease of the intestine, and in the absence of tubercle bacilli in the evacuations, was diagnosed as carcinoma, and the autopsy proved it to be a stricture of the ascending colon, caused by a cicatrix from a tubercular ulcer. During my service at the Maryland General Hospital I had a similar experience with a tumor involving the ileocecal valve, and producing an absolute stenosis. The diagnosis was carcinoma of the cecum. At autopsy a tumor as large as an orange, involving the valve, and leaving no lumen whatever, was found. Histological examination disclosed the absence of the architecture of malignant neoplasm. It did not present the appearance of tuberculous tumor, nor could any tubercle bacilli be detected in it. As the patient had a distinct history of syphilis, and a small gumma was detected in the center of the liver, it is probable that this inflammatory infiltration of the ileocecum was of syphilitic origin.*

In a masterly report on intestinal tuberculosis, Professor Nicholas Senn (" Jour. Amer. Med. Assoc.," May 21, 1898) states that he has observed the formation of chronic abscess in the ileocecal region in connection with intestinal symptoms of long standing, which he interpreted as of tubercular origin. He states that these are the cases in which, prior to the perforation of the ulcer, adhesion takes place, excluding the peritoneal cavity, and followed by the formation of a mural tubercular abscess. Intestinal strictures, ulcerations, and even catarrhs may very much simulate the tuberculous type, and yet not be histologically identical with tuberculosis. Councilman (" Johns Hopkins Hospital Reports," March, 1892) has reported a case of extensive and deep ulceration of the lower portion of the ileum complicated by stricture of the rectum, which

---

* A large ileocecal neoplasm from an ambulatory case of typhoid fever was exhibited to the Clinical Society of Maryland, November 16, 1900, by Dr. Harry T. Marshall. When I was shown the specimen it was about the size of an orange, and projected through the ileocecal valve like a beginning intussusception.

terminated in death from perforation and gangrenous periproctitis, and in which typhoid fever and tuberculosis could be safely excluded as causes. At the postmortem, ulceration of the ileum was found, with invasion of the tissues by colon bacilli. Some of the ulcers presented the appearance of an acute process, others were of a chronic nature. Numerous bacteria, both short rods and micrococci, were found in the superficial necrosed tissue, in some places extending into the cellular infiltration in the submucosa. These microbes did not seem to stand in any direct etiological connection with the pathological changes.

The chapter of investigations concerning the various forms of organisms of the colon bacillus group, their biology and pathology, is by no means closed. Perhaps the future will bring us conclusive evidence concerning the pathogenicity of certain members of this group, and that they are perhaps to be considered the cause of such types of induration as I have described in the preceding, and which can not be classed as tuberculous or carcinomatous.

Summing up critically the observations on inflammatory infiltrations of the intestinal wall, it may be said that they are, in the first place, extremely rare ; secondly, they are not due to simple chronic catarrhal enteritis ; and thirdly, that some infectious process is at the base of these abnormalities—generally tuberculosis or syphilis. Occasionally it is impossible to say even after the histological examination what the origin and etiological character of a cicatricial stricture or an inflammatory induration of the intestine may be. The clinical history and the anamnesis do not, by any means, give a sure indication in all cases.

Strictures due to stercoral ulcers that have resulted in cicatrices are considered by Nothnagel as plausible pathogenic possibilities. They generally have an annular shape, and as the stercoral ulcer always exhibits a tendency to healing, it seems thoroughly suited to produce a stricture. Of the remaining forms of intestinal ulcers, described in a separate chapter,—the embolic, thrombotic, uremic, septic ulcers,—it may be said that they do not cause strictures, because the underlying disease, of which they are simply a local expression, produces death before they can be transformed into cicatrices.

Typhoid ulcers are generally situated with their long axes parallel to the long axis of the intestine, and even in cicatrizing they would not stenose the lumen. Typhoid ulcers do not involve much of the intestine circumference; but Hochenegg and Klob have reported intestinal strictures due to typhoid ulcers. The losses of substance caused by follicular and catarrhal ulcers, as can be seen from a number of illustrations in this work, as a rule are too small to cause extensive strictures. The peptic ulcer of the duodenum on cicatrization produces a stricture in this part of the intestine whenever the ulcer heals at all. Very often the duodenum becomes dilated between the stricture and the pylorus, forming an hour-glass deformity, in which the pylorus constitutes an isthmus between the dilated stomach on one side and the dilated duodenum on the other. If the cicatrix is situated over the papilla, the opening of the biliary and pancreatic ducts may be obliterated, and great dilation of these channels ensue. Herzfelder has reported a case of rupture of the gall-bladder following its abnormal distention from this cause. Duodenal stricture from annular cicatrix is well described in the work by Samuel and W. S. Fenwick ("Ulcer of the Stomach and Duodenum," p. 45).

Strictures Due to Cicatrices from Dysenteric Ulcers.

On the authority of our countryman, Jos. J. Woodward, it may be stated that intestinal strictures from this cause practically do not occur. S. O. Habershon ("Disease of the Abdomen," London, 1862, p. 385) and J. Warburton Begbie (article on "Dysentery," Reynolds' "System of Medicine," vol. III, 1871) considered intestinal strictures resulting from dysentery a "not unfrequent" condition. The entire literature on this subject up to 1880 is given in the "Medical and Surgical History of the War of the Rebellion," by J. J. Woodward, vol. I, pp. 504 to 510. This work, in addition to being based upon and giving the results in abstract of 1,269,027 cases of acute diarrhea and 182,586 cases of chronic diarrhea, is a masterly consideration of the symptomatology, pathology, and therapy of 287,522 cases of dysentery occurring among the United States troops during the Civil War, from May, 1861, to June, 1866. Of these, 228,541 had chronic dysentery. There were 9431 deaths, of which 3855 resulted from chronic dysentery.

After a scholarly consideration of this enormous clinical material, Woodward says : " No case [of intestinal stricture] has been reported to the Surgeon-General's office, either during the war or since ; the Army Medical Museum does not possess a single specimen, nor have I found in the ' American Medical Journal ' any case substantiated by postmortem examination in which this condition is reported to have followed a flux contracted during the Civil War." With very few exceptions the foreign literature presents the same barrenness of results when examined critically for intestinal strictures of dysenteric origin, as does the American literature examined by Woodward. In the American literature, as compiled and ab-. stracted in the " Phila. Med. Jour.," since 1898, I have not been able to find a single case. There is no case of this sort reported in any of the vast amount of abstracted literature presented in Boas' "Archives of Digestive Diseases," since 1895. A case of dysenteric intestinal stricture has been described by Rokitansky ("Oesterr. Jahrbücher," Bd. xviii, 1839, S. 13). Rokitansky's description has been retained as the classical narrative of a dysenteric stricture. The patient survived the dysenteric attack for about thirty years, during which he continually suffered from various abdominal troubles, chief among which was obstinate constipation, before the occlusion became finally so complete as to cause his death. As the dysenteric process, even were it to cause stricture of the intestine, presents no pathognomonic histological evidences whereby it could be differentiated anatomically from the cicatrix resulting from any of the other forms of stenosing intestinal ulcers, it is justifiable to question the correctness of the conclusions of Rokitansky in attributing the stricture to a dysentery which had occurred thirty years prior to the patient's death. Nothnagel describes another case of a dysenteric cicatricial stricture (l. c., p. 219), which, however, is by no means an unobjectionable case, for the dysenteric cicatrix, which was diagnosed as such prior to death, was found to have developed a carcinoma. As carcinoma itself frequently causes enterostenosis, the dysenteric symptoms might have resulted from the irritation set up by the neoplasm. Treves gives a description of dysenteric strictures of the intestine, and a number of other cases are on record ; but, as Woodward suggests, a critical investigation of the literature on this subject is very necessary ; and I should add that no cases should be considered dysenteric strictures unless accompanied by evident history of dysentery, and other etiological factors, such as tuberculosis, carcinoma, and syphilis, can be excluded.

Intestinal Strictures after Traumas, Incarcerated Hernias, and Intussusceptions.

An intestinal stricture after a fall upon the abdomen has been described by Pouzet (*l. c.*). The patient died six months after the accident, in a state of collapse. He had suffered for two months prior to death from violent abdominal pains and vomiting. The jejunum was strictured 15 cm. below the duodenum by a white ring of connective tissue ½ cm. broad. As invagination frequently results from violent abdominal concussions, it is conceivable that the stricture described by Pouzet was the result of an invagination. We may dismiss the consideration of strictures resulting from the sequestration of an intussusceptum, because they are very rare, and have already been referred to in another chapter. Treves (*l. c.*) describes four cases of strictures in a portion of the ileum and jejunum which had been incarcerated. The cicatrices are supposed to have followed ulceration or circumscribed gangrene. Three of them were in the ileum and one in the jejunum.

Rectal Strictures.

These are much more frequent in women than in men, the proportion being 190 to 25. They result from the same causes as have been mentioned in connection with intestinal strictures. But there are three other causes which are not operative in the intestinal forms. These are periproctitic inflammation, hemorrhoidal ulceration, and traumas caused by the introduction of foreign bodies and the nozles of syringes and douching apparatus for administering enemata. In the last chapter of this volume, on Diseases of the Rectum, Dr. Thos. Chas. Martin has described the stricture which may be produced by chronic inflammatory thickening or abnormal development of the rectal valve (plica transversalis). The various forms of rectal ulcer have been described in a separate chapter (chap. XXI, vol. I), and the reasons assigned there explaining the preponderance of the female sex among the clinical material of rectal ulcer and stricture. The syphilitic strictures and gonorrheal strictures, or at least such as are presumed to be gonorrheal, may be said to be almost limited to the rectum. A unique cause of stricture in this location of the alimentary canal is found in the result of operation. In a paper on acquired non-malignant stricture of the rectum, W. Duff Bullard ("New York Medical Record," January 13, 1900) describes the case of a woman who had been operated upon at a large hospital for hemorrhoids, probably by Whitehead's method, and a stricture of the rectum resulted. In a second case the stricture resulted from sloughing following the injection treatment of hemorrhoids. Similarly Dr. Reuben Peterson ascribes strictures of the rectum partly to unskilful operations for hemorrhoids. He also gives an account of a tubercular stricture 1 inch above the external sphincter, in which the thickened rectal wall could be felt for some inches upward through the vagina. Nine inches of the rectum and sigmoid flexure were removed through an abdominal incision, and an anastomosis made between the upper and lower ends of the intestine by a modified Monsell method. The patient made a perfect recovery ("Jour. Amer. Med. Assoc.," February 3, 1900). These cases are mentioned because they are confirmatory of my own experience with quite a number of cases of rectal stricture, which I could attribute to no other cause than operations upon hemorrhoids. The deduction from these cases is, that operations upon hemorrhoids, or upon any abnormality of the rectum, should be performed only by experienced surgeons, and, above all things, the rectum of the cases thus operated should be examined at intervals of one month for at least one year after the operation.

Tuberculous Strictures of the Intestine.

We now come to the most frequent and interesting form of intestinal strictures, that of tubercular origin. In the chapter on Tubercular Intestinal Ulcers I have emphasized the fact that they are in the greater majority of cases of secondary origin, generally following a pulmonary tuberculosis, and due to the swallowing of infectious sputa (Klebs). According to Klebs ("Die causale Behandlung der Tuberculose," Leipzig, 1894, p. 53), the digestive apparatus is by far the most frequent portal of entry by which tubercle bacilli gain access to the organism. Opposed to this are the views of Koch expressed at the International Congress on Tuberculosis held in London during July, 1901. Concerning the recent opinions of Koch on the rarity of primary intestinal tuberculosis, and his inference that human and bovine tuberculosis are two distinct diseases, I must refer the reader to the section on Tuberculosis of the Intestines (chap. II, this volume, p. 87). Evidences of intestinal infection can be found both in the intestine itself and in the mesenteric glands ; but then there is no doubt that infection by way of the intestine may take place and no trace of ulceration, in fact no pathological alteration whatever, be discoverable anywhere in the intestinal layers (Orth, "Spec. patholog. Anatomie," Bd. 1, S. 839, and also Klebs, *l. c.*, p. 81). Orth describes extensive tuberculous caseation in enlarged mesenteric lymph-glands where no tuberculous changes could by any means be discovered in the intestines. He assumes that bacilli can enter the lymph-glands from the intestine and entirely destroy these glands without causing any change in the intestinal wall. According to Theobald Smith ("A Study of Bovine and Human Bacilli from Sputum," "Jour. of Experimental Med ," vol. III, p. 508), the march of the tubercle bacilli from the original place of infection may be concealed by reparative processes, and he even regards infection through the digestive tract as a source of pulmonary phthisis (*l. c.*, p. 509). These pathologists, therefore, suggest that the intestine may be a portal of entry for infection of the respiratory tract. If it were possible to judge of the number of mesenteric infections where the intestinal mucosa is apparently not altered, this conclusion might receive a further support.

Intestinal tuberculous ulcers may be primary or secondary. The occurrence of primary intestinal tuberculosis in adults and children has been conclusively proven by the observations of Behrens, Melchoir, and others. (See article on "Intestinal Ulceration.") Only such cases of undoubted intestinal tubercular ulcers can be accepted as primary where every trace of tuberculosis can be proved to be absent in the lungs, trachea, larynx, and genito-urinary organs. The most valuable contributions upon the importance of the tubercular process as a cause of intestinal stricture have been by surgeons. Thus, Billroth, Bouilly, Czerny, Durant, Hofmeister, Koenig, Salzer, and Schier have enriched the literature on the subject. Such ulcers are not always due to cicatricial retraction, but, as Czerny, Hofmeister, and Koenig have demonstrated, to so much secondary inflammatory induration, edema, and plastic exudation that the lumen will be narrowed and obstructed even in the absence of a cicatrix. We must therefore distinguish between the hypertrophic inflammatory type of tuberculous stricture, which is the most frequent form, and the annular or cicatricial type, which is rare. Eisenhardt, in studying 1000 postmortem examinations of tuberculous subjects, found evidences of tuberculosis in the intestinal tract in 566 cases, and only in 9 was the intestine strictured from this cause.*

Multiple Tubercular Strictures.

In all the reports of multiple strictures of the intestine which I have critically examined in the literature of the subject the evidence is quite conclusive that they are of tubercular origin. The deduction is justifiable that whenever the surgeon meets with more than one stricture in the intestinal canal he should first of all think of the tubercular origin of the condition. The vast majority of these multiple strictures are found in the ileum. In only one case (Eisenhardt, necropsy) were they found in the colon. Whenever the strictures are multiple and situated in the small intestine they are of the typical form of the cicatricial constriction. Hofmeister has (" Beiträge f. klin. Chir.," H. 3, January, 1897) collected 20 reported cases of multiple stricture of the intestine of tubercular origin. There were five cases in which there were two strictures in each patient (Eisenhardt, Esmarch, Koenig, Meyer, Voltz). Frank reported a case of three strictures; Keoberle, one of four; Trendelenburg, one of five strictures. Litten and Homén each reported a patient with six strictures; Rotter, one with seven;

---

* Clinical investigation is not competent to give reliable information concerning the relative frequency of primary intestinal tuberculosis. Histologic study of necropsy material is about the most reliable way at our command to investigate this question. For the last twelve months I have been at work at intervals in examining the digestive tracts gained at autopsy by the method used by Otto Naegeli (" Häufigkeit-Localization, etc., der Tub.," " Virchow's Archiv," Bd. CLX, S. 428), and although I have only examined a limited material (49 subjects) and the results are by no means ready for publication, it can be said that this method reveals primary intestinal tuberculosis to be of greater relative frequency than Koch admits it to be in his report (*l. c.*).

Fränkel, one with eight. A second case of Fränkel, and a second case of Koenig, and a case reported by Hofmeister, had twelve strictures. In the "Deutsche Zeitschr. f. Chir.," February, 1899, H. 5 and 6, Hans Strehl reports the case of a single woman twenty-nine years old, who had an almost immovable tumor the size of a man's fist in the ileocecal region. At operation the tumor was easily found, but there were also fourteen distinct constrictions at different parts of the intestine, so that resection offered no hope of success. The patient had pulmonary tuberculosis, tuberculous ulceration of the bowel, and tuberculous peritonitis. Nothnagel (*l. c.*, p. 262) reports several cases of this type, one of which presented three, another five, a third seven or eight tuberculous cicatricial strictures. The case of Litten, of six strictures, presented them all in a section of the ileum not exceeding ½ meter. Between these strictures the bowel was expanded into five large sacular dilations filled with liquid feces. In Trendelenburg's case five strictures were distributed over a distance of 42 cm. In a case reported by Rudolph Matas ("Phila. Med. Jour.," July 9, 1893, p. 73) there were three strictures of probable tubercular origin, contained within 13 inches (33 cm.) of the jejunum. The patient was a man forty-six years of age, who had no tuberculous history, nor any sign of disease in any part of the body but the abdomen. The entire loop, including the three strictures and the corresponding mesentery, was removed by circular enterorrhaphy, and the patient was operated April 24, 1896, and began to eat soft-boiled eggs and milk on the fourth day after operation. He left the care of the operator thirty-four days after the operation, and could eat three full meals a day without experiencing the least distress. About two years after the operation he weighed 180 pounds, which was 80 pounds more than the weight at the time of the operation. The results of surgical procedure of operation on strictures of this type, judging from the report of Hofmeister (*l. c.*), are more favorable than operations for strangulations or incarcerations. This writer has collected 83 cases of intestinal strictures of all kinds which were operated. Of these, 52 (or 62.65 per cent.) patients recovered, and of the 26 fatal cases (31.33 per cent.), death was more or less directly attributed to the operation in but 16 (or 19.3 per cent.). Operation should be encouraged at the onset of the symptoms which indicate a chronic obstruction. The phenomena of occlusion are generally ushered in by paroxysms of abdominal pain, vomiting, and obstipation. It is well not to wait for a repetition of these symptoms if they have once abated and the diagnosis of occlusion seems probable. The symptoms resulting from internal strictures of the intestine are identical with those described under enterostenoses. If they are high up in the bowel, in the ileum or jejunum, as in the case of Matas, the patient may survive for a long time without fatal permanent obstruction, owing to the liquid character of the intestinal contents in the constricted portion. In the case of Matas, the evolution of the stenotic process was unusually long, extending over twenty years, and the primary ulcerative cause, tuberculosis, had apparently completely disappeared at the time of the operation. It was one of the so-called healed tuberculoses. The patient had suffered from numerous attacks of acute obstruction brought on by plugging of the narrow orifice of the stricture by food masses. Strictures as high up as the jejunum, which evidently was the location in the case of Rudolph Matas, are extremely rare.

Diagnosis.

When the strictures are in the rectum, or even in the beginning of the sigmoid flexure, they may be diagnosed by rectal inspection, which, under proper manipulation, and with the long sigmoidoscope, will even reveal strictures in the lower part of the sigmoid. The diagnosis of strictures in other parts of the intestine is doubtful. The previous history and the condition of the stools may give some information. If the patient has had persistent constipation the clinician should think of stercoral or decubital ulcers that have resulted in a cicatrix. The visible peristalsis and plastic intestinal erections, which have been described in the chapter on Enterostenoses, are valuable clinical signs, and suggest the presence of a stricture. Whenever the cicatrices have occurred after hernias or violent external trauma the previous history will throw light not only on the etiology, but upon the nature of the stricture itself. Whenever there are undoubted symptoms of stenosis of the small intestine, in which no etiological factor can be detected, it is advisable to think first of tuberculous stricture. The differentiation between

chronic inflammatory strictures and neoplasms, particularly malignant neoplasms, is exceedingly difficult. Sometimes, when the
patients can be observed for a long time, providing the condition of
the sufferer permits this, a diagnosis is possible by exclusion, but it
will be a rare piece of good fortune. Fortunately for the treatment
of such cases of intestinal stricture, it is not always absolutely
necessary that an exact diagnosis of the cause and location of the
stenosis should be made. The mere diagnosis of stricture, when
accompanied by undoubted symptoms of an enterostenosis, calls for
operation imperatively. If there is reason to believe, from the
symptoms previously stated in the chapter on Enterostenoses, that
the stricture is in the duodenum or jejunum, the method of duodenal intubation, by a Langdon rubber tube, or the Kuhn tube including a spiral guide, will offer a means of locating the constriction.

The **symptomatology** of intestinal strictures corresponds to that
given under the heading of enterostenoses. The **treatment,** which
is essentially surgical, is given in the same chapter.

EXTERNAL CONSTRICTION OF THE INTESTINE.

External Peritonitic Strictures and Adhesions.

In the chapter on Incarcerations and Strangulations I have already
described various forms of peritoneal bands and pseudo-ligaments
in their pathological rôle of causing intestinal obstruction. In this
section the forms of intestinal impermeability will be described which
are produced by chronic circumscribed peritonitis in the absence of
strangulation or incarceration. These effects are produced by alterations in the course of the intestine, or in its lumen. The permeability is interfered with without causing circulatory disturbances.
Among the first to call attention to the abnormal adhesions of the
peritoneum, and their effects in producing intestinal obstruction, was
Virchow. In the fifth volume of his Archiv he gave the anatomical
evidence that abnormal adhesions frequently occur simultaneously.
For instance, the various curves and loops of the intestine grow together among themselves or with adjacent organs. The hepatic flexure of the colon may become adherent with the gall-bladder and the
entire biliary apparatus. The splenic flexure of the colon may become

adherent with the spleen and diaphragm, whilst the ileac or sigmoid flexure becomes agglutinated with the sexual organs, especially in women.   This form of localized peritonitic adhesions constitutes the most frequent type of this whole group of rather rare abnormalities. Treves (*l. c.*) and Nothnagel (*l. c.*) have given extensive descriptions of these conditions, of which perhaps six of the most important forms deserve mention.

1. Isolated and partial peritonitic contractions that create an enterostenosis by encircling the larger part or the entire intestine in an annular manner.   To this group belong those that have just been cited as having been first described by Virchow, under the name of "chronic mesenteric peritonitis" (mesenteritis).   The inflammation may be an extension (*a*) of an ulcerative process in the interior of the intestine, or a continuation of internal cicatricial strictures, which has already been described ; (*b*) from the neighboring organs of the intestine ; for instance, inflammation of the gall-bladder, perihepatitis, cirrhosis of the liver, perityphlitis, perisplenitis, appendicitis, and chronic inflammatory processes issuing from the female genito-urinary organs. (*c*) Virchow expressed the view that considerable damage may be done to the inner intestinal wall by the irritation of stagnating feces, and that a circumscribed peritonitis may arise therefrom.   (*d*) They may be congenital, dating from an intra-uterine peritonitis.   Willard has described a case ("Phila. Med. Times," May 5, 1883) where a pseudo-ligament at the splenic flexure had constricted the colon.   (*e*) An extremely rare form of partial peritoneal constriction without any internal intestinal lesion occurs in hernias which have been incarcerated but have been replaced or operated upon. The effects of these external localized peritonitic constrictions are the same, identically, as those produced by the chronic enterostenosis.

2. This includes the obstructions due to the adhesions of intestinal loops with each other.   A chronic peritonitis causes an agglutination between a circumscribed portion of two intestinal loops.   This may be observed both in the small and in the large intestine.   In the latter it is generally associated with coloptosis.   When two limbs of the same intestinal loop become adherent throughout their entire extent of surface, a sharp acute-angled bend or kink will develop in place of the former gradual curve.   This has been termed the "closed loop by adhesion."   But if the two limbs of the loop

are only adherent in a circumscribed spot, the graceful curve connecting the two limbs remains open, and this constitutes the so-called "open loop." The closed loop, with its sharp-angled communication, always causes an obstruction to the permeability. It is functionally as well as anatomically comparable to the external intestinal constriction. Whilst the open loop may give rise to volvulus or incarceration, it does not, as a rule, give rise to symptoms at all. The direct cause of such adhesions may be (a) compression which an intestinal loop has experienced in a hernia; (b) intestinal ulcers; (c) disease of mesenteric glands, generally of tuberculous origin. The relation of isolated partial peritonitis to visceral dislocation is difficult to understand when we are confronted with the completed process, for there may be two relations: first, the peritonitis may be primary, and have caused the dislocation, and, secondly, the peritonitis may be secondary, or caused by the dislocation. One can only judge which is the case when a fresh inflammatory process still exists. Circumscribed isolated peritonitis, which in this way causes an adhesion of one part of the colon with another, is generally associated with dilatation of the large intestine. There may also be coloptosis or abnormal elongation of the colon. In the chapter on Enteroptosis, in my work on "Diseases of the Stomach," second edition, page 708, an account is given of the various forms and types of the dislocations of the transverse colon, and Dr. J. Holmes Smith has briefly considered the anatomic aspect of these anomalies in his chapter on Anatomy of the Intestines (vol. I, chap. I). I may repeat here that abnormal elongation or dislocations of the colon may be congenital or acquired, and that the acquired types are the consequence of habitual obstipation; for the accumulation of feces must inevitably increase the weight of the colon, and lead to its descent. Acquired or congenital elongations and dislocations naturally bring the colon into approximation with remote organs, and also approximate various portions of the colon itself which are normally separated. If such approximation has taken place, catarrhal or ulcerative colitis, extending to the peritoneum, supplies the second etiological factor to produce a local adhesion.

3. Bending or curving of the intestine by isolated adhesion to another organ. These peritonitic adhesions have been found to

attach the small intestine to the transverse colon, to the uterus, or to the abdominal wall. They may be single or multiple, causing an isolated or numerous kinks in the intestine. The absolute freedom of the movement of the intestine is indispensable to its normal functioning. Whenever it is fixed in one or more places, sharp bends or kinks will inevitably develop somewhere, which, whilst they do not entirely interrupt the continuity of the lumen, nevertheless impede the progress of the feces. When such a kink has once developed, it may be aggravated by diarrhea, constipation, or sudden distention of the intestine by gases. On the other hand, there are cases in which such adhesions are found accidentally at the autopsy, having given no symptoms during life. In other cases the symptoms may be those already described under the heading of Enterostenoses. Kelling ("Arch. f. Verdauungs-Krankheiten," Bd. 1, S. 172) and Westphalen (*ibid.*, Bd. IV, S. 63) have described cases of adhesions of the transverse colon with the liver, and the resultant symptoms. On page 213, Plate 6, of this volume will be found an illustration of a case observed by myself of manifold adhesions, one of which also bound the transverse colon to the liver.

4. Manifold multiple adhesions of the intestinal loops, partly among themselves, partly with the parietal peritoneum, and partly with the solid abdominal viscera. These extensive and numerous adhesions are the result of diffuse chronic peritonitis, such as may be seen at autopsy in association with chronic, tuberculous, and carcinomatous peritonitis. This kind of peritonitis may agglutinate short sections of the intestine, or the entire ileum may be agglutinated into one immovable mass. Such adherent convolutions of the bowel may be palpated during life as a diffuse tumor, and cases are on record in which they were diagnosed as ovarian neoplasms, and laparotomy was performed for their removal. Strange to say, these most complicated of all intestinal adhesions have been known to exist without giving any intestinal symptoms. As a rule, however, symptoms do show themselves. The most frequent is constipation; the next most frequent, constipation alternating with diarrhea. The gravest symptoms are those of enterostenoses and absolute occlusion. Diffuse total adhesions of the intestine of this type are sometimes the result of operation upon the abdominal cavity. The conditions which set up these agglutinative peritonitic

adhesions after operations have as yet not been satisfactorily investigated.   I have had personal experience with two cases for which I
had advised operation for the relief of obstruction due to peritonitic
adhesions.   The adhesions were found and severed, but the autopsy
revealed in one case four, and in another case five adhesions, where
none had been discovered before.   There was no evidence of tuberculosis or carcinoma.

5. Intestinal adhesions caused by peritonitis issuing from the mesentery or the mesenteric glands.   The subject of mesenteric peritonitis
has already been touched upon in the etiology of volvulus.   The so-
called sigmoid mesenteritis causes an approximation of the two fulcrate
points of the sigmoid flexure, thus constituting one of the most frequent
causes of sigmoid volvulus.   Mesenteric peritonitis is especially
prevalent near the insertion of the cecum on the right side, and on
the left side in the mesentery of the sigmoid flexure.   It may be
circumscribed or diffuse.   When the entire mesentery is involved,
the complete small intestine becomes retracted toward the spinal
column.   Simultaneously with a chronic mesenteritis, the glands in
the mesentery may be diseased also, constituting an " *adenitis mesenterica.*"   When one or two glands are inflamed they may provoke
a circumscribed adhesive inflammation of the peritoneal covering of
one loop, fixing this loop at one spot.   There is also a chronic
peritonitis of the omentum, which I have already described in the
chapter on the Acute Occlusions.

6. Intestinal constriction caused by traction of a diverticulum.
These cases were first described by Treves.   There was no isolated
partial peritonitic adhesion, but a peculiar distortion of the intestinal
wall produced by the traction of a diverticulum, which had become
adherent to another part of the intestine, mesentery, or abdominal
wall.   The intestine thus attached by the diverticulum can not
execute its normal movements of peristalsis.   In attempting to
execute them it becomes kinked and stenosed.   The cases that
Treves described presented the symptomatology of chronic intestinal strictures during life.

Symptomatology.

This coincides with the clinical picture of enterostenoses and
occlusions.

Diagnosis.

Wherever there is a distinct clinical history of inflammation about the biliary apparatus, the appendix, the female sexual apparatus, or about the spleen, or where there is a previous history of hernia, trauma, or operations, it may lead the clinician in the direction of a correct diagnosis. External peritonitic constriction can sometimes be palpated, particularly if the abdominal walls can be brought to perfect relaxation by a hot bath or narcosis. Still the instances in which the diagnosis will prove to be correct are the exceptions, and the errors are the rule.

The **treatment** will be considered in the general chapter on Treatment of Intestinal Obstruction.

INTESTINAL COMPRESSION.

Although the lumen of the intestine is compressed in the strangulation, incarceration, volvulus, and by all forms of peritonitic bands and adhesions, these types are not considered compressions of the intestine proper. This term is limited to the mechanical weighing down of the intestinal lumen by bodies of some weight superimposed upon it. This compression is most frequently caused by carcinomas and sarcomas; also by the benign neoplasms, which may have originated in any abdominal organ, or in the mesentery, or pelvic organs. Naturally neoplasms that have arisen from one part of the intestine may compress another part; thus neoplasms of the intestine, kidney, liver, spleen, pancreas, lymph-glands, omentum, or mesentery can cause this compression. Compression of the sigmoid and rectum is most frequently caused by tumors of the uterus and ovaries. Dislocated organs which are otherwise not diseased may also cause compression; thus we meet with compression of the bowel by floating kidneys or floating spleen. Much more frequently than this complication do we find the compression by a dislocated or gravid uterus. The small intestine may be compressed by the mesentery of other loops of the ileum which have prolapsed into the pelvis (Schnitzler, "Wien. klin. Rundschau," 1895, No. 37). Similarly the duodenum may become compressed by a dilation of the stomach and consequent kinking of the pylorus.

Broadbent, Elmeyer, Kussmaul, and the author have called attention to this condition. Harrison Allen (" Anatomy ") mentions intestinal compression by aneurysm of superior mesenteric artery. The various forms of abscesses which may occur in the abdomen also play an etiological rôle in this condition. In the chapter on Volvulus I have described the compression of the limbs of the sigmoid flexure by an entire convolution of the small intestine, which may descend upon the twisted locality. The compression of the duodenum by the normal mesentery of the dislocated ileum, as described by Schnitzler, has been designated by him as " mesenteric intestinal incarceration." In order to bring about this effect, a number of abnormalities are necessary, prominent among which are relaxed abdominal walls, spinal curvature, elongation or malformation of the mesentery, and relatively low fixation of the duodenum. Those portions of the intestinal canal which are normally most immovable and fixed are most likely to be compressed. Accordingly we find that the rectum is the most frequent seat of this form of obstruction; in the first place because it is fixed within the pelvis, in the second place because it is surrounded by a bony wall, and thirdly because of its proximity to the female sexual organs, which are among the most frequent direct causes of compression. I have observed one case of rectal compression in an aged man caused by an immense hypertrophy of the prostate gland. The sigmoid flexure and the descending colon are the next most frequent seats of compression. Then follows the duodenum. The jejunum, upper ileum, and transverse colon are rarely subjected to this accident. Baimbrigge (cited from Nothnagel, *l. c.*) has described a case of acute compression of the colon by a floating spleen in which death resulted after twenty-four hours.

Symptomatology.

The symptoms of intestinal compression are usually those of a chronic enterostenosis, but the case of Baimbrigge, just cited, proves that they may also take the form of a very acute occlusion, particularly when the intestine becomes incarcerated by sudden movement of the compressing neoplasm or movable organ. The cases described by Schnitzler presented the clinical picture of acute incarceration.

Diagnosis.

The recognition of intestinal compression is possible where we can make out a neoplasm, a dislocated or floating intra-abdominal organ.   Where this is not possible the anamnesis may give utilizable hints.

PARALYSIS, SPASTIC OCCLUSION, AND MOTOR INSUFFI-
CIENCY OF THE INTESTINE.

Synonyms.—Pseudo-occlusion; Pseudo-ileus; Paralytic, Spastic, or Dynamic Ileus.

Intestinal Occlusion without Mechanical Obstruction of the Lumen.

Functional insufficiency of the peristalsis of a part or of the entire intestine, without being caused by a mechanical obstacle such as described in previous chapters, was first correctly recognized by Henrot in 1865.   In a masterly thesis on the subject ("Des pseudo-étranglements que l'on peut rapporter à la paralysie de l'intestin," Thèse de Paris, 1865) he presented the first exact representation of intestinal occlusion of this type.   Nothnagel (*l. c.*, p. 356) and Boas (*l. c.*, Inhaltsverzeichniss, S. x) speak of this condition as intestinal occlusion without any alteration of the lumen ("Ohne Beeinträchtigung des Lumen").   Perhaps they mean thereby that there is no mechanical obstacle, such as has been described in the previous chapter on Occlusion; for the lumen, as a matter of fact, is very considerably altered in all cases of intestinal paralysis.   In one condition, as in the "Gassperre," described by Leichtenstern, we may have a tremendous expansion of the intestinal lumen; and in another, as in the enterospasm, which has been described by Heidenhain ("Bericht über die Verhandlungen der deutschen Gesellschaft für Chirurgie, XXVI. Kongr.," 1897), we may have complete obliteration of the lumen by spastic contraction of the circular muscle. This has also been observed by Leichtenstern.   So the term "paralytic occlusion without alteration of the lumen" is, in my opinion, open to objection.   The significance of motor insufficiency of the intestine has been emphasized by O. Rosenbach ("Berlin. klin. Wochenschr.," 1889, No. 13 u. 14), but the original classification of Henrot, of the various conditions leading to intestinal paralysis, is still serviceable for a summary representation of this subject.

1. Intestinal Paralysis by Causes Not Directly Affecting the Intestine.—Among the etiological factors under this heading, the following conditions may be arranged : Acute orchitis, injury to the testicle, operations upon hemorrhoids, buboes, abscesses, and other inflammatory processes of the inguinal region and abdominal walls, and inflamed hydroceles. Nothnagel has observed a case after puncture of the abdominal wall for ascites, in consequence of valvular disease of the heart. Treves observed phenomena of incarceration in a child, with extreme prostration and incessant vomiting, constipation, and meteorism. A hard, very sensitive, non-replaceable tumor was found in the groin. A hernial incarceration had been diagnosed on account of this tumor, which, however, proved to be an undescended testicle. Applications of ice caused the disappearance of all the symptoms of incarceration. In the introduction to the chapter on Intestinal Occlusion I have described a number of conditions which belong under the heading of intestinal paralysis. Among others, I have there reported (see page 120) a case of a driver who had been struck in the abdomen by the shafts of an express wagon. But in this case there were anatomical changes consisting of a serous transudate, infiltrating about 8 inches of the middle ileum. This was seen at operation. At the autopsy there was no evidence of this infiltration, so that if we had not seen the intestine during the operation, but only at the postmortem table, we might have concluded that it was a case of paralytic ileus without any anatomical alteration in the intestine. The postmortem appearances are so different in these cases from the conditions observed at operation, caused pre-eminently by the cessation of arterial pressure and disappearance of disturbances caused by vascular congestion, that many cases ordinarily classed under this heading as not being associated with anatomical changes may really have presented those changes during life, but they were not demonstrable at the necropsy.

2. Intestinal Paresis from Causes Acting Directly on the Intestine, and Producing at Least a Partially Demonstrable Anatomical Lesion.—After completion of an intra-abdominal operation, intestinal resection, removal of neoplasms, etc., and the lumen has been restored, no evacuation of feces or gases may occur on the following days, in spite of re-establishment of the permeability. Meteorism develops gradually, the pulse sinks, and the patient enters a state of collapse. We have, in short, the complete clinical picture of intestinal obstruction all over again. The autopsy shows the intestine to be absolutely free from obstruction, and no sign of peritonitis. The same condition has been observed in connection with Littré's hernia, in which there is no complete obstruction of the intestinal lumen, as is well known; nevertheless the symptoms of absolute stenosis may arise under the conditions above pictured. After operations upon the female sexual organs and after reposition of incarcerated external hernias a similar pseudo-occlusion has been observed. Gall-stones of such size as to be insufficient themselves to obturate the lumen have been known to cause absolute acute intestinal occlusion. This group, which contains the cases of motor insufficiency that present the greatest interest from the standpoint of the pathological physiology of the intestine, will be more extensively considered at the end of this classification.

3. **Intestinal Paralysis Following Embolism in the Mesenteric Artery.**—This will be considered in a separate chapter.

4. **Motor Insufficiency of the Intestine Due to Pronounced Pathological Lesions.**—In the introduction to the study of intestinal occlusion, paragraph VII, this volume (p. 119), I have already stated that the most frequent cause of intestinal paralysis is peritonitis. I refer here more to the diffuse acute peritonitis than to the chronic form, for in the latter, as is evidenced in the preceding chapters, we will more frequently meet with a mechanical stenosis. Naturally, when a peritonitis has followed a perforation, the possibility of a reflex paralysis must be considered simultaneously with that caused directly by the peritonitis.

5. **Intestinal Paralysis Due to Extensive Distention by Enormous Accumulation of Gases.**—See introduction to the study of intestinal occlusion, paragraph XII, page 124, Meteorism.

6. **Motor Insufficiency Due to Habitual Constipation and Occurring in the Suprastenotic Loops.**—See introduction to intestinal occlusion, paragraphs II and X (pp. 117 and 122).

7. Intestinal Paralysis Due to Bacterial Intoxication in the Absence of Pathological Evidences of Peritonitis.

8. Pseudo-ileus in Consequence of Paralysis Occurring in the Course of Neuroses and Diseases of the Central Nervous System.—See chapter on Intestinal Neuroses.

Pathological Physiology of Intestinal Paralysis.

In considering the nature of the conditions just classified, it is necessary to distinguish carefully between motor paralysis of the intestine and arrest of the peristalsis, though the latter will have the same functional effect as a genuine paresis of the muscular fibers, and from the clinical standpoint the two will be indistinguishable. Intestinal paralysis may be brought about in two ways under the influence of the nerves : (*a*) Paralysis of the motor fibers or ganglia, causing a cessation of muscular contraction ; (*b*) reflex excitation of the inhibitory fibers for intestinal paralysis, which are found in the splanchnic nerve. The cases in groups 1 and 2 are explained theoretically by an excitation of the inhibitory nerves. In the introduction to intestinal occlusion, paragraph XI, I have cited the experiments of Goltz in which he produced arrest of the heart in diastole in a frog when the abdomen was repeatedly struck with a small rod. This experiment makes it plausible that violent centripetal irritation which originates from the nerves of the peritoneum or intestine itself may cause depression of the heart's action, bringing on the symptoms of collapse simultaneously with excitation of the inhibitory nerves for intestinal peristalsis ; *i. e.*, reflex excitation of the splanchnic may simultaneously depress the heart, thus producing a complication of symptoms corresponding to those of strangulation. This reflex inhibition of the intestinal peristalsis can naturally not be excluded in those very acute forms of peritonitis which result from perforating appendicitis and perityphlitis, and which are usually attributed to the peritonitis itself.

In the overdistention which occurs in stagnation meteorism in the suprastenotic loops, Nothnagel has found that the strongest electric current applied directly to the intestine can no longer produce any contraction. Gas resorption from the intestine is very much interfered with during peritonitis, and in the manner described contributes to the production of motor insufficiency. This gaseous distention must naturally exist for a considerable length of time before it can bring about this paresis. If it is remedied early enough, the intestine may regain its contractility. Another factor not to be overlooked is that the intestinal muscular fibers may become exhausted as a consequence of overwork, for acute peritonitis sometimes sets up an exaggerated peristalsis. So that there are many factors during acute peritonitis, all tending to produce paresis, one supplementing the other, and at times establishing a vicious circle. The case which I have cited (see introduction, paragraph VII, this volume, p. 119) of a serous transudation and edema of the intestinal wall, causing obstruction, has long ago been described by Stokes, who attributed the paralysis of the intestinal musculature observed during peritonitis to collateral edema and saturation of the intestinal wall by a serous transudate.

On the basis of a number of carefully conducted experiments, Reichel ("Darm Ausschaltung," "Centralbl. f. Chir.," 1894) has suggested that the intestinal paralysis observed after laparotomies, herniotomies, etc., is due to circumscribed infection. He demonstrates that there is a peritoneal infection without any traces of inflammatory changes or the serous covering of the intestine. I have already referred to my own experience, and given the evidence that we can not exclude the possibility of bacterial peritoneal infection in all cases where the pathologist is unable to demonstrate peritonitis. Bacteria may enter the peritoneum in two ways—during operation, and, secondly, from the intestinal lumen in consequence of changes caused by the various conditions producing obstruction. The latter is the most frequent path of infection, and explains intestinal paralysis which occurs after the bloodless replacement of external hernias. Multanowsky (Diss., St. Petersburg, 1895, in Russian) demonstrated that an interruption of the free movement of the intestinal contents of six hours suffices to permit the transmigration of bacteria through the intestinal wall, and that it is not necessary for the intestinal mucosa to be in any way necrosed to permit of this passage. The intestinal wall becomes passable not only for the colon bacillus, but for all other microorganisms which happen to be in the intestinal contents. The question of permeability of the intestinal wall for bacteria during occlusion has been answered in the affirmative by Arnd, Garré,

Bönnecken, Nepveu, Oker-Blom, Reichel, and Multanowsky.   On
the basis of their results we may assume that infection of the
abdominal cavity occurs very often and very early in case of
impermeability of the intestine.   The differences in the clinical as
well as the pathological pictures are conditioned by the quantities
and species of the various bacteria which have invaded the peritoneum.   These phenomena may vary from those of a slight transient
peritoneal irritation to that of an intestinal paralysis or acute diffuse
peritoneal sepsis.

Motor insufficiency following habitual constipation is comparable
to the paralysis which eventually supervenes in the hypertrophied
musculature in chronic stenoses, for when the coprostasis is permanent we may have a muscular hypertrophy, which is a compensatory arrangement, capable of overcoming for a long time the resistance offered by the hardened accumulated feces.   Eventually,
however, the hypertrophied muscle must become exhausted; we
have motor insufficiency, and the symptomatology of complete
occlusion results.   This occlusion may be transient or permanent.
If the muscle is simply exhausted and not degenerated, it may
recover its contractility by rest, and once more succeed in restoring
a functional peristalsis.   But if fatty degeneration has occurred in
the muscle fibers, the compensatory hypertrophy is lost altogether,
and the occlusion can not be relieved except by operation.

In the introduction to the study of intestinal occlusion, paragraph
VI, this volume, page 118, I have described blocking of the intestine by gas, the so-called "Gassperre" of Leichtenstern.   The intestinal loops which have the shortest mesentery—the duodenum
and jejunum—can not move away from the spinal column as far as
the loops which have the longest mesentery—the middle ileum;
hence the latter can rise against the anterior abdominal wall and
become immensely distended with gas in the dorsal position of the
patient; the solid and liquid contents will rather flow into the duodenum and stomach, because it is impossible for them to reach the
immensely distended loops higher up.   Leichtenstern has also
emphasized that paralysis of the musculature of the intestine is not
always a pathological entity *per se*, for it may complicate strangulations and volvulus.   A portion of the intestine may, for instance,
be incarcerated, but still not completely occluded.   But the oblitera-

tion may become complete by the supervening of paralysis.   In this instance the paralysis follows the primary or preceding incarceration.   In other instances it may come in advance and precede a strangulation,—*i. e.*, the intestinal motor insufficiency will be the first step in the pathological physiology, and a volvulus or strangulation follow upon it.

Symptomatology.

The symptoms correspond entirely to those of mechanical occlusion.   The onset may be sudden or gradual ; the symptoms severe or mild ; they may be meteorism, vomiting, suppression of fecal evacuations, and collapse.   The manner in which the impermeability is brought about during paralysis is very simple, namely this : A shorter or longer section of the intestine is paralyzed or insufficient from one or more of the causes already detailed, the sections affected are distended immensely by gas, the propelling force to move along the feces is absent, and accordingly fecal matters stagnate and accumulate in the loops above the paralytic area.   This accumulation, once having taken place, acts as a mechanical obstacle, and may also aggravate the occlusion by producing dislocation of the loops weighed down by the accumulated mass.   One of my cases is of interest in illustrating reflex pseudo-ileus :

"A female fifty years of age had suffered off and on for six months with constipation. About eight days before I was called, complete suppression of stool supervened. Castor oil and calomel and Carlsbad salts had been taken, but no evacuation had been effected. On the day before I was summoned (April 20, 1900), the patient had vomited fecal matter and was tortured by intense pains in the epigastrium radiating to the navel. Temporary relief from hot cataplasms and hypodermic injection of morphin.   April 21, 1900, in my presence the patient vomited twice and brought up material which was undoubtedly fecal.   A large colon enema brought away very little fecal matter.   The colon was entirely permeable to ileocecal valve by Langdon tube.   During lavage of the stomach for relief of the stercoraceous vomiting the duodenum was intubated and found permeable as far as the tube could reach (2 meters).   There was a period of rest after lavage, but as the symptoms of obstruction returned on the following day, operation was urged.   During the laparotomy the intestines were found everywhere permeable, but a gall-stone of the size of a hazel-nut was found in the cystic duct and 12 gall-stones in the gall-bladder, which were removed.   The patient made an uneventful recovery and was in perfect health and had regular evacuations when last seen, which was three months after the operation."

Such cases of symptomatic occlusion where laparotomy shows the lumen to be everywhere open suggest a transient, reflex; tetanic spasm of the intestinal musculature as the direct cause of the ileus. But as no one, to my knowledge, has ever seen the intestine in this condition during spastic ileus, it must not be looked upon as more than an assumption, still lacking objective clinical and experimental proof.

It is necessary to define with greater exactness what is meant by " *intestinal paralysis* " in some of these cases. This term does not imply that contractility of the muscularis is absolutely lost, but in the majority of cases it refers to a reflex excitation of the inhibitory nerves, by which the peristalsis is interrupted. Such a condition might exist,—the irritation emanating from the biliary apparatus, as in my case,—and yet no evidence of impermeability be visible at the operation.

Diagnosis.

The great similarity that this condition presents to the occlusion resulting from other conditions already described, particularly that due to cicatricial stenosis or carcinoma, and that due to peritonitis, explains the difficulties in the way of recognizing it. The general section on Diagnosis will include this subject also.

Prognosis.

This depends upon the cause. When the paralysis has resulted after surgical operation upon the abdomen, or if it is due to peritonitis, the prognosis is grave. If it is due to a reflex from rectal, ovarian, or testicular abnormalities, the paralysis may subside entirely if the primary cause is removed. So-called relative motor insufficiencies, which develop in the musculature above mechanical stenoses, have been observed to subside spontaneously and become aggravated again. This phenomenon of alternate improvement and aggravation may repeat itself frequently in benign stenosis. But eventually irreparable degenerations ensue in the compensatory hypertrophy above the stenosis. However, even here recovery is possible if the stenosis is not of a malignant nature.

The literature on the subject of Spastic Ileus has been abstracted by Dr. Edward Quintard (Amer. Gastro-enterologic Association, Session of May, 1901, Washington, D. C.).

DIAGNOSIS OF VARIOUS FORMS OF STENOSIS AND OCCLUSION OF THE INTESTINE.

There is no field in clinical pathology and diagnosis in which experience, judgment, and resourcefulness count for so much as in the diagnosis of enterostenosis and occlusion. There is no field in which the opinion of the clinician is so important. There is no field in which more weight concerning life or death can be attached to the diagnostic decision. The three cardinal objects of diagnosis are: (1) Does an enterostenosis or occlusion of the intestine actually exist? (2) What is the location of the obstruction? (3) What is the pathologic-anatomic condition causing it?

When I started to write this chapter on diagnosis I conceived the idea of presenting the clinical history of a typical case under each form of intestinal occlusion. Whilst this would no doubt have a certain advantage, it was impossible to find so-called typical cases, which should represent the symptoms representing the cardinal diagnostic features in the various forms of occlusion. In my own personal records, as well as in those of German, English, American, and French literature, it is extremely rare to find two cases exactly alike under any one type of stenosis or occlusion.

Regarding the probability with which a diagnosis can be made, I may premise that which I have to say by the following statements: (a) There are cases in which the diagnosis can be stated absolutely; (b) cases in which the diagnosis is impossible; and, between these extremes, (c) a large variety of cases in which the diagnosis can be made with more or less probability (Nothnagel). Of the possible conditions which may cause intestinal stenosis or occlusion, I have described the following:

Various forms of intestinal ulcers, chapter XXI, volume I.

Malignant neoplasms, chapter XXII, volume I.

Benign neoplasms, chapter XXII, volume I.

Volvulus and intestinal loop formation, chapter III, volume II.

Internal and herniaform incarceration of the intestine, chapter III, volume II.

Invagination or intussusception, chapter III, volume II.

Internal stricture, chapter III, volume II.

External peritonitic constriction, chapter III, volume, II.

Intestinal compression, chapter III, volume II.

Obturation of the intestine, chapter III, volume II.

Paralysis and motor insufficiency, chapter III, volume II.

In order to do justice to both the needs of the general practitioner as well as to those of the specialist, these subjects have all been described in detail, each in a special chapter; but particularly for the general practitioner a separate chapter has been compiled entitled Enterostenoses and Intestinal Occlusion, in which the sum total of clinical observation, symptomatology, pathology, diagnosis, and treatment has been given.

I. Does an Enterostenosis or Occlusion of the Intestine Actually Exist?

There are but two objective signs that permit of a positive diagnosis of obstruction: (1) When a stenosis can be felt or recognized by inspection of the rectum and sigmoid by the Martin or Kelly proctoscope or sigmoidoscope; (2) when tetanically rigid or stiffened plastic elevation of intestinal loops can be seen and palpated during attacks of intestinal colic. The symptoms and signs upon which the practitioner must depend for a diagnosis, in addition to these, are (a) obstipation, especially when associated with colic, (b) cessation of evacuation of flatus, (c) meteorism, (d) vomiting, (e) stercoraceous vomiting, (f) pain, (g) tumor, (h) leukocytosis. These cardinal symptoms may occur in diseases other than acute intestinal obstruction. They may result from peritonitis in the absence of mechanical obstruction. The various causes of peritonitis must therefore be excluded, particularly those arising from the digestive canal itself, from the biliary passages, from the genito-urinary apparatus in females, from the genito-urinary tract in males, from suppuration of infected lymph-glands, embolism of the mesenteric arteries, and also from extension of inflammatory processes through the abdominal and thoracic walls. Let us consider critically the diagnostic value of these symptoms and signs seriatim.

Obstipation, when it occurs in an individual who has always had regular intestinal evacuations and in whom we can not diagnose enteritis, sudden neurasthenia, dietetic or medicinal obstipation, should awaken a suspicion of stenosis if we can recognize causal factors in the anamnesis which are capable of producing strictures; for instance, intestinal tuberculosis or typhoid fever. Among the other conditions to be inquired into in sudden obstipation are diseases emanating from the female sexual apparatus, the bile-passages and the appendix, as well as external hernias and foreign bodies swallowed in the food.

In all cases where **attacks of colic** are associated with sudden onset of constipation the practitioner should at once methodically begin to subject his patient to a rigid examination. If in the course of the examination neoplasms or inflammatory tumors, pseudo-ligaments, evidences of chronic peritonitis, dislocations of solid abdominal organs, invagination tumor, or old hernias are found, the diagnosis becomes practically certain. Obstipation coming on with rapid weakness, anemia, and emaciation, in the absence of an assignable cause, justifies the suspicion of carcinomatous stenosis. The evacuations should be examined in all cases, and the characteristic feces of stenosis looked for; it is necessary to search for blood, pus, and mucus. Sudden obstipation and attacks of colic may occur in simple habitual constipation, where the accumulated masses of feces constitute an obstacle to the permeability. But of such importance is the symptom of obstipation that the diagnosis of stenosis is practically impossible where there are regular evacuations or where the stenosis is either so high up in the small intestine, where the contents are liquid, or when the stenosing process has not sufficiently advanced to seriously obstruct the lumen. The evacuations which occur after invagination or intussusception constitute an exception to this statement.

Conditions that may be Confused with Occlusion.—The following conditions may present identical clinical symptoms and signs as occlusions, and they have most frequently given rise to confusion in the diagnosis: Intestinal paresis after operations upon the rectum, testicle, or ovary; in a similar manner contusion of these organs or of the abdominal wall; renal or biliary colic; lead colic, flatulent colic; acute arsenic-poisoning. A number of morbid conditions in which obstipation, vomiting, and retracted abdomen are associated with delirium have been diagnosed as meningitis, when in reality an occlusion of the small intestine was present.

To Distinguish between Peritonitis and Occlusion.—As all of the symptoms mentioned can be caused by acute peritonitis, one of the most critical objects of diagnosis will be to distinguish whether the symptoms present are those of acute occlusion or peritonitis. Here the most valuable factors are the duration and the behavior of the localized pain. Peritonitis rarely develops prior to forty-eight hours after the initial symptoms of pain and vomit. In examining into the symptom of pain we must distinguish between spontaneous pain, which is present at all times, and pressure pain, which is caused only by palpation. The spontaneous pain is due to the localized process of the obstruction, as a rule, and it is generally circumscribed. The pressure pain is, as a rule, due to peritonitis, and is diffuse. If a spontaneous pain seemingly extends into a diffuse pain, and the sufferer assumes the characteristic attitude of peritoneal irritation, anxiously avoiding every voluntary movement, with legs drawn up, we may assume the development of peritonitis.

Meteorism, when it is present, may cause considerable sensitiveness to pressure, and cases of suppurative peritonitis occur in which both the localized spontaneous and diffuse or pressure pains are so slight as to be useless for diagnostic purposes. The phenomena of local and stagnation meteorism have already been sufficiently dwelt upon. If inspection, percussion, and auscultation can elicit a distinct local meteorism, a well-circumscribed, sharply distended loop, the diagnosis of strangulation or volvulus is quite certain, and peritonitis can be excluded. Diffuse general meteorism makes abdominal palpation for diagnostic purposes difficult. In the absence of every trace of intestinal peristalsis, general meteorism is very suggestive of intestinal paresis due to peritonitis.

In the differentiation between peritonitis and occlusion the *temperature* is of importance. As a rule, fever is suggestive of peritonitis if it has occurred from the very beginning of the disease. If it has developed some time after the disease, the fever can not exclude the possibility of occlusion, for in this case peritonitis may have supervened upon an occlusion.

Vomiting.—Fecal vomiting may occur in intestinal paralysis, as a consequence of peritonitis, and in consequence of fistulæ connecting the stomach and the colon, or the duodenum or jejunum and colon. In order to differentiate between a mechanical and a dynamic occlusion we must above all give attention to the anamnesis and etiology which have been stated in the chapter on motor insufficiency of the intestine. After traumas, operations upon the genital organs or rectum, reduction of hernias, laparotomies, etc., pseudo-ileus may develop. The differentiation from peritonitis has already been dwelt upon. In fistulæ which cause communication between the stomach and colon, or the jejunum and colon, we may have stercoraceous vomiting, it is true, but not obstipation and meteorism. By means of distending the rectum and colon with air or gas the stomach will be distended simultaneously if a communication exists; and again, if we fill the stomach with a solution of Burgundy-red or hematoxylin, it will pass at once into the transverse colon, and can within a minute or two be discovered in the rectum if a communication exists.

In this connection I must emphasize that vomiting, obstipation, meteorism, and pain do not in themselves by any means permit the diagnosis of occlusion. So much is evident from what has been argued in the preceding. But if the paroxysmal, localized, and visible intestinal peristalsis exists, with rigid erection of palpable and visible loops, the diagnosis of occlusion is certain. Unfortunately this sign occurs only in association with chronic stenoses; it is absent in the acute occlusions.

Leukocytosis.—The leukocyte counts are of value only if undertaken during the first forty-eight to seventy-two hours after the beginning of the occlusion symptoms. If a patient suffering from suppression of evacuations, flatus, meteorism, vomiting, and pain gives a leukocyte count of 18,000 to 20,000 after twelve hours, the diagnosis of obstruction is logical. If the symptoms become aggravated and the leukocyte count amounts to 26,000 to 28,000 after twenty-four hours, operation should not be deferred. The first studies in this country of leukocytosis and its relation to strangulation were made by Dr. Harvey Cushing (" Johns Hopkins Hospital Reports," vol. VII, 1898, p. 332, quoted from Joseph C. Bloodgood, "Blood Examinations," etc., " Md. Med. Jour.," Sept., 1901).

Liquid exudates in the peritoneum, when they can be demonstrated beyond a doubt, support the diagnosis of peritonitis. Such exudates may, however, be present and escape detection, because they may be covered by tympanitic intestinal loops. On the other hand, there is an exudate which occurs in association with interruption of the venous mesenteric circulation, during volvulus and incarceration, in the absence of peritonitis. Peritonitis does not necessarily arrest the intestinal movements in all cases ; it does so as a rule. The chapter on Intestinal Paresis gives the other causes that may lead up to this condition. The presence or absence of indican in the urine has some diagnostic significance. Indican is always present in acute peritonitis. If, therefore, indican is absent in a doubtful case, it is an argument against peritonitis, and for occlusion in the colon. But when indican is present in the urine, it speaks as well for occlusion of the small intestine as for peritonitis. Fleischer's views concerning the origin of indican in stenoses of the small and large intestine have already been given in the preceding chapters.

What is the Location of the Obstruction ?

The most fundamental question to decide here is whether the occlusion is in the small or in the large intestine. For the determination of this point Nothnagel attributes considerable importance to distention and the changes in form which the intestinal loops undergo by the accumulation of gas and liquids within them, and the plates which he gives illustrative of these appearances are indeed very instructive. He holds that the location and arrangement of the distended loops correspond, as a general rule, to their normal location. These appearances are due principally to stagnation meteorism. One of the characteristic forms of distention for the large intestine has been designated by Nothnagel "flank meteorism." This form of colon expansion can be recognized by protrusion of the lateral walls and the upper region of the abdomen. The flank meteorism may be unilateral, only extending a certain distance upward from the stenosis, when the latter is in the sigmoid flexure, or when the stenosis is higher up in the colon. It is naturally important to know the congenital or acquired possible abnormalities of the location of the colon. These may give rise to extraordinary distentions if they should be involved in an occlusion. Flank meteorism may be caused also by local meteorism in the small intestine in the absence of stenosis of the colon or sigmoid. Nothnagel cites a case where circumscribed local meteorism of the jejunum had caused distention of the lateral abdominal region, or flank.   As a rule, however, it can be said that flank meteorism is absent in stenosis of the small intestine.   A careful, painstaking study of the abdomen can not be too urgently recommended. There is no difficulty in distinguishing the distention of the colon from that of the small intestine when we are confronted with chronic enterostenosis ; but in acute occlusion, where the enormous local meteorism may develop with great rapidity, the distinction is frequently impossible.   Nothnagel also calls attention to a sign which I have already cited.   This sign can be elicited by percussion or by combined auscultation and percussion.   It consists in a change of the percussion resonance in the upper posterior lumbar region. Normally the percussion note in this region is dull, high, giving the impression of emptiness.   When the stenosis is in the sigmoid flexure or descending colon, one can frequently find this note changed to a loud and deep resonance on both sides.   But if the stenosis is in the splenic flexure or transverse colon, the change of resonance can only be made out on the right side.   In critical cases the value of this sign is indeed considerable, and is another confirmation of the great utility of skilful percussion.   Among other signs that can be made out in fortunate cases by inspection, palpation, and percussion alone are tumors and visible peristalsis. A tumor, when once seen or felt, naturally gives the very best evidence of the location of the obstruction.   The visible intestinal peristalsis and plastic rigidity are a very important indication of the localization of the occlusion.   No one who has ever seen this stormy peristalsis will ever forget the first impression of it, or mistake it for any other condition.   One must not, however, make the error of localizing the seat of the stenosis at the spot where the peristalsis ceases, for the intestinal loops which are nearest the obstacle become paralytic before others more remote therefrom. For instance, when a carcinoma is in the sigmoid flexure, the plastic rigidity and stormy peristalsis can be seen in the descending colon during the first stage of the disease ; but after the fourth or fifth day they cease in the descending and transverse colons, and can only be seen in the ascending colon.   This would lead one to presume that

the obstacle was in the hepatic flexure instead of the sigmoid
flexure.   It is important, therefore, to bear in mind the duration of
the stenotic symptoms, and if they are observed on the first day,
one is justified in localizing the obstacle at the point where the
stormy peristalsis ceases; but after the third day such localization
is inadmissible.   Unfortunately for the question of localization, this
valuable sign of plastic rigidity with stormy peristalsis is absent in
just those cases in which we should most desire a localization of
the occlusion; I mean the forms of acute occlusions—volvulus and
strangulation.

Examination of the Hernial Orifices.—*The Value of Physical
Methods of Examination, Distention of the Rectum and Colon by Air
or Water, Inspection of the Rectum and Sigmoid with the Proctoscope
or Sigmoidoscope, Sounding of the Rectum or Entire Colon by the
Langdon or Kuhn Tube.*—The hernial orifices *must* always be examined in every case of occlusion or stenosis.   " Woe to the physician," says Leube, " who fails to do this."   This " must " is
imperative.   Even the rare anatomical gates through which hernias
may possibly occur must be carefully examined to discover whether
there may not be a localized pressure pain or a swelling present.
This investigation must be done deliberately and systematically.
First the inguinal canal is examined, then the umbilical region ;
next follow the femoral region, the obturator foramen, the ischiatic
foramen, the rectum and vagina ; the entire wall of the abdomen
should carefully be palpated over for possible ventrical or lumbar
hernia.   The tiny hernias that occur in median linea alba must not
be forgotten.

Examination of the rectum by the finger alone may occasionally
instruct the clinician concerning the location of an intussusception,
stricture, or obstruction from abnormal contents.   The method first
suggested by Simon—of introducing the entire hand into the rectum
—has never appealed to my judgment as being practical.   In the
first place it requires a small hand, deep narcosis, and much time ;
then in cases in which I have tried it (two cases of sigmoid volvulus) I was not able to make out what the fingers felt.   The fingers
are so cramped within the rectum that movements are impossible.
The paralysis which supervenes upon the immense dilation of the
sphincters required in one case two weeks, in another twenty-four

days, before it was repaired.   The hand can not be introduced any
further than the wrist.   It is certainly preferable to look into the
rectum and sigmoid, and this can be readily done by the method
described by Thos. Chas. Martin, in the last chapter of this volume.

The Introduction of the Rectal Langdon Tube or Sound.—A number
of authors—A. Graser (*l. c.*), Pribram (*l. c.*), Nothnagel (*l. c.*, p.
377), and even Fitz (*l. c.*)—do not attribute much importance to rectal
and colon sounding for the location of the obstacle.   Fitz states that
he has failed to pass either the rigid or the flexible tube beyond the
sigmoid flexure in numerous attempts both on the living and dead
subject.   After repeatedly introducing the flexible tube its entire
length, it was in his experience found compactly coiled within the
rectum on passing the finger through the anus.   Treves (*l. c.*) and
Rosenheim record similar experiences.   I have elsewhere emphasized that the passage of the Langdon tube, or the Kuhn spiral
sound, through the entire colon to the ileocecal valve is practicable.
It can be proved to have reached the ileocecal valve by auscultation
over this region when air and water are alternately blown in through
the tube ; also by introducing the electro-diaphane, which can by
diaphany be observed to pass through the entire anatomical course
of the colon.   The Kuhn tube, which contains a metallic spiral of
great elasticity, can be seen by means of the Röntgen rays.
There are, of course, cases of coloptosis, where the passage of a
tube through the entire colon becomes very difficult or impossible ;
but for the determination of the permeability of the colon, intubation of this organ, in my opinion, constitutes a valuable auxiliary
to physical diagnosis.   It should be first practised on the cadaver,
and then on healthy normal persons, in order to acquire the experience and technic of introduction.   One of the adjuvant tricks, during the introduction, is to permit a stream of water of considerable
strength to issue from the end of the tube while it is being introduced, and to rotate the tube between the fingers during the introduction.   For stenosis of the rectum and sigmoid I hardly consider
the intubation necessary, because these can be seen by means of
the sigmoidoscope.   But for stenosis above the sigmoid, a cautious,
probing introduction of the rubber Langdon tube is, in my opinion,
certainly as available a method for diagnosis as distention with water
or air.

The Distention of the Colon by Air and Water.—The success of this procedure depends upon the capacity of the rectum, sigmoid, and colon. Air can be introduced by connecting the end of a long Langdon tube with the nozle of a double pair of bulbs or a pair of bellows. Illoway prefers a siphon of aerated or carbonated water. Ziemssen recommends charging the intestine alternately with 20 grams (5 drams) of bicarbonate of soda, followed by 18 grams (4½ drams) of tartaric acid. The simplest and best agent is ordinary air blown in by the bellows, which should be tried first. It will frequently give the desired information, without necessitating the distention with water, which, owing to its great weight, is itself a mechanical factor for displacing intestinal loops.

Degrees of Pressure Required.—For distention with water a large fountain syringe, or a very large Hegar funnel with a rubber tube about 10 feet long and a rectal nozle, is all that is necessary. Sometimes the water rushes in with such ease that but a few feet of pressure above the level of the rectum are necessary to accomplish distention. At other times the pressure of 10 or more feet may be necessary. It is useless to use a pressure of over 15 feet; then, also, there is no room in an ordinary dwelling where such a pressure could be obtained. Thomas (London "Lancet," 1886, 11, page 1219) has reported a case where an enema was given on the third day of obstruction, and under slight pressure. Death followed in an hour and a half. The autopsy disclosed an intussusception, and a tear was found in the sheath, and half a tumbler of water in the pelvis. High pressure should be used only in recent obstructions. In obstructions older than from three to four days, adhesions may have already formed, the severance of which may involve serious complications. In children lower degrees of pressure will produce rupture than in the adult, and the capacity of the colon is naturally much less. The quantity which the large intestine of an adult will hold with safety may be stated as 6 liters. The quantity which the large intestine of an infant may safely receive varies with the age of the child ; it can not be stated with exactness, because reliable measurements corresponding with the various periods of growth have not as yet been made. Rotch ("Boston Med. and Surg. Jour.," 1882, vol. cvi, p. 322) found that more than 17 feet of pressure were necessary to rupture the intestine of an infant after removal from the body. Forrest ("Amer. Jour. of Obstetrics," 1886, vol. XIX, p. 673), in experimenting with the colon of an infant, found that it could bear without rupture from 20 to 22 feet of pressure. For the colon of an adult he found that 30 to 37 feet of pressure were required before rupture ensued. When the object is to distend the colon with a view to determine its capacity, and perhaps immediately thereafter to relieve the obstruction, the hips of the patient should be so elevated that he will be almost inverted. The chair invented by T. C. Martin (see illustrations in chapter on Diseases of the Rectum) is admirable for this purpose if it could always be had. The patient should lie on his right side so that the fluid may more readily pass into the colon. It is advisable to give at first a small cleansing enema of one quart of warm water, to remove the fecal matter. There are, of course, stenoses of such anatomical construction that liquid irrigations from below can pass upward without apparently meeting with a hindrance. At the same time fecal matter could not pass from above. A polypus or exceptionally dry coprolith in front of a cicatricial stenosis, acting as a ball valve above the stenotic ring, might act in this way. This would give the impression of a higher seat of the stenosis than is really the case, if we should judge exclusively from the amount of liquid that has entered the bowel. In a case reported by Larrabee (" Louisville Med. News," 1881, vol. XI, 3), six quarts, it is claimed, were injected into the intestine and retained there in a case of obstruction of the ileum. It is evident that when this much fluid can be injected the obstruction can not possibly be in the colon, and must be in the small intestine. If, on the other hand, only two or three pints can be injected, as has occurred in a number of cases in my own practice, and a case in Treves' (*l. c.*, p. 398), where the rectum held but three pints, the conclusion is justifiable that the obstruction is in or at the sigmoid flexure; a larger quantity must be injected before we may conclude that the intestine above this point is passable.

In a number of cases of volvulus of the sigmoid, in which I witnessed the treatment by distention with water, the practitioners used the method in a way which gave the impression that the only object to be accomplished was to cleanse the colon. The irrigator was held but 2 or 3 feet above the rectum of the patient. Too little pressure

in using the method is as useless as too great a pressure is dangerous
(I am speaking now of the diagnostic, not the therapeutic, usefulness
of the method, and the indication then is to distend the large intestine, if possible, and without adding to the danger of the patient).
Whilst anesthesia is preferable, it is in my experience not always
necessary. In many cases forcible distention with hot water has,
in my practice, produced very evident relief in the pain while the
method was being executed. A number of objections have been
raised to the method: (a) It has been argued that the experiments
concerning the capacity of the colon are useless, because they were
made on large intestines excised from the body. (b) The objection
already advanced, that a stenosis may be passable from below, but
not from above. This I regard as an extremely rare occurrence.
Naunyn (l. c.) does not mention it at all, and Nothnagel simply
refers to it, but gives no experience of his own. Water may of
course run through a partial volvulus, a twist of 180° in one direction, on entering, and then the weight of the water which has succeeded in distending the further limb of the intestine may actually
increase the volvulus to one of 360°. These are conceivable mis-
fortunes with which we can not reckon, and which we can not foresee,
but are so extremely rare that they should not deter us from the
practice of distention for diagnostic purposes. (c) The rectum may
be filled with feces, obstructing the entrance of fluid, or it may be
so dilated as to take large quantities of water, and thus give rise to
errors of judgment. Both of these sources of error can be excluded
by inspection of the rectum and distention under negative atmospheric pressure. A cleansing enema will remove the feces. (d) It
is claimed that a part of the colon may be spasmodically contracted,
and another part meteoristically distended, which would also give
rise to error of judgment in the capacity. This condition occurs, in
my experience, only when the obstruction is in the colon itself.
Then the dilated portion is above the stenosis,—as I prefer to call
it, it is the suprastenotic portion,—and one will rarely succeed in
getting water through the stenosis. (e) The objection that the
patient's voluntary muscular efforts may resist the entrance of the
fluid is not very important, because this can be avoided by anesthesia.

Considering all of these objections critically, and judging from a
very large personal experience, I conclude that when the proper

precautions are used the exploration of the large intestine by means of forced injection is a practical and valuable diagnostic method. The question to be decided by the injection is mainly this : " Is the seat of the obstruction in the large or small intestine ? " This does not depend upon the difference of a few ounces in the quantity of fluid injected, but the value of the procedure is dependent upon wide degrees of differences, as I have pointed out before. This is the main reason why the experiments upon the excised and relaxed intestine are available for laying down the dividing-lines in determining the capacity. Extreme meteorism, should it influence the injections, can be relieved by gastric lavage, and if necessary lavage of the duodenum by the method already described. There are three very essential conditions to the success of diagnostic distention of the colon by water. (1) The injection should be made early in the course of the disease, before circulatory changes, swellings, transudations, congestions, and partial adhesions have fixed the pathological topical conditions of the bowel ; on the first or second day whenever possible. (2) About 15 feet of pressure should be used for adults, about 8 or 10 feet for infants. (3) The patient should be anesthetized. Treves recommends auscultating the ileocecal region while the forced injections are being executed. If one can detect by the ear that the liquid reaches the cecum, this would prove that the colon is permeable. Great experience and special training, however, are necessary for the interpretation of the variety of abdominal sounds to be heard in cases of intestinal obstruction.

Antiperistaltic Progress of Minute Particles from the Rectum to the Stomach.—The author's suggestions for making use of the antiperistaltic progress of minute particles of bismuth subnitrate, charcoal, or lycopodium, etc., from the rectum to the stomach for diagnostic purposes have been detailed on pages 195 and 196 this volume. My experiments with healthy human subjects show that ordinarily the particles injected into the rectum should be recognizable in the wash-water from the stomach in from eight to ten hours. In cases of obstruction this antiperistaltic progress did not take place, and bismuth and lycopodium injected into the rectum could not be found in the gastric lavage water nor in the vomited masses. (Hemmeter, " Experimentelle Studien über Antiperistaltick," etc., "Archiv für Verdauungs-krankheiten," April, 1902.) These observations are definitely available for diagnostic purposes.

The functional symptoms in the determination of the location of the obstruction are of comparatively little value. Beware of depending upon the location of *pain* as an indication of the site of the obstruction. In rare cases one has the good fortune to recognize an accurately defined, well-circumscribed pain, uniformly localized, always at the same place. This may cautiously be interpreted as pointing to the seat of the obstruction; but reliable observers—Treves, Fitz, Nothnagel, and Boas—have reported cases, and I have observed such personally, where the pain was in one side of the abdomen, say the left, and the disease in the ileocecal region; nor can it be said that the early manifestation of pain is a special indication pointing to the small intestine, for in the sigmoid volvulus the abdominal pain appears on the first day in nearly all the cases where the date was recorded.

The same skeptical conservatism is justifiable concerning the value of *vomiting* as a diagnostic indication of the location of an obstruction. It is true *fecal vomiting* is more likely to occur in obstruction of the small intestine than in that of the large, and will more promptly occur in obstructions of the ileum and jejunum than in that of the colon; it is of no importance in determining the part of the bowel affected. For instance, it occurred in 47 cases of strangulation, 14 of gall-stones, 12 of intussusception, and 5 of malignant disease or stricture, in the collection of Fitz (*l. c.*). It was present in 4 cases of stricture or tumor when the obstruction was at or below the cecum; it was noted in 4 cases of intussusception in the same region, in 2 cases of volvulus and 1 of strangulation in the large intestine. Thus in more than one-eighth of the cases of fecal vomit the acute obstruction was in the large intestine. The only deduction that can be made is that general experience with internal incarcerations of the small intestine teaches that stercoraceous vomiting is observed more frequently and earlier than in obstruction of the large intestine.

Indicanuria.—By general consensus of opinion of the prominent special workers in intestinal pathology it is agreed that excessive indicanuria indicates an occlusion of the small intestine, provided

there is no peritonitis present.   Nothnagel and a number of other
observers assert that excessive formation of indican in the urine was
not missed in any of their cases of obstruction above the ileocecal
valve. Secondly, the conditions under which excessive formation of
indican occurs aside from intestinal obstructions.   For I have seen
this excessive indicanuria in my own clinic in a variety of diseases not
associated with interference with the permeability of the intestine.
According to my experience, it is a reliable sign for the location of
the obstruction in the small intestine if considerable indicanuria
occurs on the second or third day after an acutely developing
occlusion, and in the absence of symptoms of peritonitis.   If no
appreciable increase of indican is demonstrable after the third or
fourth day, we may of course conclude that the seat of the obstruction is in the large intestine.   There are two restrictions to these
generalizations.   The first is composed of those very rare cases in
which we may have two or more simultaneous obstructions, situated
in both the small and the large intestine.   The second consists of
those cases where excessive indicanuria occurs after stenosis of the
colon of long standing, for then the backward stagnation of fecal
matter might extend up into the small intestine.   Excluding these
sources of error, peritonitis, multiple stenosis in the small intestine
and colon, and long duration of the stenosis, excessive indicanuria
in the first stage indicates an obstruction in the small intestine ; its
absence, an obstruction in the large intestine.   After longer duration of the obstruction, however, the absence of excessive indicanuria
may yet be interpreted as indicating stenosis of the large intestine,
but its presence no longer constitutes a diagnostic criterion.

The condition of the stools offers no reliable indication of the seat
of the obstruction.   If the characteristic feces of a stenosis, which
have been described in a previous chapter, are present, they speak
for an obstruction in the rectum, sigmoid, or descending colon.

Intensity and Rapidity of Symptoms.—As the small intestine has a much more abundant nervous supply, it is more liable
to produce the signs of reflex general symptoms than the large
intestine.   Moreover, those obstructions which are known to
bring about the most intense reflex nervous symptoms are more
likely to attack the small intestine than the large intestine.   Of
78 cases of strangulation collected from literature by myself,

70, or almost 90 per cent., occurred in the small intestine. Accordingly, the rapidity of the course and the intensity of the phenomena of an acute occlusion are more marked in the small intestine than in the large. Strangulations always involve the peritoneum and the mesentery, and for this reason alone they produce intense symptoms ; and as strangulations are more frequent in the small intestine, the deduction has been made that whenever the course of an acute occlusion is accompanied by violent pain, severe vomiting, and rapidly developing collapse, the seat must be in the small intestine. Reasoning inductively, we see that this conclusion is justifiable only partially on account of the nature and character of the occlusions, which are more prevalent in the small intestine. On the other hand, if the mesentery is strangulated in occlusions of the large intestine (sigmoid volvulus), we may have the same violent and stormy course as is observed in strangulations of the jejunum or ileum.

Duodenal Stenoses.—The signs which indicate a stenosis of the duodenum have already been dwelt upon in the chapter on Enterostenosis. They will differ according to the location of the stenosis, whether it is above or below the orifice of the common gall and pancreatic ducts, whether they are supra- or infrapapillary. On account of its anatomically fixed position the duodenum is more liable to compression than any other part of the intestine. Neoplasms of the liver, kidney, stomach, pancreas, and spleen may compress the lumen of this short piece of the intestine. Enlarged retroperitoneal lymphglands, neoplasms, and cicatrices in the duodenum itself, and peritonitis issuing from the biliary passages, may produce the same results. The compression of the duodenum by the mesentery of the dislocated ileum (Schnitzler) and the obturation by gall-stone have already been referred to. The symptoms of the stenoses have already been described in the chapter on Enterostenoses. The diagnosis of suprapapillary stenosis of the duodenum is practically impossible, except perhaps by intubation of the duodenum according to the method described by the author. As a rule this condition will be confounded with that of stenosis of the pylorus. In infrapapillary stenoses of the duodenum almost the entire secretion of bile and pancreatic juice finds its way into the stomach, and is generally vomited. Accordingly the stools are acholic and colorless, like those which occur in icterus. The vomiting of large masses of bile, to which Leichtenstern first called attention, is a characteristic sign ; but the outflow of bile after gastric lavage or drawing of test-meal, such as Cahn emphasized, is, in my opinion, no reliable indication of duodenal stenosis, for it can often be observed in cases where there is every reason to believe that the entire intestine is permeable, and is caused by a violent contraction of the abdominal muscles produced by the nausea during lavage and test-meal drawing. If there is much bile contained in the duodenum, this is forced into the stomach by these contractions. If a regurgitation of the mixed intestinal secretions occurs constantly and in large quantities, only then can it be interpreted as a sign of infrapapillary stenosis (Riegel, " Erkrankungen des Magens," p. 164).

Rectal Stenoses.—The location of the seat of the obstruction in the rectum has been considered in a separate chapter. In all cases of obstinate constipation, or such a condition alternating with diarrhea, containing blood, pus, and mucus, if there are hemorrhoidal veins, the rectum should be examined by inspection through the proctoscope. Dr. Thomas Chas. Martin has described this method in the article he has contributed.

Diagnostic Indications and Signs for Determining the Location.—*Résumé.*—Characteristic distentions of the intestinal loops by gas and liquid, as observed by inspection ; flank meteorism ; lumbar percussion symptom of Nothnagel ; plastic intestinal rigidity and visible intestinal peristalsis ; physical methods of diagnosis ; intubation, artificial inflation and distention, etc. ; pain, vomiting, indicanuria ; rate of onset of principal symptoms ; signs of duodenal and rectal stenosis.

What is the Pathological Nature of the Condition Causing the Obstruction ?

The determination of the anatomical nature of the process causing intestinal occlusion presents considerable difficulty, and very frequently it is impossible to recognize it. Nevertheless, an attempt should be made to determine the anatomical condition in every case, and one of the first steps, after an exhaustive anamnesis has been taken down according to the accompanying schema, is to make a careful examination of the rectum and vagina ; and a second step must be to carefully examine all the possible hernial orifices.

Onset Gradual or Abrupt.—The previous history of the patient is extremely important. Above all things, we must inquire whether the occlusion has developed suddenly or gradually. If there has been a sudden onset, we must think of incarceration, strangulation, acute invagination, obturation by foreign bodies and gall-stones, and acute peritonitis. If the onset has been gradual, we may have to deal with stricture, neoplasm, chronic invagination, or obturation by fecal tumors. A previous history of long-standing habitual constipation, occasionally alternating with diarrhea, is suggestive of fecal masses, volvulus, stricture, or neoplasm. A history of ulcerating processes, tuberculosis and syphilis, gastric or duodenal ulcer, should suggest cicatricial stricture. The age of the patient is of great importance. In children under ten years of age the only form of obstruction is acute invagination and intussusception. From the age of ten to forty we may have incarcerations as well as intussusceptions, but beyond the age of forty volvulus and knots are the most likely forms of obstruction. The distinction between volvulus, internal incarceration, and invagination, as well as acute peritonitis, presents difficulties. I have condensed the main features in the appended diagnostic schema. The prompt development of fever in an individual hitherto healthy, accompanied by pain and vomiting, speaks for primary peritonitis and against mechanical occlusion. The leukocyte count will not enable one to distinguish between these two acute conditions. Peritonitis having been excluded, the practitioner will next have to decide whether he is confronted with a case of intestinal paralysis or motor insufficiency. The diagnostic features of this condition have been emphasized in a separate chapter. This condition, as well as peritonitis, having been excluded, the four remaining states have to be differentiated, viz., strangulation, volvulus, invagination, and obturation. Rectal tenesmus, bloody stool, abdominal or rectal tumor, and age of the patient (56 per cent. of intussusception in Fitz's statistics occurred under ten years) would suggest invagination or intussusception. Forced distention by injection of warm water will afford an aid to the diagnosis between invagination and volvulus of the sigmoid. The greater the capacity of the large intestine, the more likely is the presence of intussusception than volvulus. If the obstruction is not relieved by distention of the bowel, inversion of the patient, and massage under anesthesia, and the indications point to the colon, it is probably a volvulus or an intussusception. The characteristics of invagination tumor have been described in the chapter on this subject. A very much distended, motionless loop in the left lower abdominal region is most probably the expanded limb of a sigmoid volvulus. A well-defined, localized meteorism in the epigastrium or umbilical region is suggestive of volvulus or incarceration of the small intestine. The seat of the pain is of very little utility for diagnosis. When it is in the left hypogastrium, and sharply localized, it should suggest sigmoid volvulus. If it is in the right ileocecal region, it is suggestive of ileocecal invagination. Vomiting, as elsewhere described, has little diagnostic significance, except in the case of infrapapillary duodenal stenosis, when it consists of the mixed bile, pancreatic juice, and succus entericus. The functional symptoms —diarrhea, constipation, collapse—are of no value for the determination of the nature of the occlusion. Whenever there has been a history of previous impermeability we are forced to presume a gradually developing stenosis, which has finally been completely occluded. This brings us to the consideration of slowly developing or chronic occlusions, among which we will have to differentiate between cicatricial stricture, malignant neoplasms, chronic invagination, external constriction, fecal obturation, and external compression of the intestine. The differentiation of these conditions, to which may be added strangulations by omental bands, vitelline remains, or abnormally elongated appendix, peritoneal pseudo-ligaments, incarceration in holes or slits of the mesentery, adhesions between several intestinal loops, internal hernias, with exception of the diaphragmatic hernia, loop formations among the small intestines, and occlusion by kinking and bending, is encountered by almost insurmountable difficulty. The following brief characteristics may be mentioned :

Synopsis of diagnostic indications of: I. Acute Intestinal Occlusions.

(1) Internal incarcerations and strangulations : Sudden development of symptoms; intense local pain; collapse early ; prostrating vomiting. Palpable tumor may be present, but very rarely ; if present, feels like a distended cyst, generally immovable. If there is a diaphragmatic hernia it presents the typical signs described in

a separate chapter, and is preceded usually by the history of a severe trauma. Omental hernia is indicated by pain in the mesogastrium or epigastrium; it also presents occasionally a tumor extending posteriorly to the stomach, which is not movable. Retroperitoneal hernias at times give rise to a tumor to the left of the spinal column below the stomach; retrocecal hernia is indicated by a sudden swelling in the cecal region, accompanied by symptoms of occlusion. (2) External hernias: Tumor is external to the body and hernial orifice; always palpable, but not always replaceable. (3) Strangulations and incarcerations in slits of the mesentery, kinkings, inflections, bendings: Present a history of preceding peritonitis; age under forty; sudden onset with violent pain; early vomiting; meteorism; obstipation; no tumor; most frequently occurs in the small intestine (practically 90 per cent.); colon generally free; leukocytosis high. (4) Volvulus and knot formation: Age beyond forty; preceded by habitual obstipation; paroxysms of colicky pain; local sensitiveness to pressure; distended intestinal loop can be palpated; vomiting comes on later than in previous forms; generally not fecal; meteorism pronounced; tenesmus marked; in rare instances hemorrhagic evacuation; rectum and sigmoid will not take up more than from one to three pints of water under forcible distention. (5) Acute invagination, most frequently in children and youthful individuals: Sudden onset; intermittent paroxysms of pain; tumor most frequently in the cecal region; changes its position, dimensions, and consistency; tenesmus and evacuations containing blood and mucus; vomiting; sensitiveness to pressure and meteorism not marked. Occasionally the intussusception can be palpated through the rectum, but inspection is necessary by proctoscope and rectal distention to distinguish it from carcinoma and benign neoplasms. The intussusceptum presents a depression at the side, giving somewhat the impression of the cervix of the uterus; evacuation of necrotic sections of intestine. (6) Obturations by gall-stones and foreign bodies: Anamnesis suggestive of cholelithiasis, and attacks of comparatively rapidly succeeding biliary colic; sometimes gall-stones have been vomited; gall-stone obstruction occurs in the small intestine; foreign bodies give obstruction mostly in the insane or hysterical; there are no symptoms of strangulation.

II. Chronically Developing Occlusions.

(1) Stricture: Anamnesis presents history of ulcerative processes; stercoral ulcers; tuberculosis; enteric fever. (Dysentery does not produce intestinal strictures.) History of habitual constipation, or long-continued diarrhea; evacuations may contain blood and pus; the suprastenotic loop undergoes hypertrophy, producing exaggerated peristalsis and plastic rigidity of the loop; the accumulation of the fecal matter above the stenosis is frequently palpable; the characteristic form and shape of the feces are observed with a low situation of the stricture; stenoses in the small intestine are occasionally preceded by diarrheas and sudden onset of the occlusion. (2) Chronic invagination: The course and progress of the disease show alternating improvement and aggravation. The intussusception may exist for a longer time without occlusion; then there will be a sudden development of absolute stenosis, followed again by improvement in the phenomena of occlusion, whilst those of invagination continue; discharge of necrotic intestine much rarer than in acute form; tumor which moves downward toward the rectum; repeated attacks of bloody and mucus stools with tenesmus. (3) Coprostasis and fecal tumor: Long, habitual constipation; occasionally with intercurrent diarrheas, preceded by dyspepsia and other intestinal diseases; the subjects are mostly men with old hernias, and elderly women with pendulous abdomen; other forms of obstruction must be excluded; the fecal tumor is compressible and doughy. (4) Carcinoma: The tumor is hard, nodular, increasing in size, movable in the beginning, fixed later on; the neighboring glands are secondarily involved in the later history; rare in the small intestine, more frequent in the large, consequently the phenomena of stricture of the colon or rectum are more frequent; frequently there is a history of previous attacks of a similar nature, and evacuations of blood and pus; advanced age; long-continued cachexia. (5) External compression: Floating kidney; dislocation of abdominal organs; sites most frequent are the duodenum and rectum; carcinomas or other neoplasms, or exudates, in the neighborhood of these structures.

The differentiation of the various forms of tumors—benign and malignant neoplasms, fecal tumor, invagination tumor—has already been sufficiently described, so as to enable the practitioner to command the differentiating diagnostic factors. Tumors, generally speaking, are more frequent in the large intestine. A differentiation between the various forms of tumors, the various forms of strictures, and the different types of peritoneal bands, and inflammatory processes that are capable of producing them is largely conjectural. Such diagnoses, if they are really made, can not be proved during life. An exact differentiation should, however, be attempted in all cases, even though it may be attended with numerous difficulties; in the first place because the clinician may, in individual cases, be fortunate enough to establish the exact diagnosis; and, secondly, even if he does not succeed in this, every new diagnostic study means a stepping-stone to progress and better understanding of this very difficult field of clinical investigation.

Obstructions in the Colon.

It is desirable to bear in mind that the obstruction in the large intestine was invagination or volvulus in four-fifths of the acute cases (Fitz). If the patient is under thirty years of age it is probably invagination. Presence of bloody stools, or rectal tenesmus, or rectal tumor strengthens this diagnosis, as they are not to be expected in volvulus. If the patient is over thirty years of age and there is neither tenesmus, bloody stools, nor invagination tumor, the case is probably one of volvulus, neoplasm, stricture, or strangulation. As volvulus is four times as frequent as strangulation in the colon, and about twice as frequent as tumor or stricture, we have here another aid to diagnosis. Strangulation is most frequently found above the sigmoid flexure, if it occurs in the colon at all, whilst volvulus, neoplasm, and stricture are at or below the sigmoid. (Inspection through the sigmoidoscope.)

Obstructions in the Small Intestine.

It is due to strangulation or gall-stone in nearly 90 per cent. of the cases. Gall-stone occurs after the age of forty to fifty in 84 per cent. of all cases; previous symptoms of cholelithiasis; absence of meteorism until the fourth or fifth day; occasionally a small hard tumor. Invagination occurs most frequently in early youth; the tumor is more often found than in case of gall-stone. The immediate cause of the strangulation can only exceptionally be discovered. The most frequent are peritoneal adhesions, vitelline remains, and the vermiform process.

MEDICAL TREATMENT OF THE VARIOUS FORMS OF INTESTINAL OCCLUSION.

The treatment that has hitherto been employed for the relief of various forms of intestinal occlusions has been both nonoperative, bloodless, or so-called medical treatment, and the treatment by operation. The questions of intensest interest concerning the therapeutics of these conditions are at present almost exclusively of a surgical nature. The burning questions at the bedside will be, "Shall the case be treated by bloodless, purely medical, expectant management, or shall an operation be urged?" "Can we hope for success of expectant medical treatment?" and if the case is to be treated by operation, "When shall we operate?" The answer to these questions must vary with the diagnosis and the intensity of the clinical manifestation. The first thing to decide is whether we are confronted with a slowly developing enterostenosis or an abrupt, suddenly developing occlusion. The conditions which cause slowly developing stenoses call for an operation without exception, for peritonitic adhesions, neoplasms, and cicatricial strictures can never resolve or heal spontaneously, or under the influence of internal medication. The same can be said of external compression, except perhaps the dislocated organs (floating kidney, dislocations of the uterus, etc.). If a chronic stenosis has eventuated in an absolute occlusion, it must be treated in the manner that will be described for these conditions. The chronic stenoses give the practitioner more time for deliberate consideration; he is able to make repeated examinations, and has a better opportunity to reflect upon the therapeutic course to be pursued. But in

Acute occlusions there is rarely any time given for consideration, for in the majority of cases only the first twelve or twenty-four hours give an opportunity for observing anything like characteristic symptoms. Certainly after the second day efforts at an exact diagnosis will meet with almost insurmountable difficulties: The meteorism will prevent proper palpation, the collapse and stercoraceous vomiting will so control the entire clinical picture that any other diagnostic questions except a differentiation between a mechanical occlusion and intestinal paresis in consequence of peritonitis can not be considered.

Purely medical treatment has proved successful only in a limited number of cases of group A : (1) Invagination or intussusception ; (2) a few of volvulus of the sigmoid ; (3) obturations by gall-stones and foreign bodies ; (4) occlusion following upon chronic coprostasis or stenoses.

Medical treatment has failed, as a rule, and surgical treatment is imperatively indicated, when the diagnosis points to group B : (1) Strangulations or incarcerations ; (2) the majority of cases of volvulus and loop formation ; (3) inflections, bendings, and kinkings.

It is desirable to bear in mind these two groups of obstructions in forming a conclusion as regards management of the cases. Naturally purely medical treatment can be extended longer and more consistently in group A than in group B. The first thing, then, to decide is to which of these two groups, A or B, any particular case belongs. A number of surgeons have denied absolutely the spontaneous resolution of, and also the recovery under purely medical treatment from, volvulus, strangulation, and inflection. According to these authors, such conditions require the promptest operative treatment, and no other kind of treatment should be instituted. These are the most dreaded forms of occlusion, and there can be no doubt that if medical treatment is instituted at all, it should not be continued longer than the first or second day. There are, however, a number of surgeons, but more especially clinicians, who hold that even these types are capable of spontaneous resolution or successful bloodless treatment during the first stages of the occlusion. This view is held by Boas, Nothnagel, and Curschmann in Germany, and Fitz, Osler, Tyson, and others in this country. Senn has observed spontaneous resolution of intussusception in his experimental investigations ("Annals of Surgery," 1888, vol. VII, 4). If the conditions in group B are so advanced that the incarcerations are absolutely tight and immovable, the volvulus one of 360°, and the kinkings and inflection of intestinal loops firm, medical treatment can not hope for success. But if there is only a partial volvulus of 180°, and if the incarceration is loose and movable, and the inflection not firmly fixed, then medical treatment may bring relief. The questions are justifiable, " Can we distinguish a volvulus of 180° from one of 360° ? " " Can we distinguish a loose from a tight incarceration, etc. ? " The efforts at such distinctions are, in my opinion, absolutely futile. The lighter anatomical forms may set in with the same intense strangulation symptoms as the graver forms. There is but one guiding principle for the duration of medical treatment, viz., the result of this treatment during the first twenty-four or forty-eight hours.

The indication for treatment is frequently influenced by two conditions which often call for urgent relief, independently of the anatomical nature of the process causing them. These are shock and collapse on the one hand, and intra-abdominal pressure on the other. Collapse and shock will occupy the therapeutic efforts above all other indications, because they will prevent any further treatment unless remedied; and as there are many cases of recoveries from occlusions after the intra-abdominal pressure has been relieved, one of the chief ends of therapeutics should be directed to this purpose.

The actual means of treatment are applied from three directions:

I. *Those administered or applied through the mouth and stomach:* Diet, purgatives, opium, and narcotics, metallic mercury, gastric lavage.

II. *Those applied from the rectum:* (a) Forced distentions with water; (b) air, CO_2, or hydrogen; (c) replacement of intussusceptions by a repositor; intubation of the colon; (d) rectal application of electricity; (e) administration of opium by suppositories; (f) rectal feeding in high occlusions of the small intestine.

III. *Applications direct to or through the abdominal integument:* (a) Massage; (b) electricity; (c) external hot or cold cataplasms; (d) puncture of the intestine for relief of meteorism; (e) hypodermic injections of morphin, and (f) subcutaneous injections of normal salt solution for thirst.

There is still another form of treatment, and that is general anesthesia. This is usually not considered a therapeutic method, but it can not be doubted that it really is helpful in allaying the enterospasm, tension of the abdominal muscles, and making the application of other remedial agents easier.

If I were asked what would be the most effectual curative non-operative management of a case of acute occlusion in the absence of a knowledge of its anatomical nature, I would say, "Examine and inspect all the hernial orifices, especially the rectum and vagina. If the occlusion is low down in the large intestine, give only small quantities of liquid food (albumoses, albumen, and wine). If the occlusion is in the small intestine, allow no food whatever. But (1) wash out the stomach to relieve it of stercoraceous material and prevent as much as possible further vomiting. (2) Relieve the pain by opium by the mouth in low stenosis, by the rectum in high stenosis, by hypodermic injection of morphin if it will not be retained in either of the preceding. (3) Determine the capacity of the colon by forced distention under anesthesia. This will not only throw light upon the capacity and permeability of the colon, but it was one of the most effective means outside of operative intervention for the cure of volvulus and intussusception."

I. Therapeutic Methods Applied Through the Mouth and Stomach.

The Diet.—In all acute occlusions, especially if the seat be in the small intestine, all food should be forbidden, even when the condition of the patient makes its ingestion still possible. In the majority of cases nausea and vomiting will prevent any ingestion of food. In occlusions and stenoses of the colon, however, I agree with Boas, that small quantities of liquid, readily absorbable food, egg-albumen, somatose, nutrose, and wine should be allowed; for every calorie of food material that can be given to the patient will contribute to uphold his strength. The annoying thirst can be relieved by small pieces of ice placed in the mouth of the patient, and if the stenosis is high up, much of the enemata used in the forced injections will be absorbed, or after the capacity of the colon has been determined, normal salt enemata may be given with the definite purpose of allaying thirst. When both vomiting and purging prevent the introduction of water by either end of the alimentary tract, it should be administered in the form of sterile normal salt solution, by means of subcutaneous infusion. In states of collapse with diminished arterial pressure, very soft and compressible, or even thread-like pulse which can hardly be felt, such infusions become imperative.

Purgatives are positively contraindicated in all forms of acute, subacute, and chronic occlusions, with exception of the obturation by fecal masses. If the diagnosis of fecal obstruction is not certain, it will be wise to withhold purgatives until time and exclusion of other conditions make coprostasis the most probable condition present. Heidenhain ("Deutsch. Zeitschr. f. Chir.," 1897, Bd. XLIII, S. 201) has advocated the treatment of intestinal paralysis which follows reposition of hernias or operation for occlusion by means of evacuating rectal enemata or castor oil.

Opium.—About fifteen years ago an interesting polemic arose between German surgeons and clinicians on the expediency of opium treatment in intestinal occlusions. A number of surgeons argued that the state of comparative euphoria which was brought about by opium was deceptive because the morbid alterations of the occlusion could clandestinely progress under the guise of this false improvement, and the right time for an operation be lost by procrastination. Whilst this condition actually exists, the position of the clinician is that of a helper and healer, and his duty is clear. He has no right to withhold from his patient the pain-relieving medicine in order to bring him to a better understanding of his case, and favorably dispose him to an operation. When opium is used cautiously and under careful observation, it can do no harm. The pain, the pitiable vomiting, are relieved. It may even produce a firmer pulse, prevent the phenomenon of collapse, and favor a spontaneous resolution of the obstruction. As a result of the suppression of vomiting, the secretion of urine is resumed, and the subnormal temperature of the body surface rises to the normal. According to Nothnagel, opium, by stimulating the inhibitory nerves of the intestine, exercises a calming influence upon the intestinal peristalsis. In a case reported from Kussmaul's clinic (Penzoldt and Stintzing's "Handbuch," Bd. IV, S. 596) the difference between the dangerous action of purgatives and the soothing action of opium could be observed in a striking way. It was a case of chronic invagination. Castor oil had been given, and the intussusceptum could be seen and felt descending to the anus, becoming harder and harder to the touch as it went on, and causing intolerable pains to the patient. When morphin was administered, however, not only did the pains disappear, but the tumor became unpalpable, and the invaginated portion was withdrawn. It is certain that a violent peristalsis is one of the important causative agents for certain forms of occlusion. This is especially so in

internal strangulations, invaginations, volvulus, inflection, and loop
formation.   An abnormally increased peristalsis is not only directly
blamable for the production of these conditions, but it heaps up
more and more intestinal contents against the obstruction.   Assuag-
ing and calming the excited peristalsis can therefore logically be
presumed to be of advantage in preventing an aggravation of these
conditions, even after they have already started.   Such cases as
reported from Kussmaul's clinic I have repeatedly observed in my
own practice.

   Directions for Administration of Opium.—Opium should be given
on the first day, in order to prevent the initial collapse.   The pulse
must be kept under constant observation.   Pain and vomiting will
improve, but the other grave symptoms of occlusion—suppression
of evacuation and flatus, local pressure pains, local and general
meteorism—will not give any evidence of improvement.   If the
patient is not seen until several days after the first symptoms of occlusion, the opium should not be given, unless the general condition of
the patient and the cardiac activity are good, and especially if there
are no symptoms of exaggerated peristalsis.   Personally I prefer the
denarcotized extract of opium for this purpose, because it has less of
the undesirable toxic effect of the ordinary officinal opium.   No definite rules can be laid down as to whether it should be given by
the mouth, rectum, or hypodermically.   As the absorption from
the gastro-intestinal tract is very much interfered with in these conditions, more dependence can be placed upon it if given hypodermically.   The dose of denarcotized extract of opium is ⅓ to ½
grain every three hours by the mouth, or ½ to ¾ grain in suppositories, by the rectum, repeated according to the indications and
ensuing results.   I have had cases of volvulus where one dose of
⅓ gr. denarcotized extract of opium was sufficient to allay the
pain for five hours; in others, the dose had to be repeated every
two hours.   Morphin can be given in doses of ¼ grain hypodermically every four hours.   In advanced cases the state of collapse
and the frequent feeble pulse require great caution in the use of these
drugs, but do not necessarily forbid them.   Often a collapse will
improve after opium has been administered.   The condition of the
cardiac action and pulse is the guiding criterion in this case, and if
it is at all feeble it would be wisest not to use opium at all after

the third day.   It will also be expedient to cease with the administration of opium at intervals, in order to study the clinical picture
in the absence of any misleading euphoria.   On the use and abuse
of opium see also this volume, pages 189 to 193.

Metallic Mercury.—The use of large doses of metallic mercury
for the relief of intestinal occlusion is a very ancient one.   There is
an air of medieval therapeusis about this remedy which can hardly
serve as an indorsement.   Doses ranging from 100 to 1000 grams
of solid quicksilver were given, and it was presumed that by its
weight it could force open the passage that was obstructed.   Curiously enough, the most obscure conceptions prevailed concerning
the nature of these obstructions, so that the manner of action of the
mercury was purely speculative.   Gronau described a patient to
whom 120 grams of metallic mercury were given on the seventh
day of the obstruction.   The pain continued, but it was reported
that the vomiting was checked immediately.   A week later two
copious evacuations occurred, and on the following day 11 inches
of ileum were sequestrated.   The mercury did not appear until
forty-four days after its administration.

Leichtenstern has suggested that the great weight of the mercury
may paralyze the musculature of the stomach by overdistention, and
that the cessation of vomiting, which has been interpreted as a
favorable effect of the solid mercury, may be in fact due to paresis
of the musculature.   The physician who would prescribe quicksilver at our present period would render himself liable to the
suspicion of being what the Germans call a " Quacksalber."

**Treatment of Intestinal Occlusion by a Glycerin Extract
of Animal Intestine.**—In an article entitled "L'opothérapie en-
térique dans l'occlusion intestinale" ("Revue de Chir.," Oct. 10,
1900), E. Vidal emphasizes that stercoremic infection plays an important part in causing the fatal termination of intestinal occlusion.   The
treatment should remove the obstruction, but should, as far as possible, prevent the virulent bacteria of the intestinal contents and
their toxins from infecting the general organism.   The normal intestinal wall possesses substances in its secretions which have an
antitoxic action, and if the intestinal mucosa is prevented from
exerting this action, this protective influence could be replaced by
injection of glycerin extract of a pig's intestine.   He has tried this

form of treatment in experimental obstruction produced in rabbits, as well as in two cases where obstruction had existed for a long time in human beings, and claims that the symptoms of extreme intoxication disappeared under this treatment. He recommends that this extract of intestinal mucosa should be injected before and after operations for obstruction.

Gastric Lavage.—In his experiments on the artificial production of intestinal obstruction on animals, Senn never witnessed such persistent vomiting as in man, and he attributes this difference to the fact that the animals thus experimented upon, as a rule, refused both food and drink, and that their intestinal canal, in proportion to the size of the abdominal cavity, is much shorter than in man. Gastric lavage was first recommended in the treatment of intestinal obstruction by Kussmaul ("Berlin. klin. Wochenschr.," 1884, No. 42 u. 43). By siphonage with the lavage tube the gas and liquid contents of the stomach and upper portion of the intestinal canal are evacuated, abdominal distention is diminished, and the hydrostatic pressure in the intestine above the obstruction is relieved. The accumulation of intestinal contents above the seat of obstruction acts injuriously in many ways, which have already been described in the preceding chapters. (1) It is one of the chief causes producing distention in the suprastenotic loops, (2) thereby causing violent peristalsis in these loops, (3) which gradually exhausts the strength of the patient by the pain and bringing on of persistent vomiting, (4) and leads to autointoxication by the putrefactive and fermentative changes in the semifluid intestinal accumulation. Kussmaul himself claimed for gastric lavage (1) that intra-abdominal tension was diminished, thereby securing the fundamental condition for the correction of mechanical difficulties that brought about the obstruction ; (2) that the distention of the suprastenotic loops was relieved, and thereby the pressure of the intestines against each other was diminished also ; (3) that evacuation of the accumulated contents diminished the exaggerated peristalsis.

Enormous masses are evacuated by gastric lavage in cases of intestinal obstruction, and so rapid is the transport of intestinal secretions and ingesta into the stomach that two or three hours after one gastric lavage, at which 3 or 4 liters of material were evacuated, a second lavage may bring forth a similar quantity.

This experience in a number of cases of intestinal obstruction led me to extend the lavage of the stomach, and after this organ was cleansed out, to wash out the duodenum and jejunum also, after duodenal intubation by a method first described by myself (see Hemmeter, "Diseases of the Stomach," second edition, p. 52). The upper part of the intestine, it must be understood, is very much expanded by the gases and fermenting liquids, as well as the immense serous transudation which takes place into the intestinal lumen in obstruction. The same physical laws appertain to lavage of the duodenum and jejunum as to lavage of the stomach, for we can not conceive of these loops as being cylinders presenting the same lumen throughout, but in this condition they represent a series of expanded pouches not unlike the stomach. Rehn ("Fortschritte der Med.," 1887) maintained that gastric irrigation not only evacuated the stomach of its contents, but also emptied a certain portion of the intestinal canal above the seat of the obstruction. After the abdominal cavity was opened in two cases of intestinal obstruction where this method of treatment was resorted to, he observed that a considerable portion of the contents of the dilated intestine was emptied into the stomach, and thence outwardly. It is true that gastric lavage will in this manner even relieve the duodenum and jejunum, but it will not do so at once. In my experience it generally requires three hours, under the influence of intestinal obstruction, for the stomach to become refilled after it has been once emptied by lavage. The curative effect of washing out the stomach is due to the fact that conditions of intra-abdominal pressure are created which make the resolution of the obstruction possible. The pain, and thereby abdominal tension, is relieved; eructation and vomiting are controlled; the overdistended loops, which by mutual pressure interfere with each other, are relieved of their excessive charge of gas; and by such conditions alone it is conceivable that the return of partially incarcerated, inflected, or twisted intestinal sections to their normal position may be possible. Curschmann has emphasized that the success of this treatment is especially transparent in obstructions located in the higher portions of the small intestine.

Criticism of Lavage.—From a surgical side the treatment has been criticized, and at best only admitted as a palliative means. Bardeleben ("Berlin. klin. Wochenschr.," 1885, No. 25 u. 26) asserts that there is considerable danger coincident with the employment of such a temporizing measure, as too much valuable time may be lost before a curative treatment is adopted.   Incidentally he describes a case in which gastric irrigation afforded so much relief that the operation was postponed until there was no chance of its success.   Similarly, Kuester cautions against the use of the method, particularly where the seat and cause of the obstruction can be ascertained.   The objection urged by a number of American surgeons that a deceptive euphoria is created which may induce the patient to refuse an operation does not constitute an argument against its use.   It is the duty of the physician first to use the simplest methods and those which give promise of the promptest relief.   Naturally, we can not determine *a priori* those cases in which it may lead to a cure ; but even where a cure by this method alone is out of the question, it will be of advantage, because it will arrest the vomiting and empty the stomach and upper small intestine, conditions which are absolutely indispensable to successful anesthesia should an operation be decided upon.   One should never be satisfied with one gastric irrigation, but it should be repeated every three hours.   As much as 5 liters of intestinal contents have been evacuated from the stomach during one lavage. It should be undertaken as soon as the diagnosis of obstruction is made, whether the seat and nature of the obstruction are known or not, whether an operation is contemplated or not.   The only condition contraindicating lavage is the prostration of the patient; when respiration and heart's action are already embarrassed, and the patient is in extreme collapse.   Senn ("Trans. Congress Amer. Physicians and Surgeons," vol. I, p. 49), after emptying the stomach, combines with it antiseptic irrigation, consisting of large quantities of warm solutions of salicylate and hypophosphite of soda.

II. Therapeutic Methods Applied from the Rectum.

Forced Distentions with Water.—The object which it is hoped to accomplish by the distention of the colon with water is a twofold one.   In the first place, it is expected that fecal accumulations can be softened, disintegrated, and removed, and the colon thoroughly relieved of · its contents; and secondly, it was hoped that the restitution of the obstructed bowel to its normal permeability might be aided by this distention. There can be no doubt that the first design—evacuation of fecal accumulation—can be accomplished, and if the obstruction is due to fecal impaction, or coproliths, a cure can be effected by this method alone; but how axial twists, invaginations, and incarcerations can be restored to normal permeability by colon distention is a question which is answered only by hypotheses, not by observed facts. The objections urged against the method are the following: (1) The intra-abdominal pressure is already abnormally increased in intestinal obstruction, and the injection of large quantities of water increases it still further; intra-abdominal space is still further encroached upon; the expanded loops, which are already cramped, instead of being given more space for their untwisting or resolution, are hindered still further, and the pathogenic mechanism which brought about the occlusion is rather favored than opposed. (2) The weight of the introduced water may produce atony of the colon, and exerts a strong pressure upon its walls. (3) The water which has been forced in may enter with ease through a stenosis from below upward, but owing to some valve-like fold, or a small coprolith acting like a ball-valve, it may not be able to return, thereby adding an embarrassing aggravation to the already dangerous situation. (4) Peristalsis produced in the colon by these enemata can not produce a restitution of an internal incarceration, inflection, volvulus, or loop formation. (5) The liquid can not pass beyond the ileocecal valve, the closure of which can only be overcome under anesthesia and by excessive pressure. (6) The manipulation and time required for the injection of large quantities of water into the bowel amount to an exhausting operation, and may in themselves induce collapse.

These objections, it will be readily seen, are partly theoretical. No conservative clinician expects to restore volvulus, incarceration, inflection, etc., to normal permeability by large colon injections. They are above all used for diagnostic purposes, to determine the capacity and permeability of the colon. As I have repeatedly said, one of the fundamental requisites of diagnosis is to determine whether the obstruction is in the large or small intestine, and for this purpose the forced distention of the colon by warm water is a method I can approve of, from considerable experience. Whilst it is being executed for diagnostic purposes, it may also be helpful in restoring the permeability if it is due to three conditions: (1) Coprostatic obturation; (2) obturation by gall-stones; (3) complete occlusion of a chronically developing stenosis by suprastenotic accumulation. A number of successful recoveries from ileocecal invaginations which had descended into the colon are also reported by this method. Whenever there are evidences of ulcerative processes or carcinomas which have given rise to hemorrhages, or peritonitis, or any condition which will lead to a state of the intestinal wall in which it is easily ruptured, colon distentions by water are contraindicated. The water should always be warm. The use of ice-water for these large irrigations is unjustifiable. Oil and medicated solutions have been used for the same purpose. Where water is used, from 2 to 5 quarts or liters may be necessary. Oil is particularly advantageous in fecal impaction, and then from ½ to 1 quart of olive or cotton-seed oil is allowed to run into the colon and remain there for five or six hours. Of the medicated colon irrigations, those containing soap, turpentine, or infusion of senna, are the best known.

Chlorid of Sodium Enemata.—On the basis of a number of carefully conducted experiments on animals and clinical experiences in man Nothnagel has asserted that enemata of a 5 per cent. solution of chlorid of sodium in warm water may ascend high up into the small intestine, through the ileocecal valve. Enemata not exceeding 400 c.c. in quantity may, according to him, reach the ileum. These enemata would possess the advantage that they would not increase the intra-abdominal pressure. This eminent clinician has observed the solution of physiological invagination when these salt enemata moved upward antiperistaltically and reached the invaginated portion of the intestine. Accordingly enemata containing one pint of a 5 per cent. to 8 per cent. solution of common table salt can safely be recommended after the sigmoid and descending colon have been emptied of their contents by a cleansing enema. Much discussion has taken place concerning the permeability of the ileocecal valve to the rectal injection of fluid, or to air and gases with which the colon has been distended. The literature of experiments bearing on this question has been reviewed by Senn (l. c., pp. 50 to 55), and it can not as yet be decided whether this valve is permeable to such colon injections or not. It is quite certain, however, that under physiological conditions, whilst the patient is conscious, it is impossible to force liquids through the ileocecal valve from the colon.   The Georgia surgeon, Battey, was one of the first to assert the permeability of the entire alimentary canal by enemata ("Trans. Amer. Med. Assoc.," 1878). This method, known by the name of "enteroclysis," is also recommended by Cantani ("Berlin. klin. Wochenschr.," 1892, 37) and von Genersich ("Deutsch. med. Wochenschr.," 1893, No. 41) for the treatment of Asiatic cholera.   Von Genersich has designated this lavage of the entire intestinal canal by the name of "Diaklysmos." He has injected up to 15 liters of a 1 per cent. solution of tannin into cholera patients, until profuse vomiting of the tannin solution occurred, which had been injected into the colon.   T. H. Rumph (Penzoldt and Stintzing's "Handb. d. spec. Ther.," vol. I, p. 344) has approved of this method of treatment, encouraged by the favorable results obtained by von Genersich.   The injections were made under a pressure equal to a column of water of 80 to 100 cm.*

Heschl and Bull are of the opinion that fluids can not be forced beyond the ileocecal valve in the living body.   The results of Behrens and Debierrea were not constant, though Behrens did claim to have overcome the competency of the ileocecal valve by rectal inflation of air.   Illoway ("Amer. Jour. of the Med. Sci.," vol. XLI, p. 168) had devised a force pump for the purpose of forcing water beyond the ileocecal valve, and has reported four cases of intestinal obstruction treated by this method, three of which recovered.   In his paper read before the International Medical Congress at Washington, Senn detailed a number of experiments made upon dogs to determine the extent to which the ileocecal valve was permeable to fluids forced up from below.   In three cases fluid was forced beyond the ileocecal valve, but in two of them the examination after death revealed multiple lacerations of the peritoneal coat of the large intestine, whilst the third animal sickened immediately after the experiment, and died eight days later.   These experiments left no doubt in Senn's mind that the ileocecal valve is practically impermeable to fluids forced up from below, and that it is unjustifiable to attempt to force rectal injections beyond this valve.   Senn

---

* There are distinct references to enteroclysis and the antiperistaltic movement of injections into the rectum in the writings of the Arabic physician Avenzoar (Abu Merwan Ibn Zohr), A. D. 1113 to 1162.

reports two cases of ileocolic invagination in children which he
cured by hydrostatic pressure under anesthesia and complete inversion. From the conflicting views of the various authors and
investigators cited, it is evident that the question of the permeability
or non-permeability of the ileocecal valve to water or air under
normal conditions will require further investigation. The experiments of J. Holmes Smith on this subject are given in volume I,
chapter I.

Distention with Air, Carbon Dioxid, or Hydrogen.—The
inflation of the rectum and colon with air in the treatment of intestinal obstruction is a method that has been known since Hippocratic
days. Senn ("Trans. Congress Amer. Physicians," 1888, p. 53)
has made a number of experiments with hydrogen gas to determine
by means of a mercury manometer the degree of pressure requisite
to render the ileocecal valve incompetent. He concluded that this
amount of pressure, 1 ½ to 2 ¼ pounds to the square inch, was not
sufficient to injure any of the coats of the healthy intestine.

ent portions of the gastro-intestinal canal, when in a healthy
condition and removed soon after death, did not show lacerations
under a pressure of less than 8 pounds. Senn has recommended the use of hydrogen gas for the detection of a perforation,
and also for the determination of the permeability of the entire
colon. The passage of the gas through the ileocecal valve, rendered previously incompetent by distention of the cecum, is, as a
rule, accompanied by characteristic gurgling or blowing noises,
which can be heard by applying the ear or stethoscope over the
ileocecal region. As the manipulation of the healthy, intact portion
of the intestinal canal, which is represented by the empty collapsed
loops below the obstruction, is a far less hazardous procedure than
the handling of the distended portion, Senn recommends the distention of the infrastenotic loops by hydrogen gas reaching them by
degrees, and gradual expansion with this gas from the rectum.
This method, though at first appearing to have considerable feasibility in its favor, must be very difficult of execution practically. It
will require a tube several meters in length, non-compressible, and
necessitate much manipulation during the operation after the abdomen has been opened. Quite a number of fatal cases have been
reported after insufflation. Bryant, in 20 cases collected by him in

which invaginations were treated by rectal insufflation, reports 3 cases of rupture of the bowel below the invaginated portion, whilst a fourth case, a child, died in collapse shortly after the insufflation ("Brit. Med. Jour.," Nov. 22, 1884). Knaggs similarly reported 8 cases of invagination where forcible distention of the colon by air or water was the direct cause of rupture or other serious injury ("Lancet," June 4, 1887). The insufflation of hydrogen gas, which is recommended by Senn for the detection of the location of the obstruction, and for the detection of a possible perforation, has its defects as a method; for instance, the uniform distention of the abdomen (*l. c.*, p. 57) which he cites as a sign of this perforation is in my experience often already present when the cases are first presented for examination, and may be brought about by advanced meteorism without perforation. Fitz has collected the results of the employment of injections and inflations from 1880 to 1888. It appears that there were in that period 33 cases of recovery after insufflation or injection for certain or probable invagination. In 17 cases air was inflated, in 14 water was injected, and in 2 gas had been introduced from a siphon reservoir. The treatment was used on the first day in 10 cases, on the second in 7, on the third in 4, on the fourth in 1, and on the date not given in 11 cases. He also records 11 deaths after the treatment by inflation or injection. Certain of these failures are claimed to have been due to insufficient pressure, for after death several of these intussusceptions were easily reduced. This easy reduction after death is, in my opinion, no evidence that the invagination could have been reduced with the same ease before death, for the passive congestion, the serous transudate in the intestinal coats, and the muscular enterospasm all rapidly diminish after death, and the picture at the necropsy gives but an imperfect conception of the conditions existing during life.

In conclusion I would recommend distentions of the colon by air where forcible distention with water has been tried and has given evidence of increasing the abdominal distress; for air is lighter than water, although it can not produce the cleansing effect and the thorough evacuation of the colon. Then, too, the measuring of the air or gas which is introduced requires apparatus which is not always at hand, whilst water can always be readily measured.

Intubation of the Colon.—This method has been so thoroughly described elsewhere (see p. 180, this volume) that I may pass over it very briefly at this place. The indications for intubation of the colon are : (1) The detection and location of the obstruction in the sigmoid flexure or other parts of the colon ; (2) to relieve gaseous distention of the colon, and (3) to administer high nutrient enemata in order to maintain the strength of the patient, where feeding by the mouth is impossible. According to Senn (*l. c.*), the first to advocate the use of the elastic rectal tube in this country where it was deemed necessary to make high injections was O'Bierne. Notwithstanding the arguments of Rosenheim (*l. c.*), Treves (*l. c.*), Fitz (*l. c.*), and others, I hold that the Langdon or Kuhn colon tube can be passed through the entire large intestine to the ileocecal valve, when the colon is permeable, and that it is possible to demonstrate the fact that it has reached the ileocecal valve by various methods which I have indicated elsewhere. It is certainly available for the determination of obstructions in the sigmoid and descending colon.

Replacement of Intussusceptions, etc., by a Repositor.—The repositor is generally nothing but a large bunch of soft cotton grasped by a long-handled forceps. The ileocecal invaginations can not be replaced to their normal position,—this is self-evident,—but sometimes when the beginning of the replacement was started by a repositor, it could be continued by inflations of air or water, together with the appropriate position of the patient.

Rectal Application of Electricity.—Both the faradic and galvanic currents have been employed by means of the rectal electrodes. Boudet, who uses exclusively the galvanic current, after previously filling the rectum with a liter of normal salt solution, has reported 53 cures out of 70 cases treated by this method. The negative pole is inserted into the rectum, and the positive on the abdominal wall or back. The strength of the current varies from 10 to 50 milliamperes (" Progrès médicale," 7 and 14 Févr. 1885). It is probable that the good effect of galvanism in Boudet's cases is due to the antiperistaltic ascent of the salt solution, under which, as I have described elsewhere, Nothnagel has observed the restitution of invaginations. In strangulation, incarceration, axial twist, and inflection it is not advisable to waste any time with electricity, but in invagination, coprostasis, and some obturations by gall-stone an attempt with it is rational.

Administration of Opium by Suppositories.—About ½ to ¾ grain of denarcotized extract of opium can be given in suppositories every three hours wherever the rectum is clear and opium can not be tolerated by the mouth, though in the latter case I personally always give preference to hypodermic administration of this drug. The denarcotized extract of opium may be sterilized and injected hypodermically in doses of ½ grain. It appears to act better than morphin in these cases.

Rectal feeding in high intestinal occlusions, especially where the vomiting is persistent, becomes imperative. For this purpose I prefer the Boas nutritive enema, consisting of two eggs, half a pint of milk, one gill of claret, and about a teaspoonful of salt, thoroughly mixed, warmed to body temperature, and inserted high up in the rectum.

III. Applications Direct to or through the Abdominal Wall.

Massage.—This treatment is contraindicated in all intestinal obstructions excepting that due to fecal impaction, and even in this condition it is unjustifiable if there should be any indications of peritonitis. Several cases are on record where obturating gall-stones have been pushed onward through the intestine by massage.

Electricity.—The method of application of electricity is the same as that just described—by inserting an electrode into the rectum.

External Hot or Cold Applications.—These are of assistance for the relief of the pain and sometimes of the tenesmus. If there is fever and peritonitis preference should be given to cold applications ; if the temperature is normal or subnormal, and especially if there is great pain, the hot applications should be preferred.

Puncture of the Intestine.—Puncture for the relief of dangerous distention in the suprastenotic loop is carried out in the following manner (Curschmann, " Die Behandlung des Ileus," Congr. f. innere Med., Wiesbaden, 1889): A small trocar or hypodermic needle is thoroughly sterilized and rapidly pushed into the most distended loop. The needle should be provided with a stopcock and a small rubber tube which leads to a bottle filled with a

weak solution of salicylic acid.   This bottle is also inverted in a
basin containing the same fluid.   The needle must under no conditions be held steady by the fingers after the puncture, but must be
permitted to follow the intestinal movements freely.   I have already
given a full description of the method in the general chapter on
Intestinal Occlusions, and also given the criticisms of the method in
that connection (see pages 199, 200, 201, 202, this volume), and
added a·case from my own experience where I was compelled to
use it far out in the country, with no other instruments at hand
except my pocket hypodermic syringe.   I can see no reasonable
objection to the method when performed by experienced hands,
before intestinal paralysis has set in, and as long as the peristaltic
movements of the intestine can still be felt through the abdominal
walls.   In this connection I may emphasize that J. M. T. Finney,
Naunyn (*l. c.*), and Graser (*l. c.*) advise that intestinal puncture
should be refrained from as long as a possibility of a laparotomy
is still under consideration.   In the presence of a competent
surgeon there can be no doubt of the correctness of this attitude.
Senn (*l. c.*, p. 61) is of the opinion that an intestine distended to the
extent of giving rise to distressing and dangerous intra-abdominal
pressure is always in a paretic condition, unable to expel its
contents, and whatever escapes through a needle or trocar is
expelled through the contraction of the abdominal wall.   He
asserts that puncture empties only a limited space, not more
than 6 or 8 inches on each side of the insertion of the trocar.
The objections of Senn are not applicable to the method as practised by Curschmann, for this clinician is himself opposed to intestinal puncture in cases where the intestinal wall is paretic.   Personally I would only use the method where I could still detect some
evidences of peristalsis, this being the most reliable sign that the
intestinal muscularis is still capable of contraction.   Under such
conditions my experience has been that the puncture is not attended
with any risk of extravasation.   There can be no doubt that a
laparotomy is preferable in all cases where permission is given and
where the patient is in condition to tolerate the operation.   But
there are instances of obstinate refusal on the part of the patient to
consent to a laparotomy ; there are instances where the patient is
far remote from a capable surgeon, where there is not sufficient

time to secure assistants, nurses, and anesthetics, and in such cases intestinal puncture is justifiable.

Subcutaneous injections of normal salt solutions may become urgently necessary to prevent the dangerous drying out of the tissues, undue diminution of arterial pressure, and for relief of the thirst.

SCHEMA OR SYNOPSIS FOR RECORDING CLINICAL HISTORY OF INTESTINAL OCCLUSION.

1. Date, name of patient, address, social condition, occupation. Age, sex, inherited diseases (carcinoma, tuberculosis, syphilis).
2. Previous ailments, with especial reference to the abdominal organs: Hernias, if ever strangulated; enteric fever; appendicitis; ulcers of the stomach and intestines; peritonitis; fever attending childbirth; diseases of the uterus; gall-stones; nephritic colic.
3. Previous condition of stool and digestion: Daily evacuations; constipated, diarrheic, or both alternating. Use of purgatives; passage of hard matter, gall-stones, parasites, admixtures—mucus, blood, pus, tissue fragments.
4. Present sickness: Is it the first attack or a recurrence? Origin (a cold, unsuitable nutriment, trauma).
5. Inception: Sudden, or gradual with serious derangements. Pains constant, intermittent, confined to a particular locality or diffuse.
6. Treatment hitherto: Purgatives? Which? Opium? What quantity? Food? Amount of fluid; rectal or colon enemata. What success resulting from this treatment.

PRESENT CONDITION.

1. Weight. General condition: Condition of nutrition, bodily strength, skin, color and expression of face. Tongue (dry, coated); temperature; *pulse;* breathing; perspiration; nervous system (neurasthenic, organic nervous diseases).
2. State of the abdomen: Distended in shape of barrel, symmetrically, unsymmetrically. Outer circumference; central portion. Rigid? Pliable?
3. Inspection: Are contractions noticeable at this loop? Is it possible, moreover, to see or hear any unusual motions of the intestines?
4. Percussion: Is it possible to see, feel, or determine by means of percussion the presence of a dilated, stationary intestinal loop?
5. Palpation: Is it possible to detect by means of palpation abnormal resistances? Form, size, mobility; relation of the intra-abdominal organs to each other; tumor movable with or in them; change of location with act of breathing; change of position of body.
6. Pains: Do pains exist at the time being? Spontaneous, after eating, during motions of some kind, on pressing, all over, at distinct places, constantly, at times, simultaneously with increased

peristaltic motions. Observe difference between spontaneous and pressure pain.

7. Is there belching, singultus, vomiting? When did the vomiting take place—immediately, later on, frequently? Does it occur after eating? Amount, nature of it (slimy, gally, stercoral).

8. Is the evacuation of feces and flatus suppressed? Distress before, during, or after stool? Rectal tenesmus? Is blood and viscid mucus discharged?

9. Physical examination of the abdomen : Palpation, percussion, auscultation. Extent of the hepatic and splenic dullness ; touch. Location and excursions of the diaphragm ; intestinal sounds ; metallic sounds. Are there evidences of liquid effusion of some kind into the abdominal cavity?

10. Examination of the rectum and vagina, in lying and standing postures : Hemorrhoids? Is a tumor present? Does glassy mucus together with blood adhere to the inserted proctoscope? Dislocations or neoplasms of the genital organs ; traceability, relation, and connection of other tumors with these.

11. Examination of the colon by means of distention by water and air ; flatulency.

12. Examination of the urine : Specific gravity, amount, color, albumin, indican, action of nitric acid on same (Rosenbach); coloring matter of bile. Ehrlich diazo reaction, positive or negative. To distinguish between tuberculosis and carcinoma of cecum.

After such an exacting consideration of all these matters there will surely be but a few cases remaining in which every diagnostic clue to the nature of the trouble is wanting. If, however, such a case presents itself, it will be at any rate of the greatest importance to classify it with a distinct group.

The practitioner should at least try to succeed in deciding in each case on the following important questions :

I. Is it an acute strangulation of the intestines, a continuance of which might be expected to lead to gangrene and perforation?

Mesentery involved, circulation absolutely cut off; instantaneous appearance of the entire symptoms ; incarceration shock ; severe pains ; immediate and frequent vomiting ; fixed distended loop ; diminished pulse ; cold extremities ; exudate in the abdomen.

II. Is it only a case of obturation, with a gradual accumulation of bowel contents above the obstruction? Mesenteric circulation not disturbed, nutrition of the intestinal wall partially maintained. Danger to life only by degrees due to extension, paralysis, perforation, inanition, intoxication. Occasionally unexpected acute aggravation.

In most cases irregularities of stool preceded the attack ; the inception ; slow development of the occlusion symptoms (one after the other) ; absence of appearances of collapse, as well as constant pains ; augmented peristaltic motions.

III. Ought the trouble to be interpreted as a paralytic, spastic, or pseudo-ileus, or as motor insufficiency of the intestine (intestinal palsy), particularly as a consequence of peritonitis ?

In the chapter on Intestinal Paralysis I have discussed in detail the etiology and pathogenesis of paralysis of the intestine :
 (*a*) Paralysis resulting from acute overdistention ;
 (*b*) After derangement of the circulatory system ;
 (*c*) Resulting from hernial incarceration ;
 (*d*) From direct trauma ;
 (*e*) With inflammations and ulcerations of the colon ;
 (*f*) Atony after long-standing coprostasis ;
 (*g*) The reflex paralysis accompanying diseases in the vicinity of the abdomen and colon (inflammation of bile-passages and appendix) ;
 (*h*) Following operations upon the rectum, testicle, uterus, ovaries ;
 (*i*) Following any operations upon the abdomen.
Paralysis of the colon resulting from or attending peritonitis is the most important form of all these from a practical standpoint, as far as the diagnosis of acute obstruction is concerned.   In well-defined instances the diagnosis is easy, but many times it is fraught with great difficulty, especially from the fact that peritonitis is one of the most frequent consequences of mechanical obstruction, and thus it becomes necessary to ask one's self regularly if the peritonitis in question is a primary or a secondary one, a cause or a result.   In acute primary peritonitis, particularly when occurring in the free abdominal cavity through perforation of the appendix, the symptoms are oftentimes of a similar character : sudden inception with severe pains, severe collapse, persistent and obstinate constipation, vomiting, meteorism, painful swelling, are common to both diseases.   The following factors may serve to distinguish between primary peritonitis and primary obstruction :

PERITONITIS.	OBSTRUCTION.
Generally rapid rise in temperature, very seldom the collapse temperature.	At the beginning no fever, temperature often subnormal ; later on gradual rise of temperature, particularly if there are complications.
Patient very quiet, abdomen very sensitive to the slightest pressure.	Patient restless, throws himself about very much, is in fact able to get up ; at times pressure produces relief.
Spontaneous pains gradually diminishing.	Spontaneous pains gradually increasing. Attacks frequent and more severe.

PERITONITIS.	OBSTRUCTION.
Stercoraceous vomiting rare and appearing at a later stage.	Stercoraceous vomiting from the beginning.
Meteorism from the beginning, diffuse and general.	Meteorism at first local, gradually taking a larger area.
Intestinal loops not discernible to inspection or palpation.	Intestinal loops in the shape of isolated distended cylinders discernible to the eye and hand.
No intestinal peristalsis.	Many times violent intestinal peristalsis, particularly in chronic stenoses.
Belly hard, many times as tense as a board.	Belly at first pliable, not tense.
Plentiful exudate. (Exploratory puncture, palpation.)	Little or no peritoneal exudation.
At times emission of flatus and stool.	Complete suppression of flatus and stool.
Frequently singultus.	Singultus rare.

Obstruction can readily be distinguished from the circumscribed forms of peritonitis (see pp. 173 to 175, this volume).

In the chapter on Appendicitis I have referred to cases of perityphlitis that present embarrassing resemblance to obstruction. In appendicitis and perityphlitis especial regard must be had for the rapid localization of the spontaneous and pressure pains near the region of the cecum (McBurney's point, midway between anterior superior spine and navel), the tumor, edema of the skin of the belly, paresthesia, and possibly slight contractions of the right leg. Appendicitis (see article on p. 17 this volume) may, however, present all the symptoms of acute intestinal obstruction : Sudden illness, incarceration shock, small compressible pulse, meteorism, singultus and vomiting, over the cecum a small circumscribed painful area. During the operation or after section only acutely inflamed changes in the peri- and paratyphlitic tissues and on the appendix are found. Reichel (quoted in article on intestinal paralysis, and introduction to chapter on Obstructions) interprets these cases as acute peritoneal sepsis.

LITERATURE.

1. Auvray, "Occlusion intestinale aigue par Invagination," "Gaz. des Hôpitaux," July 3, 1900.

2. Battle, W. H., "Resection of Large Intestine for Malignant Growths," London "Lancet," November 11, 1899.

3. Bayer, Carl, "Acute Intraperitoneal Effusion as a Symptom of Intestinal Obstruction," "Centralbl. f. Chir.," June 10, 1899.

4. Bell, W. Blair, "Acute Infantile Intussusception with Special Reference to Treatment by Primary Laparotomy," "Edinburgh Med. Jour.," July, 1900.

5. Bennett, W. H., "A Clinical Lecture on Some Cases of Intussusception," "Practitioner," May, 1899.

6. Bonnecken, "Virchow's Archiv," Bd. cxx.

7. Booth, Carlos C., "A Case of Resection of the Bowel for Carcinoma," "Med. Record," April 22, 1899.

8. Boudet, "Progrès Méd.," February 7 and 14, 1885.

9. Bovee, J. W., "Intestinal Obstruction from Biliary Calculi," "Virginia Med. Semi-monthly," November 10, 1899.

10. Brinton, "On Intestinal Obstruction," London, 1867.

11. Brown, C. N., "Age and Sex Factors in Intestinal Obstruction," "Virginia Med. Semi-monthly," May 25, 1900.

12. Brown, D. Dyer, and others, "Malignant and Other Obstructive Affections of Stomach and Duodenum."

13. Brown, W. L., "Strangulated Hernia through an Omental Slit," "Med. Standard," November, 1899.

14. Cadwallader, R., "Strangulation of the Intestine with Few Symptoms," "Med. Record," May 20, 1899.

15. Cathcart, Chas. W., "Acute Intestinal Obstruction," "Scottish Med. and Surg. Jour.," June, 1900.

16. Cordier, A. H., "Some Phases of Intestinal Obstruction," "Jour. Amer. Med. Assoc.," February 4, 1899.

17. Curschmann, "Deutsch. med. Wochenschr.," 1887, No. 21.

18. Curschmann, "Die Behandlung des Ileus," Congr. innere Med., Wiesbaden, 1889.

19. Douglas, Richard, "Intestinal Obstruction," "Southern Practitioner," May, 1900.

20. Eiselberg, V., "Zur radikal Operation des Volvulus und der Invagination durch die Resection," "Deutsch. med. Wochenschr.," December 7, 1899.

21. Ellsworth, R. C., "Intestinal Obstruction," "Lancet," May 27, 1889.

22. Erdmann, John F., "Intestinal Obstruction Due to Intussusception," "Annals of Surgery," February, 1900.

23. Fell, W., "Total Obstruction of Bowel Lasting Thirty-four Days," Australasian Med. Gaz.," March 20, 1899.

24. Fenwick, W. Soltau, "Hypertrophy and Dilation of Colon in Infancy," "Brit. Med. Jour.," September 1, 1900.

25. Ferrier, F., and A. Grosset, "Exclusion of the Intestine," "Revue de Chir.," August 10, 1900.

26. Fibiger, "Om tuberculose Tyndtarms strikturer og deres Forvexling med. syfilitiske Forsnevringer," "Hospitalstidende," Copenhagen, June 27, 1900.

27. Fitz, R. H., "Trans. Congr. Phys. and Surg.," vol. 1, 1888.

28. Foote, Ed. M., "Volvulus of the Sigmoid Flexure Three Times Relieved by Laparotomy," "Boston Med. and Surg. Jour.," March 9, 1899.

29. Frazier, C. H., "Acute Intestinal Obstruction of Unusual Origin; Operation; Recovery," "Phila. Med. Jour.," January 21, 1899.

30. Frentzel, "Deutsch. Zeitschr. f. Chir.," Bd. xxxiii.

31. Fürbringer, "Verhandl. des VIII. Cong. f. innere Med.," 1899.

32. Gibson, C. L., "Mortality and Treatment of Acute Intussusception, with Table of 239 Cases," "Med. Record," July 17, 1897.

33. Gibson, C. L., "The Necessary Factors in the Successful Treatment of Intussusception," "Archives of Pediatrics," February, 1900.

34. Goldspohn, A., "Two Cases of Intestinal Obstruction Following Vaginal Hysterectomy, and One after Pelvic Abscess, with a Secondary Operation in Each Case," "Medical Record," September 8, 1900.

35. Graser, "Behandlung der Darmverengerung und des Darmverschlusses," Penzoldt and Stintzing's "Handb. d. spec. Ther. innerer Krankh.," Jena, 1896.

36. Haguenot, "Memoire sur les Mouvements des intestins dans la Passion Iliaque," "Histoire de l'Academie Royale des Sciences," Paris, 1713.

37. Hand, Alfred, Jr., "Intussusception in an Infant Four Months Old, Relieved by Injection," "Archives of Pediatrics," August, 1900.

38. Harsant, W. H., "Acute Intestinal Obstruction," "Bristol Med. Chir. Jour.," England, June, 1900.

39. Hobbs, A. T., "Strangulated Hernia and Intestinal Obstruction," "Canadian Practitioner," May, 1900.

40. Hohlbeck, "Occlusion of Intestine by Meckel's Diverticulum (Drei Fälle von Darmocclusion, u. s. w.)," "Arch. f. klin. Chir.," Bd. LXI, No 2.

41. Ill, Edward J., "Intussusception of the Bowel in Children," "Amer. med. Quarterly," January, 1900.

42. Jaboulaye and Patel, "Occlusion intestinale par Bridles, etc.," "Annales de Chirurgie et d'orthopedic," June, 1900.

43. Jaffé, "Centralbl. f. d. med. Wissensch.," 1872.

44. Kammerer, Fred., "The Mortality and Treatment of Acute Intussusception," "Archives of Pediatrics," February, 1900.

45. Klubbe, "Brit. Med. Jour.," November 6, 1897.

46. Kocher, "Mittheilungen aus den Grenzgebieten der Medizin," 1898, Bd. IV, S. 2.

47. Koecke, "Adenosarcoma of the Cecum; Intussusception; Resection; Recovery," "Münch. med. Wochenschr.," January 9, 1900.

48. Koenig, "Deutsch. Zeitschr. f. Chir.," 1891.

49. Kopffgarten, von, "Tumor of the Small Intestine (Lymphangioma) Found at an Operation for Femoral Hernia," "Deutsch. Zeitschr. f. Chir.," February, 1899.

50. Kussmaul-Cahn, "Heilung von Ileus durch Magenausspulung," "Berlin. klin. Wochenschr.," 1884, No. 42 u. 43.

51. Lees, D. B., "A Case of Chronic Intestinal Obstruction; Necropsy," "Lancet," March 24, 1900.

52. Leichtenstern, "Verengerungen, Verschliessungen, und Lageveränderungen des Darms, von Ziemssens," "Handb. des spec. Pathol. u. Ther.," Bd. VII, Leipzig, 1878.

53. Lewerenz, "Ileocolic Intussusception," "Deutsch. med. Wochenschr.," February 1, 1900.

54. Lupton, Harry, "A Case of Intussusception in an Infant Ten Months Old; Laparotomy; Rapid Recovery," "Lancet," August 18, 1900.

55. McRae, Floyd W., "Acute Obstruction of the Bowels," "Jour. Amer. Med. Assoc.," May 20, 1899.

56, a. Nicoll, James H., "On the Removal of a Nevoid Tumor of the Intestine," "Brit. Med. Jour.," April 8, 1899.

56, b. Osler, Wm., article "Intestinal Obstruction," in "Practice of Med.," 3d edit.

57. Rewidzoff, P. M., "A Case of Stenosis of Duodenum Cured by Gastro-enterostomy," "Arch. f. Verdauungs-Krankheiten," October 28, 1898.

58. Richardson, Maurice H., "Acute Abdominal Symptoms Demanding Surgical Intervention," "Boston Med. and Surg. Jour.," October 26, 1899.

59. Rose, A., "New York Med. Jour.," 1900, I, p. 47.

60, a. Senn, Nicholas, "Intestinal Surgery," Chicago, 1889, p. 244.

60, b. Senn, Nicholas, "Practical Surgery," 1901, p. 737.

61. Spivak, C. D., "Medical Treatment of Intestinal Obstruction," "Jour. Amer. Med. Assoc.," May 27, 1899.

62. "Trans. of the New York State Med. Assoc.," 1898,

63. Trastour, "Bull. Général de Therapie," 1874, p. 107.

64, a. Treves, "Intestinal Obstruction," New York, 1899.

64, b. Tyson, "Practice of Med.," article "Intestinal Obstruction."

65. Whiteford, C. H., "Operative Treatment of Distended Small Intestine in Acute Obstruction and Acute Peritonitis," "Brit. Med. Jour.," April 29, 1899.

66. Ziemssen, von, "Arch. f. klin. Med.," Bd. XXXIII, H. 3 u. 4.

67. Zuppinger, "Der Darmkrebs im Knidesalter," "Wien. klin. Wochenschr.," May 3, 1900.

68. Boas, "Darmkrankheiten."

69. Nothnagel, "Erkrankungen des Darms" in his "Specielle Pathol. u. Therapie," Bd. XIV.

70. Einhorn, Max, "Diseases of the Intestines."

CHAPTER IV.

CONTUSIONS, RUPTURE, PERFORATION (TRAUMA) OF THE INTESTINE.

It is apparent that these conditions are of surgical as well as of clinical interest. Traumas which affect the abdominal wall without injuring it may lead to paralysis through direct disturbances of innervation without any anatomical changes of a macro- or microscopical nature, or cause hemorrhage in the intestinal wall, mesentery, or peritoneum, or under the most unfavorable conditions bring about rupture of the intestine. The latter occurs, according to Poland, most frequently near the lower end of the duodenum, and on the duodenojejunal flexure, which part is fixed by the muscle or suspensory ligament of the duodenum, described first by Treitz and then by Braun as a flat plate of muscle-fibers, consisting of unstriped muscular tissue which is broad at the upper end of the duodenum, narrows down to the size of a cord on its way over to the hiatus aorticus, where it disappears in the muscular tissue of the peritoneum. The fixed parts, especially the plexuses of the colon, are particularly endangered in contusions of the abdomen. It rarely happens in such cases that the injury is limited to the intestine ; usually the remaining fixed abdominal organs are affected to a mor serious extent by the effect of the traumatic changes. Several parts of the intestine may have been torn (according to MacConnac, in about 15 per cent. of all cases). Kőnig lost a patient, after having closed a traumatic rupture of his ileum by a suture, through peritonitis following fecal extravasation from rupture occurring in a part of the small intestine lying lower down in the pelvis. It may happen that the rupture of the intestine does not take place immediately after the injury, but usually a period of time, indeed weeks, after the date of the injury, when the latter has superinduced hemorrhagic infiltration and necrosis of the abdominal wall. Julien has reported a case of a girl in whom a concussion against the abdomen brought about severe abdominal phenomena with peritonitis and formation of abscesses, eventuating in necrosis of the abdominal wall, which resulted in death eight days after an unsuccessful operation and thirty days after the injury. According to Mugnier, intestinal phenomena may occur in concussions against the abdomen after a lapse of time when the injury is only a superficial one, consisting merely of slight tears and bleeding of the mucous membrane. In other traumas reported by this author the injuries affected only the muscularis and serosa. Seven to eight days afterward, or even later, diarrhea, constipation, with vomiting, and finally also peritonitis, set in. Ulcerations and necrosis develop and form the focus of agglutinating and perforating peritonitis.

Rupture of the Intestines.

Symptomatology and Diagnosis.—The clinical phenomena following severe traumas that have affected the intestines are pain, shock, pallor, feeble, small, or absent radial pulse, fainting, vomiting, and cold perspiration. In these severe cases death follows, caused by cardiac asthenia. In less grave cases recovery from the first collapse may occur as a result of resourceful treatment and nursing by rest, stimulants, warm applications or hot packing, hypodermic injections of strychnia and camphor, strong black coffee or caffein, alcohol, ether. If the patient should rally from the first shock he requires careful nursing for a long time, and must abstain from work of any kind.

Severe traumas that have caused hemorrhages into the tissues of the intestinal wall may lead either to bloody stools, enterorrhagia, or be succeeded by the signs of occlusion due to paralysis of the intestine. It is always a difficult matter to decide whether an actual rupture of the intestinal wall has taken place or not. The decision is of great importance, because a rupture of the intestine peremptorily calls for a prompt operation. Von Beck attributes great importance to the intense pain for distinguishing between rupture and contusion. This pain is so intense that the patients often faint as a result of it, and immediately enter upon a state of collapse. Von Beck (" Deutsch. Zeitschr. f. Chir.," Bd. xi and xv) emphasizes that tympanites may not develop until twenty-four hours after the accident. Against this I might urge that pronounced meteorism may develop after contusions as a result of intestinal paralysis, and I do not consider that Beck's distinction constitutes a criterion ; for in specially large perforations the abdomen may be concavely retracted and there may be no tympanites at all.   This I have twice observed after perforating typhoid ulcers and once after perforation of a duodenal ulcer.   Berndt and König have designated the appearance of severe, frequent, uncontrollable vomiting as a sign of intestinal rupture, in contradistinction to the transient vomiting occurring at rare intervals which is observed in simple intestinal contusions without rupture.

In addition to collapse the most important sign of intestinal rupture is the accumulation of a peritonitic effusion, which can be demonstrated soon after the trauma, and cessation of abdominal breathing.   In association with this there is also an intraperitoneal tympanites, giving the impression of a gas balloon in front of and above the liver.   To be sure, the liver may be displaced or twisted around so that its sharp edge points directly against the anterior abdominal wall, or the intestine may become greatly distended, thereby overlying and covering the liver.   All these possibilities must be considered, as they may give rise to confusion.

The escape of intestinal contents is soon followed, as a rule, by septic peritonitis, conditioning a grave prognosis.   There are cases, however, where a timely operation saved the patient.   When the intestines are empty at the time of the trauma, and the tear not large, the escape of fecal matter into the peritoneum and subsequent peritonitis may be prevented where the ruptured portion or the opening has been closed by close apposition of the peritoneum or omentum.   According to the experiments of Griffith, the mucosa may become everted and protrude through the tear in transverse wounds of $\frac{1}{3}$ inch.   In this manner the loss of continuity may be restored, temporarily at least, by the outward protrusion of mucosa through the fibers of the longitudinal muscular layer.   In longitudinal wounds the torn or cut circular muscle-fibers roll the peritoneum and longitudinal muscle inward, thus bringing about a temporary restoration of continuity, at least when the bowel is empty.   If the rupture did not occur suddenly, but was developed gradually from necrosis, it leads to the formation of encapsulated peritoneal abscesses containing food and fecal concretions, which may perforate through the abdominal wall or into neighboring hollow organs. The diagnosis of such an abscess, which may be made by palpation of a painful tumor accompanied by septic phenomena, and the traumatic nature of which receives support from the anamnesis, should be quickly followed by an operation. In rupture of the ascending and descending colon, retroperitoneal stercoral abscesses may form, followed by perforation through the diaphragm into the thoracic cavity. These abscesses may also break through the abdominal wall (externally). In both cases stercoral fistulæ may remain and necessitate operative closure.

Therapeutics.—As soon as intestinal rupture has been diagnosed, or its presence at least may be regarded as highly probable, with but a short time having elapsed since its occurrence, an operation should be undertaken by all means. Even collapse does not contraindicate operation if it is in the initial shock collapse and not that which comes on forty-eight hours or longer after the injury, and is due to marasmus. It is my practice to urge operation in suspected subcutaneous contusions of the intestine even if there is no positive proof of rupture; for experience has taught that an operation undertaken even when no rupture was found, benefited the patient by definitely establishing the exact state of the injury. Delay always means septic peritonitis. Von Angerer reports 9 such operations with but two recoveries ("Archiv f. klin. Chir.," Bd. LXI, H. 4).

Traumatic Rupture of Intestine by Forcible Distention.

In the section on treatment of intestinal occlusions I have described a peculiar kind of injury to the intestine, which occurs fortunately very rarely, under the excessively forcible and copious irrigation or distention of the colon by water for diagnostic or therapeutic purposes. In such cases the serosa may tear, the muscularis may yield, and the mucosa protrude through the muscularis; in fact, a genuine and complete rupture may take place, which occurs usually in a transverse, rarely in a longitudinal, direction, and mainly on the side opposite to the insertion of the mesentery. The symptoms are those of intense pains followed by an extraordinarily severe collapse, as a result of the tremendous distention of the intestine. The lesions may be only microscopic in character, requiring at least a hand lens for their detection, as they in certain of these cases consist of innumerable very minute rents on the mucosa and peritoneum. But more frequently this accident causes an actual rupture of the intestine, with a very grave prognosis.

Treatment.—With experience and proper care such an accident ought not to happen when irrigation or colon distention is practised. The practitioner may, however, have the exceptionally bad luck of encountering a patient with abnormally weak (brittle) intestinal walls (beginning amyloidosis); such a possibility can not be guarded against. The first efforts should be directed to evacuating the introduced liquids by means of a Langdon long, thick-walled colon tube. If paralysis of the intestine sets in,—and unfortunately it does so promptly, for the forcible distention is usually undertaken only for the recognition or relief of obstructions which in themselves occasionally superinduce paralysis,—then evacuation of the liquids once forced in becomes, in my opinion, a doubtful matter, and efforts at removal should be discontinued.

Strong stimulants should be used, and where severe pain has been succeeded by shock, opium should be given by the mouth, or morphin hypodermically. Where the liquid matter has not been or can not be removed, it is gradually completely absorbed, and in favorable instances an extraordinarily profuse polyuria sets in, which excretes the absorbed liquid and the excess of such as has been introduced. I have had occasion to observe one case of intestinal rupture from overdistention where serious symptoms resulted from the introduction of 5 liters of lukewarm water, and Pribram (*l. c.*) reports two similar cases where an enema had been awkwardly given from a height of 2½ meters to an elderly woman suffering from chronic obstipation. This patient died from the results of the intestinal rupture. The case observed by myself recovered under treatment by rest, diet (only somatose, white of eggs, wine and water), and opium.

The treatment of peritonitis due to contusions or rupture of the intestine is the same as that of peritonitis due to any other cause, with perhaps a more imperative demand for surgical interference. It is important also to bear in mind that incomplete tears may not give the symptoms of rupture until several days after the injury. The results of the non-operated cases, according to Petrey ("Beitr.

z. klin. Chir.," 1896, Bd. xvi, S. 545), were as follows: Of 160 cases not treated surgically, 149 terminated in death and 11 in recovery, a mortality of 93.4 per cent. Of the 11 that recovered, 10 developed a fecal abscess which had to be operated in 7 cases. These statistics include only cases in which there was absolutely no doubt about the intestinal rupture. There can be no doubt that there are cases of slight or incomplete perforation which escape a definite diagnosis, and can not be taken up in such statistics. Such cases undoubtedly heal without an operation. Of 28 cases of undoubted intestinal *contusions* treated without operation, 12 terminated fatally and 16 recovered, a mortality of 43.4 per cent. The operated cases of subcutaneous intestinal rupture gave the following results, according to Petrey: Of 42 cases operated within the first day after the injury, 14 recovered, 28 died, a mortality of 66.7 per cent. Of 18 cases operated within the first twenty-four hours, 8 recovered and 10 terminated fatally, a mortality of 45.5 per cent. Of 24 patients who were operated later than twenty-four hours after the accident, 6 recovered and 16 died, a mortality of 75 per cent.

For details of the surgical aspect of rupture of the intestine the reader is referred to text-books on intestinal surgery: "International Encyclopedia of Surgery," vol. v, p. 466; Senn's "Practical Surgery"; König, "Lehrbuch d. Chir.," etc.

Perforation of the Intestine (Gun-shot and Stab Wounds).

Perforation of the intestine, in ordinary clinical and private practice, is most often the result of ulcerative or suppurative processes in the bowel tissue itself. The perforations which result from traumas—bruises, contusions, falls, and those resulting from gunshot and stab wounds—do not occur as often in general practice, but constitute a special and distinctive part of military surgery. In the "Medical and Surgical History of the War of the Rebellion," Med. Vol., Part ii, J. J. Woodward refers to the perforation resulting from dysentery, and holds that it occurs most frequently in the cecum (*l. c.*, p. 389), but may take place in any part of the colon. A perforation of the cecum, he remarks, may be accompanied by formation of an abscess in the right iliac fossa, which may discharge into the intestine or even in rare cases through the abdominal parietes.

In 99 autopsies which he refers to (*l. c.*, p. 522) of follicular ulcerations in the chronic dysentery, perforation of the colon by ulcers was observed in only 2 cases.   In one it occurred in the transverse colon, and in the other there were several perforations just above the sigmoid flexure (*l. c.*, p. 523).   Among what he calls his undetermined cases (*l. c.*, p. 527)—namely, those that are imperfectly recorded, both as to their clinical history and postmortem appearances—there were 293 cases of this character ; the large intestine is said to have been perforated in 9 instances.   In 53 cases of acute diphtheritic dysentery (*l. c.*, p. 554), there were 11 perforations of the intestine, mostly in the cecum and transverse colon.   Some of the cases presented two perforations in the same individual.   In one case, No. 436, it is stated that there were more than 20 perforations of the colon.

Ulcerations which bring about perforation have been noticed most frequently in enteric fever (typhoid), dysentery, in the suprastenotic loops of intestinal stenoses and obstructions, in carcinoma and intestinal tuberculosis.   These latter processes may lead at first to indurated cicatricial adhesions of the intestine, and only exceptionally bring on perforation peritonitis.

The clinical phenomena of the spontaneous perforation are the same as those described in connection with the intestinal rupture mentioned in the preceding—sudden, violent pains, which, by the way, may improve with the increasing collapse, subnormal temperature or chills with high fever, intraperitoneal tympanites with a disappearance of the liver dullness by formation of a gas bladder (from escaped gas) immediately in front of the liver.   Percussion by means of the pleximeter gives a metallic resonance.

Frequently there is a serous or bloody effusion in the most dependent portions of the peritoneal cavity—a sign of peritonitis. As it is bad practice to move or lift about the patient in these grave conditions, the movability of the dullness due to the effusion can not be made out.   Tchudnowsky ("Berlin. klin. Wochenschr.," 1860, No. 20 u. 21) asserted that an amphoric respiratory murmur could be heard over the abdomen, after perforations, which was isochronic with the respiratory movements and caused by the passage of air in and out through the perforation.   It is obvious that there must be many conditions of pneumatics and acoustics that influence this phenomenon.   Although I auscultated **two** abdomens after gunshot wounds that had caused large holes in the bowel, I could not detect it, and do not consider it an available sign.

Even the disappearance of hepatic dullness is a misleading sign, for it may be produced by excessive meteorism without perforation; in this condition the liver is tilted up and over by pressure from below, and only its sharp edge left pointing toward the abdominal wall; percussion can reveal no liver dullness, so that the pulmonary resonance passed directly into the tympanitic resonance of the abdomen on the right side.

Intestinal perforation need not always be associated with meteorism; there are cases on record in which, after very large openings into the bowel, the abdomen was concavely retracted and hard as a board. This has been explained by assuming that the entrance of intestinal contents into the peritoneal cavity may act as a powerful stimulant to contraction of the abdominal muscles. This concave abdomen has been described after perforating typhoid, duodenal, and gastric ulcers; sometimes it exists only at the beginning, and later gives way to tympanites.

When the intestines are perforated by the burrowing of an extra-intestinal accumulation of pus (penetration of peri-appendicial abscess), the initial pain is wanting, and there are no signs of accumulation of gas, or formation of circumscribed gas bag in the highest portion of the peritoneum. The presence of pus in the evacuations is regarded as a reliable sign of this kind of perforation. The general condition is not seriously affected, and even a marked improvement may become evident after this escape of pus into the bowel. The general peritoneum is fortunately walled off from the abscesses which owe their origin to appendicitis, and if perforation into another portion of the bowel occurs, pain is slight and meteorism absent, because no gas can enter the peritoneum.

Nothnagel (*l. c.*, p. 441) calls attention to a sweetish aromatic odor, similar to a fruity odor, which is said to be peculiar, and not only perceived in the breath of the patient, but also in his immediate vicinity. He asserts that it was observed at his clinic not only in perforation, but also in other forms of purulent peritonitis, and suggests that it may be a phenomenon indirectly available for the diagnosis of purulent peritonitis. Its origin is not

known.   It occurred, however, when there was very little acetone
in the urine.   No mention is made whether the Gerhardt ferric
chlorid reaction was undertaken in these cases.   A solution of
liquor ferri sesquichlorati, so dilute as to have the color of Rhine
wine, is used.   Gerhardt found that many urines which contain
sugar gave a deep Burgundy red color when this solution was
added in excess.   The urine at the same time disseminates a peculiar aromatic odor, reminding one of the odor of fruit or chloroform.
The same odor is perceived in the expired air of the patient.
Such patients, in Gerhardt's opinion, are threatened with diabetic
intoxication or coma.   It is possible that during the traumas
accompanying intestinal ruptures and perforations, the pancreas
may be injured so as to produce a form of diabetes.   I suggest this simply in order to call attention to the problematical
nature of the aromatic substances that may produce the sweetish
odor of the breath to which Nothnagel calls attention.   In all such
cases of perforation the urine should be carefully tested for sugar,
and the Gerhardt reaction carried out.

Death may occur during collapse before peritonitis can be
recognized, or during the peritonitis under gradually developing
marasmus.   In rare instances previous peritonitis may produce
adhesions of such a character as to completely wall off a developing abscess.   Should this pus accumulation subsequently perforate
into the bowel or other hollow abdominal or pelvic organ, a general
peritonitis is prevented by the wall of adhesions previously formed.

Treatment.—The only hope of preserving life lies in prompt
and skilful surgical treatment—laparotomy, searching out the opening or openings, closure of same, disinfection of the peritoneum.
The medical treatment is purely symptomatic and consists of
absolute rest, abstinence from food, hypodermic injections of
strychnin, digitalin, nitroglycerin, as the indications demand.   If
pain is great, morphin should not be withheld, and ¼ grain given
hypodermically.

Modern surgical technics, especially in military surgery, can
point to a large number of recoveries after very grave intestinal
tears and perforations.   But also the records of private hospitals
are illustrative of the possibilities of prompt surgical intervention.
The records of the Hospital of the University of Maryland contain

accounts of recoveries after the intestine had been perforated in several places seriously ; in one month (1898) there were three successful laparotomies by Professor Randolph Winslow, who has also called my attention to the fact that any penetrating wound of the thorax at or below the fifth rib must be considered as a possible gunshot wound of the abdomen ; this is a diagnostic hint worth remembering.

Professor Randolph Winslow has operated 10 cases of perforation and rupture of the intestines at the Hospital of the University of Maryland, with the following results :

CASE I.—Four perforations of the small intestine, from a pistol-shot ; laparotomy ; recovery.

CASE II.—Six perforations of small intestine and three of the mesentery ; laparotomy ; death.

CASE III.—Gunshot wound of small intestine, seven perforations ; laparotomy ; death.

CASE IV.—Gunshot wound of the liver, small intestine, and mesocolon, five perforations ; laparotomy ; recovery.

CASE V.—Gunshot wound of small intestine, six perforations ; laparotomy ; recovery.

CASE VI.—Pistol wound of the first portion of the duodenum ; laparotomy ; large ragged perforation in the ascending duodenum, an inch in length ; recovery.

CASE VII.—Gunshot wound of small intestine ; laparotomy ; five perforations in small intestine and three in mesentery ; death.

CASE VIII.—Pistol wound of ileum ; laparotomy ; perforation an inch in length ; recovery.

CASE IX.—Stab wound of colon ; laparotomy ; three perforations and partial cut in another place ; recovery.

CASE X.—Gunshot wound of small intestine, rectum, and bladder ; laparotomy ; perforation of small intestine in four places ; also perforation of rectum and bladder ; death third day from pneumonia, perforations being healed and peritonitis not present.

Considering the severity of the injuries, some of which I saw personally, the percentage of recoveries (60 per cent.) is a large one.

For surgical treatment of perforated typhoid ulcers, see J. M. T. Finney, "Johns Hopkins Hospital Reports," January, 1901.

Suppurative inflammations issuing from the female genital tract are frequent causes of perforation into the intestines, or necessitate resection of portions of the intestine in the efforts to remove the original focus of the disease. Such cases fall into the sphere of the gynecologist. Dr. Thomas A. Ashby, of the University of Maryland, has described five cases of this type, all necessitating resection of the intestine, four of which recovered ("Jour. Amer. Med. Assoc.," November, 1899).

CHAPTER V.

ENTERORRHAGIA.

Synonym.—Intestinal Hemorrhages.

The escape of blood from the intestinal vessels has been described under the various diseased conditions in which it occurs—viz., intestinal ulcers, dysentery, neoplasms, invaginations, perforations, rupture, etc. Here we aim at a collective consideration of the symptoms.

Symptomatology.

The only symptom of intestinal hemorrhage is the presence of blood in the stools, and this symptom is often absent when the hemorrhage occurs in a person who has already been greatly weakened by previous illness; in such cases the blood remains in the intestines. Nothing, therefore, is more variable, more changeable, than the symptomatic appearance of intestinal hemorrhages; in its divers aspects this appearance is connected with the symptomatology of the causes which have been enumerated in other chapters above mentioned.

When the blood is not evacuated in the stools the intestinal hemorrhage has no other symptoms except those which characterize all internal hemorrhages. The patient suddenly grows pale, his face has a deathly look, his sight is clouded, veiled, and obscured, the skin becomes cold; the pulse is retarded and can hardly be detected. Afterward he experiences buzzing in the ears, nausea, vomiting, vertigo, fainting spells, all of which are symptoms which accompany great losses of blood. In such a case the real seat of the hemorrhage can be ascertained only by the detailed examinations of other morbid symptoms.

When blood is evacuated it presents itself under different aspects.

When the loss of blood is very great, the blood comes forth bright red, in the form of clots mixed with some liquid blood; in a short period of time the patient is, as it were, bathed in his own

evacuation.   These great hemorrhages are observed more especially
in those cases where an ulceration, no matter what kind it may be,
opens a blood-vessel of a rather considerable caliber.

When the flow of blood is less abundant, the blood is not immediately evacuated, but remains for a longer or shorter period of time
in the intestines, and there undergoes the digestive action of the intestinal secretions and becomes black-colored.   This is often referred
to as melena.

When the blood is poured forth in very small quantities, it is
mingled with fecal matter, to which it gives a dark color, and the
appearance of tar.

In the microscopic examination of the blood-containing stools, one
finds the red globules, some of them modified, some swollen, partly
discolored, and in course of destruction, or already completely
destroyed.   The blood-corpuscles after a few days are transformed
into masses of hemoglobin more or less voluminous.

The microscopic examination of the fecal matter furnishes indications from which one may foretell a subsequent intestinal hemorrhage.   In the typhoid affections Nothnagel found that the microscope showed small particles of blood in the fecal matter from
twelve to thirty-six hours before a considerable intestinal hemorrhage.   The probability of a venous intestinal hemorrhage is still
greater when one can perceive bloody streaks in the evacuations with
the naked eye.

The physical examination of the abdomen ought to be made with
the greatest precaution, because any excessive pressure upon the
abdominal wall, and also any imprudent movement, may cause a
hemorrhage or the recurrence of one.   In my own practice I have
observed a fatal hemorrhage from the performance of abdominal
massage, undertaken by a bold masseuse, without my permission, on
a case of dysentery.

It is asserted by Courtois-Suffit that one may detect a muffled
sound in the abdomen when the hemorrhage remains internal.   This
is observed, however, only when the blood accumulation in the intestines has taken on considerable proportions.   I have never been
able to confirm this observation.

Occasionally after a hemorrhage, edema and even a slight transient albuminuria are observed.   These phenomena should be attrib-

uted to the serious anemic condition which is the result of the hemorrhage.

In newborn children the intestinal hemorrhage is of a special character, and deserves particular mention. (See Hemmeter, "Diseases of the Stomach," on Melena Neonatorum, second edition, p. 685.) Since very often it can not be attributed to any *one* unmistakable cause, it is less well known in its objective characteristics. Very often it is preceded by various precursors—paleness of the skin, fall in the temperature, retardation of the pulse, depression of the fontanels, and an increasing apathy—indications of internal hemorrhages. Afterward the bloody evacuation appears, which sometimes is preceded by blood-vomiting. The blood is of varying coloration, sometimes dark, sometimes light, and occasionally pouring forth so abundantly as to stain the swaddling clothes. Frequently it consists of a single bloody evacuation, or this may be followed by discharge of a fluid which contains but little blood. In other cases, however, the hemorrhages are repeated and even last several days. From this a state of increasing blood-impoverishment results, which carries off the infants. In all cases melena neonatorum is a very grave symptom.

In the other intestinal hemorrhages the secondary symptoms are variable, and must be described with their causes.

Pathologic Anatomy.

This may be reduced to a statement of the essential conditions. The contents of the intestine contain blood ; occasionally one finds it in the form of red, black, and spongy clots, which mold themselves to the shape of the intestinal canal until they even assume its form (blood-clot cylinders) ; sometimes also they are soft masses very similar to tar and having an offensive smell. The wall of the digestive tube has a varying appearance ; it may be pale, anemic, or it may also in places show bloody extravasations and ulcerations. If these latter are the cause of the hemorrhage, thrombosis of the blood-vessels may be found, or one may discover, rising from the bottom of the ulcer, a watery or colored liquid which takes its origin from the mesenteric artery. The other organs are frequently very much discolored. If considerable hemorrhages have occurred several times, one may often detect fatty degeneration of the heart, the liver, the kidneys, the pancreas, and the glandular cells of the intestines and of the stomach.

The remaining pathological features have been detailed under the consideration of various intestinal diseases in the course of which enterorrhagia may occur.

Diagnosis.

First, Differential Diagnosis.—When blood is not evacuated with the stools one can not do more than suspect an intestinal hemorrhage. If blood is evacuated, however, its various appearances may cause one to believe that a hemorrhage is present.

In very severe constipation it may happen that the fecal matter has a brownish-black appearance, which should suggest the presence of blood. The doubt ought to yield on microscopic and chemic examination. A large quantity of bile may give the evacuations a brownish-black appearance, as if they contained blood. The stools may also have a dark color because the patient has used preparations containing iron or bismuth.

The same is true if one finds in the evacuations red fruits or certain berries which have not been digested. The Boas stool sieve is an excellent means for dissipating all these doubts, it being sufficient to wash the evacuation with water. If the blood is really present, the water takes on a bloody tint. The blood-corpuscles may be detected by the microscopic examination before placing the stool in the sieve.

Second, Diagnosis of the Location of the Hemorrhage.— The color of the blood is frequently a very valuable source of indication for the seat of the hemorrhage. Unless the hemorrhage was very violent, the blood is rarely bright red after it has had to pass through a certain length of the intestine. The case is entirely different, however, when the lesion is situated in the lower portion of the intestines, in the colon or in the sigmoid flexure, or in the rectum. In such cases inspection by proctoscope will reveal the location of the source of the hemorrhage. (See chapter on Diseases of the Rectum.) According to the pathological conditions which one finds, one can often ascertain the location of the hemorrhage. After severe burns one naturally thinks of the duodenum ; if the patient is a sufferer from dysentery, the first thought is of the large intestine. Finally, blood may pass out from the anus and yet not take its origin from the intestines. In such cases the hemorrhages may come from the nose, the pharynx, lungs, esophagus, or the stomach. Epistaxis and operations for hare-lip may produce pseudo-hemorrhagic evacuations in infants.

Third, Etiological Diagnosis.—*Etiology, Pathology, Symptomatic Value.*—As a rule, the intestinal hemorrhages are observed more frequently in men than in women. They occur very rarely in infancy, and when they do appear in new-born children they constitute a class of diseases by themselves. In such cases we have to do with a septic infection, or the so-called melena of the new-born.

From a standpoint of the origin of the blood we may separate intestinal hemorrhages into three classes—arterial, venous, and capillary. Hemorrhages which are simply capillary may frequently be very abundant, and may show themselves under circumstances where, on account of the presence of intestinal ulcers of large size, one might be led to assume a hemorrhage of larger blood-vessels.

Kennedy maintains that intestinal hemorrhages are due more frequently to an excessive hyperemia of the mucosa than to the opening of the larger blood-vessels into the ulcers. In my experience venous hyperemia is not a frequent cause of ulcer.

Intestinal hemorrhages may be due to quite a number of causes.

Anomalies of the Intestinal Contents.—It is not at all rare that a persistent constipation causes an intestinal hemorrhage when the masses of the fecal matter, if excessively voluminous and hardened, mechanically irritate and wound the intestinal mucosa. The hemorrhage which is thus produced is not very considerable; it usually starts from the large intestine, in the shape of points and streaks of blood, which cover the surfaces of the condensed fecal matter.

Foreign bodies which have been swallowed may also produce the same result. Henoch relates a case where a man had an intestinal hemorrhage every time he ate thrushes. The reason was that he swallowed the bones too, and these, not being dissolved in the intestines, wounded the mucosa.

Intestinal hemorrhages may also be produced by *poisonings*. We must add here that the excessive use of purgatives may be compared to a poisoning.

Intestinal hemorrhage may also be produced by *parasites*. Among these, the most important is the duodenal anchylostomum. This parasite fixes itself firmly on the intestinal mucosa, perforates it, and occasionally penetrates into blood-vessels. The anemia thus caused may be diagnosed by the minute study of the conditions under which it is produced. (See chapter on Intestinal Parasites.) It will be easy to recognize its cause by the serious state of anemia which characterizes it, an anemia which resembles the pernicious progressive anemia, and which exists in the endemic state. If any doubt still exists, it will be necessary to look for the anchylostomum eggs in the fecal matter (use stool-sieve).

Local Affections of the Abdominal Wall.—The intestinal hemorrhages which may be due to traumas have been considered in a separate chapter. In such cases it is not difficult to determine the origin ; it is, so to speak, before our very eyes. Enoch and Wilms thus observed a transient intestinal hemorrhage appearing after a herniotomy. This probably was due to the attempts at reduction of the intestinal loops. The introduction of foreign bodies into the rectum may also produce the same effect. Of all the causes of intestinal hemorrhage, ulcerations of the walls of the intestine are most important. The diagnosis of these conditions is given in a separate chapter.

In hemorrhages occurring in the course of ulcers, of ulcerated tumors, and of foreign bodies, we have to deal with a direct rupture of the blood-vessels, whether they be arterial or venous.

Typhoid Fever.—In the epidemics of typhoid fever the frequency of intestinal hemorrhage is variable ; the average figure given most frequently is 5 per cent. This percentage of frequency is that which my records of cases at the University of Maryland Hospital show for typhoid fever. It is extremely rare in children. The hemorrhage is produced at two distinctly separate periods of the disease. Either it appears at the beginning of the disease, and, in such a case, is usually of very little importance, or it appears in the course of the second or third week. In the latter case it is at the same time more violent and has a considerably greater symptomatic value. It is almost always accompanied by general and grave phenomena ; as the fever continues in its course, the hemorrhage is signaled by a sudden and distinct lowering of the temperature ; the thermometer falls two or three degrees. Occasionally one observes together with the hemorrhage either a very pronounced coldness in the limbs or a surprising diminution in the severity of the cerebral symptoms and the delirium. This, however, is only a momentary calm, since the symptoms of the typhoid fever soon reappear. The danger of perforation after severe intestinal hemorrhages is very great. This intestinal hemorrhage is always a very grave occurrence, in spite of the opinion, which is supported by Trousseau, that it need not be considered an unfavorable symptom. The opinion as to its gravity must be determined more especially by the period in which it appears, whether its appearance is early in the course of the fever, or late.

Tuberculous Enteritis.—In this disease the intestinal hemorrhage is *not a frequent* accident. The evacuations may contain blood without our being able to attribute to this phenomenon the name of intestinal hemorrhage. There are, nevertheless, cases where abundant intestinal hemorrhage with immediate grave symptoms exists. Trousseau and Courtois-Suffit assert that these complications are observed more especially in the course of acute tuberculosis. They are observed also quite frequently in chronic tuberculosis. Etiologically they are recognized by the symptomatic retinue which they complicate—namely, long-continued diarrhea, emaciation, and chronic tuberculous cachexia, with its pulmonary manifestations clearly in evidence.

Dysentery.—Hemorrhages as they occur in dysentery have been described in a separate chapter. The special character of the evacuations in dysentery enables us to recognize them immediately. In this disease, when the intestinal ulcerations have become established, the evacuations become bloody ; besides mucous matter they contain pure blood, also membranes and necrotic tissue. The patients suffer from tenesmus, gripings, and may have fifty stools in twenty-four hours.

Simple (Peptic) Duodenal Ulcer.—This form of peptic ulcer has been considered in all its clinical and pathological details in a separate chapter. Most frequently the loss of blood is sudden and very abundant ; it manifests itself, on its first appearance, a short time after meals. The patient is afflicted with great discomfort, suffering from more or less violent colic, and occasionally presenting the symptoms of dystrypsia. The blood may be vomited or may not show itself except in the evacuations; in the latter case it may appear suddenly, because the duodenal ulcer hemorrhages are often profuse. The patient then evacuates a quantity of black fecal matter, often quite large, and at the same time shows the symptoms of an internal intestinal hemorrhage—namely, paleness and discoloration of the integuments. This special behavior of the disease, joined to the classic symptoms of duodenal ulcer, symptoms which are already manifest or which will commence after the intestinal hemorrhage, will render the diagnosis easy and certain. (See Ulcer of the Stomach, "Diseases of the Stomach," second edition, p. 486, and Ulcer of the Duodenum of a separate chapter, p. 594, vol. I, "Diseases of the Intestines.")

Cancer and Sarcoma of the Intestine.—In this disease melena is a frequent symptom. If the neoplasm is situated in the lower section of the intestine and if the hemorrhage is abundant, the blood usually retains its bright red color. Besides, it always accompanies a series of symptoms which indicate its origin and nature—namely, pains in the abdomen, signs of stenosis, and palpable tumor.

Hemorrhoids.—Hemorrhoids occur very frequently, but may easily be recognized as to their origin. The character of the hemorrhoidal flow, the visual examination of the varicose projection, do not permit one to make an error. In the great majority of cases the losses of blood are not very abundant, and permit of a favorable prognosis. We must not, however, forget that occasionally they are very severe, and a state of anemia which may become alarming may be one of the consequences.

Polypus of the Rectum.—The evacuations often have the appearance of slimy, mucous stools, tinged with blood, and resembling currant jelly. Occasionally, also, one observes hemorrhages of the rectum which are so abundant that they cause great anemia in the patient. No other cause can occasion such abundant hemorrhages in children, and consequently its symptomatic value is considerable. When the polypus protrudes from the anus the diagnosis is certain. Rectal inspection by proctoscope should never be omitted. (See chapter on Diseases of the Rectum.)

Frequently the intestinal hemorrhages are the consequence of an inflammation (congestion) of the mucosa. In general the hemorrhages due to this cause have very little importance. According to Leube, they are frequently observed in the enteritis which is common among the aged. They are comparatively frequent in the inflammations of the mucosa which are the results of burns of the skin. Beyer describes one case where an intestinal hemorrhage occurred at the time when the patient had erysipelas in his face. It is a well-known fact that cutaneous burns and erysipelas may both cause ulcerations of the intestines in an analogous manner. The enterorrhagia which has been observed in amyloidosis is described in a separate chapter.

Intestinal Hemorrhage in Consequence of Congestion of the Portal Vein System—Hepatic Cirrhosis.—According to Grainger-Stewart, amyloid degeneration of the intestinal blood-vessels often produces intestinal hemorrhages. They may also be observed in connection with the emboli of the superior and also of the inferior mesenteric artery, in the obstructions of the main branch of the portal vein, chronic affections of the liver, hepatic cirrhosis, and cancers. In the last-mentioned cases the hemorrhages constitute a serious complication, which may become a rapid cause of death. They frequently precede ascites; that is to say, they are observed at a period when it is difficult to form a diagnosis of hepatic cirrhosis. These facts may be explained by the hypothesis that a congestion in the system of the portal vein is present. The vasomotor system of the abdomen has a special function, or at any rate an influence by virtue of which, through the agency of a complex mechanism of innervation, a congestion of quite a different intensity from that which appears in other vascular districts is occasionally observed. In the healthy subject this congestion will not give occasion for a hemorrhage, because the liver has the power of distending and taking up considerable quantities of blood, which can very easily be passed from the system of the portal vein to the intestinal venous system, and *vice versa*. If, however, the liver is cirrhosed, it loses its elasticity and contracts the path of the flow into the vena cava. If we therefore suppose that under these conditions a congestion in the portal vein system occurs, this congestion may distend it to such a degree that the vein or its radicles may burst—that is to say, a hemorrhage is caused (Debove and Courtois-Suffit).

The stagnation of the abdominal veins in chronic diseases of the heart and lungs is also capable of causing intestinal hemorrhages. These are easy to diagnose if they appear with the symptomatic indications of the original disease.

Intestinal hemorrhages occur very frequently in the course of numerous *infectious* diseases ; they may, however, easily be recognized by means of the febrile symptoms which either accompany or precede them.   The enterorrhagias occurring in dysentery, enteric fever, tuberculosis, and syphilis are directly due to ulcerating processes, and have been described.

Intestinal hemorrhages occasionally occur in *intermittent fevers.* According to Frerichs' opinion, they are caused by embolic obstructions of the branches of the portal vein.   Although I have treated a large number of patients suffering from malaria, and have personally lived in malarious districts for half a year at a time, I have never observed enterorrhagia attributable to this infection.

In enteric fever losses of blood have been observed on several occasions without there being present any ulceration of the mucosa. Murchison has observed this occurrence six times in 7000 cases of typhus, and Russell has seen it three times in 4000 cases.

It seldom happens that intestinal hemorrhages are encountered in the course of *Asiatic cholera.*   When they do occur, they almost invariably are a very bad symptom and give an unfavorable prognosis.

Yellow Fever.—The intestinal hemorrhages which occur in yellow fever are due to two conditions—viz., one is a pathological alteration in the composition of the blood, both of its solid and liquid constituents, whereby it can no longer clot as perfectly as normal blood, and, secondly, by the development of intestinal ulcers, as I have observed in a number of histological studies undertaken on the intestines of subjects dead with yellow fever. Councilman has described characteristic appearances in the liver-cells which he believes are distinct, and regions of necrosis which are abundant in bacteria have been found in the liver.   The intestinal ulcers in yellow fever may be due to the general congestion and catarrhal swelling.   At present no definite decision can be reached concerning the exact pathogenesis of these lesions.   They are extremely rare, since I have examined a number of intestines sent to me by Southern colleagues without having discovered them.

Melena of the New-born.—For an account of melena neonatorum see the author's work on "Diseases of the Stomach," second edition, page 685. Ebstein and Klebs are of the opinion that the gastro-intestinal hemorrhages of the new-born may be of infectious origin. The melena of new-born babes does not take its origin from a single anatomical process, and its causes may be widely different. Many theories have been advanced and many causes assigned as predisposing toward this disease, but this proves that no one of these causes is sufficient in itself. Very frequently the children who are attacked by this disease are well developed, and born of healthy parents. The melena has also been attributed to improper confinement, especially, according to Eichhorst, a confinement which has lasted too long or which has been artificially terminated; also the premature ligation of the umbilical cord. As already mentioned, one very important cause is the infection of the new-born children, and it is necessary, from this point of view, to emphasize a form of infectious icterus which frequently is accompanied by various kinds of hemorrhages (Winkel's disease).

In all these cases the prognosis is very unfavorable; the mortality may even reach as high as 50 per cent. If the hemorrhages have continued for more than thirty-six hours, it is exceptional that a cure can be effected. In other respects the prognosis depends upon the character of the melena; the puerperal and ulcerated form of the disease almost always ends fatally.

Intestinal hemorrhages are encountered also in those having a congenital tendency to hemorrhage, hemophilia, hemorrhagic diathesis, in the disease of Werlhof; also in scurvy, in uremia, and in hemorrhagic purpura.

Treatment.

When the hemorrhage has set in.—Absolute quiet, in bed. Nourishment, iced milk and cold beverages.

Applications of ice to the abdominal wall.

Subcutaneous injections of ergotin or ergotol, and especially of morphin, are useful in suitable cases. In cases of amyloidosis or thrombosis or embolism of the mesenteric artery or vein, as well as in the enterrorhagias occurring as results of hepatic cirrhosis, ergot has proved useless in my experience. Subcutaneous injections of normal salt solution are sometimes necessary to restore normal blood pressure. If a state of collapse exists, the strength should be sustained with alcoholic wines, and, if need be, with subcutaneous injections of ether.

The various forms of enterorrhagia in which surgical treatment becomes imperative have been considered in separate chapters, where the special treatment is given under each type.

The medical treatment of enterorrhagia has also been given in previous chapters where the varying pathogenesis is narrated, and also in the chapter on Intestinal Parasites.

CHAPTER VI.

SURGICAL TREATMENT OF APPENDICITIS.

THE CLINICAL ASPECTS OF INTESTINAL SURGERY.

Introduction.—A large number of pathological conditions of the intestine call for surgical interference at once, inasmuch as medicinal treatment is of no utility whatever in their management. Such are, for instance, the perforating ulcers in any part of the intestinal tract, the benign and malignant neoplasms, the diverticula of Meckel, actinomycosis of the intestine, etc. It can not be properly considered the object of this work to give an account of all the possible abnormalities which demand operative treatment, and to describe the technic requisite thereto, and the various methods that are eligible for the purpose of accomplishing the objects in view. The main object of this chapter is to point out the indications for surgical intervention, to emphasize the signs and symptoms that should guide the general practitioner in the transference of his cases from purely expectant treatment to the care of the surgeon. I shall accordingly consider only the indications for surgical treatment of benign and malignant neoplasms, of appendicitis and perityphlitis, and of the manifold forms of intestinal occlusion. The reason being that in these conditions there is always more or less of debatable territory between the domains of internal medicine and those of surgery, which, according to the prevailing indications in any particular case, may at one time be conceded to the clinician, at another time to the surgeon. The pathological states just mentioned represent the most important territories about the variable boundary-line ("Grenzgebieten") between medicine and surgery.

A number of surgeons have announced the view that there is no purely medical, nonoperative treatment for appendicitis (Deaver,[*] Finney, Murphy, Dieulafoy, etc., the latter a clinician). This conception of the therapeutics of inflammations of the vermiform appen-

---

[*] First edition, "Treatise on Appendicitis" (see p. 395 for opinions in his second edition).

dix has, however, not as yet found widespread approval, and indeed an exact knowledge of the pathology of this process not only makes it rational to expect that certain forms of it should be amenable to purely expectant treatment, but in a number of types this line of conduct is the only one to be pursued.   For appendicitis is not always one and the same pathologic-anatomical condition, but it is a name given to a variety of conditions, some of which are not even associated with the formation of ulcers, or even with the development of pus ; and which do not progress beyond a stage of simple catarrhal inflammation.   From a critical study of the literature of the subject and considerable personal experience I am of the opinion that eight essentially different types of disease may be classified under the heading of appendicitis.   This classification is based partly upon the clinical history and partly upon the pathological anatomy. It is not possible to diagnose at the bedside all the classes as outlined.   I believe that it is possible to distinguish simple catarrhal appendicitis, as long as it remains in this stage, from the other forms.   The pathologic-anatomical element enters into the classification of the types with abscess formation and perforation, groups III and IV.   In the following I shall endeavor to give the diagnostic factors by which a recognition of even these two groups is made possible.   The remaining six groups—appendicular colic, catarrhal appendicitis, appendicitis associated with occlusion, peracute appendicitis with peritonitis from the incipiency and gangrene of the vermiform process, the returning, relapsing, and chronic types—should, as a rule, present no difficulties of diagnosis.   These classes may be designated as follows :

(I) Appendicular colic ; (II) simple catarrhal appendicitis ; (III) ulcerative appendicitis with inflammatory edematous infiltration of the abdominal musculature, localized peritonitis, with or without a pus focus in the appendix.   This type may terminate in resolution and recovery ; there may be spontaneous resorption of the small abscesses, with improvement of all the symptoms ; but, on the other hand, the cases may progress gradually or suddenly into the next type.   (IV) Appendicitis with undoubted abscess formation, with presence of marked leukocytosis and high temperatures.   Exploratory puncture, as advocated and practised by a number of German clinicians, always gives evidence of pus, but, if carried out at all, it should only be done if operation is to immediately follow upon the puncture. It is not recommended. Abscess formation can be recognized without the puncture. There may be in this case development of subphrenic abscess, pylephlebitis, and liver abscess formation. (V) Appendicitis associated with intestinal occlusion; (VI) peracute appendicitis with the clinical picture of grave diffuse peritonitis from the incipiency and gangrene of the vermiform process; (VII) returning and relapsing appendicitis; (VIII) chronic appendicitis.

NATURE, CONCEPT, AND COURSE OF THESE VARIOUS FORMS.

I. Appendicular Colic.

There are undoubted cases of slight pain in the ileocecal region with or without fever, localized at or about McBurney's point, which must be considered as resulting from a disease of the appendix. The appendix, in those cases in which it can be palpated by Edebohls' method of palpation, is not found enlarged, or very slightly so, and the attacks are characterized by alternate improvement and exacerbation. This condition has been interestingly described by Talamon ("La colique appendiculaire"), who distinguishes it carefully from the plastic forms of appendicitis, as well as from the chronic forms and the relapsing and returning type. The anatomical conditions underlying this state are in all probability either a catarrhal condition of the appendix, a very slight adhesion with or without abnormal position, or a concretion with or without a stricture of the vermiform process. Appendicular colic may occur in people who have never had an attack of appendicitis or perityphlitis, but it is more frequent in individuals who have had either one of these diseases, occurring especially during convalescence. This form of appendicular colic may be due to stagnation of the contents of the cecum, associated with gaseous distention, because such events are sometimes observed to follow obstipation with some degree of regularity, and to subside upon the administration of enemata or purges. Meteorism, sensitiveness to pressure, and cutaneous hyperesthesia over the cecal region may be present. Such attacks should be interpreted as premonitions, and not be passed over as a trivial condition, for they are sometimes, after they have been repeated on three or four occasions, followed by typical suppurative appendicitis.

II. Simple or Catarrhal Appendicitis.

This is a condition of inflammation of the vermiform process in which the pathological histology of enteritis exists in the appendix. It is presumed that there is, as a rule, no ulceration present, though this is naturally very difficult to determine clinically. Leukocytosis is not present. Whilst appendicular colic requires nothing but strict dieting, hot cataplasms, and a few small doses of morphin if the pain is violent, catarrhal appendicitis requires stricter dieting, and absolute rest in bed. But this form, like type I, heals as a rule without leaving any evil consequences. On the other hand, if neglected, it may develop into the typical suppurative appendicitis. The fever in both I and II rarely requires special treatment, but the pain and the vomiting, if present, should be controlled. Mild diarrhea need cause no anxiety, but when it becomes severe, indicative of a stormy peristalsis, opium should not be spared. After the attack of catarrhal appendicitis is over, semisolid and liquid diet and two or three weeks' rest are advisable. It need hardly be emphasized that cases of groups I and II recover not by virtue of any medicament or system of treatment, but by the "vis medicatrix naturæ," favored by rest and diet.

III. Ulcerative Appendicitis with Exudation.

In these types the fever is moderately high, the ileocecal pains severe ; vomiting is generally present ; cloudy and high-colored urine ; after a few diarrheic passages strong distention of the abdomen follows. After the first day there is distinct peritoneal irritation and a palpable resistance in the ileocecal region. The skin is not reddened over the induration, but may be intensely sensitive. In some debilitated individuals the pains may be sufficiently severe to bring on collapse. Pressure over the ileocecal region does not relieve, but aggravates the pain. If the patient at once begins treatment, adheres to a strict diet, and maintains absolute rest, the tumor during the following days (the second or third day) gradually increases in size, and projects above Poupart's ligament, and almost reaches the median linea alba, on a line a few centimeters above the anterior superior spine of the ilium. The greatest dimensions of this tumor are reached on the third or fourth day. After that the fever diminishes, and the tumor may actually at once begin to diminish in size, though at first very slowly. Fever may have disappeared entirely in a few days, but the tumor will take much longer to become reduced to a size where it can no longer be palpated. This fever is sometimes spoken of as *lytic*, because it relates to "*lysis*," or solution of the solid products of exudation.

In most cases the fever has disappeared in from five to eight days, but there are types in which, with the best of care, as outlined above, the course of the disease may extend over a period of three weeks. The evacuations are, as a rule, suppressed, but flatus may pass. I have found diarrhea present in exceptional cases. In the entire literature on the subject concerning this type, diarrhea is given as a symptom in from 7 to 15 per cent. of all cases, and constipation was present in from 63 to 82 per cent. The pathological conditions underlying this clinical picture are a hyperemic swelling and ulceration of the appendix with or without fecal concretions. In most of these cases there is an actual pus focus present in or about the appendix. The various loops of the intestines may be agglutinated by fibrinous peritonitis. The tumor mass is also partly made up by stagnating intestinal contents, the indurated omentums as well as the congested visceral and parietal peritoneum.

Certain clinicians (Fitz, Borchardt, Sahli) separate the tumor into an extraperitoneal envelop and an intraperitoneal nucleus, which is generally considered to be of a purulent nature. According to Treves (*l. c.*), the pus may be absent after two or three weeks of acute inflammation, and in confirmation of this assertion he cites the case of a girl fifteen years old, upon whom he operated for appendicitis after twenty-two days of fever. On incising the induration he found no pus, and the patient recovered. The presence or absence of pus in the beginning of these cases is very difficult to determine, and small pus foci may escape macroscopic detection entirely even after the tumor is incised, and, on the other hand, there are cases in which the operation which was undertaken for grave symptoms on the second day disclosed an accumulation of pus.

In the previously described types of appendicitis—the appendicular colic and the simple catarrhal type—resolution and restoration to integrity occur in the great majority of cases; and even in this third type of ulcerative appendicitis with small pus foci and exudates there is no reason why complete resorption should not take place, provided there is no perforation of the vermiform process. According to my experience, there is no reason why spontaneous restitution should not occur even if there are small pus foci present; for cases have been reported, and I have observed them in my own practice, where exploratory puncture gave evidence of the presence of pus, but none was found at an operation undertaken fourteen days afterward. The bacteria which are contained within encapsulated abscesses perish, the pus becomes sterile, and the pus-corpuscles undergo fatty degeneration. Small pus foci may be absorbed, and in large ones the pus is condensed, thickened, and surrounded by thick fibrinous walls. It is not probable that large abscesses heal spontaneously in this way. If such abscesses heal at all it is because they have evacuated their contents into one or another of the hollow structures of the abdomen, through the appendix itself, the colon, the bladder, vagina, or rectum. Such sudden evacuations of pus are marked by rapid disappearance of the fever, and generally by a rapid improvement. If, however, the evacuated pus sets up a new inflammation elsewhere, there may be aggravation of the general phenomena. As a rule, however, cases of this third group, which may already be designated as cases of perityphlitis with tumor formation, belong to the favorable types and generally heal spontaneously. Pribram gives an account of a hundred cases of this type which entered his clinic, and among which there were only 3 which gave evidence of abscess formation; these 3 were operated. Of the remaining 97 cases, 94 recovered spontaneously and but 3 died. Of these 3 fatal abscesses, 1 was complicated with interstitial hepatitis, and the 2 others with pulmonary tuberculosis.

Statistics from hospitals are not as valuable for the deduction of conclusions regarding the future history of this type, particularly if we desire to ascertain whether they continue free from relapses, as are statistics from private practice. In a report of the German Surgical Congress, 1889, Kümmel tabulated 850 cases of appendicitis which he had observed during his hospital service. Of these, 619 recovered without operation. This proportion of 72 per cent. of recoveries under purely medical treatment represents very nearly the proportions given by Talamon (*l. c.*), who asserts that only 25 per cent. of the cases of this type justify surgical intervention.

. In private practice the results are still better, as these patients can afford better treatment, better diet, longer rest, and more careful general attention. Besides, it is not a matter of such great difficulty to follow up their future history for the purpose of tracing out any possible relapses; whereas in hospital practice by far the great majority of cases are not seen again.

This group III is the one concerning which there has been most discussion between clinicians and surgeons as to the question concerning the matter of treatment, whether it should be surgical or purely medical. In the following I shall attempt to emphasize the clinical indications and signs which are available for deciding this point. Every case treated medically and recovered from, and remaining free from relapses for three or more years, must inevitably strengthen the belief in the usefulness and effectiveness of nonoperative methods in these cases ; and every case that rapidly becomes worse and imperatively demands operation, will give support to the views of extreme surgical advocates—i. e., that all cases should be operated upon. It is to be regretted that many important features of the previous history are not narrated in the reports. Authors speak simply of "appendicitis" in the majority of cases, without describing its special character. In a general way it can be stated that more cases of this class III are treated by operations in hospitals than in private practice. Pribram (Ebstein u. Schwalbe, "Handb. d. prak. Med.," Bd. ii, S. 710) has followed up the future history of 21 cases operated on in the hospital, of which 8 (or more than 33 per cent.) had relapses. Kleinwächter, in formulating the statistics in Biermer's clinic, discovered that these hospital cases gave a future history of relapses in 20 per cent. of the cases. Pribram states that in private practice relapses are much rarer. Personally I have collected 32 cases of appendicitis, which occurred in private practice between the years 1889 and 1891. Of these, 9 recovered after operation, and 23 after purely medical treatment. Of the 9 operated, all were well six years after the date of the operation. Of the 23 that recovered after medical treatment, 2 had relapses within the first five years, but the relapses were again recovered from without operation, and the patients were capable of attending to their business.

French Opinions.—In France the discussion on the proper

treatment of appendicitis received an impetus in 1898 from the articles of Dieulafoy, which appeared in " La Presse Médicale," 1898, and in the "Bulletin de l'académie de Médicine," Paris, 1899, vol. XLI, in which this clinician expressed himself as an enthusiastic champion of surgical intervention. At the meeting of the French Société de Chirurgie (see " Revue de Chir.," 1898, p. 769) Poirier claimed that in all cases of appendicitis surgical intervention was proper. Broca and Potherat agreed with him, while Tuffier and Quénu held more moderate views concerning operation. At a meeting of the Congrès Français de Chirurgie, October 16 to 21, 1899, the discussion on appendicitis manifested a change from the radical views of Poirier. Roux was opposed to immediate operation. Larger insisted that the great majority of cases get well under purely medical treatment. At the Academie de Médicine, in January, 1899, a curious result was arrived at, inasmuch as the physicians, with Dieulafoy at their head, insisted that appendicitis ought to be operated at the earliest possible moment, whilst the surgeons, led by Tilleaux, considered that many cases justified a waiting policy, and medical treatment was quite sufficient, especially in first attacks.* From the French reports it would appear that the majority of the prominent surgeons and many of the clinicians favor prompt and invariable operation, and have little confidence in medical treatment.

German Views.—The German surgeons and clinicians are strikingly at variance with the French and American. In the "Twentieth Century Practice of Medicine," vol. IX, Ewald expresses the opinion that 90 or 91 per cent. of all cases of appendicitis, taken in the widest sense, recover without any operation. He favors a treatment by rest, liquid nourishment in small amounts, opium, and local external treatment. Czerny (" Progressive Med.," June, 1899, 130) admits that the first attack of appendicitis belongs to the physician. He recognizes that it may subside without complication, and there may be no further indication for surgical intervention. The cases in which alarming symptoms due to perforation and abscess formation recur demand operation. Hertzog

---

* This entire French discussion in the various societies has been ably abstracted by Dr. H. H. Young in the " Maryland Medical Journal," for April, 1900.

("Zeitschr. f. klin. Med.," Bd. xxxvi, 1899, S. 247) reports 285 cases of appendicitis treated by medical means; of these, there were 249 cases of circumscribed perityphlitis, with 4 deaths, a mortality of 1.6 per cent.; and 36 cases of diffuse perityphlitis with diffuse peritonitis, with 36 deaths. The total mortality in this series was therefore 14 per cent.

These views, together with those of Kümmel, Rotter, Sonnenburg, and Braun, stated elsewhere in this article, suffice to evidence the conservative tendency among the German surgeons.

English Opinions.—The English surgeons are, as a rule, believers in conservatism, though not quite to the same degree as the Germans. Treves, to whom the credit of introducing the operation for chronic appendicitis in the interval is due, later on wrote the article on appendicitis in "Allbutt's System of Medicine," vol. iv, p. 906, in which he states that there is absolutely no feature of the initial symptoms of the attack to enable the surgeon to foretell the advent of suppuration—an assertion which, in my opinion, disregards the diagnostic value of the leukocytosis, the characteristic fever coincident with the formation of pus in the abdomen, and the development of fluctuating tumor. Yet these signs may not be present altogether as initial signs, and then Treves' conclusions would be correct. A painstaking study of the general condition of the patient, of the pulse, temperature, leukocytosis, combined with repeated and thorough examination of the abdomen, including bimanual examination with one or two fingers in the rectum, will, in the majority of cases, inform the physician whether pus is developing or not, and this is really the most important sign. For the development of pus means that the surgeon should visit the patient, together with the physician, every day. Treves favors the use of medical measures first; he is no opponent of morphin and hot fomentations. Even Moullin (London "Lancet," December, 1899, p. 1657), who is an advocate of radical and prompt operation, concedes that there is a certain proportion of appendicitis patients who show improvement before thirty-six hours have passed, and he does not propose to operate upon these. He asserts that relapses occur in about 60 per cent. of nonoperated cases, which is surprisingly high according to experiences I have gained at Baltimore.

American Opinions.—Beck ("New York Med. Jour.," 1898)

expresses the opinion that the safest treatment consists in the early removal of the appendix; that patients who are cured under medical treatment would also have recovered under operative treatment; that the use of opium is rational after the diagnosis is made. Deaver ("Appendicitis," second edition) is an emphatic advocate of prompt removal of the appendix even in the absence of pus. He condemns the use of morphia and opium, and sanctions the use of castor oil or calomel. H. A. Hare ("Jour. Amer. Med. Assoc.," vol. XXXI, p. 330) expresses the view that some cases are operative and some are amenable to medical treatment. His article is of importance because it calls attention to the great variations that the disease may present, and because it defines the use of opium—namely, for the palliation of pain until the diagnosis is clear, and not to relieve pain entirely or to produce sleep. Coley ("Progressive Med.," January, 1899) does not believe that the advocates of operating immediately have by any means proved their case, and that there is undoubtedly a growing tendency among representative surgeons of the world toward conservatism in the treatment of acute appendicitis, and that this is fully warranted by the facts at present at our command. Harschar ("Jour. Amer. Med. Assoc.," 1898, vol. XXXI) expresses the belief that a considerable number of cases seen in the first attack are either aborted by medical treatment or subside spontaneously at the end of twenty-four hours, and that of these the majority have no recurrence. The advantage and the weight of opinion, if we may judge from the reports during the past year, are on the side of waiting this short period (twenty-four to thirty-six hours), except in fulminant cases. In this class there is general agreement in favor of immediate operation.

The tendency toward conservatism among the American surgeons was most noticeable in two important papers published by Richardson, one in the "Boston Med. and Surg. Jour.," 1898 (Richardson and Brewster), and the other in the "Amer. Jour. of the Med. Sci.," December, 1899. Richardson in the last paper expresses his views as follows: "As a rule, the appendix should be removed if the diagnosis is made in the first few hours of the attack. After the early hours (twenty-four) the operation is advisable (1) if the symptoms are severe, and especially if they are increasing in severity; (2) if the symptoms recur after marked improvement; (3) if the

symptoms, though moderate, do not improve.   The wisdom of
operation is questionable (1) in severe cases in which an extensive
peritonitis is successfully localized, and the patient is improving;
(2) in cases which are at a critical stage, and which can not successfully undergo the slightest shock."   Then he asks: "Should the
appendix be removed in every case?   It should not be removed
(1) in localized abscesses with firm walls; (2) when the patient's
strength does not permit long search."   Richardson's mortality for
acute cases which were operated is 21.7 per cent., while under
medical treatment this surgeon reports a mortality of only 16.4 per.
cent.   W. S. Halsted, in a private conversation with the author,
expressed himself in favor of tiding over the acute cases to a time
when intervention is most sure to be successful.   In brief, he prefers
the operation in the interim, whenever possible.   W. W. Keen
("Transactions of the Medical Society of the State of New York,"
February, 1891) classifies five forms of appendicitis: (1) A mild
form corresponding to the simple catarrhal appendicitis; (2) perforative appendicitis with peritonitis; (3) perforated appendix with
abscess formation; (4) chronic appendicitis; (5) recurrent appendi-
icitis.*   This eminent surgeon uses the following words with regard
to the mild forms : "That the mild forms are frequent is proved by
the statistics of Toft, Hektoen, and Fitz; so frequent, indeed, that
we must assume that nearly one-third of all adults have had one or
more attacks. . . .   This very frequency has been urged by
some as a reason for frequent operative interference.   *To my mind
it argues precisely the reverse.*   If appendicitis can be recovered from
without abscess and without operation, it is to my mind the strongest
reason why, on general principles, *we should deem that an operation
on this class of cases is by no means often to be done.*"

In April, 1900, the "Maryland Medical Journal" submitted the
two following questions to an equal number of representative
American surgeons and clinicians:

" 1. Given a case of appendicitis: What are the absolute indications for operation ?

" 2. Given another case of appendicitis: How do you recognize
the favorable moment for surgical intervention ?"

---

* This comes very near the classification suggested by myself at the beginning of this
chapter.

Some of the surgeons who answered formulated the conditions for operation without apparently considering that it would be of interest to describe the characteristics of cases in which surgical treatment could be safely delayed.   From some opinions it is not possible to conclude whether they believe that appendicitis will get well, in certain cases, by the natural curative powers of the organism. Robert T. Morris, of New York, Herman Mynter, of Buffalo, Frederick H. Packard, of Philadelphia, perhaps J. C. Wilson, of Philadelphia, advocate prompt operation in all cases at any stage. Robt. Abbey, of New York, would delay operation until convalescence from the first attack, provided the patient can be kept under close observation, and within immediate reach of surgery. Nicholas Senn and Roswell Park do not express themselves concerning the possibility of recovery without operation.   The clinicians, as a rule, are conservative.   Answers were received from Fitz, Alfred Stengel, W. Gilman Thompson, and Fred'k C. Shattuck.   Fitz states that the physician should give each patient a chance to recover from the immediate attack without an operation, since the great majority of attacks are mild, and the least risk from operation is taken when the appendix is removed while there are no symptoms of active inflammation.   Immediate operation, according to him, is called for when the sudden onset of intense abdominal pain and exquisite tenderness is associated in the course of a few hours with a rapid pulse, elevated temperature, and retracted abdominal wall.   This condition is indicative of a certain degree of shock.   In a private letter to the author Fitz expresses the opinion that nearly three-fourths of the cases can recover safely under medical treatment.   The immediate surgical treatment applies to the remaining fourth, and remote surgical treatment also to about one-half of all the cases, to prevent the discomforts and dangers of chronic appendicitis. (This letter was received January 23, 1901.)

For the rest of the views collected in this symposium the reader is referred to the original article, "Maryland Med. Jour.," April, 1900.

Rotter, in giving the proportion of spontaneous cures to that of recoveries after operation, gives the following figures :   In 192 cases of appendicitis and circumscribed perityphlitis he had 82 per cent. of spontaneous recoveries.   Thirty-two cases were operated, of which 2 died, a mortality of 6 per cent. Of 159 cases not treated by operation, only 3 died, mortality 1.9 per cent. The total mortality was 2.6 per cent. Sahli's figures are based upon 4593 cases compiled from private practice in Switzerland. The physicians reporting their cases included reference concerning returns and relapses in persons who had spontaneously recovered from appendicitis and perityphlitis. As a result of this collective investigation Sahli has calculated 20.8 per cent. relapses. Most relapses occur within one year after the primary attack, and recurrences that take place later than three years after the first attack should not be considered relapses or returns. Nothnagel speaks of "*Recidiven*" after nine and even after eighteen years—in my opinion a debatable application of the term "relapse." Sonnenburg, Lenander, and Kümmel have emphasized the fact that these relapses are most common in appendicitis patients who have never had a perforation of the vermiform process. Kümmel gives the history and pathologic-anatomical state of 55 cases operated for relapse. The appendix was not perforated in 33 and perforated in 22 of these. In 27 of the 33 cases that had not undergone perforation there had been either simple chronic catarrhal inflammation with hypertrophy of the muscularis, and the characteristic changes in the mucosa, or there was chronic inflammation with formation of ulcers or stricture (but no perforation).

In the second edition of his "Treatise on Appendicitis," Dr. John B. Deaver concedes a wider latitude to the utility of expectant treatment in acute cases than in the first edition. The chapter on Treatment in the first edition started off with the conclusion that there was but one course to pursue, and that was to remove the appendix as soon as the diagnosis was made (first edition, p. 116). This sentence and that on page 122—viz., that the appendix should be removed in the beginning of the attack, that appendicitis is a surgical affection and should be treated as such—gave the impression that Dr. Deaver did not acknowledge such a thing as expectant or nonsurgical treatment in acute cases of simple appendicitis. In the second edition, page 235, he concedes a larger degree of usefulness to expectant treatment in those acute cases which at the onset do not bear the imprint of great seriousness, and which show marked improvement at the end of twenty-four hours following the institution of medical treatment, and continue to present steady improvement until evident convalescence is fully established.   Many of these patients, he admits, apparently recover entirely, but he doubts that their appendices have returned to the normal condition.   "It is not really necessary," he continues, "that all these patients should be subjected to immediate operation, provided the attack be the first from which they have suffered, and the operation could not be performed under the most favorable circumstances."   The medical treatment that he practises consists of diet; local applications to the right lower abdominal quadrant, consisting of an ice-bag ; laxatives, of which his choice is castor oil, calomel, or Rochelle salts; enemata; and, above all, absolute rest in bed.   He is strongly opposed to the use of opium, because in his opinion it masks the symptoms, favors retention in the appendix and intestines, causes distention of the bowel, depresses the gastric, renal, hepatic, pulmonary, and cutaneous functions, whereby the elimination of waste products is impeded, increases nausea, and because it decreases the antibacterial functions of the blood and the antitoxic power of the lymphatics.   Notwithstanding all these objections, there is an imperative duty confronting the practitioner in every case of appendicitis in which there is much pain.   That duty is to relieve the pain.   If this can be done by local applications, by suppositories of asafetida, so much the better; but if these expedients do not succeed, morphin should not be withheld.   (See p. 331, vol. I, and p. 191, vol. II.)   In my experience, I have, as a rule, succeeded in relieving the pain by such small doses of morphin ($\frac{1}{6}$ grain hypodermically) that none of the objectionable side-effects which Deaver describes were observed. To bring on these results which constitute his objections the patient must be brought under the effect of opium by large doses.   I doubt whether less than 4 grains of opium during the day can effect such conditions.   It will, however, be best not to use opium at all, but very small doses of morphin, sufficient to take the keen edge from the intense pain.   Such patients will still have pain enough to keep them mindful of their perilous state, but the suffering will be bearable.

Can we determine clinically whether a perforation of the appendix has taken place or not?   Which are the indications that justify the conclusion that the peri-appendicial or perityphlitic tumor contains pus?   These are two distinct questions, for the presence or absence of perforation does not necessarily coincide with the presence or absence of pus. Whilst it is perfectly logical, and as a rule not misleading, to presume the presence of pus in all cases where the appendix has become perforated, it is by no means correct to *exclude* the presence of pus in the tumor when there is no perforation. With perforation of the appendix we invariably have pus formation. With appendix not perforated we may also have pus formation ; for the infectious agency may find its way through the wall of the appendix not only by the opening of a perforation, but also by way of the lymph channels, when there is no perforation. This occurs in the so-called suppurative and gangrenous appendicitis, where the structures of the organ are so loosened that bacteria may permeate it almost with the same ease as if there were a direct opening. The cardinal symptoms and signs indicative of both pus formation and perforation have been formulated as follows : (1) Sudden onset of appendicitis with marked fever and intense symptoms ; (2) acute pain in the right iliac region ; (3) rapid development of a painful resistance, usually without a trace of fluctuation ; (4) fever usually preceded by chills ; (5) a rising leukocytosis ; (6) vomiting combined with diarrhea or constipation ; (7) very active sympathetic involvement of the general constitution. On closer consideration it can not escape the critical observer that this representation corresponds to the clinical picture of every acute intense perityphlitis, and Sahli has remarked that although one finds pus at all operations undertaken in cases as characterized by Sonnenburg, it is not because these clinical pictures constitute characteristic indications for the presence of pus, but because every perityphlitic tumor following these acute symptoms contains a purulent nucleus. There is, in my opinion, no absolute clinical criterion for the presence or absence of perforation.

Coming now to the question as regards the presence or absence of pus, there are but three absolutely reliable signs and symptoms which make the presence of pus extremely probable. These are : (1) Distinct fluctuation in the perityphlitic tumor, by abdominal or combined abdominal and rectal examination ; (2) positive result of exploratory puncture ; (3) continued high fever, in the absence of the Widal reaction for enteric fever. Concerning the value, utility, and advisability of abdominal puncture I have spoken elsewhere.

Roux says that it is sometimes dangerous, frequently without result, and always superfluous. In doubtful cases it would be a great support for the correct diagnosis if pus could invariably be demonstrated in this way. But experience teaches that pus can not be aspirated at times when the operation showed it to be present. When the physician finds a tumor which gives distinct fluctuation under the conditions above mentioned, there can be no doubt that the perityphlitic tumor is a pus-filled abscess. But there are other cases which undoubtedly occur, where even at the operation the perityphlitic tumor presents itself as nothing but a circumscribed serous or serofibrinous exudation. Such tumors, of course, do not present fluctuation as a rule, but only a more or less hard resistance. As many solid tumors in the ileocecal region which have such a resistance and no fluctuation may contain a central pus focus, the distinction here becomes indeed difficult. If a solid tumor without fluctuation is accompanied by continued high fever, the conclusion that it contains a pus nucleus is justifiable. By continued fever I do not mean a fever remaining approximately at the same degree, but simply the presence of fever after five to ten days, whether it be remittent, intermittent, or continuous. I have already stated elsewhere that a comparatively low temperature, and even absence of fever, does not necessarily contraindicate the presence of pus. For this reason the study of the course of the temperature has but a limited and relative diagnostic value for the determination of pus in perityphlitic tumors. All we can say is that, as a rule, in the majority of cases high continued fever speaks for the presence of pus in perityphlitic tumors, although they present no signs of fluctuation.

As the cases of group III are intimately correlated with those of group IV, in which there is always an undoubted abscess formation, I will consider the treatment of the two conjointly, after emphasizing the clinical features of the fourth group.

Group IV.

A limited number of the cases, as described in group III, of ulcerative appendicitis with exudates and small pus foci, do not recover after the first or second week, but the fever continues uninterruptedly, or there may be a temporary remission of the fever, after which it sets in again with pains and vomiting. The induration or the tumor becomes larger, the epidermis over it is slightly red, and an indistinct fluctuation can be made out within the indurated mass. On examination through the rectum or the vagina it may be possible to palpate a well-circumscribed, spherical or ovoid, or a diffusely outlined tumor, which is very sensitive to pressure, and generally gives evidence of distinct fluctuation. The inflammatory edema of the cecal region increases after the first week instead of diminishing. If the abscess is well encapsulated there may be no fever at all. Such cases are rare, and are merely mentioned to guard against the exclusion of pus formation simply because there is no fever. These are the cases in which Borchardt, Curschmann, Fränkel, Körte, Fürbringer, and Renvers recommend intestinal puncture in order to ascertain the presence or absence of pus. In cases where operation is contemplated, exploratory puncture has been sanctioned after its dangers have been explained to the patient, but its use should be positively restricted to such cases. In my opinion exploratory puncture can be omitted altogether in that event, for the laparotomy will give better information. Keen, Sonnenburg, Roux, Finney, and Karewski are opposed to it altogether. The presence of pus can, as a rule, be determined without exploratory puncture by careful study of the temperature curves, the evidence of a strong leukocytosis, and the results of abdominal palpation, especially when combined with examination through the vagina or rectum.

Subphrenic Abscess.—In extreme cases of abscess formation, when the pains radiate toward the loins, where the skin becomes edematous, and there is great sensitiveness over the hepatic region, the excursions on the right side becoming difficult and painful, and when a marked dullness can be made out above the liver in the absence of respiratory murmur, we must suspect the development of a subphrenic abscess. Under these conditions Curschmann and von Leyden have described the formation of a pleuritic exudation on the right side with rusty or bloody sputum. Under renewed chills a particularly violent attack of coughing may bring forth a large quantity of offensive pus, after which rapid improvement of the physical signs and symptoms may set in.

Infection of Biliary Apparatus.—In other cases pyemic fever, chills, and great emaciation may be associated with jaundice ; the liver rapidly increases in size, the spleen also, and the patients may be subject to diarrheas containing purulent admixtures ; this whole group of symptoms suggesting that an infection of the biliary vessels has taken place by way of the mesenteric veins, and most probably formation of abscess in the liver.   I have already described a similar condition in the chapter on Dysentery as an extension of the dysenteric infection to the liver.   Among 257 cases of appendicitis Fitz has observed 11 cases of involvement of the liver.

Condition of the Kidneys and Urine.—The amount of urine secreted in twenty-four hours is considerably diminished, often not exceeding 300 c.c.; but even if not as low as this the urine is very dark, and contains a strong sediment of urates.   The amount of indican and aromatic ethereal sulphates is excessive.   These two factors are generally proportionate to the quantity of pus that is present.   Albumin and albumoses are, in my experience, very frequently present, and even the morphological elements of the kidney may be found after sedimentation.   This is not always a good reason for stating a grave prognosis, for all the abnormal constituents may disappear and the urine return to the normal condition as the suppurative condition improves or is recovered from.

The cases of groups III and IV will be treated by "armed expectancy" or surgically according to the conclusions reached as regards the presence or absence of perforation and pus. If the onset is not stormy and the development of the symptoms not rapid ; if the fever becomes gradually less without the use of antifebrile medicines ; if there is no marked induration, and if, although a tumor be evident, it presents no fluctuation, the practitioner will be justified in continuing purely medical means of treatment—that is, by absolute rest, strictest dieting, small doses of morphin hypodermically for pain ; if necessary, small rectal enema of lukewarm water for the evacuations, not exceeding one pint; avoidance of purgatives and antifebrile medicines. Salol in doses of 5 grams and salicylate of soda in doses of 15 grains, three times a day, in my opinion, have a distinctly beneficial effect upon the systemic and local pyemic processes, and as they are very good intestinal disinfectants, there is no reason why they should not be tried. If the size of the exudation and the temperature decrease gradually, let there be no other treatment " *simplex sigillum veri.*"

The simpler the treatment, the better.   Very large exudates sometimes are resorbed in a surprisingly short time; and if the general condition is good, one should not disturb the favorable progress
of the case.   The sudden decrease of a very large exudate, with
abrupt sinking of the temperature, should create a suspicion that an
abscess has broken through into the intestine, and such cases should
be treated with special attention.   But this accident, as far as I am
able to determine from the literature of the subject, occurs only in
very large abscesses where fluctuation could be determined prior to
the breaking through of the pus accumulation.

If, however, the presence of pus is unmistakably recognizable,—
severe intense symptoms, high and continued fever, tumor with
fluctuation and leukocytosis (Pribram sanctions the demonstration
of pus by exploratory puncture),—operative treatment should be
at once undertaken.   The object of this chapter, as it is written
by a clinician and not a surgeon, is simply to state the indications,
and not enter upon the consideration of the technic, but to give
the clinician an idea of the gravity of the complications associated
with operations during the height of the attack, and the differences
of opinion which exist among surgeons themselves concerning the
question whether there should be at once a radical operation,—
i. e., whether the cause of the whole trouble, the appendix, should be
immediately removed after opening and draining the abscess, or
whether this removal is to be postponed until the acute symptoms
have subsided and the patient has at least partially recovered from
the effects of the pain, fever, exhaustion, and insomnia; I consider
it instructive to quote the following divergent opinions : Fowler (" A
Treatise on Appendicitis," 1894, p. 134), Murphy, Deaver, Poirier,
and J. M. T. Finney are in favor of immediate and prompt radical
operation with immediate removal of the diseased appendix.
Richardson, H. Braun, Körte, Schede, and Rotter consider that the
simple incision and drainage of the abscess is sufficient for the first
operation, and that the removal of the appendix should be postponed for the reasons described above.   It may not be considered as
going too far into the surgical side of the question if it is explained
why certain surgeons hesitate in removing the appendix immediately.
In the first place, it is sometimes very difficult to even find the appendix ; and, secondly, even if it were found, its removal during the

presence of an acute inflammation with loosening of the peri-appendicial and peri-cecal tissues is a serious matter. When the pus accumulation has been large, the recognition of a partially gangrenous vermiform process in the wall of the abscess is usually impossible, because it is bound down and covered by protecting adhesions. These latter form a protecting wall against peritoneal infection, and separation of these adhesions during the first operation means to throw open the peritoneum to an infection from which it has hitherto escaped by good fortune. H. Braun (Ebstein u. Schwalbe's "Handb. d. prakt. Med.," Bd. ii, S. 1178) considers the extirpation of the appendix under such conditions as unnecessary and dangerous. Many of the large abscesses are not smooth, well-defined cavities, but contain numerous diverticula and recesses, sometimes necessitating several incisions into the perityphlitic tumor.

Referring once more to the precedent of a perforation in the formation of perityphlitic pus accumulation, which was discussed in the preceding, and the undoubted occurrence of such pus tumors where no perforation had ever taken place, I should add that the majority of cases of abscess are no doubt due to perforation, but that it is not always possible to discover the perforation at the operation, because it may have become healed over or covered by adhesions, so as to be unrecognizable. This may be the explanation of a case reported by Dr. Ela, in the "Boston Med. and Surg. Jour.," February 6, 1890, which he designated as typho-enteritis, and in which he held that the appendix was normal; but Fitz doubted it ("Boston Med. and Surg. Jour.," vol. cxxii, p. 167), because it was adherent, and a fecal mass the size of a dried bean was found in the cavity of the abscess, which fecal masses are usually molded in the appendix.

The confidence in the correctness of clinical judgment will be strengthened by the results of nonoperative treatment in classes I and II, and will receive similar support by a recommendation of surgical intervention in groups IV, V, VI, VII, and VIII. The much-disputed groups concerning which the most discussion has taken place are those embraced under headings III and IV. A number of surgeons have asserted that appendicitis and perityphlitis are always conditions calling for surgical intervention. One might conclude from this extreme view, which Nothnagel characterizes as "operative fanaticism," that most cases of these diseases perished in the pre-antiseptic surgical period—a conclusion which is by no means borne out by a critical investigation of postmortem statistics.   One of the few statistics of autopsy on this special point—the frequency of disease of the appendix—will be found in "Nordiskt. Med. Arch.," VII, VIII, by Tofft.   In 300 postmortem examinations the appendix was found normal in 190, and more or less diseased in 110.   I have not been able to examine this article critically in the original, which is in the Scandinavian language, but the term "more or less diseased" conveys but an indefinite impression.   A much larger amount of autopsy material for this same point in question has been examined in Vienna.   In twenty-seven years 44,940 necropsies were made in the Vienna Pathological Institute.   Twenty of these twenty-seven years fall upon the period of 1870 to 1889, in which, according to Edebohls (*l. c.*), relatively few operations for appendicitis and perityphlitis were undertaken.   In this enormous number of autopsies death was attributable to perityphlitis and peritonitis depending upon this condition in only 148 cases—that is, 0.3 per cent.   These figures from one of the most reliable and accurate authorities on the subject constitute a convincing argument against the assertion that appendicitis unless operated proves fatal.   The number of conservative surgeons who oppose the surgical treatment of appendicitis by principle in every case is increasing.   The treatment, it is admitted by them, should in the majority of cases of group III be along purely medical lines in the beginning at least, and in many cases even throughout the further course of the disease.   On the other hand, the most able clinicians,—Osler, Nothnagel, Fitz,—with whom I agree, are of the opinion *that surgical intervention should not only be undertaken as a last resort, but that operation should take place much more frequently than hitherto, but after more precise and more clearcut indications.*

Those in favor of operation at all times and under all conditions argue that it is impossible to say in any concrete case whether perforation has occurred or not ; that simple appendicitis rarely heals completely ; that there is always danger of relapse, which may bring the patient into a dangerous condition ; that the danger may clandestinely lurk in the abdomen after spontaneous cures of appendicitis, and later on these inflammatory residues may cause hepatic and subphrenic abscesses. Concerning the frequency of relapses, I have already given the statistics of Nothnagel, placing them at about 20 per cent. The American writers place the relapses at from 40 to 50 per cent. My own experience is expressed by saying that relapses occur in only one-third of the cases studied with regard to future history. There are indeed very rare, insidious cases which begin apparently in an innocent manner. The pain may be violent at the beginning, but soon becomes bearable ; the pulse does not exceed 100, and the temperature 101.5° F. There is no evidence of an inflammatory tumor; the general condition is good. The practitioner has every right to expect a favorable termination under purely medical treatment. Suddenly, on the third or fourth day, a perforation resulting from an acute gangrene of the appendix occurs, with septic peritonitis, and the patient sinks into a state of collapse— all this without any premonitory sign of change in the clinical phenomena. Who will presume to have been able to give the unfailing advice to the managing practitioner in such a case ? This clinical picture is given by such a master of diagnosis as Nothnagel, and he concludes that unless one operates by principle in every case, such an accident as just pictured can not be avoided. And I may add that in my own experience such fulminating cases were not always averted even where the surgeon was present and ready to act from the onset. Fortunately, accidents of this type are extremely rare, and they can not persuade clinicians with analytical minds and critical judgment to become adherents of the ultrasurgical treatment of appendicitis in all cases.

It is very gratifying to be able to state that most operative statistics are favorable. The results of many surgeons indicate no death whatever from operation. Most of such operations are undertaken after very precise indications ; and even then death may result as a direct consequence of the operation. Willy Meyer gives the percentage of deaths directly attributable to operation as 2 per cent. These are based upon American statistics. Then there are other unpleasant results and complications of operation,—abdominal fistulæ, hernias, insufficiency of the abdominal recti muscles,—all of which, when summated, are of sufficient importance to merit quotation when the rare cases of unexpected fatal termination of simple catarrhal appendicitis are cited by some surgeons in criticism of the purely medical treatment of this condition.

Borchardt and Körte have formulated the indications for surgical operation in the following manner : If the temperature remains high longer than four or five days in spite of proper treatment (rest, diet, small doses of opium, no antifebrile medicines), and any detectable exudate growing larger presents the symptoms of abscess (fluctuation), and the general condition during this time remains bad or even grows worse. They argue *that if every case of acute appendicitis is operated, many useless operations will be performed, and notwithstanding the operation, it will be found impossible to cure all cases of perityphlitis.* These remarks by two German surgeons, and those of the most conservative American surgeons quoted elsewhere, merit careful consideration by those who would operate in all cases and at all periods. After a perityphlitic abscess has been incised the condition, as a rule, results in a cure in from four to six weeks. But there may be relapses in exceptional cases ; for small pus recesses may remain behind concealed among the adhesions, and later on set up a new inflammation.

V. Appendicitis with the Symptoms of Acute Intestinal Occlusion.

This condition demands prompt surgical interference, and should be treated according to the principles laid down in the chapter on the Surgical Treatment of Intestinal Occlusion. Unfortunately, when appendicitis gives rise to the symptoms of ileus, it does so by first setting up a diffuse peritonitis. We are then confronted with a condition corresponding with intestinal paralysis (see chapter on this subject). If the symptoms of complete suppression of evacuations and flatus, meteorism, severe collapse, feculent vomiting, and perhaps plastic rigidity of the intestinal loops, in addition to intensified peristalsis, are due to diffuse secondary peritonitis, originating from an appendicitis, operation will be of no avail, but in my experience rather aggravates the condition and hastens the fatal issue. But then the same symptoms of occlusion may be caused by direct compression of a fixed intestinal loop on the part of the tumefied appendicial and peri-appendicial structures. The small intestine, as well as the large intestine or the rectum, may be subject to such com-

pression.   As a rule, such symptoms of occlusion begin several
weeks after the onset of the disease, when we have every reason to
presume that the resorption of the exudate is actively proceeding.
Here the intestinal impermeability is probably due to inflection
caused by freshly formed pseudo-ligaments.   Ewald (" Diseases of
the Intestines," " Twentieth Century Practice of Medicine," vol. ix,
1897) calls attention to those extraordinary cases of appendicitis
which from the very beginning present the symptoms of pronounced
intestinal occlusion.   One of the cases described by him exhibited
fecal contents in the stomach at an early lavage, and death followed
under severe cerebral symptoms on the third day.   The autopsy
showed a light inflammation of the cecum and phlegmonous psoas
abscess.   Angerer, Hartley, Lenander, Ranschoff, and Peyrot are
of the opinion that intense appendicitis may produce the clinical
picture of intestinal occlusion in the entire absence of peritonitis, or
at least when but very limited areas of local peritonitis can be discovered.   If the diagnosis can be made and the occlusion is due to
the condition mentioned by Ewald ("Discussion on Typhlitis,"
"Verhandl. d. XIII. Congress f. innere Med.," Wiesbaden, 1895),
then a cure is possible.   At all events, it is clear that purely medical treatment can accomplish very little under such conditions.

VI. Appendicitis with the Clinical Picture of Diffuse Peri-
   tonitis.

That such a condition is not amenable to purely medical treatment must be evident to every thinking clinician.   The next question will be, " Is it amenable to surgical treatment?"   Notwithstanding that a large number of these unfortunate patients die in
spite of laparotomy, and although the fatal termination is in some
cases hastened by the operation itself and the narcosis, about the
only hope they have is from laparotomy.   The most favorable results from operation are seen in those forms of peritonitis which are
due to perforation.   The laparotomy must be undertaken immediately after the perforation is recognized.   No time should be lost.
Laparotomy produces the most favorable results when undertaken
for the subacute and chronic fibrinopurulent forms of peritonitis ;
and the most unfavorable results—so unfavorable, indeed, that the
opinion has been expressed by competent clinicians that these cases

should not be operated at all—are met with in the acute septic forms of peritonitis. The patients afflicted with these forms are under the depressing influence of an intense general autointoxication, to which the fatal termination is directly attributable ; for the pathological changes found in the peritoneum itself or about the appendix are frequently not considerable, and can by no means explain the gravity of the clinical picture. The great feebleness of the heart's action is one of the main features of these forms, and contraindicates the narcosis. It is surprising to learn the fact that cases of this type have recovered spontaneously by the recuperative powers of the organism, after operation had been declined by surgeons on account of the apparent hopelessness of the situation.

VII. Returning and Relapsing Forms.

The distinction between what have been designated as returning and relapsing forms has been made in the clinical consideration of appendicitis. The only means of preventing relapses is the radical removal of the appendix, and the proper time for this is in the intervals between the attacks, when there is no fever. There are considerable technical advantages to be gained from an operation at this period. Attempts at radical operations during the acute process of inflammation are more dangerous, and the seeking out of the appendix presents greater difficulties, because the tissues are congested, swollen, loosened by diffuse serous infiltration, and very fragile. Radical operation during the height of the acute attack sometimes necessitates drainage of the abscess cavity, which in turn may involve the formation of an abdominal fistula. In the interval between the attacks—not earlier, say, than five weeks after the acute attack—the appendix is found with greater ease, and the danger of infecting the peritoneum is less. In 80 per cent. of the cases operated for relapses Treves found perforations of the appendix. This is sufficient evidence to justify the operation in the intervals, which has been, as a rule, followed by very favorable results. It must be mentioned, however, that relapses have been observed even after the radical removal of the appendix.

VIII. Chronic Appendicitis.

This term is applied to those cases in which the ileocecal distress

never ceases, and there are no intervals of freedom from pain.   In
such cases, after an attempt has been made with medical treatment,
and a course of hot baths, extending about one month, has been
tried without improvement, the pains and complaints still continuing, the safest means of regaining health and comfort is the radical
removal of the appendix.

So we can sum up as follows :

1. Operative treatment is not indicated in all cases of appendicitis.   Most cases of groups I, II, and III heal spontaneously,
and 60 to 70 per cent. of these types without relapses.

2. Operation is indicated when the presence of an abscess can
be made probable by the diagnostic features already outlined.

3. The removal of the appendix, preferably in the intervals
between the attacks, is indicated when there are reasons to believe
that we are confronted with (*a*) the presence of concretions in the
vermiform process, (*b*) perforation, (*c*) repeated relapses, (*d*) chronic
appendicitis.

4. In cases of peritoneal sepsis the operation is useless, but
might be undertaken if there is the least doubt of the correctness
of the diagnosis.

5. Diffuse peritonitis can be treated successfully only by operation.

6. Intestinal occlusion in association with appendicitis should be
treated according to the principles laid down in the chapter on the
Surgical Treatment of Intestinal Occlusions.

The most recent German contribution to the subject of surgery
of appendicitis is the fourth edition of Eduard Sonnenburg's
"Pathologie und Therapie der Perityphlitis," Leipzig, 1900.   In his
former editions Sonnenburg contended that *simple catarrhal appendicitis* could not be diagnosticated, but in this edition his further
experience has convinced him that the diagnosis of this condition *can
be made with absolute certainty*.   He describes cases in which the
attacks immediately begin with severe symptoms, not preceded by a
preliminary attack of catarrhal appendicitis.   These he conceives to
be circumscribed purulent peritonitis, in consequence of perforation
of the vermiform appendix, and argues that the preceding or beginning stages—*i. e.*, the advance attacks of simple catarrhal appendi-

citis—have passed unnoticed, or have been misinterpreted. This eminent surgeon individualizes with admirable precision between the cases to be selected for operation, and distinguishes the treatment of the attacks from the treatment of the disease itself. He favors meeting the attacks by expectant treatment—diet, morphin injections, and hot moist compresses. He argues that the operation in the attack will never become popular on account of its great difficulty. If, however, there is no decided change for the better after four or five days, under close observation of the pulse, temperature, and general condition, he does not hesitate to operate even during the attack. He cautions against the stubborn adherence to the doctrine that a tumor should be demonstrable by palpation and percussion, in order to justify an operation (*l. c.*, S. 250). His deductions are as follows:

1. The operation during the free interval is to be preferred to that during the attack.

2. Simple appendicitis (appendicular colic and simple catarrhal appendicitis) rarely constitutes an indication for operation during the attack.

3. Perforating appendicitis calls for operation during the attack, and strict selection of the cases.

4. Gangrenous appendicitis must be operated during the attack, and early.

5. Perforating and gangrenous appendicitis with complications imperatively calls for operation.

The following mortality after his operations is indicative of his results:

50 cases of simple appendicitis, with 2.0 per cent. mortality.	
232 " " perforating " " 21.5 " "	
99 " " gangrenous " " 28.0 " "	
179 " operated in the interval, " 0.5 "	

From a critical consideration of the large number of opinions quoted in the preceding, the first impression which the clinician will gain is that "experience is fallacious and judgment is difficult" (Hippocrates). The next conclusion that can be reached is that the treatment of appendicitis in its stages, as designated in groups III and IV especially, is by no means a settled matter.

Personal Practice.—Speaking strictly for myself, I should like to emphasize that I would not hesitate a moment to transfer at once each and every case of appendicitis to the surgeon if the reported experiences and results of operative treatment, and the advice of various surgeons the world over, showed only an approximate or a reasonable degree of uniformity, and if they could demonstrate as many perfect recoveries without relapses in the mild forms of acute cases as have been gained by the course which Tuffier designates as "armed expectancy." Richardson's statistics demonstrate a mortality of 21.7 per cent. for acute cases that were operated, and only 16.4 per cent. for acute cases under conservative treatment, and confirm my opinion. It is a great pleasure to learn of the statistics of many surgeons as being almost entirely free from fatal cases, and of many others in whom the fatal cases were presented in such a condition that a recovery was recognized as impossible the minute the abdomen was opened. These operations are done in modern hospitals, where the surgeon has at his command an ample number of trained assistants, trained nurses, and sterilizing apparatus ; but our advice concerning surgical treatment must be applicable not only to the perfected conditions of a modern hospital, but to all emergencies of private, and particularly country, practice. The great majority of writers on the subject of surgery of the appendix are surgeons of exceptional experience. The results would no doubt be far from being as favorable were the injunctions for operative treatment to be followed out by all physicians and surgeons, particularly those that are remote from modern clinics.

Let the practitioner associate an experienced surgeon with himself in every case of appendicitis, even the simplest and mildest; let the patient be seen three to four times daily; let the temperature, the pulse, the pains, the rigidity of the abdominal muscles, and the growth of any inflammatory indurations be closely watched ; the leukocytes counted every six hours ; give no food on the first day ; give no medicines except a little morphin (gr. ⅙) if the pain is severe. It is a most important duty to relieve suffering, and it can be done by doses that will not frustrate the efforts of diagnosis. Let it not be forgotten that it is the *vis medicatrix naturæ which cures appendicitis, and not the medical treatment.* A high initial *temperature* and even a chill or two need not frighten the physician. But if the temperature is 102.5° to 103° F. on the third day, let the surgeon prepare for operation. A sudden rise in leukocytosis should prompt this even on the second day. If the temperature sinks very gradually from the third day onward, and the general condition of the patient appears favorable, operation can still be delayed. The longer the case has lasted, the lower will be the degree of fever that should be considered as indicative for operation. For instance, on the sixth day a fever of 102° F. should make a laparotomy justifiable. While fever of the degrees mentioned constitutes an indication for operation, comparatively low temperatures by no means contraindicate the operation. There are cases of acute diffuse peritonitis in which the temperature may rapidly sink. Here, however, there are other diagnostic signs which call for operation.

The Pulse.

I have spoken of the characteristics of the pulse in inflammatory conditions of the abdomen, in the chapter on Treatment of Intestinal Occlusions. The pulse of appendicitis which would cause the physician anxiety might be characterized as a jerky, irritable, or snappy pulse, particularly if it exceeds 120 beats in a minute. While grave changes of an inflammatory nature in the cecal region can not occur without alterations of the pulse and temperature, they may be transacted without aggravating the pain.

Tumor.

The growth of the tumor can only be controlled by frequent examinations. It is my rule not to palpate an appendicial tumor more than once a day. If more frequent examinations are desired, let them be very superficial and executed with the flat surface of the hand. Meddlesome and frequent palpation may set up an extension of the suppurative process, or even press out fecal contents into the peritoneum through an existing perforation. When the tumor is deeply hidden in the cecal or pelvic tissue, one examination per day by combined rectal or vaginal and abdominal palpation is justifiable.

Leukocytosis.

The leukocytosis in appendicitis corresponds roughly to the degree of temperature. It is rarely of absolute diagnostic value without the other clinical signs spoken of in the preceding. A leukocytosis above 20,000 on the first or second day is suggestive of general peritonitis. A leukocytosis above 20,000 after the first week or ten days may be taken to indicate a local abscess (Greenough).

The significance of the white blood-cell count will vary according to the day after the initial symptoms on which it is undertaken and according to the presence or absence of peritonitis. For diffuse peritonitis, after it has been established forty-eight to seventy-two hours, may effect a condition in which the general constitution is unable to bring about a high leukocytosis. For instance, we may have a case of appendicitis which on the second day presents a leukocytosis of only 6000 to 10,000. The suppurative process becomes aggravated, breaks through the appendix, and causes a septic peritonitis. The blood count on this day will show at or after the perforation a leukocytosis of 20,000 to 25,000, perhaps more. But if the case is not operated, the patient gradually becoming more septic, we may find on the fourth or fifth day a leukocyte count of only 5000 to 6000. These are fatal cases, as a rule. A low leukocytosis is by no means a contraindication to operation, if the fever continues high, the pulse rapid but full enough to justify the step, and the other symptoms of pus formation are present. But a sudden rise of leukocytosis, say from 6000 or 8000 to 18,000 or 20,000 and above, with these symptoms just referred to present, is considered as an imperative call for exploratory laparotomy. Whether or not a sudden rise in leukocytosis, as stated, should be interpreted as an indication for operation even in the absence of local symptoms and fever, can not be dogmatically stated at present; but in general terms a leukocytosis is an indication for operation ; its absence does not speak against it.

Appendicitis is a disease in which clinical and surgical efforts at diagnosis and treatment are to be wedded. The subject has not sufficiently matured for dogmatic conclusions as to which treatment does the most good in the beginning of acute cases. We need many more statistics by conservative men, arranged and corrected with critical judgment, and conservative analysis of the cases, to settle these questions. But if the two branches of practical medicine will be wedded, it will not be "for better or for worse," but only for better.

Statistics of necropsies of appendicitis, in addition to those mentioned in this article, have been given by Leudet ("Arch. gén. de Méd.," Paris, 1859, vol. II, pp. 139, 315), Finnell ("Med. Record," New York, 1869, vol. IV, p. 66), Toft ("Dissertatio de fabricâ et functione processus vermiformis," Groningue, 1840, p. 24), Fitz ("Amer. Jour. of the Med. Sci.," Philadelphia, 1886, n. s., vol. XCII, pp. 321–346), Einhorn ("Münch. med. Wochenschr.," 1891, Bd. XXXVIII, S. 121, 140), Wallis ("Hygiea," Stockholm, 1892, Bd. LIV, S. 578–595), Ribbert ("Arch. f. Path. Anat.," etc., Berlin, 1893, Bd. CXXXII, S. 66–90), and Robinson ("Med. Record," New York, 1895, vol. XLVIII, p. 373). Kleinwaechter ("Mitt. a. d. Grenzgeb. d. Med. u. Chir.," Jena, 1896, Bd. I, S. 727, 728) and With ("Peritonitis appendicularis, etc.," Kjobenh., 1897, 8vo) have furnished statistics regarding the duration of appendicitis under medical treatment, while Sands ("Ann. Anat. and Surg. Soc.," Brooklyn, New York, 1880, vol. II, pp. 249–270) and Fitz ("Boston Med. and Surg. Jour.," 1890, vol. CXXII, 619) investigated the mortality under medical and under surgical treatment. McBurney ("Med. Record," New York, 1895, vol. XLVII, pp. 385–390) presents personal statistics of operations for appendicitis in the presence of diffuse septic peritonitis. Von Mayer ("Rev. méd. de la Suisse rom.," Genève, 1898, vol. XVIII, pp. 285–299) gives us a very unique, practical, and interesting study of 75 operative cases of chronic appendicitis. Of these, 33 presented clinical symptoms corresponding to the lesions found, 32 presented no clinical symptoms, and 10 had severe symptoms with no lesions. Statistics of operative cases, with mortality, have been published by Clay ("New Orleans Med. and Surg. Jour.," 1878–79, vol. VI, pp. 196–216), Bull ("Med. Record," New York, 1894, vol. XLV, pp. 385–389), MacDonald ("Trans. Assoc. Amer. Obst. and Gynec.," Philadelphia, 1895, vol. VII, pp. 131–144), Murphy ("Jour. Amer. Med. Assoc.," Chicago, 1894, vol. XXII, pp. 302, 347, 387, 423), Johnson ("Jour. Amer. Med. Assoc.," Chicago, 1896, vol. XXVI, pp. 1202–1206), Kuemmell ("Berlin. klin. Wochenschr.," 1898, Bd, xxxv, S. 321–328), Sonnenburg ("Mitt. a. d. Grenzgeb. d. Med. u. Chir.," Jena, 1898, Bd.

III, S. 1–21,) Deaver (" New Orleans Med. and Surg. Jour.," 1898–99, vol. LI, pp. 443–445), Halliday (" Brit. Med. Jour.," London, 1898, vol. I, p. 1195), etc.

OPERATIVE TREATMENT OF INTESTINAL OBSTRUCTION.

According to Max Bartels (" Die Medicin der Naturvölker," " Ethnological Contributions to the Aboriginal History of Medicine," S. 305), abdominal surgery was first practised among the aboriginal races of North America, and Bancroft reports on an abdominal section performed by an Oncanagan Indian. Bartels gives a detailed descriptian of a cesarean section executed by a Chippewa Indian upon his pregnant wife. Both the wife and the child were saved. But setting aside this aboriginal surgery, to which little scientific but only historical importance can be attributed, abdominal surgery was founded and developed on American soil, and much of the newer advancement in the operative treatment of intra-abdominal diseases is due to the genius and perseverance of American surgery. It would lead me too far to even only refer to the work of McDowell, Sims, Battey, Gross, and the later and more modern surgeons, W. W. Keen, McBurney, Richardson, Murphy, Halsted, W. F. Weir, Senn, Deaver, Finney, and numerous others. But it is my duty to emphasize that in abdominal surgery the American operators have been pioneers. They have set the pace and others have followed. They have not been mere imitators, and from the evidence of the scientific spirit which moves them we are justified in hoping for future beneficent development in this field of medicine.

A number of surgeons have claimed that all cases of mechanical intestinal obstruction should be submitted to operation, and that it is a doubtful and risky expedient to procrastinate by purely medical treatment. The position taken by these men at first sight seems logical enough, for even under the very best statistics purely medical treatment is credited with 33 per cent. of cures of the total number of cases treated in this manner. So that clinicians must shoulder a responsibility of 66 per cent., or two-thirds of the fatal cases of the total number treated. If the consensus of the opinion of leading internal clinicians could be ascertained, they would no doubt gladly transfer all cases of intestinal obstruction to the surgeon, if it were not for the fact that laparotomy in itself is a very serious procedure and does not show much better results apparently than expectant treatment.   This difference, however, is probably more apparent than real, as we shall presently see.   The manipulation and searching through of the injured intestinal loops, the extruding of the distended bowel through the abdominal wound, the reflex depression upon the circulatory and nervous system—all these conditions introduce into the clinical picture a number of new factors, which may eventuate as gravely as the disease itself.   Septic infection and peritonitis can, it is true, be to a large extent prevented by the surgeon.   Unfortunately there are not only serious differences of opinion as regards the indications for operation in intestinal obstruction, between internal clinicians and surgeons, but among surgeons themselves.   Statistics concerning the results of both operative and purely medical treatment are largely unreliable, because they lack that critical conservatism which should state all the details of the clinical history and treatment, even that which would not exactly reflect to the glory of the physician or surgeon.   A conservative critical review of these statistics is still urgently desirable.   According to Goltdammer, Curschmann, and Fürbringer, the mortality of intestinal obstruction treated by purely medical means varies from 65 to 70 per cent.; and according to Ashhurst, F. Curtis, Treves, Poppert, Naunyn, Schramm, and Obalinski, the mortality of obstruction treated by laparotomy varies from 60 to 70 per cent.   The most most recent figures, those of Chas. L. Gibson (*l. c.*), give a mortality of 47 per cent. for operations for intestinal obstruction.   For obturations it is 47 per cent., for strangulations 67 per cent.   Kocher ("Mitt. a. d. Grenzgeb.," Bd. IV, 1898, S. 2), whose results are reckoned among the best, has a mortality of 38 per cent. for all cases of intestinal obstruction treated by operation.   This surprising mortality in spite of modern antiseptic surgery is explainable by the pathological changes which the intestines undergo with great rapidity in obstructions.   Most surgeons admit that the manipulation and surgical procedure necessary for the relief of obstruction would be tolerated by healthy individuals without any attendant risks.   Schede has stated that not 5 per cent. of deaths would result from such procedures executed on normal intestines. But in occlusion forty-eight hours suffice to bring on a condition in which the simplest operation, such as the severance of a peritoneal band, will be likely to terminate the case fatally.

In group B (see résumé of clinical chapter on obstructions, p. 333), strangulations or incarcerations, the majority of cases of volvulus and loop formation, inflections, bendings, and kinkings (classified on page 310), there are two factors which above all others control the success of operations for intestinal occlusion : **First, the definiteness and accuracy of the diagnosis.** Nothing so much enhances the success of the surgeon as a consciousness of a reliable knowledge of the seat and the nature of the occlusion. This will enable him to have a clear view and understanding of the object to be accomplished by the operation. **The second important factor is the time at which the operation is undertaken.** The **sooner** it is undertaken *after the diagnosis of obstruction is first made, the more favorable will be the result.* Naunyn (*l. c.*) has compiled the results of operation on 288 cases of intestinal occlusion. The recoveries, when the operation took place during the first forty-eight hours, amounted to 75 per cent. If the operation took place from the third day on, the recoveries sank to 35 to 45 per cent. The unfavorable results are due to pathological alterations which the intestinal wall had undergone in consequence of circulatory disturbances. The epithelium of the mucosa is destroyed, and microorganisms invade the peritoneum. In addition to this we have autointoxication from the absorption of the products of intestinal putrefaction.

It is not my intention to outline the surgical conduct of the cases, but simply to furnish a few guiding lines to the general practitioner in his difficult decision concerning the question how long he shall persist in purely medical treatment and when to insist on an operation. In this connection it is expedient to advise the general practitioner that the instruction of the patient himself, as well as his relatives, in the critical condition of the disease, is imperative. There is always considerable time lost in the hesitation of the patient to consent to an operation, but if the physician has made the probability of an operation a familiar idea to the sufferer from the beginning, no valuable time will be lost when the critical hour for the decision on the laparotomy has arrived.   How long shall the practitioner treat his cases by purely medical means? This question is answered differently according to the state of the diagnosis. Two conditions may exist : (*a*) Either the diagnosis is clear during the first two days, or (*b*) the diagnosis is obscure.   (*a*) *If the diagnosis is clear during the first two days, and the seat as well as the anatomic nature of the occlusion is recognized, then the purely medical treatment should not be continued longer than forty-eight hours* (Nothnagel, Boas, Naunyn).   If the bloodless methods of treatment which I have enumerated have been applied in a methodical and energetic manner for two days without success, laparotomy should be undertaken immediately at the end of the second day in most of the anatomic forms of mechanical occlusion. (*b*) *The diagnosis is obscure.   What course is the practitioner to pursue?* Cases in which the *diagnosis is obscure*, as they come under observation, are of two classes : First, those with an *intensely acute and rapid course*, in which the patients enter upon a state of collapse in a surprisingly short time.   As these cases almost always terminate fatally, they should in my opinion be *operated on at once*, for every life that is saved in this manner is a gain and a gift, pure and simple.   *Secondly, the diagnosis is obscure*, but the *course is moderate*, the symptoms not severe.   Here purely medical treatment should be extended to two days.   Gastric lavage, colon distention, and opium may often bring relief, but simultaneously there should be a constant control of the cardiac action and the general condition and strength of the patient.   Such a sufferer should have the trained nurse at his side continuously, and should be visited by the physician every three hours.

In this connection it is also important to distinguish between symptoms of strangulation, which are characterized chiefly by grave symptoms of collapse and depression of the heart's action, and the symptoms of simple occlusion, where collapse is not marked and the heart's action is in a fairly good condition.   The condition of the *pulse* is the best indication of the state of the heart.   The " *tactus eruditus* " of the physician can here, in many instances, suffice to judge the period at which medical treatment must cease and surgical treatment begin.   The characteristic of the pulse may be designated as (1) frequency or rate, (2) tension, (3) fullness, (4) the height, or impulse.   If the frequency or rate is moderate, the tension, fullness, and height considerable, we are confronted with only moderate occlusion symptoms, as a rule, even though there may be stercoral vomiting and much distention of the abdomen.   But if the rate or frequency increases, together with a reduction of the tension and fullness, especially if there are other symptoms of collapse, then we are confronted with a condition of strangulation, an indication for prompt operation.

Occasionally the practitioner is not called to attend a case until several days after the first appearance of the occlusion.   As the diagnosis can be distinctly made only during the first two days, it must naturally be more or less obscure in these cases.   Continuous vomiting, intolerable pains, insomnia, lack of nutrition, and often intense autointoxication from the intestine, have reduced them to a condition where they can hardly stand an extensive operation.   On the other hand, if they are not operated, they will inevitably die. What is to be done?   If the general condition, as evidenced by a fair condition of the heart, gives hope that they can stand a laparotomy, this should be undertaken as the only chance they have of surviving the attack.   Very frequently the establishment of an artificial anus is the extremest operative measure such a patient can stand.   The criticism I have given in the preceding, concerning the reliability of statistics on the results of medical and operative treatment respectively, is supported by the discovery that in many of them cases of simple peritonitis and perityphlitis and appendicitis are included among intestinal occlusions.   A thorough and very critical classification of this entire clinical material would probably bring to light many other defects, such as errors in the duration of the occlusion, in the age of the patient, or in the exact nature of the pathological conditions causing them.

Boas (*l. c.*, p. 461) arrives at the conclusion that purely medical treatment and surgical treatment may show an equal number of successes and equal dangers, and it becomes the duty of the physician to decide in each individual case which method of treatment offers the best prospects of cure.   My personal experience at our clinic at the University of Maryland and the results of other large hospitals in the United States from which I could collect information lead me to differ from this conclusion.   It is true the statistics of

Chas. L. Gibson (*l. c.*) give a mortality of 67 per cent. for strangulations, but then the mortality for all operations for intestinal obstructions was only 47 per cent.   Above all, we must not forget that Gibson's statistics are not American statistics exclusively, but collected from the entire literature of the subject, and suffering from the same defects which I have previously specified as found in the statistics of other countries.   H. Zeidler (" Mitt. a. d. Grenzgeb.," Bd. v, S. 608) also gives the same number of recoveries and fatalities under medical as well as surgical treatment.   The figures, however, upon which these statistics are based date back to the beginning of antiseptic surgery, at which time the diagnosis of intestinal occlusion was by no means as advanced as it is at the present day, and the clinicians did not transfer their intestinal occlusions to the surgeon until all internal methods of treatment had been exhausted and the cases were all in an advanced stage of the disease.   Therefore the comparatively mediocre results of surgical treatment are explained by the fact that the operations were undertaken too late.   It is true that some invaginations, some forms of enterostenoses or obturations by gall-stones or coproliths, can be successfully treated and cured by purely medical treatment.   Curshmann (" Deutsch. med. Wochenschr.," 1887, No. 21) even claims to have produced cures of inflections, incarcerations by bands and volvulus, by this method, and in some cases was able to support his arguments by the results of autopsies.   All these things may be true and are admitted.   It is also undeniable that laparotomy is no innocent procedure.   That does not change any of the deductions which I have previously made—*namely, that in all strangulations or incarcerations, volvulus or knot formations, inflections, bendings and kinking, and invaginations medical treatment should not be prolonged over forty-eight hours.*   In enterospasm and all obturations purely medical treatment may be somewhat prolonged according to special indications.

Are shock and peritonitis contraindications against operation? Shock and collapse may be met with immediately at the onset of the occlusion, when this should be designated as the incarceration shock, and toward the end of the disease from gradual exhaustion of the vital powers.   This is the collapse, coming on as the disease progresses, from vomiting, pain, insomnia, and lack of food.   The incarceration shock which comes on with the initial symptoms of

the disease is caused reflexly by the act of the incarceration itself.
So far from being a contraindication to operation, it is actually an
urgent indication for prompt surgical procedure.   Many times the
action of the heart is observed to improve the minute the abdomen
is opened, and especially immediately after the strangulating agency
is removed.   The collapse which comes on at the end of the disease is a different condition.   It means exhaustion.   The majority
of these patients will come to grief under an operation.   But then,
that is their only hope.   Every such case which is luckily brought
over the effect of an operation is practically a human being lifted
out of the grave.   It must be left to the judgment of the surgeon
to decide whether he shall yet operate or not.

Peritonitis.

If the peritonitis is restricted, it does not constitute a special contraindication to operation.   Many operations are undertaken when
a circumscribed peritonitis exists, and the cases result in recovery.
Such small areas of peritonitis can in fact rarely be diagnosed.   But
when the peritonitis is diffuse, the operation becomes hazardous.

An operation, when once decided upon, places the further conduct of the case in the hands of the operator.   Therefore the
question of the kind of operation to be performed can not be considered one of the objects of this chapter.   But for the instruction
of the general practitioner I may state that the selection between
an artificial anus,—an intestinal fistula communicating with the
exterior,—on the one hand, and a laparotomy involving searching
through the intestine for the cause of the impermeability, and the
subsequent removal of it, is also of interest to the internal clinician,
because the question rests not only upon his diagnosis, but also
upon the power of endurance of the patient, of which he often is
the only judge.   In a general way it can be said that the artificial
anus is indicated in a number of forms of obturation, when the
position and kind of the obstruction are known.   But in all forms
of strangulation, incarceration, invagination, volvulus, and in some
forms of obturation in which there is no special diagnosis of the
obstruction, laparotomy and seeking out of the cause of the impermeability are indicated.   Artificial anus, intestinal fistula, or
enterostomy has in my experience been but a makeshift, justifiable
only when the strength of the patient did not permit of a laparot-

omy; or when a laparotomy had been performed, and, after careful searching, the obstacle could not be found. After all, laparotomy and seeking out the cause of the obstruction are the course indicated both by practical experience as well as theoretical considerations (Nothnagel). The results of laparotomy are the more favorable when the surgeon is enabled to proceed directly toward the seat of the obstacle. In 39 laparotomies undertaken for the relief of internal obstructions by peritoneal bands and adhesions, as a consequence of external hernias,—which most frequently permit of a direct conclusion as to the seat of the obstruction,—Naunyn has tabulated 28 recoveries, or 72 per cent.

Treatment of Individual Forms of Obstruction.

Strangulations and Incarcerations.—If the diagnosis is clear, the physician may consume from twenty-four to forty-eight hours by the medical treatment outlined in the preceding, and unless decided recovery follows, an operation must be undertaken.

Inflections.—The distinction between the inflections and internal incarcerations and strangulations meets with insurmountable difficulties, and therefore the kinkings, bendings, and inflections should be treated as are the incarcerations and strangulations.

Invaginations and Intussusceptions.—(1) Acute; (2) chronic.

1. Acute.—Although such an excellent surgeon as Rydygier himself recommends a trial of the bloodless medical treatment for invagination ("Deutsch. Zeitschr. f. Chir.," 1896, Bd. XLII), this should not be extended over twenty-four hours, for the far better results of early operation are evident from the best of the statistics. The most recent statistical compilation is that by Chas. L. Gibson, of which I have quoted the following tables ("Annals of Surgery," October, 1900). According to the tables of this author, the mortality of the first six days after the beginning of the symptoms of invagination was the following: First day, 37 per cent.; second day, 39 per cent.; third day, 61 per cent.; fourth day, 67 per cent.; fifth day, 73 per cent.; sixth day, 75 per cent. Here, then, the guiding rule will be : Medical treatment no longer than for twenty-four hours.

The following tables concerning the operative results on 500 cases of various forms of intestinal obstruction are taken from the article by Dr. Charles L. Gibson (*l. c.*) :

TABLE I.—RESULTS BY DAYS.

(The figures on the left of each column represent cures; those on the right, in italic type, deaths.)

Days.	1.	2.	3.	4.	5.	6.	7.	8.	9.	10.	11.	12.	13.	14.	3 Weeks.	4 Weeks.	Not Stated.
Bands,	3	2 *12*	4 *19*	5 *23*	11 *11*	6 *11*	4 *7*	8 *5*	8 *5*	6	1 *1*	2 *2*	3	1 *1*	1 *6*	0 *2*	5 *1*
Intussusceptions,	22 *13*	14 *13*	20 *5*	10 *4*	11 *4*	3 *5*	4 *5*	4 *3*	3 *0*	0 *0*	1 *0*	1 *0*	0 *0*	0 *0*	4 *1*	3 *0*	8 *10*
Volvulus,	3 *8*	8	6 *7*	9 *7*	8 *8*	3 *7*	4 *3*	2 *7*	1 *1*	2	1	0	0	1 *1*	1	0	4 *3*
Meckel's diverticulum,	1 *0*	2	2	2 *6*	4 *4*	0 *3*	1 *3*	0	1	3	0	0	0	0	0	0	0 *1*
Gall-stones,	1 *1*	1 *1*	2	3 *2*	4 *3*	3	5	1	0	0	1 *0*	0	0	0 *1*	0	0	1 *4*
Openings,	1 *0*	3 *5*	5 *3*	3 *3*	0 *1*	5 *1*	5 *1*	0 *0*	0	0	0 *0*	0 *0*	0 *0*	0 *0*	1 *0*	1 *0*	0 *1*
Foreign bodies,	0 *0*	0 *1*	0 *1*	1 *2*	1 *3*	1 *0*	1 *0*	0 *1*	0	3	0 *0*	0 *0*	0 *0*	0 *0*	1 *0*	0	0
Miscellaneous,	1 *0*	0 *3*	1 *0*	1 *0*	0 *1*	1 *2*	0 *1*	0 *1*	0 *0*	1	0 *0*	1 *0*	0 *0*	1 *0*	0	0	3
Hernias,	12 *0*	45 *14*	45 *23*	30 *17*	24 *16*	12 *13*	7 *2*	14 *10*	1 *1*	6	2 *1*	2 *0*	0 *0*	1 *1*	2 *2*	0	30 *11*
Total,	44 *19*	94 *65*	68 *78*	54 *60*	57 *28*	65 *24*	22 *28*	32 *28*	8 *17*	21	36	53	45	11 *10*	3 *4*		48 *34*
Grand total mortality, per cent,	29	31	42	42	49	60	49	54	67	44							
Mortality for intestinal obstruction alone, per cent,	35	38	47	44	56	63	54	63	61	47							

TABLE II.—MORTALITY OF THE DIFFERENT VARIETIES OF OBSTRUCTION.

	20 Per Cent.	25 Per Cent.	30 Per Cent.	35 Per Cent.	40 Per Cent.	45 Per Cent.	50 Per Cent.	55 Per Cent.	60 Per Cent.
For intestinal obstruction alone, .									
For all one thousand cases, . . .									
. .									
. . .									
Openings, ...									
Gall-stones, ...									
Meckel's diverticulum, ...									
Volvulus, ...									
Intussusception, ...									
Bands, ...									
Hernia, ...									
Foreign bodies, ...									

TABLE III.—INTUSSUSCEPTION, ONE HUNDRED AND EIGHTY-SEVEN CASES; MORTALITY AND CONDITION BY DAYS.

Day.	Died.	Cured.	Total.	Mortality, Per Cent.	Reduction.	Artificial Anus, Per Cent.		Resection, Per Cent.		Various.	Per Cent. Reducible.
1st, ...	13	22	35	37	33	. .		2	6	. .	94
2d, ...	14	22	36	39	30	3	8	3	8	. .	83
3d, ...	20	13	33	61	20	4	12	9	27	1	61
4th, ...	10	5	15	67	6	3	20	5	33	. .	40
5th, ...	11	4	15	73	7	5	33	2	13	2	47
6th, ...	3	1	4	75	2	. .		1	25	. .	50
7th, ...	5	4	9	. .	5	1		3	33	. .	. .
8th, ...	3	4	7	. .	4	2		1		. .	. .
10th, ...	3	. .	3	. .	. .	2		1		. .	. .
11th, ...	. .	1	1	. .	1	. .		. .		. .	. .
12th, ...	1	1	2	. .	1	1		. .		. .	. .
14th, ...	1	. .	1	. .	1	. .		. .		. .	. .
3d week, ...	1	4	5	. .	3	2		. .		1	. .
4th week, ...	. .	3	3	. .	1	. .		1		1	. .
Not stated, . .	10	8	18	. .	12	1		4		5	. .
Total, . . .	95	92	187	51	126	24		32			

TABLE IV.—DIVISION OF CASES ACCORDING TO AGE.

	UNDER 1 YEAR.	1-10.	10-20.	20-30.	30-40.	40-50.	50-60.	60-70.	70-80.	80-90.	90-100.
Number of cases,	81	73	55	87	70	73	58	50	21	4	1
Per cent., total number of cases,	14	14	10	15	12	14	10	9	4	..	..
" males,	70	73	67	76	65	47	38	56	65	..	..
" mortality,	47	50	49	47	23	56	33	54	38	..	..
" bands,	..	4	38	40	43	33	31	28	14	50	..
" intussusception,	100	40	23	16	11	4	5	8	5	..	..
:: volvulus,	..	8	12	11	25	26	31	28	38	..	..
" Meckel's diverticulum,	..	5	3	16	5	1	5	..	..	25	..
·· openings,	..	6	11	10	5	9	1	6	5	..	..
" gall-stones,	..	..	..	..	1	8	13	26	33	25	..
" foreign bodies,	..	18	2	2	1	4	1	2	5	..	..

TABLE V.—DIVISION OF CASES ACCORDING TO SEX.

	MALES.	FEMALES.	MORTALITY, MALES.	MORTALITY, FEMALES.
			Per Cent.	Per Cent.
Total,	472	410	53	37
Per cent. of obstruction cases,	65	35	54	33
" of hernia cases,	34	66	28	40
" of intussusception,	72	28	45	56
:: of bands,	58	42	40	30
" of volvulus,	64	36	65	39
" of Meckel's diverticulum,	78	22	65	33
" of openings,	52	48	63	35
" of gall-stones,	24	66	33	53
" of foreign bodies,	43	57	..	..

Intussusceptions.—If the diagnosis of intussusception is sure, which in many cases offers no great difficulties (dysenteric, offensive hemorrhagic evacuations, or even stools consisting of blood alone, and a cylindrical-shaped tumor), it is left to the surgeon's discretion whether he shall perform an operation immediately or not. In small children, if internal therapeutics have had no good result, an early operation is advisable, because in them the disease usually proceeds more rapidly. According to the statistics of Chas. L. Gibson, just quoted on previous pages ("Annals of Surgery," October and November, 1900), laparotomy gives more favorable results in such cases when the intussusception may yet be replaced than when a resection is necessary. In adults there is no such imperative need for haste in operating, because in them the disease occasionally results favorably without operation; the intestine in cases not far advanced becomes permeable for a while. It happens in exceptional cases when no adhesions have formed, that intussusceptions may be restored to the normal state even a long time after their first occurrence. Schramm has reported such a replacement eighteen days after, and Czerny a similar one six months after the first beginning of the abnormality. Wilson withdrew an intussusception after seventeen days of obstructive symptoms, and the patient recovered (" Transylvania Jour. Med.," 1835, vol. VIII, p. 486). Although in the table of 500 cases of intestinal obstruction which I have collected from literature 32 per cent., or nearly one-third, of the cases of intussusception recovered under purely medical treatment, it is in my opinion a bad policy to anticipate such a recovery. Many times it is associated with the sequestration of an intestinal slough, which in the later history eventually leads to death from annular strictures. Peritonitis and the formation of bands also follow intestinal sloughing. Lanceus has reported a slough of 3 feet of the ileum ("Rev. Med.," Buenos Ayres; Canad. "Lancet," 1880, vol. XIII, p. 360).

Gibson believes that although the means of purely medical treatment constitute a valuable aid, and should be the first choice under certain conditions, " it is almost a misfortune that there should be a means of relief, as owing to its ill-judged use it costs many lives by delay and illusions as to its effects."

2. *Chronic Invagination.*—Most authors agree that the bloodless method of treatment may be applied for a longer time in these forms of invagination. However, they may here also be easily overdone. The changes in the neck of the intussusceptum may be such that forced colon irrigations may easily cause intestinal rupture. Rydygier's (*l. c.*) statistics of operative treatment of chronic invaginations give a rather low mortality—only 24 per cent. Therefore it is wise not to extend medical treatment longer than four or five days.

Volvulus.—The diagnosis of the location and nature of the obstruction is not difficult in this case. Therefore the surgeon will have no difficulty in finding the seat of the trouble after laparotomy. The clinician may then occupy two or three days with his efforts to produce a solution of the twist. This is especially recommended by Naunyn, who favors an individualizing plan of treatment in these cases, and advocates the operation only in severe cases giving evidence of strangulation symptoms. Nothnagel favors a prompter operation whenever the diagnosis of volvulus is clear, no matter whether the course is an intensely acute one or one of moderate severity.

Intestinal Paralysis.—This may be surgical or purely medical. Surgical treatment may become necessary where the motor insufficiency of the intestine is due to complications resulting from external hernias, or inflamed and undescended testicle. The form of intestinal paralysis which follows upon traumas, peritonitis, and intra-abdominal operations baffles every kind of treatment. The intestine may be stimulated by enemata or purges ; massage, electtricity, and hydropathic applications are sometimes followed by apparently favorable results for a short while. Intestinal puncture may relieve the meteorism, but is a hazardous undertaking if the intestine is paralyzed. The most favorable form of motor intestinal insufficiency is that which is due to fecal obturation. This type can generally be overcome by the methods of treatment already outlined. The same can be said of the reflex intestinal paralysis, which is due to removable causes—for instance, orchitis, salpingitis, inflammatory conditions about the biliary passages, appendix, ovaries, etc. A number of spontaneous recoveries from intestinal paralysis have been reported, and I have personally observed what was apparently a grave case of paralysis of the intestine associated with sudden dilation of the transverse colon, and which followed an operation for the removal of gall-stones, recover completely after it had existed for six days. The treatment consisted of castor oil by the mouth, lavage of the stomach and colon, hypodermic injections of sterile olive oil and strychnin, and the application of a strong faradic current to both the rectum and the abdominal wall simultaneously.

Intestinal Obturation Caused by Gall-stones.—The operative results have not been very satisfactory hitherto in these cases. Therefore the indications in favor of an operation must be weighed with extreme care in gall-stone occlusion, and the individual features of the case carefully considered. If we can detect a slow downward movement of the stone in the small intestine, and if it causes no lesions of the intestinal wall (ulcers, bleedings, and peritonitic irritation), we may quietly await the result, since the prospects for a spontaneous cure are not bad. If the stone remains a long time at one place, if the symptoms of occlusion are very severe, if a violent pain is felt at the seat of the stone, and if blood is found in the evacuations, an operation may finally become necessary.

Obturation Caused by Foreign Bodies.—Foreign bodies usually stick fast in the intestine only when the intestinal lumen is stenosed at any point. If we can find out that the swallowed foreign body was pointed, angular, or sharp-edged, an operation is advisable on account of greater intestinal lesions and of perforation. If the appearance and size of the foreign body are not known, the indications in favor of an operation and the choice of the time are the same as in chronic intestinal stenosis, which we have already discussed.

Naunyn has rendered the task of the physician much easier by rendering the indications for an operation more precise in the various kinds of intestinal occlusion. In spite of this, however, the task is still a very difficult one, on account of the exceedingly difficult differential diagnosis and the varying course of the disease, which may differ considerably even in those cases of intestinal occlusion which are due to the same causes. If the physician wishes to do justice to his task he must carefully weigh the reasons for and against an operation, and cautiously consider each individual circumstance in the case before him. If he does this he will usually succeed in solving his problem.

In the more severe cases of intestinal occlusion, where an early operation is imperatively necessary, it is very advisable for the physician, unless he be himself a trained surgeon, to call in an experienced surgeon as soon as the diagnosis of intestinal occlusion is certain, so that they may observe and treat the patient together. This is hardly ever practicable in the country, but in the larger cities and towns it may generally be done. If such early conjoint treatment and observation are carried out, the clinician will avoid the reproach of the operator that he had not seen his case early enough and was unable to familiarize himself with the collateral conditions, the state of the heart, kidneys, etc., which are so essential to a successful laparotomy.

In such cases it is still a frequent occurrence that the surgeon is forced to rely entirely on the statements of the physician in charge, who in turn is liable to error, and may have based his treatment on false deductions.   The discussion and the interchange of opinions between the surgeon and the physician are of advantage not only to the patient, but also to the practitioners themselves.   If they have determined on the necessity of an operation, it is of course entirely within the sphere of the surgeon alone to say what kind of operation it is to be—whether he shall construct a preternatural anus or perform the radical operation.   The formation of an artificial anus was recommended thirty years ago by Fräntzel, and later also by experienced surgeons.   It has the advantage over the radical operation in that it can usually be carried out more easily.   In more recent times it has been performed by prominent surgeons, and especially in those cases in which it was impossible to locate the seat of the occlusion.   It has also been observed repeatedly that soon after its construction the feces passed off by the natural way, and that there remained nothing to be done exept to close the artificial anus (Schede).   In many cases, however, the decision, whether an artificial anus is to be constructed or whether the radical operation is to be performed must be made after laparotomy.   In regard to various methods of operating on intestinal occlusions, the student is referred to the text-books on surgery.

Relapses after Operation for Intestinal Obstruction.

Whilst operation may remove the direct cause of an impermeability, it can not destroy the changes or effects of chronic peritonitis; so that after the severance of adhesions or bands renewed obstruction may occur months after the operation by the development of new adhesions.   Fortunately these accidents are rare, and as a rule relapses after operations for intestinal obstructions are the exception.

This does not apply to the volvulus of the sigmoid flexure, which has shown a strong tendency toward relapses even after operation. Surgical treatment may untwist the loop and return it to its normal position, but it can not always remove the predisposing cause,— viz., the elongated and narrow mesentery of the sigmoid flexure,—

which may be still further contracted by a local mesenteritis, making the two ends of the loop almost parallel, free at one end, but fixed at the other. Obalinski was obliged to repeat laparotomy for volvulus of the sigmoid twice within four months ("Arch. f. klin. Chir.," Bd. XLVIII, 1894). Braun has reported two relapses in a similar case. Roser ("Centralbl. f. Chir.," 1883, No. 43) reports loss of a patient by a relapse. Roux ("Centralbl. f. Chir.," 1894, No. 37) performed three laparotomies on the same patient for sigmoid volvulus. Trojanoff (quoted by Zeidler) and Sklifossowsky ("Chir. Annal.," Bd. II, S. 92, Russian) had to operate a second time for relapse. H. Zeidler ("Mitt. a. d. Grenzgeb.;" Bd. v, S. 631) reports a similar case. A number of operations have been suggested with the special object in view of preventing these relapses. Senn ("Exper. Beitr. z. Darmchir.," Basel, 1892) proposed shortening the mesocolon by a fold parallel to the axis of the bowel. Winiwater produced an entero-anastomosis between the limbs of the sigmoid. Trojanoff did a similar operation. Braun sewed the sigmoid to the inner side of the left lateral abdominal wall. Nussbaum suggested sewing it to the wall of the pelvis. Roser proposed sewing the mesentery of the sigmoid to the peritoneum of the lateral abdominal wall. These surgical plans to prevent relapses of volvulus of the sigmoid are mentioned simply to emphasize the gravity of these recurrences. In my own experience I have had two cases of relapses of sigmoid volvulus after operation. It is very desirable that some precautions should be taken during the operation to prevent occurrence of relapses.

THE CLINICAL ASPECTS FOR OPERATIVE TREATMENT OF CHRONIC ENTEROSTENOSES.

Operative treatment of the chronic enterostenoses should always aim at the radical removal of the cause of the stenosis. The surgical methods and their modifications that aim at a restoration of the permeability of the intestinal channel are so numerous that I have restricted this consideration to the fundamental types of operations which are in common use to-day. For the etiology and pathology of enterostenoses and their various types I refer to the chapters on Enterostenosis, Benign and Malignant Neoplasms,

Intestinal Occlusions, Appendicitis, Omphalomesenteric Remains, Intestinal Ulcers, Cicatrices and their Consequences, etc. The simplest operative procedure for the relief of stenosis is *simple incision and subsequent intestinal suture*, which is carried out for the removal of an obturating gall-stone, foreign body, or polypus. Among the other simple operations might be mentioned *disinvagination* of old forms of intussusception. Certain forms of slight stenoses can be cured by the so-called *enteroplastic operation*, according to the principles described by Heineke-Mikulicz for strictures of the pylorus. (See Hemmeter's "Diseases of the Stomach," second edition, p. 363.) The liberation of an intestine from compressing or inflecting adhesions is occasionally also one of the simpler operations, though in exceptional conditions it may become a very complicated surgical procedure. The great majority of enterostenoses demand the execution of two typical major operations : (1) *Entero-anastomosis* or *entero-enterostomy;* (2) *enterectomy* or *intestinal resection*. Entero-anastomosis aims at the restoration of the permeability of the canal by establishing an artificial communication or fistula between the supra- and the infrastenotic loop, leaving the cause of the stenosis untouched. Enterectomy removes the stenosed area completely, and restores the natural conditions for the onward movement of the intestinal contents. If we are confronted simply by a technical obstacle of a benign type—for instance, an inseparable adhesion—both operations accomplish their object with equal effectiveness. The entero-anastomosis has the advantage that it restores the permeability where the radical removal of the stenosed section can not be executed for technical reasons. It is an easier and less dangerous operation. But intestinal resection—enterectomy—is the only operation which can remove the entire diseased area. There is a third operation which is a transitional form between these two operations just considered—viz., exclusion of the diseased area by severing it from the remaining intestine, but permitting it to continue in connection with the mesentery, and not removing it from the abdominal cavity. The intestinal portions above and below the obstacle are united by suture, and the loops belonging to the excluded obstructing portion are brought into union with themselves or made to open externally. Experience teaches that after these operations a radical and enduring cure has resulted in many cases; in others a longer or shorter period of improvement has followed.

Results of Enterectomy.—In 50 cases of intestinal resection for simple stricture reported by Hofmeister ("Beitr. z. klin. Chir.," Bd. xvii), the following immediate results are given: 34 (68 per cent.) recovered, 15 (30 per cent.) terminated fatally; in one case the surgeon had to confine himself to exploratory laparotomy. In 13 cases operated for multiple stenoses the same surgeon reports 5 recoveries, 3 exploratory laparotomies, and 5 deaths. These statistics suffer from the objection that they are not the individual experiences of the author, but compiled from various sources. Von Schiller has reported the results of operations executed at Czerny's clinic within four years for occlusions due to chronic intestinal diseases. There were 15 resections, 8 for malignant neoplasm, 5 for tuberculosis, 1 for actinomycosis, and 1 for chronic invagination. Of these, 9 cases recovered and 6 died, a mortality of 40 per cent. ("Beitr. z. klin. Chir.," Bd. xvii).

Results of Entero-anastomosis.—In the paper just quoted by Schiller, there were 10 cases of this operation, 3 for malignant tumors, 3 for tuberculosis, 3 for chronic invagination, and 1 for incomplete volvulus. Seven cases recovered and 3 ended fatally, a mortality of 30 per cent. Von Eiselsberg (Langenbeck's "Arch. f. klin. Chir.," Bd. liv) performed 3 simple entero-anastomoses and 3 complete intestinal exclusions, in 1896, without losing a single case. All of Hofmeister's 5 cases of simple entero-anastomosis recovered. Entero-anastomosis, in its cause and consequences, is an analogous operation to gastro-enterostomy (concerning the statistics of which see Hemmeter, "Diseases of the Stomach," second edition, pp. 361, 362). In complicated cases of enterostenosis the operation at times becomes arrested after the abdomen is opened, amounting only to an exploratory laparotomy. Further operation being impossible of execution, either because the intestines are balled up into such a tight knot by inseparable adhesions that their liberation without producing severe lesions is impossible, or because the surgeon is confronted by multiple stenoses, distributed over such a wide area of the intestine that an exclusion or resection of the diseased district is simply hazardous. These conditions are fortunately rare, and, as a rule, only met with in very advanced and

inveterate cases.   The cases where a total resection of the stenosed
area or the formation of an artificial by-way is absolutely impossible are so rare that they are generally reported as surgical
curiosities.   In a paper on the "Obstructive Diseases of the
Lower Ileum," Bristowe ("Amer. Jour. of the Med. Sci.," February, 1891) has reported 5 cases of stenosis of the ileum, of which
4 died of inanition without having been given the opportunity
for relief by rational surgical aid.   In the fifth case an operation
was undertaken which went no further than an exploratory laparotomy, because the malignant nature of the disease became apparent.   Bristowe expresses himself as a determined opponent of
operation, in spite of the discouraging result of expectant treatment
and the open confession that this form of therapy must be inevitably
followed by a fatal termination in these cases.*   Although I admit
that the technical difficulties of operation for enterostenosis may be
very grave, it is doubtful whether the internal clinician is a competent
judge of the possibility or impossibility of executing a successful operation.   The results of Halsted, Keen, Senn, Weir, Park, McBurney,
and a large number of other Americans, as well as of the German
surgeons who have been cited in various parts of this chapter, will
serve to give an idea of the almost insurmountable difficulties which
modern surgeons have surmounted with admirable success.   When
the operations are undertaken for chronic enterostenosis of a benign
type, the patients recover in the great majority of cases ; but patients
afflicted with malignant intestinal diseases are naturally unfavorable
subjects for restitution to integrity.   As an individual afflicted with
malignant stenosis must inevitably perish, every attempt to save
such a patient by operative procedure or to relieve his symptoms
for a longer period is justifiable.   To quote again from the statistics of Schiller (*l. c.*) from Czerny's clinic at Heidelberg, 1 case of

---

* At the end of his paper Dr. Bristowe states that he might recommend exploratory laparotomy, but doubts that there will be any favorable results therefrom.   In his estimation
the autopsies of his cases proved that a radical operation had no prospects of success for
technical reasons.   The reader is referred to the original paper for the details of the
necropsy, which I believe will convince the conservative clinician that this writer has by
no means proved the impossibility of executing a successful operation in 3 of his cases.
The third case, that of a man sixty-four years old, with adhesions 2 inches above the
ileocecal valve, there producing an angular inflection, impresses me as having been
indeed a very favorable case for operation.

intestinal sarcoma continued in perfect health for ten years and six months after the operation, 2 cases of carcinoma continued well for five and a half years, and a third case for three and a quarter years.

The results of operation for tuberculous stricture give to these an intermediate position between the malignant and benign stenoses. A review of the surgical procedures for the operative treatment of tubercular strictures and their relative value is given in an excellent paper by Rudolph Matas ("Phila. Med. Jour.," July 9, 1898). Of 50 complete resections for tuberculous strictures tabulated by this author, including cases in which an artificial anus was left after incision, there were 34 cures (68 per cent.) and 15 deaths (30 per cent). Almost as good results have been obtained by entero-anastomosis.

The German results of operation for chronic enterostenoses are given in a paper by Dr. Sklodowski ("Mitt. a. d. Grenzgeb.," 1900, Bd. v, S. 329).* Also in an "Inaugural Dissertation" by Kurt Tietze ("Ueber die totale Darm ausschaltung," Leipzig, 1899).

Length of Intestine which Can Be Resected without Danger to Life.—From the experiments of Nicholas Senn, abstracted in his "Practical Surgery," pages 800–802, and of Trzebicky ("Przeglad Chirurgic," 1894, Tom I, Zesz 4) on dogs, the organism will survive the removal of one-half of the small intestine, not including the duodenum; two-thirds of the intestine, when removed, destroys the chemistry and mechanism of digestion to such a degree as to make life impossible. This author has compiled 9 cases of extensive intestinal resection in the human being, the length of the resected portion varying from 100 to 200 cm. (39 ½ to 79 inches). Of these, 5 cases recovered, including one of Kocher, of 208 cm. (82 ¼ inches), and one of Koeberle, of 205 cm. Dr. T. A. Ashby resected 26 inches of intestine at the University of Maryland Hospital, making an end-to-end anastomosis with a Murphy button and

---

* Both Sklodowski (*l. c.*, p. 396) and Matas (*l. c.*, p. 78) speak of a re-establishment of fecal "circulation," a confusing term, which should be eliminated from the literature of intestinal surgery, because there is no such thing as circulation of feces. There is a normal downward peristaltic movement, and under pathological conditions an abnormal antiperistaltic movement of the fecal matter. But a circulation of feces, which includes the return of the moving substance to the original starting-point, is a physiological impossibility.

removing tubes and ovaries from which the suppurative inflammation had started.   The case recovered and was well one year after the operation (" Jour. Amer. Med. Assoc.," November 11, 1899). In a case * operated at the Johns Hopkins Hospital, Baltimore, by Dr. J. Mitchell, the measurement of the resected portion was stated to be 9 feet of small intestine.   The case was one of embolism of the mesenteric artery.   To my knowledge this is the longest piece of intestine that has been resected.

THE SURGICAL TREATMENT OF INTESTINAL NEOPLASMS.
(A) MALIGNANT NEOPLASMS, CARCINOMA, AND SARCOMA.
(B) BENIGN NEOPLASMS.

As there is no successful internal treatment of malignant neoplasms, all that the practitioner can accomplish is the symptomatic relief of pain, intestinal hemorrhage, tenesmus, obstipation, and peritonitis.   The only way to accomplish anything like permanent relief is by operation.   It will be the duty of the clinician, also, to establish the diagnosis.   Is he confronted with a case of intestinal carcinoma?   In which part of the intestine is it located?   Are there any adhesions or metastases?   The great difficulty lies in the task to transfer to the surgeon cases that have been diagnosed sufficiently early to permit of radical extirpation of the neoplasm.   Unfortunately the early diagnosis of intestinal carcinoma, in the present state of our knowledge, is simply impossible.   In most cases an absolute diagnosis can only be made by exploratory laparotomy. It is encouraging to note that the remote results of operations undertaken with a view to extirpate intestinal carcinomas are improving from year to year.   The surgical treatment of the rectal carcinoma has been described in a separate chapter.   Sarcomas of the small intestine rapidly become inoperable owing to adhesions with adjacent intestinal loops or organs, and owing to metastases in the mesenteric and retroperitoneal lymph-glands.   In 1899 Siegel reported that sarcoma of the small intestine was the indication for resection in but 5 cases up to that year.   Only one of these patients lived one year after the operation.   In 2 cases the later history was not observed, and 1 case died of metastases three weeks after the

---

* The case terminated fatally.

operation. Czerny, however, reports a more favorable result in a female patient whom he first operated for an ovarian sarcoma and 5 years later for an alveolar sarcoma of the small intestine. She was still in perfect health six years after the second operation.

The Carcinomas of the Large Intestine.—This history and statistics of the work of American surgeons on this subject is given in the special works stated at the end of this chapter. In addition to the figures designating the most frequent location of cancers in the large intestine which I have already given (see pp. 680 and 683, vol. 1), I might add the following of Leichtenstern. Of 121 carcinomas of the large intestine, 42 were in the sigmoid, 32 in the cecum, 30 in the transverse colon, hepatic and splenic flexures, 11 in the descending colon, and 6 in the ascending colon. As late as 1880 Péan recommended enterotomy above the obstacle as the only surgical procedure to be advocated for the relief of the symptoms caused by intestinal cancer, and in 1883 Mydel recommended the artificial anus for one year in order to prevent a relapse of stenotic symptoms. Both of these opinions have been superseded by the results of resection. At the German Surgical Congress, held at Berlin, April, 1900, Körte, in an article on "The Operative Treatment of Malignant Tumors of the Large Intestine," presented a number of patients and demonstrated specimens of carcinoma of the large intestine which he had removed. He has operated, in all, in 54 cases ; the oldest patient was eighty-four years old, and 9 patients were in the thirties. The site of the tumor was the sigmoid flexure in 19 cases ; it was ileocecal in 15 cases. The most important symptom is passage of blood and mucus in the stools and the early occurrence of intestinal stenosis from annular tumors. It was possible to perform the radical operation in 19 of his 54 patients. Five of the patients which were presented remained well from three to eight and one-half years after operation. As a palliative operation enterostomy is preferable to entero-anastomosis.

Wölfler's statistics ("Berlin. klin. Wochenschr.," 1896, No. 24) show a mortality of 39.5 per cent. for all forms of intestinal resections, but for resections undertaken specifically for intestinal carcinoma the mortality was 54 per cent. This difference emphasizes the influence which the nature of the malignant disease exerts upon the result of the operation. In 1890 Billroth (Tenth International

Congress of Medicine, Berlin, 1891) reported a mortality of 50 per cent., and in 1892 Czerny a mortality of 50 per cent. On the other hand, there is a possibility of considerable prolongation of life, as shown by the results of Wölfler's operations, 7 of whose patients lived four years, and 15 lived from one and one-half to three and one-half years after resection for carcinoma, without return of the disease. It is known of individual cases that from eight to seventeen years have elapsed after operation in comparatively good health of the patient.

The Surgery of Benign Neoplasms.—The benign neoplasms, described in a separate chapter, call for operative treatment only when they give rise to symptoms of enterostenosis or occlusion. Steiner has reported 15 cases of intestinal myomas operated for this purpose, 2 of which terminated fatally; 9 were located in the small intestine, 7 of which were removed by resection, and 2 by enterotomy and extirpation with subsequent intestinal suture. Four myomas were in the rectum, 3 of which were cured by ligating the pedicle, and 1 by executing Kraske's operation. All of the 13 cases operated by Steiner ("Beitr. z. klin. Chir.," Bd. XXII, S. 1) recovered. Lipomas of the small intestine seem especially liable to produce invagination. Hiller ("Ueber Darm-Lipoma," "Beitr. z. klin. Chir.," 1899, Bd. XXIV, S. 509) reports that in 20 patients with intestinal lipoma, intussusception was observed 9 times.

The treatment of benign neoplasms of the rectum has been considered in a separate chapter. It is important to note that the results of artificial anus, for the relief of symptoms due to benign neoplasms, are as a rule very unfavorable, whereas results of resection give a fair prospect of an enduring recovery. As far as the clinician is concerned, his duty can be formulated by the statement that benign intestinal neoplasms will, as a rule, not be recognized until they give rise to symptoms of stenosis, and as it is not the object of this treatise to enter into the technic of the operation, but simply to point out the indications thereto, an exhaustive consideration of the surgery of these types of new growths can not be considered as properly within the domain of this chapter.

For further reference concerning the technic, etc., the reader is referred to the following works on intestinal surgery : E. Albert,

"Lehrbuch d. spec. Chir."; Dennis, "System of Surgery"; Kocher, "Text-book on Surgery"; Koenig, "Lehrbuch d. spec. Chir."; Keith, "Text-book of Abdominal Surgery"; Roswell Park, "Surgery by American Authors"; Maylard, "Surgery of Alimentary Canal"; Greig Smith, "Abdominal Surgery"; Treves, "Manual of Operative Surgery"; Wharton and Curtis, "Practice of Surgery"; Lilienthal, "Imperative Surgery"; Nicholas Senn, "Text-book of Surgery and Surgical Treatment"; "Intestinal Occlusions," "Trans. Amer. Assoc. Phys.," *l. c.;* also N. Senn, "Practical Surgery," Phila., 1901.

The American literature on intestinal surgery is considerable, but not all is equally meritorious. As the most prominent weekly medical journals bring brief abstracts of the surgical publications the world over, it is no longer necessary to attempt a compilation of these in a text-book of this character.   It would lead me too far to attempt it.   For example, my stenographer has tabulated sixty articles on intestinal surgery from volume IV, 1899, of the "Philadelphia Medical Journal."

CHAPTER VII.

INTESTINAL ATROPHY.

Atrophic degeneration of the intestinal wall, while it may involve all the layers, exerts its grave influences by the atrophy of the mucosa and muscularis. The condition has almost exclusively a pathological interest only, for excepting the atrophy of the mucosa of the large intestine it can not be diagnosed; especially so when it is confined to the small intestine. In my work on "Diseases of the Stomach," second edition, p. 850, I have given the pathological histology of atrophy of the stomach in the chapter on Achylia Gastrica. Intestinal atrophy is always the consequence of other diseases. Some authors have recognized a chronic atrophic enteritis analogous to chronic atrophic gastritis. Exact histological investigations that are associated with complete clinical histories are extremely rare. The subject was first systematically studied by Nothnagel ("Zeitschr. f. klin. Med.," 1882, Bd. IV, S. 422, and also "Beitr. z. Physiol. u. Pathol. d. Darms," 1884). Later on Scheimpflug ("Zeitschr. f. klin. Med.," 1885, Bd. IX, S. 40) confirmed the results of Nothnagel. A circumscribed inflammatory atrophy of the intestinal mucosa was found in 80 per cent. of all cadavers that were examined by Nothnagel. It occurred most frequently in the large intestine, especially in the cecum. Scheimpflug gives the following figures: Atrophied areas were found in the cecum in 96 per cent., in the ascending colon 66 per cent., in the middle ileum 64 per cent., in the lower ileum 62 per cent., in the transverse colon 58 per cent., in the descending colon 43 per cent., in the superior ileum 25 per cent., and in the duodenum 0 per cent. The extent of the atrophy was very variable, occurring partly only in small islands, partly in extensive and continuous districts. Jürgens ("Berlin. klin. Wochenschr.," 1882, No. 23 u. 28), Blaschko ("Virchow's Archiv," Bd. XCIV), Sasaki ("Virchow's Archiv," Bd. XLIII), Klebs ("Handb. d. path. Anatomie"), Kundrat, Leube, and Werber are among the most prominent contributors to this field of special pathology.

It will be expedient to consider separately the changes in the various layers of the intestinal wall.

State of the Columnar Surface Epithelium.

It is a common experience at autopsies to find the intestinal epithelium separated from the mucous membrane in consequence of cadaveric changes even when the remaining layers are in a perfectly normal condition.   Undoubtedly this separation and destruction of the columnar epithelium may also take place at a still earlier period when the intestines have been inflamed.   The postmortem loss of columnar epithelium occurs very rapidly.   I have found it separated in various isolated areas when the autopsy was made within two hours after death.   I remember a case where there was extensive destruction of the columnar epithelium found during a necropsy of a man dead from an accident.   The examination was made while the body was still warm, perhaps an hour to an hour and a half after death.   Much of the epithelium was intact, but that there should have been any detachment at all is an indication of the rapidity of this process.   J. J. Woodward (*l. c.*, p. 326) had already emphasized that the loss of epithelium observed in most of his autopsy records was a postmortem change.*   Nothnagel has made control examinations of intestines of dogs, and has arrived at the same conclusion.

The Mucosa.

Only the advanced stage of atrophy can be recognized by the naked eye, by the absence of the normal velvety appearance which is imparted to the surface by the villi.   Atrophies of the mucosa in the large intestine are also difficult of recognition macroscopically ; the microscope is necessary to decide the presence or absence of atrophy.   One of the most evident effects of atrophy is a reduction in the breadth of the mucosa, which occurs with the increasing diminution in size and degeneration of the cells, accompanied by a corresponding atrophy of the glands, which become shorter and smaller.   The intercellular supporting tissue of the mucosa also participates in the atrophic process, thereby contributing to the

---

* These autopsies were on bodies of soldiers dead from diarrhea and dysentery during the Civil War, 1861–65.

general reduction of the breadth of the mocosa, which may be so
far atrophied that no trace of its former existence is left except a
very small border of fibrous connective tissue overlying the muscularis mucosæ.   The destruction of the glands may occur as the result
of two different processes, according to Nothnagel : (1) The gland-
cells are gradually loosened more and more and forced toward the
lumen of the intestine.   The loosening is brought about by a swelling
of the interstitial tissue and the accumulation of round cells.   They
are then lifted up and pushed out of their normal situation, and cut
off from their normal blood supply.   (2) When a catarrh takes the
more chronic course, the proliferating connective tissue chokes off
the glandular tubules in their lower portion, separating them from
the upper portion, and eventually causes their complete atrophy
during the progressive fibrous metamorphosis of the tissue.   Under
certain conditions cystic dilations of the glands may be formed,
and preserve part of the gland structure—though in a modified
state—for some time.

Inflammatory atrophy of the mucosa is not always necessarily
the result of chronic intestinal catarrh.   Nothnagel has failed to
find glandular structures and villi in extensive districts of the
mucosa in a child five years old, that had been sick only four days
with a severe attack of vomiting and diarrhea (gastro-enteritis?), and
he observed the same in many other cases of acute catarrh.   He
suggests that the development of the loosening and degeneration
of the glandular tissue requires a more acute onset of the process,
and that it does not develop when the process is a slow one from
the beginning.   He holds, then, that the atrophy of the mucosa is
by no means a regular consequence of the enteritis or colitis, though
there is a definite pathogenetic relation between this atrophy and the
catarrhal inflammatory processes.   He does not believe that there
is an etiological connection between atrophy and changes in the
nervous apparatus of the intestine.

**Measurements of the Breadths of the Various Layers and
Structures in the Intestinal Wall—Normal, Hypertrophic,
and Atrophic.**

The length of the glands in the colon mucosa in adults is
normally from 0.370 to 0.5 mm. ; in atrophy, from 0.25 to 0.1, 0.04,

and even 0.012 mm.   The submucosa in the small intestine has a breadth of 0.25 to 0.60 mm.; in the large intestine the submucosa has a breadth of 0.5 to 0.75 mm.   A pathological increase in thickness may be accepted when the dimensions for greater distances amount to the following : In the small intestine, 0.8 to 1.0 mm.; in the large intestine, 1.0 mm. or more.   An atrophy may be diagnosed when the thickness in the small intestine is but 0.2 mm., in the large intestine 0.3 mm. or less.   The following figures are indicative of variations in the muscularis.   The normal breadth for the colon, not including the teniæ, for very young children is 0.25 to 0.375 mm.; children several years old, 0.5 mm.; adults, 0.6 to 1.0 mm.   When the muscularis exceeds 1.0 mm. in breadth, we may assume a hypertrophy; when it is less than 0.5 or 0.6 mm., an atrophy is probable.   Normal dimensions for the small intestine of adults are from 0.3 to 0.7 mm. for the muscularis.   It is not safe to depend upon a measurement of the thickness of the entire intestinal wall, for I have personally seen cases which in micrometric measurement appeared normal when the entire breadth of the intestinal wall was measured.   In one such case, however, there was a distinct atrophy of the mucosa when measured alone, but the loss of breadth in the mucosa was made up by an increase in the submucosa.   The results of ten measurements of different places, taken in the average, were the following in this specimen: mucosa, 0.2 mm.; submucosa, 1.2 mm.; muscularis, 1.7 mm.; peritoneum, 0.1 mm.

The Muscular Layer.

The atrophy of the muscular layer is by no means always proportional to that in the mucous layer.   A number of pathologists (Klebs, *l. c.*) have asserted that atrophy of the intestinal muscularis may occur in pathological conditions that bring on general cachexia, —for instance, phthisis, carcinoma, exhausting suppurations, enteric fever,—as a result of which state the atrophic muscle bundles are separated from each other, and thereby become more distinctly visible.   Even traumatic rupture of the intestine has been attributed to this atrophy of the muscularis.   After a careful investigation of this subject, Nothnagel has not been able to confirm this view.   He has in some cases found an independent muscular atrophy when the intestine was otherwise normal, and is disposed to attribute this to a congenital hypoplasia. Partial atrophies of the muscularis occur in hernias and diverticular expansions of the intestinal wall. The hypoplasia of the muscularis, referred to in the preceding, occasionally constitutes the anatomical basis for persistent obstipation. It is important to bear in mind that occasionally a slight hypertrophy of the muscularis may be found in connection with chronic intestinal catarrh, without atrophy of the mucosa. Even when the mucosa is atrophied, there need not necessarily be an atrophy of the muscularis, though in the majority of these cases the breadth of the muscular layer is somewhat beneath the normal dimension. No cause can be assigned for the production of intestinal muscular atrophy.

A few words about the follicles and the submucosa. The statements of the various observers who have studied intestinal atrophy (Baginsky, Kundrath, Werber, Hervieux, Lambl) concerning the condition of the follicles differ widely. Baginsky describes them as being deficient in cells and atrophied. Some of the others give an account of a hypertrophy, and still others of an atrophy. Nothnagel has never been able to confirm an isolated atrophy of the follicular apparatus; even when the mucosa is in an extreme state of atrophy the solitary and agminated follicles may be well preserved in size and number. In very rare cases he has been able to find the follicles in an undoubted condition of atrophy.

Concerning the **submucosa**, it may be said that pronounced atrophy is one of the greatest scarcities, even when the mucosa is in a state of advanced atrophy from the rectum to the upper jejunum. In one of my cases the width of the submucosa was 1.2 mm. in ten different localities, about one foot apart, while the mucosa was only 0.2 mm. in width.

Fatty Degeneration of the Muscularis.

That the diminution in breadth of the muscularis is not always due to an atrophy pure and simple has been demonstrated by E. Wagner ("Arch. d. Heilk.," Bd. 11, 1861), who discovered fatty degeneration in the intestinal musculature in 10 out of 400 necropsies, mostly phthisical and alcoholic subjects. Nothnagel (*l. c.*, p.

135) found this fatty degeneration in only 3 male subjects out of a material of 50 cases carefully examined by microscopic investigation. Two of his cases occurred also in drinkers. He could not establish any closer connection between this fatty degeneration and catarrhal atrophies of the mucosa. Scheimpflug has found this degeneration after poisoning by arsenic ; and Orth has found it after chronic peritonitis. Furneaux-Jordan attributes great importance to the fatty degeneration of the intestinal muscularis, to which he assigns the production of not only persistent obstipation, but also of death as a result of intestinal occlusion in consequence of the inability of the muscularis to contract ("Brit. Med. Jour.," 1879, vol. I, p. 621). He found this condition most frequently in fat persons with tremendous bellies, and in persons presenting evidences of such degeneration in other organs.

PROGRESSIVE GASTRO-INTESTINAL ATROPHY—ATROPHIC AND DEGENERATIVE CHANGES IN THE NERVE PLEXUSES OF THE INTESTINE—ATROPHIA GASTRO-INTESTINALIS PROGRESSIVA.

A condition in which the mesenteric plexus, the muscularis, and finally even the nerves and vessels of the mesentery, undergo fatty granular degeneration and atrophy has been described by Jurgens (*l. c.*). He regards it as an independent morbid condition of rather frequent occurrence, and capable of producing death under phenomena of collapse and shock. It is asserted to be in some etiological relation with Addison's disease. Blaschko (*l. c.*) found degeneration of the ganglia of Meissner's and Auerbach's plexuses and their connecting fibers in two cases. In one of these, a female alcoholic subject, there was also a fatty degeneration of the muscularis. Orth (*l. c.*, p. 856), whilst recognizing isolated degenerations in the muscularis of the colon, even such scattered through the small intestine and stomach, is very conservative in assigning them as secondary to nerve degenerations. The ganglia and intestinal nerves are frequently subject to swelling, formation of vacuoles, degeneration and atrophies during acute infectious diseases, especially after acute diseases of the nervous central organ ; accordingly Orth cautions against attributing intestinal muscular atrophies to preliminary degenerations in the mesenteric plexuses. The investigations of

Scheimpflug demonstrated histo-pathological degenerations in the intestinal nervous apparatus, after tuberculous meningitis, croupous pneumonia, acute yellow atrophy of the liver, acute arsenical poisoning, and after various prolonged diseases leading to general marasmus. So that it would indeed seem that the plexuses of Meissner and Auerbach, and their connecting paths, are rather frequently the seat of degeneration. Whether or not there is time for the production of secondary degeneration and atrophy of the muscularis in such a complex pathological condition, and whether the atrophy of the muscularis when it does occur, is due to absence of trophic influences, as a result of disease of the intestinal plexuses, or whether it may not be directly due to the fundamental disease occurring simultaneously with the degeneration of the nerve ganglia, are questions which I am not able to decide in the light of our present knowledge. Certainly the evidence so far furnished by the investigators cited does not convince me that atrophy of the intestinal muscularis is secondary and attributable to atrophy of the plexuses of Meissner and Auerbach.

Clinical History.

As the two layers which are predominantly affected in intestinal atrophy are the mucosa and the muscularis, a clinical history could only be evolved from the interference with or the absence of the functions of these structures. The principal function of the mucosa is that of resorption. The other two functions are protection from invasion of intestinal bacteria, which is executed by the columnar epithelium, and secretion of the succus entericus. The digestive power of the latter is not very considerable, because the only digestive agent which is contained in it is an amylolytic ferment, of which there is plenty in the saliva and pancreatic juice. We can not, therefore, judge of the existence of an atrophy of the mucosa of the small intestine by any determinable reduction of the digestive power, since this is mostly carried out by the pancreatic and gastric secretions. Above and beyond this there is great doubt whether the intestinal epithelia, the follicles and villi, can be subject to atrophy without extensive degenerations throughout the mucosa. The function of the muscularis—that of peristalsis—must naturally be affected when there is a muscular atrophy. This, however, escapes diagnostic detection, for obstipation due to muscular inactivity occurs also in enteritis and colitis. Of course it is in this case not due to atrophy or degeneration. Atrophy of the mucosa in localized areas—for instance, the cecum—escapes detection entirely. The marasmus observed in tabes mesenterica of infants has been attributed to the loss of absorption in consequence of atrophy of the entire intestinal mucosa, and the cases of complete intestinal atrophy of adults were also distinguished by advanced cachexia. But this could not be attributed exclusively to the intestinal atrophy, because other complicating diseases, such as leukemia, existed simultaneously.

Atrophy of the mucosa of the colon can, under certain conditions, be diagnosed. The two principal features that are characteristic of this condition are found in the stools. First, they are peculiarly soft and mushy, although there is only one stool a day. Secondly, they do not contain any admixture of mucus, as is found to be characteristic of catarrh of the colon. The mushy consistency is due to the larger percentage of liquid contained in the stool in consequence of the lessened absorption of water by the atrophic mucosa. As a rule the stools become thickened in the colon by condensation as a result of absorption of the liquid constituents. Only in colitis are the stools thin and diarrheic ; but then they are more numerous and contain much mucus. The absence of mucus in the stools of atrophy of the colon mucosa is a result of destruction of the glands of Lieberkühn. I should add that these two signs (mushy stool and absence of mucus, with only one movement a day) occur only when the entire large intestine has lost its mucosa by atrophy. Even a very small healthy portion of mucosa, when, for instance, that of the sigmoid flexure and rectum is spared, may effect sufficient condensation of the colon contents and sufficient secretion of mucus to produce an apparently normal stool—*i. e.*, one containing an admixture of mucus and being of firm consistency.

There is no special **treatment** for intestinal atrophy ; the process itself can not be influenced. The diet should be that of chronic enteritis.

CHAPTER VIII.

ABNORMALITIES OF FORM AND POSITION.

Idiopathic Dilation of the Colon.

Nature and Concept.—By idiopathic dilation of the colon is meant an abnormal primary enlargement not consequent or dependent upon any disease or recognized pathological condition. The disease may be congenital, producing symptoms soon after birth, or acquired. In the cases which are designated as congenital, the absolute evidence for assigning a congenital cause is frequently lacking ; they are designated in this way for want of a better reason to assign for the dilation. In a number of the patients reported in the literature of this subject the dilation began at such an interval after birth as to render the congenital origin very doubtful. They are therefore considered as acquired.

Etiology.—The etiology of congenital dilation of the colon is not known. Judging from the cases reported in literature, there are two varieties of infantile dilation of the colon : (1) Colectasia due to some abnormal development, the result of malformation of the colon, sigmoid, or rectum, existing at birth and at once producing its symptoms. As this is naturally a secondary dilation, the term "idiopathic" does not apply to it. (2) Colectasia producing its symptoms within weeks or months after birth, giving no evidence of any malformation or any other abnormality of the large intestine, and which therefore can logically be called idiopathic dilation. Fitz ("Amer. Jour. of the Med. Sci.," 1899, vol. cxviii, p. 132) characterizes the term "congenital idiopathic" dilation of the colon as a misnomer. As a matter of fact, it is evident from the above classification that one type only is congenital in the exact sense of the term, and that type is not idiopathic, but secondary to some abnormality in the colon, sigmoid, or rectum. Infantile dilation of the colon may be congenital or idiopathic, but not both. Treves (London "Lancet," 1898, vol. 1, 276) has suggested that all cases of so-called idiopathic dilation in young children are due to congenital defects in the terminal part of the bowel; that there is, therefore, in all these cases an actual mechanical obstruction, and that the dilation of the bowel is not idiopathic. In support of this view he describes a patient, a child, with dilation secondary to congenital stenosis of the large intestine. He successfully removed not only the descending colon, but also that part of the large intestine corresponding to the sigmoid flexure and rectum, down to the anus. This tube was represented by a rigid cylinder, which, though pervious, was solid looking, 8 or 9 inches long, and had constituted the obstruction. The cases of Atkin (*l. c.*), Dodd (*l. c.*), Formad (*l. c.*), Osler ("Archives of Pediatrics," 1893, vol. x, p. 111), Walker (*l. c.*), and Rolleston and Haward ("Transactions of the Clinical Society of London," 1896) support this opinion of Mr. Treves. In one of Osler's cases an operation was performed by Halsted, during which the sigmoid flexure was found twisted upon itself, but not so as to cause any obstruction. The sigmoid flexure measured 45 cm. (17⅝ inches) in circumference, and its walls were much thickened; there was no evidence of stricture or impaction. An artificial anus was made, fluid feces and gas escaped, the distention was entirely relieved, and the case recovered. There was no return of symptoms for several years. The case was then lost sight of. The second of Osler's cases (*ibid.*) was supposed to be a genuine idiopathic dilation of the colon, but autopsy two years later showed a stenosis of the sigmoid flexure.

In my work on "Diseases of the Stomach," I have described inflections of the duodenum producing absolute or relative stenosis of the passage immediately beyond the pylorus, and giving rise to secondary dilation of the stomach. The kinking of the duodenum became evident only when the stomach was filled, and was readily overlooked when the organ was empty (see "Diseases of the Stomach," second edition, p. 660). Familiarity with the anatomical course and structure of the colon in infants makes it evident that such a mechanical obstruction due to inflection may be readily produced in the infantile colon by distention with gas or liquids. Rosengart ("Die Pathogenese der Enteroptose," "Zeitschr. f. diet. u. physikal. Therapie," Bd. 1, S. 215) has dissected a number of infants, and maintains that soon after birth there is no such thing as the transverse colon, but that the ascending and transverse colon merge into one straight line, ascend diagonally from the cecum in the right lower abdomen, directly across the splenic flexure.   Dr. J. Holmes Smith and myself have dissected a number of full-term infants at the University of Maryland, and we have been able to confirm Rosengart's findings in a number of cases (see " Diseases of the Stomach," second edition, p. 706).   It is possible that such a condition of normal inflection might be overlooked at a laparotomy or even a necropsy unless especial attention was directed to it, and the colon distended artificially in order to observe the effects of experimental dilation upon the possible inflection.   This may explain part of the cases in which positively nothing abnormal was discovered at laparotomy or the autopsy.   Other congenital cases may be due to imperfect development of the muscularis of the colon; still others to abnormal or imperfect innervation of the colon.   Indeed, some of the cases bear a striking resemblance to the intestinal paralysis described in another chapter.   Even the hypertrophy of the intestinal walls, which has been described in a number of cases, would not contradict this interpretation, for in the suprastenotic compensatory hypertrophy in the intestine of adults we also have an increase in the thickness of the muscular layer, and notwithstanding this, paralysis may develop ; i. e., either functional paralysis from overwork, which may be temporarily recovered from, or complete paralysis due to degeneration of the hypertrophied muscle.   Colitis can not be assigned a place in the etiology unless it can be demonstrated to have existed sufficiently long to have produced atrophy of the muscularis of the colon, an occurrence not very likely in neonats.   J. P. Crozer Griffith ("Amer. Jour. of the Med. Sci.," September, 1900) applies the term congenital not only to actual dilations present at birth, but also to a congenital tendency toward early dilation, a state which, while not demonstrable anatomically at birth, is conceived to be a fundamental infirmity inclining to dilation of the colon as the child becomes older, a condition which this author believes to be much more common than the actual dilation present at birth.   Griffith has reviewed the entire literature of the subject up to date, and reported two new cases, one from his own experience, in which right inguinal colotomy was done by John Ashhurst, Jr.; and a second which he saw in the clinic of Dr. Wm. Pepper.

As regards the various types of the congenital form, he defines three varieties: (*a*) Those in which the children suffer from earliest infancy, as soon as food begins to enter the colon ; they then rapidly grow worse ; (*b*) others with a less intense type, who had sufficient power to resist the distention some time, although showing great ineffectiveness of the expulsive powers at all times ; (*c*) cases which had periods of improvement, in which the distention largely disappeared, although the imperfect condition of the colon remained, and relapse occurred in nearly every instance.   It is evident from this classification that children of types (*b*) and (*c*) may grow up, and especially those of type (*c*), who may reach adult life ; so that it is conceivable that an adult having a dilation of the colon may have been born with the condition that Griffith specifies as " a tendency to dilation."   It makes it possible that colon dilations in the adult may not always be acquired.   Whatever may be the underlying causes of the idiopathic cases, the active cause is deficient peristalsis, which gradually leads to an accumulation of fecal matter and consequent dilation of the transverse colon and sigmoid flexure. As a result the main symptoms will be constipation and abdominal meteorism.   It is also conceivable that distention of the lower portion of the large intestine, especially the sigmoid flexure, may cause a twist or infantile volvulus, as was found in one of the cases reported by Osler.   The anatomy of the infantile sigmoid and colon (Henke, "Topographische Anatomie des Menschen," Berlin, 1884), their peculiar course and length, make the facility with which they may become mechanically inflected or twisted intelligible.   A distinction between congenital dilation (secondary) and those occurring in early childhood which are idiopathic is manifestly impossible without satisfactory necropsies ; and even a necropsy will not always show the condition that existed during life.   In the introductory chapter to the intestinal occlusions I have given a description of stenotic conditions observed during life at laparotomies, which could not be made out at the necropsy.   Unfortunately there is much diffuseness and uncertainty in the literature of the subject concerning the definition of the terms "idiopathic" and "congenital."   What is required in order to clear up the subject are careful investigations by experienced pathological anatomists into the anatomical and histological state of the entire intestinal tract from the mouth to the

II—29

anus ; measurements of the lengths of the various portions of the intestine, of the mesocolon ; serial sections of the walls of the colon, and sigmoid and rectum, at various localities ; of the intestinal nerves and ganglia ; injection of the blood- and lymph-vessels.   In fact, one can not be surprised at the absence of satisfactory knowledge concerning the pathogenesis of the condition, when in the entire literature there is no evidence that any one has systematically investigated it from the above standpoints.

Idiopathic Dilation of Adult Life.—In the compilation of the literature referred to, J. P. Crozer Griffith (*l. c.*) has tabulated 24 cases which he considers congenital, using at the same time the term "idiopathic," which, however, does not conform to the interpretation which Fitz (*l. c.*) gives to this designation.   The conception of the latter impresses me as the more correct one.   For instance, in Griffith's list of what he calls congenital idiopathic dilations—the term to which Fitz takes exception—is included Martin's case ("Montreal Med. Jour.," 1897, vol. xxv, p. 697), in which there was a partial narrowing of the lower portion of the sigmoid flexure through possible thickening of the mesocolon. Quite a number of these cases—those of Osler, Mya, Generisch— presented considerable thickening of the walls of the colon.   A hypertrophy of the wall of the large intestine occurs, in my experience, only in cases of chronic stenoses, as a result of the continued efforts of the bowel to overcome the obstruction, or in consequence of hypertrophic colitis.   It is a condition that can not be present at birth, because one of the essential requisites to its development is overwork of the muscularis, which can not have taken place as long as no food entered the bowel.   Compensatory hypertrophy, therefore, is strongly suggestive of a chronic obstruction, even when the evidence thereof can not be detected.   Of the congenital forms, there were, according to Griffith, only three which reached adult life—those of Peacock, Formad, and Hichens. Among the 29 cases compiled by him as not congenital, 16 are among adults.   This list may be swelled to 18 by a case reported in Fitz's paper (*l. c.*), from the practice of Dr. F. B. Harrington, of Boston.   If it is difficult to ascertain whether the condition is congenital or not in a child, it must be much more difficult to arrive at a conclusion concerning this point from the history of an adult.

Personally I should be inclined to consider every case with marked hypertrophy of the wall of the colon as acquired, because compensatory hypertrophy, as explained above, is always secondary to some obstruction. Formad's case, however, a man aged twenty-nine years, had been afflicted with constipation since the second year of his age. At the age of twenty he became a museum freak on account of the enormous distention of his abdomen, and was known as the "balloon man." The abdomen was constantly increasing in size, and measured 220 cm. (86½ inches). The whole colon, especially the transverse, was found distended with gas and semi-liquid feces at the autopsy, measuring 25 to 76 cm. (10 to 30 inches) in circumference. There were no thickening of the wall, no kinking or stricture, no impaction, no abnormalities in the rectum or small intestine. The illustration on page 452, from Tyson's "Practice of Medicine," second edition, illustrates the comparative size of the colon in Formad's case.

Richardson's patient ("Trans. Amer. Surg. Assoc.," 1897, vol. xv, p. 585) was a man forty-seven years of age, who had been in good health until the age of forty, when obstipation became evident and increased in severity. Symptoms of acute obstruction developed, and a semi-volvulus of the sigmoid flexure was found, corrected, and stitched to the abdominal wall. Five months later a second attack of acute obstruction occurred, and the sigmoid was again found twisted. It was then resected successfully, and the patient recovered completely. The case which Fitz reports was a lady thirty-seven years of age, who traced her infirmity back to her fifteenth year, when she suffered from attacks of weakness two or three times a year. She was admitted to the Massachusetts General Hospital, November, 1898. For eighteen months previous to the date of her admission she had been unable to work, and was confined to bed a couple of months at a time on four or five different occasions. The abdomen began to enlarge, and there was more or less pain in the right iliac fossa, where there was a sensation as of a lump. The waist was small, the epigastrium flat, but below the navel the abdomen was uniformly distended, tense and tympanitic to a marked degree. Urine negative; 68 per cent. of hemoglobin, 5,000,616 red corpuscles, 13,400 leukocytes three hours after dinner. The stomach had a capacity of 25 ounces of

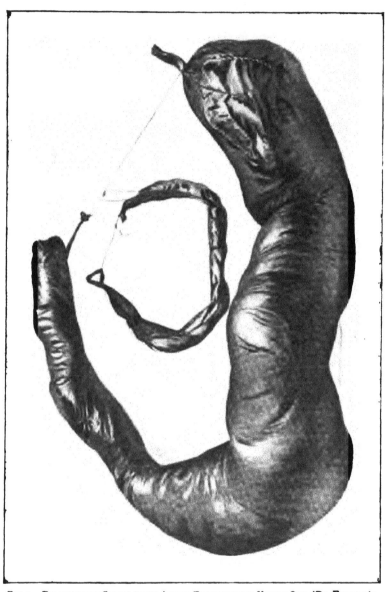

FIG. 9.—DILATION OF COLON FROM ADULT TWENTY-NINE YEARS OLD (DR FORMAD'S CASE).—(*From Tyson's " Practice of Medicine.*")
(For description see text, p. 451.)

water; free HCl and lactic acid were present (composition of test-meal and quantitative figures not given).   She was informed of the probable cause of her condition, and the doubt of any permanent relief except by surgical procedure.   Dr. C. B. Porter exposed the greatly enlarged sigmoid flexure at a laparotomy.   It was apparent that there was neither an organic stricture nor fecal impaction, and as the pain had been referred to the right iliac region, and the appendix was closely attached to the abdominal wall, it was removed with the hope of relieving the pain.   The operation was recovered from, but gave no permanent relief.   She returned to the hospital for the purpose of having a portion of the colon resected.   Dr. M. H. Richardson removed the enlarged sigmoid flexure, which represented the chief constituent of the abdominal swelling, although there was some dilation of the rectum and descending colon. Convalescence has progressed favorably without interruption.   In the report of this case Fitz emphasizes the relation of idiopathic dilation of the colon to phantom tumor, because the abdominal distention resembles a tumor and even disappears under anesthesia. The case of Formad and that of Fitz exhibit the features of idiopathic dilation of the colon free from any obvious congenital peculiarities, the only prominent factor in the etiology being antecedent chronic obstipation, but no fecal impaction.   In numerous of the remaining cases which occurred in adults there was a direct cause to which the colon dilation was attributable.   Any stricture, ulcer, neoplasm, or any one of the many types of occlusion, any type of the inflammations which may invade the intestine, would be sufficient, in my estimation, to stamp the case as one of secondary dilation, and exclude it from the idiopathic type, even if these pathological changes did not occur in the colon, sigmoid, or rectum, but in some part of the small intestine.   Thus a stricture resulting from ulcer in the ileum might reflexly cause an enterospasm in the colon or sigmoid.   The latter could not be discovered at the autopsy, which would reveal nothing but the primary source of irritation in the small intestine.

Symptomatology.—The two main symptoms are obstipation and meteorism.   In the majority of cases the obstipation dates from birth, or at least within a few days after birth.   This was the case in 22 of the patients of the subjoined synopsis.   In other cases several weeks or months are recorded as having elapsed before the obstipation began. In a few of them—Fütter's, for instance—there is no history of constipation. In a number of cases attacks of diarrhea are recorded, and it appears that in several of them the diarrhea was terminal. Abdominal distention developed contemporaneously with the constipation in the great majority of cases. The pathogenesis of meteorism has been dwelt upon in the chapter on Enterostenosis, where it has been emphasized that it is not always due to the accumulation of gases resulting from fermentation of the intestinal contents, but that its most important cause is the disturbance in the mesenteric circulation. We have there distinguished between local and stagnation meteorism. In none of the reported clinical histories have I been able to discover that such a distinction had been made, or whether the plastic rigidity of the intestinal loops had been observed in any case. These observations would naturally throw considerable light upon the nature of the process, particularly whether it was due to stenosis or intestinal paralysis. The tympanites seem always to have been very marked, and it is asserted to have depended largely upon the degree of obstipation. It was capable of being relieved, and in most cases a decided diminution in the size of the abdomen was effected by enemata and purgatives; the evacuation of the gases through a rectal tube often gave relief. Visible peristaltic movements in the distended colon were frequently perceived through the thin abdominal walls, but plastic erection of the loops ("Darmsteifung") is not reported in any of the cases. Vomiting has not been a very frequent symptom. Spontaneous pain and pressure pain were either absent or only slightly marked; they are especially mentioned only in the cases which survived the first two years of life, and who developed a tendency to relapses.

Character of the Stools.—The description of the stools as given in the reports varies considerably. Above all, I could not discover any statement corresponding to the characteristics of the so-called stenotic feces. The stools rather indicate a motor insufficiency or paralysis of the colon, and not a stenosis or an obturation by coprostasis. Henoch mentions the observation that the insertion of a rectal tube always brought away soft feces. At autopsies the intestinal contents have nearly always been found in a semisolid state;

only exceptionally were the evacuations hard or scybalous. Hirsch-sprung reported a case in which there had been no stools since birth; yet the finger introduced into the rectum produced a discharge of a stream of meconium. The following table gives the ages and sex of 26 cases, in which there was no evidence of stenosis or obstruction, and which may therefore be considered as idiopathic. A number of the cases—those of Peacock, Bristowe, Hughes, Hadden, Generisch—presented ulcerations of the bowel at the autopsy. As no specific statements concerning the histologic nature of these ulcers accompany these reports, it is difficult to determine whether the ulcers are the cause or the result of the dilation and obstipation. The muscular hypertrophy, however, which was present in very many of the cases, though not in that of Formad which is pictured in the text, can logically be looked upon as a secondary compensatory effort. Cases presenting anatomical alterations of this character will always constitute a doubtful class, because both conditions—ulcer and hypertrophy—are capable of producing the clinical picture of enterospasm, and yet no evidence of the latter could be found at autopsy. In 26 cases of the subjoined table, 5 were females and 21 males, 20 occurred under the age of twelve years, 16 were at the age of eight years or under.

TABLE OF AGES AND SEX.

Bristowe ("Brit. Med. Jour.," 1885, vol. I, p. 1086), ...	female,	8 yrs.
Cheadle ("Lancet," 1886, vol. II, p. 1117), ...	male,	3 yrs.
Fitz ("Amer. Jour. of the Med. Sci.," 1889, p. 135, ...	female,	37 yrs.
Formad ("Univ. Med. Mag.," 1892, vol. IV, p. 625), . . .	male,	29 yrs.
Fütterer ("Virchow's Archiv," 1886, Bd. CVI, S. 555), . . .	male,	14 yrs.
Gee ("St. Bartholomew's Hosp. Reports," 1884, vol. XX, p. 191),	male,	4½ yrs.
" (ibid.), ...	male,	4 yrs.
Generisch ("Jahrb. f. Kinderheilk.," 1894, Bd. XXXVII, S. 91),	female,	1¼ yrs.
Griffith ("Amer. Jour. of the Med. Sci.," September, 1899), .	male,	2 yrs. 11 mos.
Hadden ("Internat. Clinics," 1893, vol. IV, p. 53), ...	male,	11 weeks.
Harrington (reported by Fitz, l. c., p. 133), ...	male,	40 yrs.
Henoch ("Beitr. z. Kinderheilk.," 1861, S. 123), ...	male,	1¼ yrs.
Hichens ("Lancet," 1898, vol. II, p. 1121), ...	male,	20 yrs.
Hirschsprung ("Jahrb. f. Kinderheilk.," 1888, Bd. XXVII, S. 1; "Pädiat. Arbeiten," "Henoch's Festschr.," 1890, S. 78), ...	male,	8 mos.
" (ibid.), ...	male,	7 mos.
"	male,	2½ mos.
"	male,	10 yrs.

Hobbs and de Richemond ("La méd. moderne," 1898, vol. IX,
    p. 652), ... female,   2½ yrs.
Hughes ("Trans. Path. Soc. of Phila.," 1887, vol. XIII, p. 40), male,   3 yrs.
Martin ("Montreal Med. Jour.," 1897, vol. XXV, p. 697), . male,   3½ yrs.
Mya ("Lo Sperimentale," 1894, vol. XLVIII, p. 215), . . . female,   2½ mos.
    " (ibid.), ... male,   5½ mos.
Osler ("Archives of Pediatrics," 1893, vol. X, p. 111), . . . male,   10 yrs.
Peacock ("Trans. Path. Soc. of London," 1872, vol. XXIII,
    p. 104), ... male,   28 yrs.
Rolleston and Haward ("Trans. Clinical Soc. of London,"
    1896, vol. XXIX, p. 201), ... male,   12 yrs.
Walker and Griffith ("Brit. Med. Jour.," 1893, vol. II, p. 230), male,   11 yrs.

Prognosis.—From the accompanying statistics it is very evident that the prognosis is grave. Of 26 cases, 19 are known to have terminated fatally. Only 3 patients—those of Fitz, Cheadle, and Osler—are known to have recovered: Fitz's case after resection of the dilated sigmoid flexure, by Richardson; Cheadle's case recovered under medical treatment; and Osler's after the establishment of an artificial anus by Halsted. The four remaining non-fatal cases disappeared from observation.

Diagnosis.—The diagnosis is evident from the symptoms enumerated, the age of the patient, constipation, and the distention. Often the diagnosis can be made on inspection, the distended colon being outlined through the abdominal wall. Examination of the rectum by finger or small proctoscope should in no case be omitted. As Griffith emphasizes, a sharp diagnostic line between idiopathic and obstructive congenital cases can not always be made out. Electrodiaphany of the colon may be executed in doubtful cases.

Treatment.—The treatment may be medical or surgical. The purely medical treatment consists of the use of laxatives, enemata, massage, electricity, and strychnin. One of the cases, that of Hughes, is reported to have been made worse by enemata. The use of the rectal tube for the evacuation of gases is a simple procedure, and often brings great comfort to the patient. If the tube be of the Langdon type, it may give information of the course and permeability of the colon. Puncture of the intestine with a fine trocar was executed in the cases of Hirschsprung, Hobbs and Richemond, and Martin. If the cases do not improve after a week's trial of purely medical means, they should be subjected to exploratory laparotomy. Fitz's case of resection of the sigmoid recovered, as also the case reported by Osler, in which Halsted made an artificial anus. The case of Griffith, in which an artificial anus was made, terminated fatally, and death was attributed to the exhaustion of the patient, the operation having been undertaken too late. The brilliant operation undertaken by Treves in a case of secondary congenital dilation due to stenosis resulted in recovery.

LITERATURE.

I. IDIOPATHIC DILATIONS OF THE COLON.

1. Bertie, "La Pediatria," 1894, vol. III, pp. 136, 161 ; "Contributo alla causuistica della dilatazione congenita del colon," "Pediatrica," Firenze, 1895, vol. III, pp. 136, 161, 1 Plate.

2. Bristowe, "Brit. Med. Jour.," 1885, vol. I, p. 1086.

3. Cheadle, W. B., "Idiopathic Dilation of the Colon," "Lancet," London, 1898, vol. I, p. 399; "Lancet," London, 1886, vol. II, p. 1117.

4. Fitz, "Amer. Jour. of the Med. Sci.," 1899, vol CXVIII, p. 132.

5. Formad, "Univ. Med. Mag.," 1892, vol. IV, p. 625.

6. Fütterer, "Virchow's Archiv," 1886, Bd. CVI, S. 555.

7. Gee, "St. Bartholomew's Hospital Reports," 1884, vol. XX, p. 19.

8. Generisch, "Jahrb. f. Kinderheilk.," 1894, Bd. XXXVII, S. 91 ; "Avastagbel veleszuletett tagulassa es tul tengesse" ("Congenital Dilation and Hypertrophy of the Colon"), "Orvosi hetil," Budapest, 1893, Bd. XXXVII, 583, 596; also translation (abstract), "Pest. med.-chir. Presse," Budapest, 1894, Bd. XXX, S. 51, 56.

9. Hadden, "Internat. Clinics," 1893, vol. IV, p. 53.

10. Henoch, "Beitr. z. Kinderheilk.," 1861, S. 123.

11. Herringham, W. P., and Clark, W. B., "A Case of Idiopathic Dilation of the Sigmoid Flexure," "St. Bartholomew's Hospital Reports," London, 1895, vol. XXXI, pp. 57–62 ; also abstract, "Lancet," London, 1894, vol. II, p. 1281 ; also abstract, "Brit. Med. Jour.," London, 1894, vol. II, p. 1240.

12. Hichens, "Lancet," 1898, vol. II, p. 1121.

13. Hirschsprung, "Stuhltragheit Neugeborener in Folge von Dilatation und Hypertrophie des Colons," "Jahrb. f. Kinderheilk.," Leipzig, 1887, n. f. Bd. XXVII, S. 1–7 ; "Jahrb. f. Kinderheilk.," 1888, Bd. XXVII, S. 1 ; "Pädiat. Arbeiten," "Henoch's Festschr.," 1890, S. 78.

14. Hobbs and de Richemond, "La méd moderne," 1898, vol. IX, p. 652.

15. Howden, R., "A Case of Marked Distention of Transverse and Descending Parts of the Colon," "Jour. Anat. and Phys.," London, 1897 and 1898, vol. XXXII, pp.67–75.

16. Hughes, "Trans. Patholog. Soc. of Phila.," 1887, vol. XIII, p. 40.

17. Jewell, J. S., "Neurol. Review," Chicago, 1886, vol. I, pp. 218–226.

18. Martin, "Montreal Med. Jour.," 1897, vol. XXV, p. 697.

19. Money, A., and Paget, S., "A Case of So-called Idiopathic Dilation of the Colon," "Trans. Clin. Soc. of London," 1887–88, vol. XXI, pp. 103, 106 ; also abstract, "Lancet," London, 1888, vol. I, p. 221 ; also abstract, "Brit. Med. Jour.," London, 1888, vol. I, p. 246; also abstract, "Med. Press. and Circ.," London, 1888, n. s., vol. XIV, p. 110.

20. Mya, G., "Lo Sperimentale," 1894, vol. XLVIII, p. 215.

21. Osler, W., "On Dilation of the Colon in Young Children," "Archives of Pediatrics," New York, 1893, vol. X, p. 111; also reprint; also "J. H. U. Bulletin," Baltimore, 1893, vol. LV, pp. 41–93.

22. Peacock, "Trans. Pathol. Soc. of London," 1872, vol. XXIII, p. 104.

23. Rissler, J., "Wtvidgning af colon tranversum somorsak till ileus; laparatomi; helsa" ("Dilation of the Colon Transversum as the Cause of Ileus; Laparotomy; Recovery"), "Hygiea," Stockholm, 1896, vol. LVIII, pt. 2, p. 659.

24. Rolleston and Haward, "Trans. Clin. Soc. of London," 1896, vol. XXIX, p. 201.

25. Walker and Griffith, "Brit. Med. Jour.," 1893, vol. II, p. 230.

II. DISPLACEMENTS AND SECONDARY DILATIONS OF THE COLON.

1. Banks, "Dublin Jour. Med. Sci.," 1846, vol. I, p. 235.

2. Chapman, "Brit. Med. Jour.," 1878, vol. I, p. 566.

3. Ebers, "Hufeland's Jour.," August, 1836, vol. LXXXIII, p. 62.

4. Eisenhart, "Centralbl. f. d. innere Med.," 1894, S. 1153.

5. Favilla, "Gazetta medica di Milano," 1846, vol. V, p. 213.

6. Gay, "Trans. Pathol. Soc. of London," 1854, vol. V, p. 174.

7. Goodhart, "Trans. Clin. Soc. of London," 1881, vol. XIV, p. 84.

8. Harrington, "Chicago Med. Jour. and Exam.," 1878, vol. XXXVI, p. 400.

9. Herringham and Clarke, "St. Bartholomew's Hospital Reports," 1895, vol. XXXI, p. 57.

10. Kennedy, "Med. Press and Circ.," London, 1883, n. s., vol. XXXVI, p. 149.

11. Lacave, "Verhandl. van het Genootschap ter Bevord der Geness en Heilkunde te Amsterdam," II. Deel, I. Stuck, 1858, 7.

12. Lespinasse, "Jour. de Med. de Bordeaux," 1888–89, vol. XVIII, p. 427.

13. Lewitt, "Chicago Med. Jour.," 1867, vol. XXIV, p. 359.

14. Little and Callaway, "Trans. Pathol. Soc. of London," 1851, vol. III, p. 106.

15. Money and Paget, "Trans. Clin. Soc. of London," 1888, vol. XXI, p. 103.

16. Morris, "Brit. Med. Jour.," 1886, vol. II, p. 1211.

17. Noorden, von, "Münch. med. Wochenschr," 1895, Bd. XLII, S. 598.

18. Oulmont, "Bull. Soc. Anat. de Par.," 1842, vol. XVII, p. 336.

19. Parry, "Posthumous Works," vol. II, p. 380.

20. Pennato, P., "Rivene ta di sc. med.," Venezia, 1887, vol. VI, p. 486.

21. Pippinskold, "Finska tak sallsk handl Helsingfors," 1880, XXII, 410.

22. Rissler, J., "Hygiea," Stockholm, 1896, vol. LVIII, pt. 2, p. 659.

23. Strahan, "Lancet," 1893, vol. II, p. 1245.

24. Thomas, C. H., "Cincinnati Lancet-Clinic," 1883, n. s., vol. XI, p. 573; also "Illust. M. and S.," New York, 1883, vol. II, p. 194; also reprint; also "Maryland Med. Jour.," Balt., 1883, p. 588; also "Polyclinic," Philadelphia, 1883, vol. I; p. 85; also "Proc. Phila. Co. Med. Soc.," Philadelphia, 1883, vol. VI, p. 79; also "Boston Med. and Surg. Jour.," 1884, vol. CXI; also "Med. and Surg. Reporter," 1884, vol. I, p. 75; also "New York Med. Jour.," 1884, vol. XXXIX, p. 25.

25. Trastour, E., "J. de med. de l'ouest," Nantes, 1880, vol. XIV, p. 8–33; "Gaz. med. de Nantes," 1884, vol. III, p. 81.

26. Vulpian, "Gaz. d. Hôpitaux," 1877, p. 75.

27. Wallman, "Virchow's Archiv," Bd. XIV, S. 202.

28. Wells, "Trans. of the Society for the Improvement of Medical and Surgical Knowledge," 1812, vol. III, p. 158.

INTESTINAL DIVERTICULA. PERSISTENT OMPHALOMESEN-TERIC (VITELLINE) REMAINS. INTESTINAL DUPLICA-TIONS.

A diverticulum of the intestine is usually a sacculation of the ileum due to non-obliteration of the vitelline duct. Diverticula represent offshoots or extensions from the normal channel of the bowel, and may be congenital or acquired. Congenital diverticula are composed of all the layers of the intestinal wall, but the acquired diverticula only of the mucosa and serosa, one of which is usually protruded through a slit in the muscularis. The congenital forms are also known as true and the acquired as false diverticula. This classification is not invariable, for there are exceptional forms of the acquired type in which the diverticulum is composed of all the layers of the intestinal wall. The first description and illustration of this abnormality was given in 1701 by Ruysch ("Thesaurus anatomicus," 1701, p. 283), and its origin from the omphalo-enteric duct was suggested by Morgagni ("The Seats and Causes of Diseases," 1769, vol. II, p. 141). We are indebted to Meckel, however, for the first logical explanation of the manner in which this embryonic malformation arises, and for having emphasized its importance in the etiology of abdominal diseases.

Congenital Diverticula.—I have already dwelt upon the views of Meckel in the general chapter on the Enterostenoses, and also in the chapter on the Acute and Chronic Intestinal Occlusions—Ileus, this volume. The reader is referred to these chapters for the pathological relations of the so-called diverticulum of Meckel. It is usually situated ½ to 1 meter (12 inches to 3 feet) above the ileocecal valve. In exceptional cases it was found very close to the ileocecal valve—5 cm. above it—and in other cases it was found in the jejunum. Lobstein and Wrisberg have observed a connection of the vitelline duct with the duodenum, according to Meckel (Reil u. Autenrieth, "Arch. f. Physiol.," 1809, Bd. IX, S. 428). The length of the diverticulum of Meckel varies from 1 inch to 4 inches on the average (3 to 10 cm.). Cases have been reported in which it was 10 inches (25 cm.) long. Its wall corresponds exactly to that of the ileum in histological structure, containing Lieberkühn's glands and Peyer's patches. As a rule, the diverticulum arises from the convex side of the intestine, opposite to the insertion of the mesentery. If it is situated in close proximity to this insertion it may possess its own mesenteriolum. If the diverticulum is closed toward the intestinal lumen, cystic dilations may develop, due to retention of the secretions. These are known as enterocystomas. Roth has found the cylindrical cells in such an enterocystoma lined with cilia ("Virchow's Archiv," Bd. LXXXVI, S. 371; see also literature, Orth's "Specielle pathologische Anatomie," vol. I, p. 771). In rare instances the diverticulum establishes an open communication between the ileum and the external abdominal surface, terminating in a small opening at the umbilicus, through which the intestinal contents may escape. In the chapter on Strangulations and Incarcerations the mechanism is pictured by which the Meckel diverticula may give rise to those forms of intestinal obstruction. It is generally not as wide throughout its course as it is at its place of origin from the ileum, and the bulbous or globular termination at its free end is due either to the accumulation of contents or a hernia-like protuberance of the mucosa or submucosa through the muscularis. The terminal end is, as a rule, free, and only exceptionally adherent at the umbilicus. As a result of inflammatory adhesion, the distal end may become attached to any place within the abdominal cavity with which its length permits it to come into contact. Its most frequent location for attachment is the mesentery. Other locations are at any part of the small intestine, cecum, colon, pelvic viscera, inner abdominal wall, omentum. Fitz ("Amer. Jour. of the Med. Sci.," 1884, p. 30), in a masterly contribution, has called attention to the rôle played by this abnormality in the causation of obstruction, cyst formation, and intestinal duplication, the so-called double cecums (Lockwood) and double colon (Scheiber, "Oesterr. med. Jahrb.," H. 2; also "Jahresb. von Virchow u. Hirsch," 1875, Bd. I, S. 79). Andrau ("Treatise on Pathology") refers to a case mentioned by Brugoni, in which two colons sprang from a single cecum and reunited at the rectum. The literature on duplication of the intestine is reviewed in the article by Fitz, above cited, and the view advanced that one of the two tubes is, as a rule, a diverticulum.

In a case of intestinal obstruction occurring in my private practice, the cause of the ileus was found at operation to be a Meckel diverticulum 2 inches long, which had become inverted and pro-

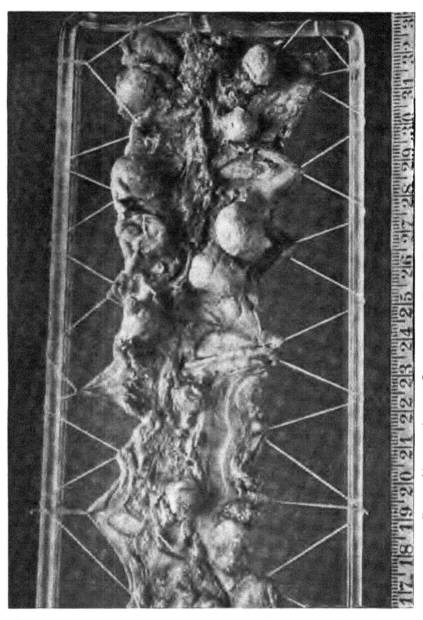

Fig. 10.—Multiple Acquired Diverticula of Colon. View from Peritoneal Surface.

461

truded into the ileum 18 inches from the ileocecal valve. A mass of hard fecal matter held it in its position and completed the stenosis. There were evidences of enterospasm at the laparotomy. Resection of the diverticulum was performed and the patient recovered.

Acquired Diverticula.—The acquired diverticula are herniaform protuberances of the mucosa and serosa in which the muscularis is absent. In exceptional cases all the intestinal layers were represented, but the term hernias of the mucosa, as applied by Rokitansky, is insufficient, because it does not mention the serosa, which is included in all forms. They usually occur on the side of the intestine where the mesentery is inserted, generally being surrounded by the two sheaths of the mesentery. As a rule, they occur in larger numbers, and are only exceptionally isolated. They vary from the size of a pea to that of a large orange, and are usually of a spherical or cylindrical shape. Wallmann ("Virchow's Archiv," Bd. xiv) has observed 9 of them in the colon, and Hansemann ("Virchow's Archiv," Bd. cxliv) has described 400 diverticula in one case in which they were most frequent in the jejunum and upper ileum, whereas the lower ileum, cecum, and colon were comparatively free ; the sigmoid, however, was very closely crowded with these protuberances. Generally they are more frequent in the large intestine and rectum than in the jejunum, ileum, and duodenum. It is interesting to note that even in the vermiform process small diverticula have been observed. Acquired malformations of this kind may, as a rule, be considered under two headings: (1) Pulsion diverticula, due to pressure upon the wall of the intestine from within, and (2) traction diverticula, which are due to drawing upon the intestinal wall from the outside. One of the conditions for the development of the pulsion diverticula is a place or spot where there is a lessened resistance in the intestinal wall. These spots are found to be at the transition of the mesenteric vessels into the intestinal wall. A case showing the intimate connection between the bloodvessels and the paths through which the false diverticula protrude is described by Martin H. Fisher ("Jour. of Exper. Med.," vol. v, p. 332). He also presents the illustration of a false diverticulum of the appendix (*ibid.*, plate xxiv), and gives a graphic description of the microscopic appearance of the development of the protrusion.

The literature of this subject is compiled in this article. Pulsion diverticula are most frequently found in the colon, where, as is well known, there are small protuberances present normally. Their origin here has been attributed to persistent obstipation. Pulsion diverticula have been described after obturation from gall-stone and in the suprastenotic changes which occur in obstruction. The traction diverticula are small funnel-shaped pouches caused by retraction of chronic localized peritonitis or mesenteritis by cicatrices in the wall of the intestine itself, or by inflammatory processes in adjacent organs. They have been observed after atrophy of the pancreas, and Birch-Hirschfeld described a case of traction diverticulum in which pseudo-ligamentous retractions of the mesentery were attached to the apex of the protuberance. Hanau, Hansemann, Grasberger, and Klebs have described the relation of the mucous hernias or protuberances of the intestine to the places of exit of the mesenteric veins. Such protuberances of the mucosa along the venous sheaths could be produced experimentally by increased intra-intestinal pressure. Acquired diverticula may give rise to stercoral ulcers, perforation, and peritonitis in rare cases; otherwise they have little clinical significance and escape recognition during life. Nothnagel (*l. c.*, p. 254) has described a case which was diagnosed either as sarcoma of the intestine or peritoneal tuberculosis with tubercular stricture. At the autopsy both conditions were found; but what interests us here specially is the formation of diverticula of a semiglobular shape at the places where the larger neoplasms were located.

Displacements of the Intestine. Enteroptosis. Coloptosis.

The subject of enteroptosis, or dislocations and misplacements of the intestine, has already been fully considered in the author's work on " Diseases of the Stomach," second edition, pages 695 to 732, because it was impossible to give a correct representation of gastroptosis alone without at the same time going into the pathogenesis of dislocations of the intestine. The displacements of the colon have also been considered in that chapter, page 724. In the chapter on the Anatomy and Histology of the Intestine (vol. 1, p. 17), Dr. J. Holmes Smith has considered these abnormalities from the anatomic standpoint. The reader is referred to these two articles for a more explicit statement of these conditions. Among the older writers who have considered this subject are Annesley, Esquirol, Fleischmann (1815), de Häen, Ruysch. Morgagni also has distinct references to these abnormalities of position. The dislocations which have been caused by peritonitic adhesions were first described accurately by Virchow ("Virchow's Archiv," 1853, Bd. v, S. 281). The historical references on dislocations of the abdominal viscera and the various publications of Ewald, Meinert, and Landau, in Germany, and Glénard and others, in France, have been referred to in the work on "Diseases of the Stomach," pages 698 to 700. In 1885 Glénard, in a rather schematic and fantastic publication, which nevertheless was a presentation of careful clinical observation, forwarded the idea that the descent of the right or hepatic flexure of the colon, followed by dislocation of the transverse colon, was the primary disturbance in enteroptosis. When the hepatic flexure of the colon has sunk, the right half of the transverse colon follows up to the place where it is connected with the pyloric end of the stomach by the tense gastrocolic ligament; here the colon becomes kinked or inflected, and stagnation of contents results. The prestenotic part of the colon becomes dilated, but the part beyond the stenosis contracts, so that it can be felt as a tense cord. This is an inflection with stagnation meteorism and no local meteorism. Ewald confirmed the clinical observations of Glénard, in the main, but does not agree with him on the etiology. The palpable colon beyond the stenosis which Glénard designated as " cord colique transverse " is considered by Ewald to be the pancreas. Recent investigations by Kelling, Kuttner, Hertz, Metlzing, Langenhand, Schwedt, and Rosengart have attempted to clear up the subject of the pathogenesis of dislocations of the intestine, by experimental investigation, but the three publications to which we are, above all others, indebted for a clearer intelligence and more comprehensive representation of this subject, are by Leichtenstern (von Ziemssen's "Handbuch," Bd. vii, 2. aufl., S. 509), Curschmann ("Deutsch. Arch. f. klin. Med.," 1894, Bd. liii, S. 1), Fleiner ("Münch. med. Wochenschr.," 1895, No. 42–45). Abnormalities of position may occur in both the small and the large intestine, but as the former is only brought about by inflections, kinkings, compressions, and herniaform dislocations, the abnormalities of position of the small intestine have accordingly been considered under these headings in other chapters, and I will here limit myself to the consideration of abnormalities of position of the colon.

Intestinal displacements may be acquired or congenital. Acquired abnormalities of position, size, and capacity have been considered in the author's work on " Diseases of the Stomach," and in the chapter on idiopathic dilation of the colon. The theory of Rosengart ("Zeitschr. f. Diät. u. physikal. Therapie," Bd. 1, S. 220) advances the view that (1) the congenital enteroptosis is the persistence of the fetal situation of all or of a part of the abdominal viscera; (2) acquired enteroptosis is the gradual retrograde development from the normal to the congenital or fetal position. The views of Langerhans have already been cited in the article in my work on "Diseases of the Stomach." Leichtenstern (*l. c.*) gives a sketch of four principal causes of coloptosis: (1) The most frequent is failure of the cecum to descend into the right iliac fossa; it remains posterior to and in contact with the liver; (2) defective development of the muscular ligaments of the colon, which results in excessive length of the large intestine, because it is not brought together by the muscular contractions; (3) disproportion between a deficient fetal development of the abdominal cavity, on the one hand, and excessive development in length of the colon oh the other; (4) abnormal development in the length of the mesentery, permitting of excessive movability of the colon, and consequently of the formation of abnormal flexures.

Congenital Abnormalities of Position and Form.—Curschmann (*l. c.*) describes the following congenital variations of displacements of the large intestine:

1. In the cecum and ascending colon, (*a*) whilst the cecum is attached in its normal position, excessive development of the ascending mesocolon may give rise to actual loop formation in the ascending colon, a genuine volvulus; (*b*) enlargement and elongation of the cecum, taking in also the beginning of the ascending colon, and giving rise to twists and rotation around the longitudinal axis of the cecum, with eventual intestinal occlusion; (*c*) inflection and kinking of the cecum, being thrown back toward the liver covering a corresponding portion of the ascending colon; the vermiform process may thus come in contact with the edge of the liver, or even extend beneath it; these cases, which Curschmann describes in an interesting clinical history, should they develop appendicitis, may present all the clinical signs of cholelithiasis; (d) persistence of the cecum or appendix in contact or posterior to the liver; the ascending colon is shortened or absent entirely. This places the vermiform process in juxtaposition to the biliary passages, and if there should be any appendicial or peri-appendicial inflammation, the differential diagnosis from cholelithiasis would be extremely difficult.

2. *Transverse Colon and Flexures.* — (a) Either the hepatic or splenic flexure may be absent, but the colon be abnormally short; (b) one or the other of these flexures is wanting; the colon, however, is abnormally long. When the flexures are wanting and the colon abnormally short, the ascending colon runs from the ileocecal region on the right, upward toward the middle and posterior portion of the abdomen and underneath the liver. There is either no transverse colon at all or a very short one, which immediately passes over into the descending colon in the left lower and outer abdominal region. A similar description is given by Rosengart (*l. c.*) of the course of the ascending colon in the neonat. (See article on Enteroptosis in author's "Diseases of the Stomach," second edition, *l. c.*) When the flexures are absent and the colon is abnormally elongated, the transverse colon is replaced by an immense loop or several loops with closely approximated limbs, which generally cover the anterior portion of the abdomen and are also anterior to the liver. This condition necessarily replaces the normal anterior liver dullness by a loud tympanitic resonance; the normal hepatic dullness, however, can still be made out on the lateral and posterior abdominal region. Sometimes the liver exhibits a permanent groove with an indurated and thickened peritoneal lining, representing the bed in which the loop of the colon rested.

3. *Descending Colon and Sigmoid Flexure.* — (a) Abnormal elongation of the loops of the sigmoid flexure. Such abnormally long sigmoid loops are, as a rule, found in the middle of the abdomen, their long axes parallel to the linea alba. They may extend up into the vault of the diaphragm, and cover over the stomach, the left lobe, and part of the right lobe of the liver. Under such conditions it happens that the region which is normally occupied when the sigmoid and descending colon are of regular size

is now superimposed by loops of small intestine.   This necessarily brings about the following change under pathologic conditions : The entire abdomen may be tympanitic by distended sigmoid
loops, and the lower and outer portions of the left inferior abdominal region will not give any evidence of meteorism, because in this
place the loops of small intestine lie anteriorly.   (*b*) Persistence
of the relatively long sigmoid flexure of the infant in adults.   This
is fortunately a rare condition, as Curschmann found it only 15
times in 233 autopsies.   (*c*) Double sigmoid loops.   This must be
an equally rare condition.   I have not found it once in 180 autopsies examined especially for the purpose.   (*d*) Occurrence of an
abnormally strong loop between the lower limb of the sigmoid
flexure and the beginning of the rectum.   Curschmann calls attention to the fact that this abnormal loop and the cecum may come
into juxtaposition in the right iliac fossa ; thus the beginning and
end of the colon are in contact with each other,—a most embarrassing abnormality when it should become necessary to make an
artificial anus under such conditions, for the mistake is very easily
made that the lowermost end of the colon could be sewed into the
abdominal orifice and thus the large intestine opened below the
point of occlusion.

Acquired Abnormalities of Position and Form.—According
to Fleiner (*l. c.*), disturbances in the location of the colon are traceable to abnormal inflections and kinks, which produce a disturbance
of the movement of the feces.   He ascribes these abnormalities in
part to a condition of atonic obstipation, and as some of the etiological factors he cites a number of agencies which exert increased
pressure upon individual sections of the colon ; for instance, corsets,
belts, an attitude during work which inclines the body too much
forward, sedentary habits of life.   This author has cited a number
of very interesting clinical histories illustrating the difficulty with
which such cases are differentiated from cholelithiasis.   In addition
to the functional disturbances mentioned, organic changes in the
intestinal wall may supervene.   Thus we may be confronted with
catarrhal changes, expressing themselves clinically in diarrhea or
constipation alternating with diarrhea, and occasionally only the
symptom of constipation is present in connection with membranous
colitis.   This condition of visceral dislocations with colicky pains,

or pains corresponding to what has been described as enteralgia, has received much attention from French authors, and is liable to be confounded with hepatic and renal colic, intercostal neuralgia, the crises of tabes, and duodenal ulcer.

These abnormalities of position, when they occur in association with neurasthenia gastrica or intestinalia, are, in my experience, very perplexing problems for diagnosis.   When such patients complain for months and years of extreme pain in localized areas of the abdomen, and examination of the feces, analysis of test-meals, blood, and urine, and physical examination of the abdomen and rectum reveal no positive abnormal indications, the physician has seemingly struck his "pons asinorum."   The symptoms, in addition to pain, are feeling of pressure, distention and fullness in the stomach, intestinal colic, conditions of the bowels as described in the preceding, flatulence, more frequently constipation, loss of will power, loss of weight, depression of spirit, incapacity for decided mental or physical exertion.   Boas correctly observes that a large number of physicians, without going into detailed examination of the viscera, falsely interpret these symptoms as the expression either of anemia, gastric or intestinal catarrh, or sometimes of hysteria alone ; then they order preparations of iron ; or when they expect gastro-intestinal catarrh, purgatives or bismuth preparations are given, sometimes with intestinal antiseptics (so called) ; and when they suspect hysteria the prescriptions call for bromids, valerian, and asafetida.   These are the cases which most frequently drift into the hands of the specialist with wrong diagnoses.   Yet I see no reason why a correct diagnosis in at least a large number of such cases should not be made.   I am now speaking only of those types of acquired dislocations of the stomach and colon which are due to atony and acquired inflections partially traceable to obstipation, and not due to those forms which Curschmann has so minutely described, and to which I have referred in the preceding—namely, of congenitally abnormal formations and dislocations as well as elongations of the colon.   The main object to bear in mind in the acquired types described by Fleiner is to determine the size and location of the stomach and transverse colon.   This can be done in the great majority of cases by distention with air ; either distending each individually by air, or first the stomach with air and then the colon thereafter with water.   The course of the colon may also be made out in many cases by electrodiaphany.   When it is intended to illuminate the colon and map out its course by this method, the position and size of the stomach should be determined first.   The same limitations and restrictions apply to the method when used for the determination of the anatomic course of the colon as have been referred to in connection with illumination of the stomach.   I used it first in 1891 for transillumination of the colon, and demonstrated it to the Clinical Society of Maryland in that year.   In 1892 Heryng and Reichmann published the first account of transillumination of the colon by this method.   (See article on Electrodiaphany, "Diseases of the Stomach," second edition, pp. 104–112.)   In 1898 Boas and Levi-Dorn described a method by which the course of the intestine could be traced out by means of the Röntgen rays and the skiagraph.   The patient was given a capsule filled with chemically pure bismuth subnitrate, and the course of the capsule observed on the fluoroscope.   The method has not been applied to a sufficiently large clinical material to permit of any deductions concerning its diagnostic value.   Dr. M. K. Kassabian, of Philadelphia, has kindly presented us with a skiagraph which illustrates the possibilities of this method for locating individual portions of the intestine (see Plate 7, p. 285).   If the enteroptosis, coloptosis, and gastroptosis can be determined in this way, the treatment outlined in the chapter on Enteroptosis, in the author's book on "Diseases of the Stomach," second edition, pages 726–730, should be undertaken and continued for at least three to four months.   If after this trial of purely medical treatment there is no very decided improvement, the case should be considered from the surgical aspect, whether or not a replacement of the dislocated organs, and attachment in their normal position, is possible by operation.   The colon is most frequently dislocated by the weight of accumulated fecal contents, and by the weight of neoplasms, to which perhaps coprostasis has supervened, adding to the bulk which the intestine has to carry.   If the colon has, in addition to these abnormalities, a long mesentery, the dislocation will occur so much more readily.   The dislocations of the colon to which Virchow first called attention were those due to circumscribed peritonitis, generally producing an adhesion at a remote place from its normal location.

Abnormal elongation and position of the colon need not necessarily give rise to symptoms during life. I have observed a number
of cases of exceedingly great elongation of the colon, in which
there had not been even the sign of obstipation during life. In
other instances the abnormal elongation may be the cause of
volvulus, loop formation, and incarceration. The greatest significance is attached to these abnormalities from the diagnostic standpoint; if, for instance, the loops have covered the liver in such a
way as to prevent the elicitation of the normal liver dullness by
percussion, the difficulty of diagnosing a pathological reduction
of the size of the liver is very great. I have already pointed out
that when the appendix is located underneath the liver a possible
appendicitis may be confounded with cholelithiasis and perforating
gall-stones. To this is added the further complication that the
recognition of these abnormalities in size, form, and location
presents insurmountable difficulties if a volvulus, an inflection, or
peritonitic adhesion has occurred.

Treatment.—The treatment of these abnormalities varies with
their nature and the underlying cause. Sometimes the Weir
Mitchell rest cure, associated with hydrotherapy, electricity, and
massage, is of marked assistance in restoring health. In all cases
a properly adjusted abdominal bandage should be worn. Obstipation calls for special treatment. Strychnin and a readily assimilable
form of iron (ferratin) are frequently decidedly beneficial. Whenever three months of medical treatment produce no decided benefits, gastropexy, gastrorrhaphy, colonopexy, or resection of part of
the elongated colon, should be considered.

Dr. H. W. Lincoln is enthusiastic in recommending a plaster
bandage applied to the lower abdomen in such a way as not
to contain too much of the plaster, which would be too heavy and
too rigid ("New York Med. Record," January 12, 1901, p. 69).
They are made of narrow strips of zinc plaster, 2 or 3 inches wide,
which are applied over the abdomen, reaching around to the back.
I have used these bandages, and the patients accredit to them a
decided benefit. Unfortunately, they can not be readily removed,
and therefore they interfere with daily applications of electricity to
the abdomen, should this be considered necessary.

CHAPTER IX.

DISEASES OF THE INTESTINAL BLOOD-VESSELS.

I. Embolism and Thrombosis of the Mesenteric Artery.—II. Embolism and Thrombosis of the Mesenteric Vein.—III. Venous Congestion of the Intestine.—IV. Dilation of the Hemorrhoidal Veins.

EMBOLISM AND THROMBOSIS OF THE MESENTERIC ARTERY.

Plates 8, 9, 10, and 11, showing the distribution and topography of the mesenteric vessels, should be consulted where the text refers to the anatomy of these structures.

The intestinal vessels may become the seat of disease resulting in embolism and thrombosis from the same pathological conditions that cause these abnormalities elsewhere. There are, however, two constitutional diseases which may specifically affect the intestinal blood-vessels ; these are syphilis and amyloidosis. Embolism and thrombosis of the mesenteric artery are extremely rare conditions, as I could collect only 40 cases, two of which are not published in literature, but occurred one at the Johns Hopkins Hospital, and one in my own clinical practice. Faber ("Deutsch. Arch. f. klin. Med.," Bd. xvi) and Litten ("Virchow's Arch.," Bd. LXIII, and "Deutsch. med. Wochenschr.," 1889, No. 8) had collected 20 cases up to the year 1875. The first three cases were reported by Virchow, to whom the science of pathology is indebted for the first concept and description of the embolic and thrombotic processes. The occlusion of the mesenteric artery, in the great majority of these cases, occurred by an embolism—*i. e.*, by a plug of blood fibrin or other material brought with the current from a distant part of the circulation, and forming an obstruction at its place of lodgment. Only in exceptional cases did the occlusion come about by an autochthonous thrombus ("*autochthonous*," meaning formed in the place where it was found). The origin of the embolus was traced to three different sources. The majority of them originated in the heart, where endocarditis with valvular disease or thrombi were found ; next most frequently the place of origin was a focus of atheromatous degeneration of the aorta. In rare cases the embolus had its origin in the pulmonary vein, where clots had been formed as a result of gangrenous pulmonary infarctions. Litten (*l. c.*) has described two cases, and Firket and Malvoz (cited by Nothnagel, *l. c.*, p. 454) have described one case of autochthonous thrombosis of the mesenteric artery ; but in the latter case there is some doubt as regards the autochthonous nature of the thrombus, because the subject gave evidence of atheromatous degeneration not only in the mesenteric artery, but also in the aorta and endocardium. In the cases thus far reported in literature the superior mesenteric artery is most frequently occluded. The inferior mesentery is occluded but rarely. Only two cases of the latter have been reported, and reference to them can be found in the article by Litten (*l. c.*). One of these cases occurred in the experience of Gerhardt, but it was complicated by a simultaneous plugging up of the superior mesenteric artery. The other case was reported by Hegar, and constitutes an uncomplicated obturation of the inferior mesenteric artery. The mucosa of the colon, sigmoid, and rectum was infiltrated, congested, and presented numerous superficial blood extravasations of variable size. There was no necrosis or hemorrhagic infarction of the mucosa.

Thrombotic or embolic occlusion of the superior mesenteric artery occurs in three main types or variations : (1) Either the main trunk of the artery may be occluded near its origin from the aorta, or (2) one of the larger branches may be obturated ; finally (3) one of the smaller branches, or one of the very finest terminal branches, may be obturated. As the obturating process is usually secondary to endarteritis somewhere else, or to cardiac valvular disease, it is frequently observed that hemorrhagic infarcts of other organs, particularly of the spleen and kidneys, occurs contemporaneously with embolism of the intestinal vessels. According to Cohnheim, hemorrhagic infarcts can occur only in endarteries, or terminal arteries—*i. e.*, in vessels from which the establishment of a collateral circulation is anatomically impossible. The mesenteric arteries, however, are not terminal in the sense of Cohnheim. It is interesting to emphasize in this connection that one of the most extensive anastomoses in the body is formed by the

PLATE 8.

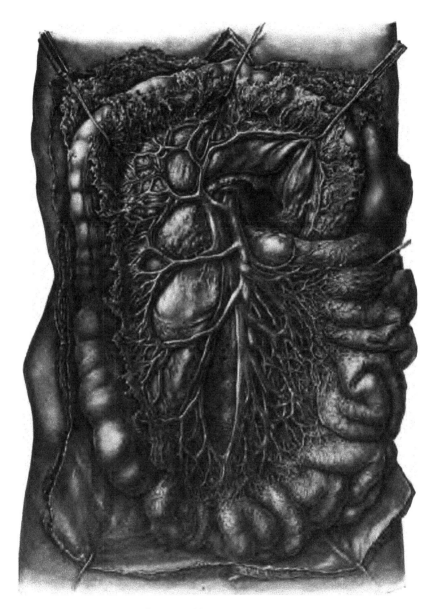

SUPERIOR MESENTERIC VESSELS.

The transverse colon is drawn up, great omentum removed, to show the superior mesenteric artery and vein and their distribution. The cecum and ascending colon are recognizable to the lower left of the drawing, and the coils of the ileum to the lower right.—(*From Deaver's "Surgical Anatomy."*)

left colic artery (which arises from the inferior mesenteric) with the median colic artery (arising from the superior mesenteric). In addition to this, the superior mesenteric communicates above with the celiac by means of the gastro-duodenal branch. It therefore requires an explanation of the mechanism of the tremendous circulatory disturbances which obturation of the superior mesenteric artery can bring about in spite of this apparently complete anastomosis. This has been furnished by the experiments of Litten (*l. c.*), which demonstrated that the superior mesenteric artery is a terminal or end-artery at least functionally, if not anatomically. It is true the entire immense vascular territory of this vessel can be injected and filled up from the aorta by way of the anastomoses just mentioned after the main stem has been ligated; but in the living human being or animal different conditions of pressure control the distribution of the circulating blood. When the superior mesenteric artery is ligated or obturated in the living animal, the blood pressure in its enormous circulatory territory becomes equal to zero, and the relatively small amount of blood which can flow in from the collateral branches—the inferior mesenteric and the pancreatico-duodenal—does not nearly suffice to raise it. What now happens is an inflow of blood from the portal vein's territory. This has a somewhat higher positive pressure than that from the collateral circulation before mentioned, and produces a venous hyperemia, with infarction of the tissues with venous blood and necrosis. Referring to the three main types of obturation, that of type (1)—plugging up the superior mesenteric near its origin from the aorta (see Plate 8)—involves the entire small intestine with the exception of the superior horizontal portion and the middle portion of the duodenum, and in addition the cecum, ascending and transverse colon. When one of the main branches of the artery is obturated we have a varying pathological picture according to the district which this branch supplies. This is relatively the most frequent form, and affects the ileum and lower jejunum most often. Whilst the types thus far considered affect either the entire small intestine or at least large parts of it, the parts invaded are, as a rule, connected, and represent one long continuous pathological alteration. But when a number of smaller branches are obturated, the areas of hemorrhagic infarction, venous hyperemia, edema and necrosis may be separated by apparently healthy districts. Cases in which the entire small intestine, cecum, ascending and transverse colon were affected in continuity have been described by Oppolzer ("Allgemein. Wien. med. Zeitschr.," 1858, 1862, and 1864), Faber (*l. c.*), and Kaufmann ("Virchow's Archiv," Bd. cxvi). Typical cases of embolism of the smaller arteries, in which diseased portions of the intestine were separated by healthy portions, were described by Firket and Malvoz (*l. c.*). When the very smallest arterial branches of the mesenteric artery are obturated, those which are contained within the structure of the intestinal wall itself, a pathological condition ensues which corresponds to the embolic and thrombotic ulcers which have been described in another chapter. In a case which I observed personally, one of the larger branches of the superior mesenteric was obturated by an embolus in a male patient afflicted with arterial sclerosis and with calcareous deposits upon the valves of the heart. Five and a half feet of the lower ileum were in a state of edema, venous congestion, and partial necrosis. The mucosa presented numerous areas of superficial necrosis, was of a greasy brownish-gray color, and was readily detached by a stream of water running from an ordinary hydrant, upon which it was tied for the purpose of cleansing the intestine of its contents. Numerous ulcers were found, especially in the lower portion of the ileum, some of them penetrating to the serosa. The intestinal lumen was filled with extravasated blood of a tarry consistency. The walls of the intestine were immensely thickened, the tissue loose and pulpy, and replete with a liquid the chemical nature of which corresponded to a mixture of serum and small amounts of blood. All of the arteries in the intestine were empty and contracted. The veins of the intestinal wall, of the peritoneum, and of the mesentery corresponding to the obturated district were enormously congested. On the peritoneal surface of the intestine, as well as in the mesentery and omentum, were numerous small extravasations of blood. The individual intestinal loops were covered with recent formations of fibrin, and there was a sero-sanguinolent peritonitic exudation. This case had presented itself with the symptoms of intestinal obstruction, and died before preparations could be made for operation.

Symptomatology.

The cases of obturation of the mesenteric arteries are so rare, and

PLATE 9.

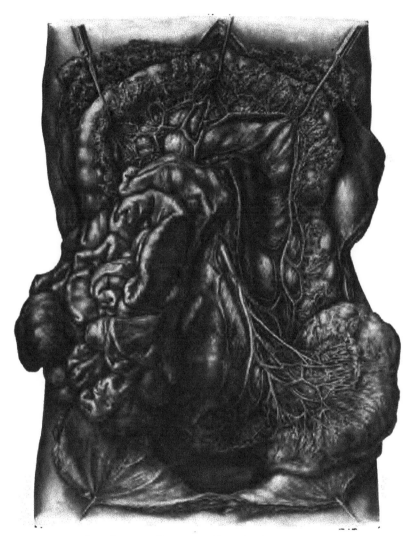

INFERIOR MESENTERIC VESSELS. ASPECT A.

The transverse colon is drawn up and the small intestine pulled aside. In the lower center of the illustration a few vertebræ are recognizable. To the right and left of these, the right and left common iliac artery. To the lower right, the inferior mesenteric artery and sigmoid colon are evident. Above, the transverse colon extends across the upper abdomen, and below, a glimpse into pelvic fossa.—(*From Deaver's "Surgical Anatomy."*)

present such great variations in their symptomatology, that an exhaustive or even a typical clinical picture of the condition can not be given. Whilst the pathological picture, as a rule, corresponds to that which I have just given in a case observed personally, the clinical pictures of the various cases that have the same pathological substratum by no means agree. Whether the cases are due to embolism or to autochthonous thrombosis, the onset is usually very sudden. The clinical situation is controlled by two conditions ; namely, either intestinal hemorrhages or intestinal occlusion. If the initial symptoms occurred in the midst of an already existing pathological condition of another character, it is easily understood how they may have passed by unnoticed. The principal symptoms are pain, both spontaneous and pressure pain, vomiting, intestinal hemorrhage, and occlusion. The pains are colicky, may be located in any part of the abdomen, or occupy the entire abdomen. Whilst the belly is sensitive to pressure, the spontaneous pains are more or less continuous, and are ascribable to peritonitis. As a rule the cases present a distinct initial colicky pain and a subsequent peritonitic pain, but there are clear cases in which both were absent. The intestinal hemorrhage is either contained in the stools, which may be regular, or there may be a more or less continuous flow of clear blood from the anus. The stools then have the odor of carrion, and a dark brown or tarry appearance. In the case which I saw the amount of blood evacuated was excessive ; one stool, which apparently consisted of a solid clot, filled the entire bed pan, the subsequent capacity of which, as measured by water, amounted to two quarts. In the chapter on Enterorrhagia I have referred to other symptoms of profuse intestinal hemorrhage, which may be present even when the blood is not evacuated by the anus. Such symptoms—namely, sudden reduction of the temperature and appearance of collapse—are observed in this condition. The cases which run along under the symptomatology of acute occlusions are very perplexing. Nothnagel (*l. c.*) and Kaufmann (*l. c.*) described cases of this kind. The case which I observed in my practice presented the typical symptoms of acute occlusion. Nothnagel refers to two other such cases which were reported to him, and I know of at least one other case, which was described to me by Dr. J. M. T. Finney, of Baltimore. It is evident that when complete suppression of feces and flatus exists, with sudden acute abdominal pain, and no sign of intestinal hemorrhage, the diagnosis of occlusion is very likely to be made. There may even be fecal vomiting. The occlusion is attributed to an intestinal paralysis caused partially by the penetrating vascular and structural changes which the bowel must undergo, and also by the peritonitis.

Diagnosis.

The diagnosis is based upon the symptoms narrated in the preceding, and upon the demonstration of a source for the embolism. As I have already remarked, an absence of such a source does not negative the diagnosis of obturation of the mesenteric arteries, because the embolus may have originated in an autochthonous manner, or from an atheroma of the aorta which can not be demonstrated. Sometimes emboli exist in other arteries simultaneously. These are happy cases for diagnosis, but rare ones. The most significant signs are (a) excessive enterorrhagia, in the absence of previous symptoms pointing to intestinal disease, no indications pointing to independent lesions of the bowel, nor interference with the venous circulation; (b) intense colicky pains; (c) fall of the body-temperature; (d) evidences of exudation and tympanitic distention. So the clinician must seek for evidences of valvular disease, endocarditis, and arterial sclerosis. In the case which I have observed, described in the preceding, there was almost complete loss of vision, due no doubt to an embolism of the central artery of the retina; so that in all cases in which there is any suggestion of hemorrhagic infarctions of the kidney, together with optic disturbances and the symptoms referred to in the preceding, careful ophthalmoscopic examination of the fundus of the eye should be carried out. If the embolus is infectious, its clinical history is marked by chills and rigors. If the diagnostic factors mentioned in the preceding—(a), (b), (c), and (d)—are presented together, the diagnosis can be positively made; but if any one of them is wanting, particularly if there is no sign of intestinal hemorrhage, the diagnosis is impossible. Probably the nearest to a recognition of the correct state of affairs that will be made is the diagnosis of intestinal obstruction.

PLATE 10.

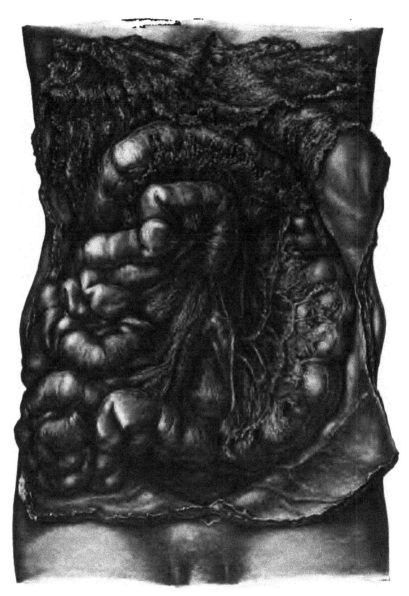

INFERIOR MESENTERIC VESSELS. ASPECT B.

The transverse colon is drawn up, small intestines pulled aside. In the center of the illustration a few vertebræ are visible, and to the right and left of these, the right and left common iliac artery. To the lower right of the illustration, the distribution of the inferior mesenteric artery to the descending colon is evident. Very little of the sigmoid flexure is apparent in this illustration.—(*From Deaver's "Surgical Anatomy."*)

Course and Prognosis.

This pathological condition is, as a rule, fatal, death being caused in from twenty-four to forty-eight hours by acute anemia and collapse. In exceptional cases the duration is sufficiently long for the development of acute peritonitis and intestinal occlusions dependent thereon. When one reflects upon the gravity of the pathological changes, it is surprising that recoveries should be possible at all, particularly when the main stem of the artery or one of the larger branches is obturated; however, cases of undoubted recovery have been described by Cohn, Moos ("Virchow's Archiv," Bd. XLI), and Virchow. In the latter case this great pathologist described the superior mesenteric artery as being transformed into a hard and rigid cord, and obturated by a large adherent and dry clot, projecting as far as the aorta. There were no changes in the jejunum or ileum. Cohn's case was an embolic obturation of the colic branch of the superior mesenteric. The slate-gray discolored transverse colon presented the remnants of a former hemorrhage in the shape of numerous ocher-colored spots. It does not seem probable that recovery can occur when the main branch of the artery is occluded; at least none of the cases thus far reported gives the satisfactory pathological evidence for that conclusion. If, however, the obturated arterial district is not very extensive, or even if it occurs in one of the larger branches, not suddenly, but very gradually, so that the collateral circulation has time to develop and conduct into the deprived district a requisite amount of blood, then the possibility of recovery is not excluded.

Treatment.

Even if the diagnosis can be made, the treatment remains purely symptomatic. The main effort should be directed toward maintaining the strength of the patient by hypodermic injection of strychnin and stimulants, controlling the hemorrhage by application of ice-bags and the hypodermic injection of ergotol, and relieving pain by hypodermic injection of morphin.

THROMBOSIS OF THE MESENTERIC VEIN.

In a previous chapter I have given the clinical picture which results when the intestinal veins are compressed or occluded in circumscribed obstruction of the intestine, in incarceration, strangulation, invagination, and volvulus. The pressure suffices to compress the thin-walled vein, but not the more resistant walls of the artery. As a consequence of this the arteries keep on pumping new blood into the strangulated parts, whilst the veins can lead none away. An enormous congestion results, and dilation of all veins, which extends to the capillaries; the intestinal portion involved becomes dark or blackish-red, and is immensely thickened by the accumulation of blood and serous transudation. All this has been more minutely described in chapter III, page 115, this volume. But when the mesenteric veins become obturated by a thrombus, circulatory disturbances of a similar character occur, but uncomplicated by contemporaneous occlusion of the intestine. Under such conditions one observes a more or less extensive dark red discoloration of the intestine, which becomes thickened, tough, and puffy. The thickening occurs particularly in the submucosa. In the most extensive infarction the beginning of the necrosis is recognizable first at the tips of the valvulæ conniventes. The anatomical picture is very similar to that resulting from obturation of the mesenteric arteries. In some cases there may be peritonitis, with or without a hemorrhagic exudate. The hemorrhagic infarction is not a venous hyperemia, but due to an arterial congestion. Such cases have been described by Eisenlohr ("Jahrb. d. Hamburg Stattskrankenanstalten," Jahrgang 2, 1890), Grawitz ("Virchow's Archiv," Bd. cx), and Pilliet ("Progrès méd.," 1890, No. 25). The primary causes of the thrombosis of the mesenteric veins are not recognizable from the cases thus far reported, but it seems probable, from the descriptions of the observers cited, that a pre-existing intestinal disease is one of the conditions, and that this process extends to the root branches of the mesenteric veins. Eisenlohr's and Pilliet's cases had symptoms of intestinal disease, diarrhea, etc. Pilliet especially suggests the existence of a mycotic intestinal disease, whilst Grawitz presented the history of a case occurring during malarial cachexia, with chronic splenic tumor, and the eventual thrombosis of the pancreatic and superior mesenteric

PLATE ii.

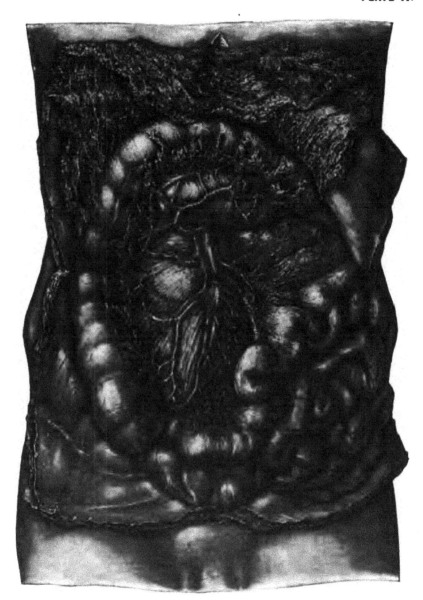

RIGHT SIDE OF MESENTERY, CECUM, AND ASCENDING COLON.
The great omentum is pulled up to show the transverse colon and mesenteric vessels.

veins.   In some cases the thrombosis begins in the peripheral branches of the mesenteric vein, originating in the intestine, and extending upward in these.   It does not begin in the trunk of the portal vein.   Alexander ("Thrombose der Pfortader u. ihrer Aeste," "Berlin. klin. Wochenschr.," 1856, No. 4) described a case in which a primary thrombosis of the portal vein extended far into the roots of this vein, even up to their very origin.   It may be a question of doubt as to which was the primary thrombosis in these cases, that of the mesenteric veins situated in the intestines, or that of the trunk of the portal vein.   The primary seat of the thrombosis may be located in the portal vein if the mesenteric veins are found greatly dilated and in addition other radicals of the portal vein are affected.

Symptomatology.

The clinical picture closely resembles that of thrombosis of the mesenteric artery.   It may also present itself essentially in two types —that of intestinal hemorrhage and that of intestinal obstruction. In the case described by Grawitz there were appearances of grave enteritis, with enterorrhagia and violent abdominal pain, so that the diagnosis of abdominal typhoid or enteric fever with perforation was considered probable.   The clinical differentiation of thrombosis of the mesenteric artery and that of the mesenteric vein, in my opinion, meets with insurmountable difficulty.   The suggestion that a preexisting intestinal disease or lesion speaks for mesenteric vein thrombosis, and that a source for an embolus, such as heart disease or arterial atheroma, speaks for arterial embolus, is misleading ; for in the arterial thrombosis a previous intestinal disease may exist also, and cardiac disease is not necessarily excluded in thrombosis of the mesenteric vein.

Treatment.

Even though correctly diagnosed there can be no methodical treatment of these conditions.

PERIARTERITIS NODOSA INTESTINALIS.

Kussmaul and Maier have described a disease of the intestinal arteries under this name which runs its course with the following symptomatology : Diarrheas, colics, tenesmus, intestinal muscular paralysis, albuminuria, and marasmus.   The walls of the arteries give the histological evidences of arteritis.   The ileum and the beginning of the colon were found ulcerated.   Such a periarteritis is sometimes observed in advanced general and intestinal syphilis. The condition is preeminently of pathological interest.

VENOUS HYPEREMIA OF THE INTESTINES.

Elsewhere I have pointed out that the amount of blood in the intestine is usually found to be very small at autopsies.   This was especially the case when the cardiac tonicity was very low for a considerable time prior to death.   In the introduction to the chapter on Enterostenoses and Occlusion, I have also described cases where I have observed an intense exudative inflammation of the peritoneum and the serous surface of the bowel during laparotomy, and still at the autopsy no trace of inflammation or hyperemia could be discovered.   We must not, therefore, always assume in cases of hepatic cirrhosis or cardiac disease, which have given rise to intestinal symptoms, that there was no hyperemia during life because we can not discover any at the autopsy.   The tendency of the intestine to evacuate its blood during and after death may have effaced every trace of the hyperemia.

Venous hyperemia of the intestine is due to obstruction to the venous circulation.   The two paths which are most frequently obstructed are the portal vein, the impediment being here offered by hepatic cirrhosis, and the inferior vena cava, where the venous current is obstructed by cardiac and pulmonary diseases.   As a rule, other organs which are comprised in the radicals of the portal vein, or influenced by backward congestions of blood originating in the heart, also show simultaneous evidences of venous hyperemia. During hyperemia the intestine is edematous, swollen, and infiltrated.   This edematous condition, which is accompanied by a dark blue, cyanotic discoloration and dilation of the veins of the serosa, submucosa, and mucosa, does not extend uniformly over the entire bowel, but affects the large intestine whilst the small intestine is but slightly altered, and *vice versa*.   The dilations of the hemorrhoidal veins have been described in the chapter on Rectal Diseases, by Dr. Thomas Charles Martin.   Congestive dark discol-

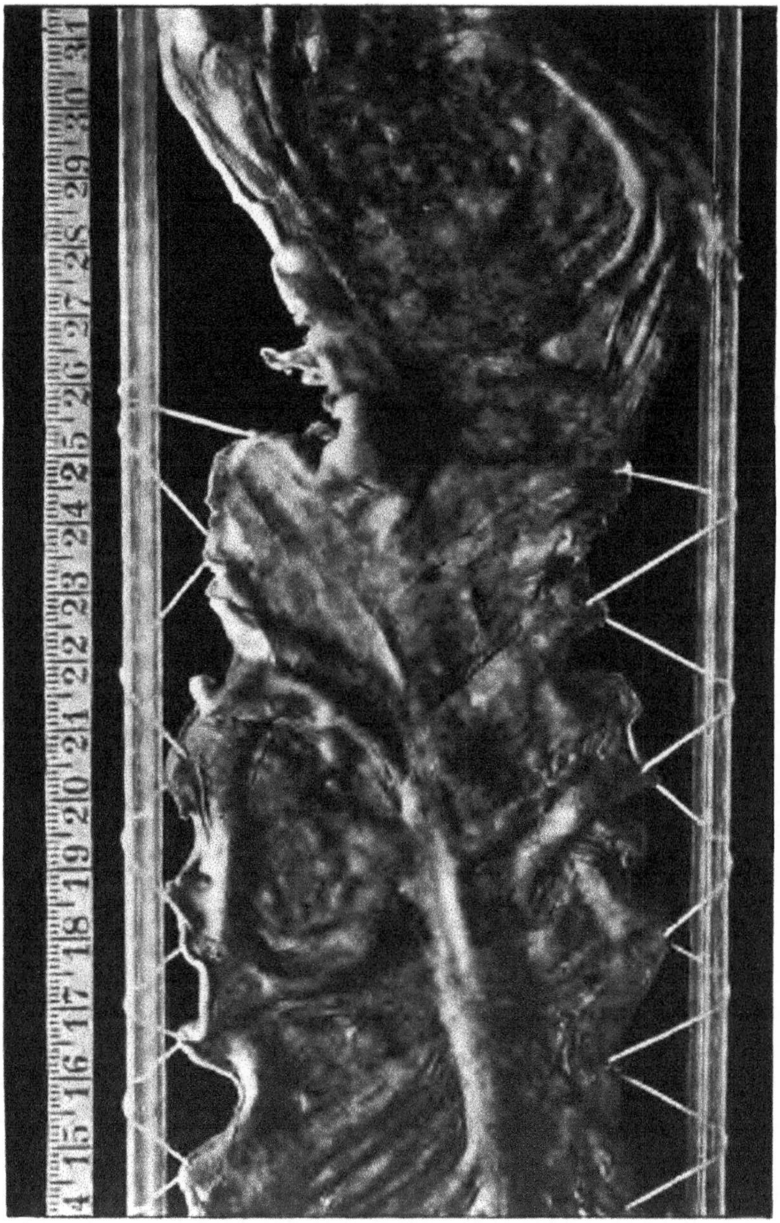

FIG. 11.—CHRONIC PASSIVE CONGESTION OF COLON.

orations of the intestine occur in some forms of poisoning, especially in poisoning by carbon monoxid; and according to Klebs, in death after recent diabetes, with demonstrable changes in the celiac plexus.   The passive venous congestion as a result of cardiac, pulmonary, or hepatic disease may cause dilation of the intestinal veins, but rarely any varicose dilations, such as are found at the cardiac end of the esophagus and in the lower rectum.   In a case of profuse hematemesis in a young man twenty years of age, which I.saw with Dr. Edward A. Smith, there were simultaneous excessive losses of blood from the stomach by emesis and from the bowel; the stools had a tarry consistency.   The liver was normal to percussion and palpation.   The young man denied having ever indulged in the use of alcohol, and there being no history of past infections, we excluded the possibility of hepatic cirrhosis.   The gastric hemorrhage being uncontrollable, I advised an operation for supposed gastric ulcer.   At the laparotomy, by Dr. J. M. T. Finney, no ulcer could be detected in the stomach.   Twenty-four hours after the operation the case terminated fatally.   At the autopsy we found a cirrhotic liver, a bunch of hugely dilated veins in the cardia, one of which had perforated, and another bundle of varicose veins in the pylorus reaching down into the horizontal portion of the duodenum.   This case illustrates how closely hemorrhage from esophageal piles in hepatic cirrhosis (Osler) may simulate hematemesis from gastric ulcer when the first-named condition occurs in the young and the hepatic cirrhosis can not be recognized.   Experimental ligation of the inferior vena cava and of the portal vein can not reproduce exactly the condition of venous hyperemia, because in all experiments this state must be brought on suddenly and abruptly, whereas the disease process itself is one that develops slowly. Accordingly any deductions from experiments as to whether stagnation of the blood in the intestine after these ligations causes increased peristalsis or arrest of peristalsis can not be applied to the clinical picture of this abnormality.   Nothnagel assumes that the nervous apparatus of the intestine is damaged by the insufficient supply of normal oxygen in the blood, and in this he recognizes the cause of the obstipation, which is the most frequent functional disturbance observed.   Venous hyperemia of the intestine may or may not induce enteritis.   It is a common experience to observe the intestine of individuals dead from heart disease in a state of passive venous hyperemia, but at the same time no evidences of catarrh can be detected even microscopically. There are, however, other undoubted cases where the histological evidences of enteritis are unmistakable after venous hyperemia of this kind.

DILATION OF THE HEMORRHOIDAL VEINS (PHLEBEC-TASIA ; HEMORRHOIDALIS).

Hemorrhoids and dilation of the rectal veins are considered from the clinical aspect in a separate chapter. It will suffice here to add simply a few remarks concerning their pathogenesis. This condition is produced by stagnations occurring as a result of valvular disease or diseases of the myocardium, pulmonary emphysema, compression of the lung by spinal curvatures, thrombosis of the inferior vena cava, interference with the portal circulation, hepatic cirrhosis, syphilis, carcinoma, pylephlebitis, etc. Anything which reduces the lumen of the pelvic canal may bring about an ectasis of the rectal vein, more especially habitual obstipation with the accompanying accumulation of fecal masses in the rectum, advanced obesity, and intra-abdominal, especially omental, accumulation of fat which mechanically obstructs the return flow of the blood through the pelvic veins. (This occurs more especially when simultaneous excessive ingestion of food and drink has increased the pressure in the portal artery.) The gravid uterus and displace-
· ments as well as neoplasms of this organ, ovarian tumors, act in an analogous manner. It is claimed that certain intoxications may produce venous dilations in the rectum ; alcohol, strong black coffee, and tea are accused of this deleterious influence, but if they can exert such an influence,—which in my opinion is not clearly demonstrated,—they do so either by favoring obstipation or weakening the circulation. In certain families there seems to be a hereditary predisposition to the formation of hemorrhoids. In the work of Georg Ernst Stahl * ("On the Hemorrhoidal Conditions," etc., 1698) they were not looked upon as a local disease of the rectal veins, but as a constitutional dyscrasia ; and even in later literature

---

* Georg Ernst Stahl, "De vena portæ porta malorum hypochondriaco-splenetico-hysterico-colico-hæmorrhoidariorum."

the so-called hemorrhoidal dyscrasia was frequently associated with another hypothetical conception—that of the abdominal plethora.

The dilation of the rectal veins is dependent upon purely localized and mechanical conditions. Von Recklinghausen argues that the deciding factor for the explanation of the accumulation of blood in the rectal veins is to be sought in gravity. No matter in what position the body is,—standing, sitting, or lying,—the blood in the hemorrhoidal veins must flow upward from a lower position, against the force of gravity. This is the principal factor in the pathogenesis. All others mentioned are simply aggravating causes. Frerichs was of the opinion that hemorrhoidal varices were by no means frequently found in hepatic cirrhosis—an opinion in which Nothnagel, Sappey, Thierfelder, Monneret, and Damaschino concurred. This view is supported by the fact that while hepatic cirrhosis and cardiac insufficiency do cause pathological increase of pressure in the venous system, this increase is exerted uniformly over so large a circulatory territory that it can not be especially localized upon the hemorrhoidal veins. In addition to gravity, the next most important etiological factor is a weakened circulation; and as this is most frequently observed in individuals showing slight energy of the motor apparatus, especially those who are accustomed to an abundant diet and a sedentary habit of life, which must lead to defective metabolism, we find that hemorrhoids are not so frequent in plethoric individuals as was supposed, but rather in subjects afflicted with a debilitated circulation, whether they are plethoric or not. In a recent investigation Georg Reinbach has advanced the argument that hemorrhoids are not always due to a dilation of already existing veins, but to new formation of veins. He does not mean by this an inflammatory proliferation, but the development of a genuine blood-vessel neoplasm, a venous angioma, which of course may be accompanied by the signs of venous hyperemia and inflammation. This reminds of the suggestions of Allingham ("Diseases of the Rectum," New York, 1883), who distinguished between venous, capillary, and arterial hemorrhoidal knots. There can be no doubt that arterial telangiectases occur in the rectum, but they should be held separate and distinct from hemorrhoids. It is also conceivable, as Bardeleben has pointed out, that large hemorrhoidal varices may force up arterial branches from the submucosa during the progress of their enlargement, or that two or more varicosities in becoming confluent may include an artery, thus transforming it into an integral part of a hemorrhoidal tumor.

The clinical pathology and complications and treatment of hemorrhoidal dilations have been treated in the chapter on Diseases of the Rectum.

AMYLOIDOSIS OF THE INTESTINE.

Synonym.—Amyloid Degeneration of the Intestinal Vessels.

Nature and Concept.

Amyloidosis of the intestine is a peculiar degeneration or infiltration of the intestinal tissue with a translucent albuminoid material, which takes a temporary reddish-brown color when treated with a dilute solution of iodin, and, further, becomes violet or blue when treated with sulphuric acid. Methyl violet and other blue anilin dyes impart to it a rose-red color. It attacks most frequently the kidneys, spleen, and liver, the intestine being the fourth in order of frequency. Amyloidosis of the intestine is always a secondary disease consequent upon some other well-known primary affection, prominent among which the following have been recognized : chronic suppuration of bone, syphilis, tuberculosis, malarial cachexia; in brief, any chronic process, especially suppurative process, eventuating in exhaustion and loss of the secretions and tissue juices. Among these conditions may be mentioned chronic dysenteries or diarrheas, chronic gastric ulcers with exhausting hemorrhages, bronchial blennorrhea in association with bronchiectasy, chronic parenchymatous nephritis, gout, leukemia ; in extremely rare cases the intestine itself was the organ primarily affected. Orth (*l. c.*, p. 857) has examined such a case where the intestines were in a state of amyloid degeneration and none of the other organs was affected, but could assign no cause for this localization of the amyloidosis. Intestinal amyloidosis was first described by Virchow, who in fact was the first to call attention to this condition in a scientific way (" Ueber dem Gang der amyloiden Degeneration," " Virchow's Archiv," Bd. VIII, 1865, S. 364; also "Die cellular Pathologie," Berlin, 1858, S. 340), although H. Meckel (" Annalen des Charité-Krankenhauses," Jahrg. IV, H. 2, Berlin, 1853, S. 264) had observed the characteristic iodin reaction in both the large and small intestine prior to Virchow. The villi are frequently wanting in advanced cases, as they are very liable to atrophy and detachment in this condition.

Amyloidosis of the Intestinal Blood-vessels.

This form of degeneration affects the blood-vessels, especially the capillaries and smallest arteries, and occasionally the veins, in advance of any other intestinal structures; and therefore it can logically be classed among the diseases affecting the intestinal vessels. In fact, Virchow regarded it as almost exclusively limited to the minute arterioles, especially those of the superficial layers of the submucosa and the villi, but stated that it could be traced also along the capillaries given off from these vessels, for a short distance. It is now known that not only the vessels throughout the intestinal walls—i. e., in all the layers—may be affected, but, according to Friedreich ("Virchow's Archiv," Bd. xi, 1857, S. 387; also Bd. xiii, 1858, S. 498), the degeneration may even be demonstrated in the mesenteric vessels. When an intestine is examined by the naked eye in this condition, the mucous membrane presents an extremely pale appearance, is somewhat thickened and exceptionally translucent; otherwise little alteration can be detected. When iodin is applied to a small portion of the bowel, numerous reddish or brownish points make their appearance, being situated on the general surface of the mucosa, which stains yellow. The reddish-brown points are the intestinal villi the minute vessels of which have undergone amyloidosis. Similarly the affected vessels in other situations assume the characteristic color with iodin. In the smaller arterioles it is particularly the muscular stratum which becomes amyloid, the degeneration always beginning in the tunica media. The capillaries and minute arterioles are predominantly affected; occasionally also the veins. The intestinal blood-vessels are often diseased alone; next most frequently we find the degeneration in the blood-vessels, and at the same time in the muscularis mucosæ. In still other cases it is the longitudinal and circular muscular layers, together with the vessels contained in them, which are degenerated. The follicles and Peyer's patches are, as a rule, free from amyloidosis. This can also be said of the tissue of the mucosa proper, the glands, and the glandular epithelium. The epithelium itself is very rarely subject to this degeneration. Hayem has mentioned the occurrence of amyloid concretion in the follicles in cases which were secondary to chronic caries and necrosis of bones (M. G. Hayem, " Note sur la dégénérescence amyloid du tube digestif," " Compte Rendu des séances de la Soc. de Biologie," November, 1865, 4me série, T. II, p. 191). He found the condition in five out of forty scrofulous children with chronic suppuration of the bones, and discovered in some an almost exclusive degeneration of the follicles, as opposed to the more common form of the primary and almost exclusive degeneration of the vessels.

As amyloidosis causes a thickening and rigidity of the intestinal vessels, it is natural that it must produce serious disturbance in the nutrition and the functions of the intestine. The relations to inflammatory conditions of the intestinal mucosa are less obvious. In the chapter on Intestinal Ulcers I have described the characteristic losses of substance which are observed in association with intestinal amyloidosis, which, according to Hayem and others, are the consequences of this form of degeneration. Kyber ("Virchow's Archiv," Bd. LXXXI) does not admit the etiological relations between amyloid disease of the intestinal vessels and formation of ulcers, but regards these as simple catarrhal ulcers.

Symptomatology.

The clinical history of amyloidosis does not present many symptoms.

Diarrhea is the only symptom of importance. It is usually very protracted and obstinate. The stools, however, do not present anything characteristic. This symptom is attributed by some to the injured absorptive power of the mucosa, preventing the resorption of liquids and maintaining the intestinal contents in a fluid state. Cohnheim, on the contrary, explains the diarrhea by an abnormal exchange of osmosis of liquids through the diseased capillary walls. Traube explains the liquid and frequent discharges by the anemia of the intestinal wall, citing the experiment of Schiff, in which violent peristalsis followed upon compression of the abdominal aorta. This experiment, however, is not applicable to the explanation of the anemia in amyloidosis, which comes on very gradually, whereas that following compression of the aorta comes on very suddenly.

During our Civil War, Wm. Aitken ("Science and Practice of Medicine," third Amer. edit., Philadelphia, 1872, vol. II, p. 682) claimed to have repeatedly seen soldiers dead of diarrhea in the hospital at Netley, in whom the entire alimentary canal was in a state of extreme amyloidosis. J. J. Woodward ("Medical and Surgical History of the Rebellion," part II, p. 333) had also observed amyloid degeneration in the intestinal arterioles, capillaries, and villi of the small intestine, and also in the submucosa of both the large and the small intestine. He had also observed that in small arteries in the vicinity of tubercular ulcers this amyloid degeneration was manifested by glassy swelling of the intima and indistinctness of the nuclei of the muscular coat, and he had also produced the characteristic reaction by iodin (*l. c.*, p. 596).

In an epidemic of 48 cases of dysentery at Bay View Asylum, Baltimore, I could obtain undoubted amyloid reaction in the intestines of two cases at autopsy.

Pain.—In uncomplicated intestinal amyloidosis neither pressure nor spontaneous pain in the abdomen has been noted.

Hemorrhage.—T. Grainger Stewart attributed importance to the occurrence of hemorrhage in intestinal amyloid disease ("Brit. and Foreign Med.-Chir. Rev.," vol. XLI, 1868, p. 201). In this paper he presents the details of 3 cases of intestinal amyloidosis, all of which were syphilitic, but presented no bone disease. Previously intestinal hemorrhage had been observed by Hayem (*l. c.*) and Wilson Fox ("Brit. and Foreign Med.-Chir. Rev.," vol. XXXVIII, 1866). T. G. Stewart asserts that the hemorrhage may occur without any lesion of the intestinal mucosa, and attributes it to abnormal fragility of the blood-vessels. He does not regard it as a necessarily dangerous accident, remarking that the hemorrhage sometimes comes and goes for years without markedly depressing the vital powers. In the literature on this subject I have not been able to ascertain with definiteness the relative frequency of intestinal hemorrhage as a symptom of amyloidosis. Traube ("Gesammelte Beiträge," Bd. III, 1878) and Nothnagel (*l. c.*) hold that the evacuations of simple amyloidosis are not bloody. In eight reports in which any reference was made to this symptom, five state that the evacuations may be hemorrhagic, and three maintain that they are not hemorrhagic. Evidently this does not permit of any exact deduction available for diagnosis. Nothnagel is so positive, however, on the absence of blood, that he cites it as a diagnostic support when diarrhea is present, without pain, together with the etiological moments which have been cited in the preceding. In the two cases of dysentery to which I have referred, and which gave evidence of amyloid degeneration, blood had existed in the stools off and on for two months in one and six weeks in another case. No history of syphilis could be elicited.

Diagnosis.

From what has been stated in the preceding it is evident that the diagnosis of intestinal amyloid degeneration is difficult. The clinician might think of this condition when protracted and obstinate diarrhea exists in the absence of abdominal pain of any kind, and when there is a simultaneous enlargement of the liver and spleen, together with albuminuria. Even then there is no certainty as to the recognition of this disease. Possibly direct inspection of the rectum and sigmoid, as described by Dr. T. C. Martin, in the chapter on Diseases of the Rectum, would permit of a recognition of the marked anemia of these parts, and if need be a minute portion of the surface of the sigmoid or rectum could be removed with the curet for chemical and microscopical examination. The very small wound left on the mucosa could be closed by iodoform collodion. This is the only means that suggests itself to me for making a reliable diagnosis, particularly as all the other symptoms cited in the preceding may be produced by catarrhal and tubercular intestinal ulcers.

Prognosis.

The disease is always fatal, but, as remarked by T. Grainger Stewart, it may exist for years without depressing the vital powers. There is no telling, however, how long it may have existed before a case presents itself for treatment of the graver symptoms. Therefore the prognosis should always be stated as unfavorable.

Treatment.

There is no successful treatment of amyloidosis. The three aims of the treatment should be to maintain the strength of the patient, combat the primary disease (syphilis, tuberculosis, bone necrosis), and check the diarrhea. The latter is best accomplished by regulating the diet, which should be that given in the chapter on Diarrhea. For the profuse liquid evacuations opium, bismuth subnitrate, and bismuth subgallate, also bismuth salicylate and tannate, are sometimes effective. Bismutose (a combination of bismuth and proteose, partially soluble) should be applicable in this condition, as it is non-toxic and effective in thickening the feces. Salol, tannigen, and tannalbin may be employed. There are cases, however, in which the diarrhea is uncontrollable and baffles all treatment.

INFLUENCE OF INTESTINAL AFFECTIONS UPON THE BLOOD.

The effect of abnormal conditions of the blood and blood-vessels on the nutrition of the intestines has been described in a number of the preceding chapters.

The work thus far done upon the blood in diseases of the intestines has proved as yet, with a few exceptions, of no diagnostic importance; but these exceptions are extremely important, and we can not, therefore, agree with Herz (" Störungen des Verdauungs-apparates," etc.) when he says that neither the determination of the number or the quality of the blood-cells nor the specific gravity nor the alkalinity of the blood has a differential diagnostic value as between the different forms of digestive disease or between these and disease of other organs. Under the head of leukocytosis it will be seen that the white cell count is of decided value not only from a diagnostic, but also from a therapeutic standpoint. This has been emphasized in the chapter on Intestinal Obstruction and Appendicitis. The changes in the red cells brought about by diseased conditions of the intestines are often very marked and merit some attention here.

Action of Purgatives.—The classic investigations of Mathew Hay ("Jour. of Anat. and Physiol.," vol. XVI, 1882, p. 430) show that the action of saline cathartics is to cause a temporary increase in the number of red corpuscles in the cubic millimeter of blood, due to a concentration of the blood. A man thirty-three years of age was given a concentrated solution of Glauber's salt: 21.3 grams of sodium sulphate in 85 c.c. of water. The following changes occurred .

At 3.25 o'clock,	. . . . 4,850,000 corpuscles per cu. mm.
" 3.38 "	. . . . 5,025,000 " " "
" 4.15 "	. . . . 6,540,000 " " "
" 4.55 "	. . . . 6,190,000 " " "
" 5.20 "	. . . . 6,610,000 " " "
" 6.00 "	. . . . 5,710,000 " " "
" 6.45 "	. . . . 5,140,000 " " "
" 7.40 "	. . . . 4,930,000 " " "

This table shows the action of the salts in extracting the fluid from the blood, which fluid is, however, rapidly replaced from the tissues. Hay has also shown that the amount of fluid withdrawn is greater the more concentrated the salt solution. Grawitz has obtained the same results with sulphate of magnesium. A girl was given 15 grams of this salt in 50 c.c. of water. In fifty-five minutes thereafter the specific gravity of the blood had increased from 1050.5 to 1053.9. Two hours later the specific gravity had declined to 1051.6.

In simple diarrheas as the result of chilling of the body surface and in nervous diarrhea the changes of the blood are similar to those caused by the action of cathartics. On the other hand, chronic diarrhea causes no marked changes in the quality of the blood. In dysenteries the serum of the blood loses a portion of its albumin, so that its specific gravity is diminished instead of increased as in acute diarrheas. (See chap. xx, p. 515, vol. I.)

Anemia.

Anemia as the result of intestinal disease is of common occurrence both from loss of blood and as an accompaniment of the disturbance in nutrition to which the intestinal affections often give rise. Anemia may occur as the result of hemorrhage from any large loss or from repeated losses in smaller amounts, as from hemorrhoids. Less frequently the anemia is the result of loss, not of the blood itself, but of the blood plasma. In dysentery the impoverishment of the blood is due not only to the loss of blood cells, but also, and often to a greater extent, to the loss of serum albumin from the blood, as Fr. Osterlein has shown. Von Jaksch was able to demonstrate the presence of large amounts of serum albumin in the feces of a chlorotic woman. Herz also found large amounts in the diarrheic stools of a patient who was taking a minimum amount of nourishment, which led to a very severe anemia. The condition of the intestine itself seems to play a decided rôle beyond that of allowing the loss of the constituents of the blood. Thus Pavy ascribes to the intestinal glands an important part in the formation of blood. Forcheimer also looks upon the intestinal mucosa as one of the places where hemoglobin is formed. In investigations on rabbits he found the blood in the mesenteric veins to be 18 per cent. richer in hemoglobin than the mesenteric arteries; and that the blood of individuals was decidedly richer in hemoglobin after eating than before. Should Forcheimer's theory prove correct, the existence of the anemia which is so frequently an accompaniment of diffuse intestinal disease will receive a further explanation. We are as yet not in a position to speak with certainty of a hematopoietic function of the intestinal mucous membrane, as the insufficient absorption of nourishment in these conditions undoubtedly is an important factor; but the theory is plausible and undoubtedly merits further investigation. It explains those cases of chlorosis where, in spite of the exhibition of large amounts of easily assimilated food, the condition persists. The action of intestinal parasites upon the blood has been much studied. They are recognized to be the cause of anemic conditions often severe in character. This may be due to the repeated loss of blood, as occurs in anchylostomum duodenale, to the loss of nutriment caused by the parasite, to reflex nervous influence, and, finally, to toxic substances formed by the parasites. The anchylostomum duodenale and bothriocephalus latus often give rise to a severe progressive anemia. (See chapter on Intestinal Parasites.) O. Schaumann has reported 72 cases of bothriocephalus infection accompanied by severe anemia. Often a progressive deterioration of the blood was observed, followed by a prompt improvement after the expulsion of the parasite. As shown by him, Fr. Muller, and Askanazy, the same conditions of the blood are met with as in pernicious anemia: the marked poikilocytosis, polychromatophilia, normoblasts, and megaloblasts. The cause is supposed to be the toxic effect of the material thrown off by the worm. The anemia accompanying the tapeworm commonly found in this country (the tænia mediocanellata), the lumbricoid worm, and the oxyuris is often marked, but not usually severe. In a fatal case of ascaris lumbricoides reported by Demme the blood count was as low as 1,650,000 per cu. mm. Intestinal autointoxication has been ascribed as a cause of anemia, especially of chlorosis. Nothnagel looks upon it as an etiological factor in some cases where putrefaction of stagnating fecal masses, and the consequent absorption of toxic substances, occurs. But the urine does not show in this disease an increase of those substances which are usually increased in autointoxication. Another view is that of Bunge, who thinks that as the result of intestinal putrefaction hydrogen sulphid is formed, which combines with the iron present in the food to form unabsorbable compounds, thereby robbing the system of its normal supply. This is as yet pure hypothesis. The demonstration of an anemia in connection with an intestinal disease is of course of no diagnostic value, as it differs in no way from the anemias due to other diseases.

Leukocytosis.

It is in those intestinal affections which belong both to the physician and surgeon that the examination of the blood is of greatest interest. The determination of the presence or absence of leukocytosis, and its degree if present, is of value, not only as an aid to diagnosis, but often as an indication of the method of treatment. By the presence of leukocytosis we are often enabled to distinguish appendicitis from a number of affections with which it may be confounded. In intestinal, biliary, and renal colic, and in the various forms of neuralgia that simulate appendicitis, there is no increase in the number of white cells, while in appendicitis it is absent only when the inflammation is catarrhal in character, or in those extremely grave forms where the symptoms are severe and the resistant powers of the individual are feeble. Cabot has added a third condition : viz., where there is an abscess very thoroughly walled off; in other words, the absence of leukocytosis (less than 10,000 per cu. mm.) in a case of appendicitis with mild symptoms indicates either a catarrhal form or a thoroughly walled off abscess ; if accompanied by severe symptoms it indicates a grave condition with feeble resistance, and renders the prognosis grave. From a therapeutic standpoint we may say that the presence of a marked increase in the number of white blood-cells is an indication for surgical intervention. While it is not possible in the present state of our knowledge to set down any exact figures which may act as an infallible guide for operation, yet a persistent, and especially an increasing, leukocytosis renders it advisable.   In cases of leukocytosis of 20,000 or over in the first few days of appendicitis operation is indicated. The absence of a leukocytosis does not indicate that operation is not necessary.

Marked leukocytosis, involving especially a decided increase in the number of eosinophiles, has been found in all forms of intestinal parasites.   Leichtenstern found the proportion of eosinophiles as high as 72 per cent. in anchylostomiasis, and 34 per cent. in tænia mediocanellata.   The number was especially great where Charcot-Leyden crystals were present in the feces.

The gastro-intestinal diseases in which an etiological relation to pre-existing abnormality in the structure and composition of the blood has been attempted are mainly gastric ulcer occurring in chlorosis (see Hemmeter, " Diseases of Stomach," 2d edition) and the atonic obstipation of chlorotic patients ; this has been considered in chapter XVI, vol. I.

CHAPTER X.

INTESTINAL NEUROSES, NERVOUS DISEASES OF THE INTESTINES.

To this category all those pathological conditions of the intestine belong which are not caused by demonstrable anatomical changes, but by irregularities in the functions of the motor, sensory, and secretory intestinal nerves, without any apparent histological substratum. Just as the nervous diseases of the stomach, so also those of the intestines may be divided into three great classes: (1) Motor, (2) sensory, and (3) secretory neuroses. Under each of these we may distinguish two sub-classes, one of which is characterized by a morbid increase in nervous irritability (state of excitation), the other by a decrease or even a suspension of the nervous irritability (state of depression). The intestine, just like the stomach, is very rich in nervous apparatus (see chapter on Anatomy of Intestines), which is in direct or indirect communication not only with the brain and spinal cord, but also with the nerves of many other organs. Exciting or depressing impulses may reach the intestine from the blood, the intestinal mucosa, and from numerous other portions of the body. Consequently the conditions are very favorable for the development of neuroses, which must be traced back either to a decrease or to an increase of the irritability of the intestinal nerves. The recognition and differentiation of the anatomical diseases are often very difficult. Differentiation is still more difficult when we have to exclude with certainty all pathologic-anatomical changes and to trace back the disease symptoms to functional disturbances of the intestinal nerves alone. The difficulty in correct judgment and recognition of intestinal neuroses becomes evident by the fact that great gaps still exist in our knowledge of the anatomy and physiology of the intestinal nerves and of the symptomatology of the individual neuroses. This is due to the fact that the attention of clinicians has been directed to intes-

tinal neuroses only for the last few years.   Of the intestinal
nerves, the motor fibers and their relation to peristalsis are best
known, thanks to the investigations of Nothnagel, F. P. Mall,
Braam-Houkgeest, and others.   Numerous observations made
during intestinal diseases show that the intestine undoubtedly possesses sensory nerves.   This is about all that is known about
them ; their exact course is still doubtful, although it is very probable that the splanchnics contain the sensory fibers.   In the same
way we can only form conjectures as to the nature of the secretory nerves.   Moreau, and afterward Hanan, carried out an experiment which has often been cited as a proof of the existence
of secretory nerves.   It consisted of the ligation of an intestinal loop
and the section of all nerves leading to it externally.   Under such
conditions the loop was filled with a liquid, which was pronounced
to be succus entericus, because it contained a diastatic ferment. We
may, however, make the following objection to this conclusion,
namely, that the diastatic ferment had remained behind in the intestinal loop from the last digestion, and that the mucosa had retained it, and that all secretions and fluid from the animal body
contain diastatic ferment.   Fleischer thinks that there is a much
better argument for the existence of secretory intestinal nerves in
the observations made by Quincke, Demant, and Masslof, both in
men and in animals ; that a great secretion of intestinal juice could
be observed in the lower sections of the intestines, some time after
the introduction of the food into the stomach, but long before the
passage of the chyme over into the intestines.   He thinks that this
can be explained only by the assumption that the secretory intestinal nerves were excited reflexly by the gastric nerves. (See vol. 1,
p. 53.)

The introduction to the chapter on Neuroses of the Stomach
(Hemmeter, " Diseases of the Stomach," second edition, p. 733)
presents also the physiology and etiology of intestinal neuroses, together with the hypotheses concerning their nature, cause, and
characteristic phenomena.   Here also are described the combined
neuroses, and their relation to the diseases of other organs.   This
account, in its important physiological and pathological facts, applies also to intestinal neuroses.

In spite of the great gaps which at the present time still exist in our knowledge of intestinal neuroses, an attempt will nevertheless be made to describe their various symptoms, and also to include all their clinical phenomena, as far as possible. We shall consider first the motor neuroses, because they are most frequently observed, and therefore best known; second, the sensory neuroses; and, finally, secretory neuroses.

MOTOR NEUROSES OF THE INTESTINE.

Motor neuroses of the intestine are traceable either to an increase or to a decrease or even suspension of the normal excitability of the motor nerves. Nervous diarrhea and atony, the principal representatives of the two forms of motor neurosis, have already been considered in the sections on diarrhea and constipation respectively. We shall therefore have to discuss the rarer forms of motor neurosis —that is, enterospasm, proctospasm (see chapter on Diseases of the Rectum), peristaltic unrest, paralysis of the intestinal muscularis and of the sphincters.

Enterospasm.

Nature and Description.—Enterospasm is caused by simultaneous tonic contractions of the longitudinal and the circular muscularis of the intestines or of individual sections of the same. These contractions may continue for a long or short period of time. Under normal conditions the contractions of the longitudinal intestinal muscularis alternate with those of the circular muscularis. During the contractions of the longitudinal layer the circular layer is relaxed; when contractions of the former cease, the circular fibers contract. The occurrence of peristaltic movements of the intestines is dependent upon the periodic alternation of the contractions of the longitudinal and the circular muscularis. (See chapter on Peristalsis.) According to the most recent view (Ehrmann), the longitudinal muscularis is innervated by excito-motor fibers of the splanchnic nerve, and by inhibitory fibers in the vagus; the circular muscularis is innervated by excito-motor fibers in the vagus and by inhibitory fibers of the splanchnic. On this assumption the alternation in the contractions could easily be explained, if we presuppose an alternating excitation of the splanchnic and the vagus. If this theory is correct, the simultaneous spastic contractions of the longitudinal and the circular intestinal muscularis which cause enterospasm are due either to an increase in the irritability of those fibers of both the splanchnic and vagus which cause contractions of the intestinal muscularis, or to a decrease in the irritability in both sets of the inhibitory nerves. In either case the motor impulse flowing to the intestinal muscularis is stronger than the inhibitory impulse. Contemporaneous spastic contractions of the longitudinal and the circular muscularis of the intestines may also occur if the irritability of the sensory intestinal nerves is increased or if these nerves are affected by exceptionally strong irritants. This is proved by observations made during intestinal colic. In the former case, however, the contractions are always accompanied by more or less severe subjective complaints and pains. Enterospasm, therefore, can be differentiated with certainty from colic only in those rare cases where pain is absent, and where it consequently is the result of a motor neurosis alone. If, however, pains occur in the further course of the enterospasm, we are justified in assuming that at first only a motor neurosis existed, and that the sensory nerves became affected later on. This frequently occurs also in other neuroses. If the enterospasm extends over the entire intestine, or even the greater portion of it, as for instance the small intestine, the abdomen may present a boat-shaped concavity, which is absent in those cases in which the enterospasm is confined to single, smaller sections of the intestine, as for example the large intestine. The latter cases are much more frequent than the former. In both cases there is usually a persistent stool retention, which may last for days. The feces usually show the same changes in their form which are observed in a stenosis and in long-continued inanition, and which have been described in the chapter on Enterostenoses. Occasionally enterospasm is complicated with proctospasm. (See Disease of the Rectum.)

Nothnagel (*l. c.*, p. 482) doubts the existence of enterospasm as an independent functional neurosis, and suggests that strictly speaking it is not a morbid entity, not a neurosis "sui generis." Enterospasm does not stand out with sufficient independence from the symptomatology of neurasthenia, hysteria, and hypochondria to merit classification as a distinct intestinal neurosis, according to this eminent

author.   Whilst primary spastic conditions of the intestinal muscularis are indeed very rare, there is no doubt in my mind that they
do occur; at least I have had opportunity to observe three cases
on different occasions, which after the most critical study I could
not consider in any other light than that of functional enterospasm.

Clinical History.—C. G.; student; age nineteen; both parents
living; both neuropathic; heart and lungs normal; urine negative;
complains of violent paroxysms of pain radiating from the umbilicus to
right anterior superior spine of ileum.   Attacks come on about once in
ten days.   Obstipation for five years.   Rectum and sigmoid normal to
inspection.   On the day before and during the attack, either no evacuations at all or small worm-like threads of normal feces.   Attacks of pain
last for an hour at a time; then comes a brief interval of rest, relief,
and relaxation, after which pain returns.   Test meal: Free HCl $= 72$;
combined HCl $= 10$; total acidity $= 84$.   Hyperchlorhydria.   Stomach
normal in position and size.   During attacks patient must remain in bed.
Abdomen much retracted.   In the intervals between the attacks the patient
is well, except for obstipation, pyrosis, and headaches.   On several occasions during the enterospasm no fecal evacuation occurred for seven days.
Treatment: Magnes. usta, Sod. bicarb., and Ext. belladonnæ for hyperchlorhydria; denarcotized extract of opium for the pain, by suppositories;
hot cataplasms to abdomen.   Under this treatment the attacks were, as a
rule, relieved in one or two days.   After he had been observed in four
paroxysms, he consented to a course of five weeks' treatment of his hyperchlorhydria by a method first suggested by Biedert and Langerman—
namely, local gastric irrigation with alkaline solutions, followed by a
solution of tannin ($\frac{1}{2}$ per cent.) (see Hemmeter, "Diseases of the
Stomach," second edition, p. 833), with proper diet and galvanic electricity to abdomen.   Ten months have elapsed since this treatment, and
he has had no return of his enterospasm.   In this patient the entero- .
spasm seemed directly dependent upon the hyperchlorhydria.
    The second case was that of a female patient, thirty-four years of age,
also of neurasthenic extraction.   The gastric contents showed hyperacidity: Free HCl $= 64$; total acidity $= 72$.   She had frequent attacks
of enterospasm, alternating at times with attacks of pneumatosis.   (See
Hemmeter, "Diseases of the Stomach," second edition, p. 755.)   During
the attacks of enterospasm, which lasted four to five days, she felt strong
desire for stool, but could not evacuate any fecal matter.   The rectum
and sigmoid were normal to proctoscopic inspection.   The abdomen,
during the attack, was considerably sunken in, but the abdominal recti
muscles were not tense, so that the fingers could readily palpate through
them.   But occasionally there was an induration palpable in the right
ileocecal region, corresponding to the appendix.   On one occasion this
tumor was examined by me personally, and on percussion gave a deep,
loud, tympanitic resonance.   On another occasion the tumor was not in
the ileocecal region, but apparently in the transverse colon, and peristaltic

waves could be felt traveling through it. I considered the case one of enterospasm, because of the absence of evidence of any other demonstrable disease, excepting a retroflexion of the uterus. At times there were signs of such pronounced and distressing symptoms from pylorospasm that a colleague, into whose hands the case drifted, considered it a pyloric carcinoma. One year after I had first seen the patient, her relatives requested me to attend an operation upon her, undertaken with the view of removing an inflamed appendix. After laparotomy, by an experienced and dexterous surgeon, nothing abnormal could be detected in the abdomen; ovaries normal; appendix, gall-bladder, cecum, and sigmoid flexure normal; spleen, liver, and kidneys normal; stomach normal. Inasmuch as her most distressing symptoms had recently been due to a pylorospasm, a pyloroplastic operation, according to Heinecke and Mikulicz, was performed. The patient recovered from the operation. Eight months have passed since then, during which I have visited the patient once. She still suffers from attacks of enterospasm, occasionally alternating with pneumatosis. As she has not returned to me for treatment, I am not able to tell what effect a treatment would have such as was applied in the previous case.

Cherchevsky ("Contribution à la pathologie des névroses intestinales," "Révue de Méd.," 1883) has reported a case in which there was stercoraceous vomiting, and a piece of formed fecal matter 8 cm. long, it is claimed, was vomited. The condition is called by this author "ileus nervosus." In a case described by Talma ("Deutsch. Archiv f. klin. Med.," Bd. LXIX) there were also attacks of gastric colic associated with vomiting.

Etiology.—Enterospasm is not found as often in men as in women, especially in those who have become very nervous and irritable as a result of previous disease (especially uterine troubles). It often accompanies basal meningitis in its first stage, and also other diseases of the central nervous system, where pressure is exerted upon the pons and the medulla oblongata. It also accompanies chronic lead-poisoning. As a complication of this disease, enterospasm usually extends over the entire intestine, or at least over a large portion of the small intestine. The more usual form of enterospasm, where it is confined to single sections of the intestine (especially the large intestine), generally attacks nervous, irritable persons, and sufferers from hysteria and neurasthenia. It occurs in such persons especially when chance causes irritate the intestine, such as ingestion of highly seasoned foods and the administration of drastic purges. In many cases enterospasm occurs

secondarily as an accompaniment of colitis. In such cases, especially if the patient is slow in putting himself under treatment, we
usually can not decide definitely whether the colitis is the cause or
the result of the enterospasm, or if both occurred simultaneously.
If the enterospasm lasts for some time, the stagnating fecal masses
and gases irritate the intestinal mucosa intensely, so that the conditions for the development of colitis are very favorable in enterospasm.

Symptomatology.—In the general enterospasm accompanying
basilar meningitis, in other diseases of the central nervous system,
and also in chronic lead-poisoning, the abdomen usually presents a
boat-shaped or trough-like, concave depression of its anterior wall.
This depression is even much greater than after long-continued
inanition, in which state the empty intestine, on account of its
elasticity, contracts only moderately; whereas in intense enterospasm the intestinal lumen is often entirely obliterated. In the
more usual form of enterospasm, where the disease is confined to
single, smaller sections of the intestine, the boat-shaped depression
is not present. Indeed, the abdomen may even become asymmetrically distended at circumscribed places, where atonic intestinal loops
excessively distended by feces and gases are situated above the
spastically contracted intestinal loops. The atony of the intestinal
loops lying immediately above and adjoining the contracted sections—suprastenotic loops—and the resultant distention by feces
and gases may probably be explained by the fact that the muscularis
loses its energy after having vainly striven to remove the obstruction to the passage of the feces. When this occurs, the intestinal
wall can offer no further resistance (just as in advanced organic
stenosis), and it is excessively distended by gases and accumulating
feces. The chyme and the feces can be carried downward only by
the peristaltic motions of the intestines. (See section on Peristalsis.)
These in turn are dependent upon the alternating contractions of
the longitudinal and circular muscularis, which cease in their
normal regularity when enterospasm sets in. In general enterospasm the intestinal lumen is extensively contracted; in circumscribed enterospasm it is contracted only at various places by the
tonic contractions of the circular muscularis. Persistent stool retention must inevitably follow this condition in both forms of entero-

spasm; when it occurs in circumscribed enterospasm, it is called spastic constipation.   The stools are often retained for several days at a time.   If purges are administered, the feces pass off only in slight quantities and with frequent pains.   If enterospasm is complicated with proctospasm, such as sometimes happens, defecation is completely checked.   Finally, the feces are evacuated in the form of flattened strip-like bands of various lengths, or cylinders as thick as lead-pencils; sometimes the feces appear as small globules like sheep dung, which were formed in the haustra or sacculi of the colon.   But as similar forms of feces may also be found in intestinal steriosis, atony, and inanition, they point to enterospasm only when the aforesaid conditions are excluded.   The feces always appear in bands, strips, or thin cylinders, and have a dark brown instead of a light yellow color, when they have been retained a long time in the intestine during enterospasm.

Pain.—Enterospasm usually, but not always, causes pains. These are oppressive, straining, constricting, pinching, and sometimes even cramp colic.   Sometimes they are felt exclusively in the umbilical or in the left hypogastric region; at other times they may have their location at other parts of the abdomen.   They are usually increased by pressure on the abdominal walls and by bodily exertions.   After copious evacuations have taken place, the pains usually either cease entirely for a time, or grow very much less. The defecation is often accompanied by painful sensations.   The enterospasm occurs in paroxysms, which continue for a varying length of time.   In many patients they occur at night, robbing their sleep.   If the attacks last for some time, and quickly succeed one another, and if they are accompanied by colicky pains, the general health and state of nutrition may be seriously impaired.

Diagnosis.—General secondary enterospasm accompanying basilary meningitis, lead-poisoning, etc., can be recognized easily and with certainty if it has not been accompanied by pains from the onset: the abdomen is concavely depressed (boat-shaped concavity), the feces present the formative changes described above, and other symptoms of the fundamental disease are also present. If the enterospasm is accompanied by pains from the onset, it can not be distinguished from colic, especially if the latter is found as a complication of the same diseases as are known to be etiological to enterospasm. The diagnosis of the circumscribed form often presents greater difficulties than that of the general enterospasm, since the characteristic boat-shaped depression is wanting. These difficulties, however, may be overcome if the stools are inspected frequently, if other symptoms of neurasthenia and hysteria are present, and if it can be determined by anamnesis that strong irritants had affected the intestine previously.

Prognosis.—The prognosis is favorable if the cause can be recognized and removed, although enterospasm is a very obstinate and troublesome disease. It may be cured by a careful mode of living, by the protection of the intestine against pernicious influences, and by rational therapeutics, to be outlined.

Therapeutics.—The treatment of enterospasm must naturally attempt the removal or improvement of the mental and neurotic disease. It usually is best to start the treatment in the severe cases by prescribing denarcotized extract of opium (gr. ¼), tinct. belladonnæ (gtt. 10) either alone or together with opium, or subcutaneous injections of morphin. This relieves the cramp and ameliorates or removes the pains altogether.

If no evacuations take place after this, one should endeavor to cause them by giving mild purgatives,—castor oil, senna, citrate of magnesia—and by lukewarm water enemata; or, still better, by oil enemata, which often yield good results. Drastic purges, cold enemata, massage, and faradic electricity do no good, in my opinion, but often do damage and increase the suffering. The galvanic current (25 milliamperes) applied to spine and abdomen by large plates sometimes relieves the pain. Priessnitz bandages at night can be recommended. Hot external applications to the abdomen are always indicated. Strong bodily exertions must be avoided. After meals it is extremely desirable that patients should take a rest for several hours (in the dorsal position). Only easily digested food should be prescribed, based on analysis of the gastric contents, not only during the paroxysms of enterospasm, but also when these have subsided. Besides this, care should be taken to render the evacuations regular. If the enterospasm is the consequence of extreme nervousness, neurasthenia, etc., this will require special treatment.

PERISTALTIC UNREST OF THE INTESTINES.

Nature, Description, Etiology, and Symptomatology.—The normal intestinal movements, by which the chyme and the feces are passed downward during digestion, are neither visible nor perceptible. If they can be distinctly perceived through the abdominal walls (provided they are not too thick), it is a sure indication that they are considerably increased. An increase in the intestinal peristalsis may be caused by strong irritants, which originate in the blood or the intestinal mucosa and affect the nerves, or by an increase in the excitability of the sensory or motor nerves of the intestines. In the discussion of certain anatomical diseases of the intestines, — such as diarrhea, chronic stenosis, occlusions, catarrhs, —we have also learned that they very often cause a very great increase in the peristalsis, especially if they are accompanied by advanced decomposition and fermentation of the intestinal contents, together with excessive formation of gas. This increase, however, may also be caused by purely functional disturbances of the sensory and motor intestinal nerves, without any objective anatomical changes in the intestine to be detected. If this increase in the peristalsis continues a long time, or if it occurs in paroxysms, which frequently recur after longer or shorter intervals, it is called *peristaltic unrest*. When this is caused by an increased excitability of the sensory intestinal nerves, it will be accompanied by subjective complaints, such as unpleasant sensations of swaying to and fro, contractions and unrest of the intestinal loops, and sometimes even cramp-like pains. Besides these symptoms, it may cause swashing, rumbling, gurgling noises, which are loud enough to be heard not only by the patient, but by persons in the immediate neighborhood. If the excitability of the motor nerves alone is increased, while that of the sensory nerves remains normal, the subjective complaints may not be perceptible. In such cases the noises, starting from the intestines, and the stool retention are the only symptoms of the disease. If the peristaltic unrest sets in at night, the noises alone may prevent sleep even if there are no subjective complaints. There are cases in which the exceedingly active and disagreeable movements last continuously even after intestinal digestion is completed, and they are also accompanied by severe pains. This form of peristaltic unrest may be dependent upon a combined sensory and motor neurosis. Peristaltic unrest of the intestine is associated fairly often with a similar condition of the stomach.

Peristaltic unrest is usually met with in nervous, hysterical, and hypochondriacal persons. However, it also occurs in otherwise perfectly healthy persons, in whom there is not the slightest trace of neurasthenia. In women it often sets in during the menstruation period or during pregnancy. In some persons it is caused by certain highly seasoned or difficultly digestible foods. It may also be caused by the excessive use of tobacco, by psychic excitement, excessive mental work, etc. French authors have attributed it to tight lacing. In many cases no apparent reason can be discovered for it.

We might expect that, as a result of the increased motility of the intestine in peristaltic unrest, its contents ought to be excreted more rapidly, and that the stool ought to be more frequent than usual, and of a thin pulpy or watery consistency. The exact opposite is usually observed in most of the cases of peristaltic unrest—namely, persistent stool retention. Therefore it is probable that the peristaltic unrest is restricted to the small intestine alone, and that the movements of the large intestine are still more sluggish than usual. Fleischer suggests the possibility that the effect of the exaggerated peristalsis of the intestine may be counteracted by those antiperistaltic movements which may appear under certain abnormal conditions. However, normal peristaltic and antiperistaltic movements can not occur in the same section of the intestine at the same time; and if they occur in different sections,—that is, if there be normal downward peristalsis in one section and antiperistaltic movements in another section below it,—a fecal accumulation must result where the two movements collide. But if the two forms work in a diverging direction,—that is, toward the stomach and upper loops, and toward the rectum and lower loops,—the phenomenon of stercoraceous vomiting may occur. This theory seems to be supported by the observation that in peristaltic unrest evil-smelling eructation and even stercoraceous vomiting may occasionally appear.

In my work on "Diseases of the Stomach" I have pointed out how some of the so-called gastric neuroses may, by thorough and systematic histological investigation, yet be proved to be due to anatomical alterations in the gastric mucosa, and also given the microscopic evidence that at least one form of hyperchlorhydria is due to pathological increase of the oxyntic cells. (Hemmeter, "Histologie d. Magendrüsen bei Hyperacidität," "Archiv f. Verdauungs-Krankh.," Bd. LV, S. 23.) Similarly methodical investigation may succeed in demonstrating an anatomical substratum for one or more of the intestinal neuroses. The anatomical alterations in the nervous plexuses of the intestines (plexuses of Auerbach and Meissner), described by Blaschko, Sasaki, Scheimpflug, and Jürgens, have not as yet been brought into distinct etiological relations with the motor intestinal neuroses.

Emminghaus ("Münch. med. Wochenschr.," 1894, No. 5 und 6) has described two cases which are interesting in this connection. The first was that of a female patient who had for years suffered from intractable constipation. At the necropsy an old pleuritic cicatricial induration was found on the right side, presenting a tough, glistening, white, very circumscribed appearance, and corresponding accurately to the region of the right major splanchnic nerve. This nerve showed marked reduction in the number of nerve bundles in comparison with the left splanchnic. Whilst the latter showed four large and fourteen small, entirely intact bundles on cross-section, the diseased right splanchnic showed but four large and two small ones. In a second case, in which habitual constipation gave way to a slight diarrhea three weeks before death, a fibrino-purulent exudation, walled off in the right pleura, covered the origin of the splanchnic. Here, too, the right splanchnic gave the histological evidences of advanced atrophy.

Diagnosis.—In cases where the intestinal movements can be distinctly perceived and felt through the abdominal walls, the diagnosis of peristaltic unrest is very easy. Usually it is not very difficult to determine the nervous nature of the disease, because other nervous symptoms are usually present; the paroxysmal appearance of the disease and the influence of certain accidental causes also argue for the existence of a neurosis in certain cases. Those anatomical changes of the intestine which may cause an increase of the peristalsis can usually be recognized with certainty or excluded.

The **prognosis** is favorable.

Therapeutics.—In the less severe cases the disease can usually be cured by a non-irritating, easily digested diet, by a regulation of the stools by mild purgatives, rest, and hot external cataplasms. If the disease is more obstinate, and is accompanied by cramp-like pains and other complaints, opium is advisable, also tinct. belladonnæ, (10 drops at a dose), morph. mur. in small quantities. Stronger doses are to be avoided on account of the existence of constipation. If the peristaltic unrest also occurs at night, and prevents sleep, a hypnotic should be administered, such as bromid of strontium with chloral hydrate, or sulfonal, because the nervousness, and together with it the peristaltic unrest, may easily increase as a result of the insomnia. If this unrest is only a partial symptom of general nervousness, one must endeavor to exert a quieting and sedative influence over the entire nervous system by means of well-known hydropathic and electric (galvanic current) applications. Some-times a combination of strontium, ammonium, and sodium bromid acts very satisfactorily, or arsenic preparations. In an exceedingly annoying and obstinate case of peristaltic unrest which had been unsuccessfully treated by a number of European specialists, a per-manent improvement was effected by the following :

 ℞. Tinct. valerian. ammon., ... ʒ x
  Strontium bromid, ... ʒ iv
  Liquor of the arsenite of potassium, ... 50 drops
  Denarcotized extr. of opium, ... gr. ij
  Elixir simpl., q. s. . . . . ℥ vj.   M.
 Sig.—One tablespoonful 3 or 4 times daily.
 Together with this, calcined magnesia and carbonate of soda for the relief of a marked gastric hyperacidity were used.

If a distinct uric acid diathesis can be made out, warm alkaline baths have been very helpful in my experience.

Paralysis of the Intestinal Muscularis.

This condition has already been described in association with the subject of intestinal obstruction. But for the purpose of complete-ness to the representation of the intestinal neuroses, a short reca-pitulation is in order.

Paralysis of the intestinal muscularis may either extend over the entire organ or may confine itself to individual sections of the same ; in either case it causes a complete stoppage of the passage of the feces. It frequently is only a partial symptom or a resultant appearance of numerous anatomical diseases of the intestines and of other abdominal organs.   Thus it may be observed, for instance, in stenoses, in the various forms of occlusion, in those inflammations of the intestines which lead to extensive ulcerations and consequent cicatricial stenoses (enteritis, tuberculosis, enteric fever, peritonitis). Dysentery, according to Woodward (*l. c.*), does not cause intestinal stenoses.   These diseases usually cause intestinal paralysis by first causing an excessive increase in the peristalsis in the loops above the obstruction.   After this has existed for a varying period of time, the muscularis becomes exhausted.   The intestinal walls are then excessively distended by the accumulated masses of feces and gases ; the muscularis finally is paralyzed.   If the excessive distention of the intestinal walls and their muscularis lasts for a long time, the paresis may become irreparable.   The development of intestinal paresis from the intestinal atony, causing persistent constipation and coprostasis, is a rare occurrence, usually requiring a long time.   It is usually the result of the gradual hyperdistention of the intestinal walls by gases and by the accumulated and condensed fecal masses, which occasionally close the intestinal lumen entirely (coprostatic obstruction).

Intestinal paralysis usually sets in quite suddenly, without any increase in the peristalsis having been previously detected, both in general peritonitis and in severe traumatic injuries to the intestinal walls (for instance, hernial incarcerations and hernial operations), that cause great disturbances in the circulation, and an edematous infiltration of the intestinal walls.

Intestinal paralysis is caused much more rarely by the fact that inhibitory impulses may be transferred from a disease focus outside of the intestine itself (abscess formation of the inguinal glands or of the abdominal walls, contusions of the testicles, inflammatory hydrocele) to the motor centers of the intestines, and thus cause an arrest of the intestinal movements (Henrot).   (See chapter on Motor Insufficiency of the Intestine.)

Intestinal paralysis may occur also in other diseases, such as tabes, myelitis, meningitis, tumors of the brain, and certain psychoses—hypochondria, melancholia, hysteria.

After intestinal paralysis has set in, the passage of feces and flatus ceases entirely.   The intestine is inflated meteorically.   Vomiting sets in, which finally becomes stercoraceous. If, however, the paralysis has set in very suddenly, the vomiting may be absent.

Prognosis.—If a long time has elapsed since the start of the intestinal paralysis, there is little hope that the muscularis will recover completely and perform its functions again, even if the causes of the paralysis have been removed. The prognosis is most favorable in those cases in which the intestinal paralysis is the result of excessive fatigue of the muscularis, and of overdistention by accumulated feces and gases, in the absence of any anatomical disease of the intestinal wall and its peritoneum. If one succeeds in removing the stagnating feces and the intestinal gases artificially, then the intestinal muscularis usually recovers very quickly, even if the intestinal lumen is somewhat contracted at any one place.

Therapeutics.—The fundamental disease must first be considered in the treatment. If this permits the application of electricity and massage, then these are especially to be recommended. One should endeavor to cause a thorough evacuation of the accumulated fecal masses and gases by copious enemata of warm water, or of ℥viij of olive or cotton-seed oil. These oils should be thoroughly washed by shaking them repeatedly with pure water.* Drastic purges are entirely useless if the intestinal muscularis is completely paralyzed.

Insufficiency or Paralysis of the Sphincters.

Paralysis of the sphincters is always a secondary disease. It is observed most frequently as a result of long-continued organic diseases of the rectum, such as proctitis, hemorrhoids, ulcer processes, stricture, tuberculosis, syphilis, carcinoma, enlarged prostate. In these diseases the paralysis is brought about in very much the same way as the paralysis of the intestinal muscularis, which has just been described. At first spastic contractions of the sphincters are caused, which lead to fatigue, and finally a complete paralysis of the muscularis. If obstinate constipation exists at the same time, or if the passage of the urine is hindered from any reason, the appearance of the paralysis may be hastened, because the frequent,

---

* Almost all imported olive oil is American cotton-seed oil that has been purified and relabeled in France and Spain.

violent straining makes great demands upon the sphincters, and more especially upon the external sphincter. Insufficiency or paralysis of the sphincters in rare instances is caused by extension of the inflammatory or ulcerative processes from the rectum to the anus, and thence inward to the muscularis. An edematous infiltration or partial destruction of the muscular fibers may then render them incapable of performing their functions. The paralysis may also occur independently of anatomical diseases of the intestines, as in many affections of the brain and spinal cord, where the patient may lose the power to contract his external sphincter. If it is only a case of fatigue or partial paresis of the sphincters, the patient can usually retain gases and semi-solid feces completely when he remains quiet; during violent bodily exertions, coughing, sneezing, or straining during urination, a small portion of the feces will pass out, however, especially if they be thin, pulpy, or watery.

If the sphincters are completely paralyzed, gases and feces pass off against the patient's will, even during rest (*incontinentia alvi*). If the paralysis is the result of proctitis, hemorrhoids, strictures, cancer, etc., a bloody, mucous mass frequently protrudes from the open anus continuously, macerating and attacking the skin in the neighborhood of the anus, giving rise to peri-anal dermatitis.

Diagnosis.—Paralysis of the sphincters can be recognized without difficulty. The anus is open, and the anal folds are smoothed out. One can penetrate into the rectum easily with two and even three fingers. If one wants to ascertain whether the disease is purely nervous, or if it is dependent upon anatomical diseases, a thorough examination of the rectum must be made with the proctoscope. (See chapter on Diseases of the Rectum.) It is perhaps best to emphasize again that intussusceptions may also paralyze the sphincters, as soon as the intussuceptum has penetrated into the rectum.

The **prognosis** must naturally vary with the nature of the underlying disease. If incurable diseases are at the basis of the paralysis, the prognosis is unfavorable. Sphincter paresis from a neurotic condition or from exhaustion is amenable to rational treatment.

Therapeutics.—The treatment must naturally vary with the cause. (See Diseases of the Rectum.) It is especially necessary to cause a thorough emptying of the colon several times a day by means of enemata; in paresis of the sphincters all accumulation of condensed feces in the rectum should be prevented. Patients whose urination is hindered from any reason, and in whom the frequent, severe straining has caused a paresis of the external sphincter, should be taught to draw off the urine by means of a catheter.

Electricity and massage, and subcutaneous injections of strychnin nitrate (gr. $\frac{1}{36} = 0.0001-0.0015$ per dose) in the folds of the anus, have been recommended and are frequently effective.

SENSORY NEUROSES OF THE INTESTINES.

Introductory Remarks.—Sensory neuroses are theoretically explained by either an increase or a decrease or even complete suppression of the normal excitability of the sensory intestinal nerves. Of these two forms of neurosis only the former has any great practical interest. It is dependent upon the increased irritability of the sensory nerves, and is represented by the fairly frequent enteralgia (colic) and the rarer hypogastric neuralgia. The other form, which is caused by the decrease or suspension of the excitability of the sensory nerves,—an anesthesia of the intestines,—possesses only a theoretical interest, because it usually evades detection, except in one case which will be mentioned later. It is well known that the excitation of the sensory intestinal nerves by means of chemical and mechanical irritants during intestinal digestion causes no sensations which reach consciousness. We can therefore easily understand why the absence of that excitation as a result of functional disturbances in the sensory nerves may not be recognized. There is an exception to this in the case of the sensory rectal nerves. When the feces pass into the rectum, they irritate the rectal nerves mechanically, and their entrance can be felt distinctly. The excitation of these nerves then causes a desire to evacuate. If the excitability of the rectal nerves has been decreased as a result of diseases of the spinal cord, or of long-continued fecal accumulation in the rectum, by which its walls are excessively distended, then the patients do not feel the entrance of the feces into the rectum and their passage through the anus, and, as a result, there is no desire for stool. If the excitability of the sensory rectal nerves has become entirely extinct, the innervation of the sphincters, which under normal conditions is reflexly caused by their excitation, no longer takes place, and the sphincters are not closed.   If the patient has also lost the power of contracting his external sphincter, the feces are passed off involuntarily, and the patient has his attention directed to the evacuation only by the smell and the soiled condition of the clothing.

Enteralgia, Mesenteric Neuralgia.

Nature, Description, and Etiology.—Nothnagel correctly objects to classifying "colic" with sensory neuroses of the intestines, because it is always a secondary phenomenon produced by tetanic intestinal contractions.*   No more should colic be considered a sensory neurosis of the intestines than cramps of the calves (which are pathogenetically analogous to colic) should be considered a neurosis of the ischiatic nerve.   Under normal conditions the digestive processes cause no sensations which reach consciousness.   Even after excessive meals the very active intestinal peristalsis occurring during intestinal digestion is, as a rule, not noticed.   On the other hand, disagreeble sensations of oppression, tension, and fullness in the abdomen, or even more or less violent intestinal pains, may be caused by exceptionally strong irritants under a normal excitability of the sensory intestinal nerves, or by the usual digestive irritation, if the excitation is morbidly increased.   These irritants may develop in the intestinal lumen or reach the nerves through the blood.   This intestinal pain reaches its greatest intensity when both of these factors are present simultaneously—that is, both local (intestinal) and systemic (circulatory) irritants.

Enteralgia may also be caused by inflammatory processes of the intestinal walls, especially if they lead to the formation of ulcers. This form of enteralgia naturally can not be considered a neurosis ; only those forms in which no anatomical alterations can be found deserve classification under this heading.   If the irritations ·which affect the sensory intestinal nerves are very strong, or if the excitability of the latter is considerably increased, the intestinal pain is accompanied by spastic contractions of the muscularis, which may extend over the larger part of the intestine (as, for instance, in lead

---

* Intestinal colic or enterodynia has been described in chapter XVI, page 394, vol. I.

colic) or may confine themselves to single sections. They are hardly ever absent in the more severe cases of enteralgia, and on that account constitute an important symptom. The spastic contractions of the intestinal muscularis may both increase the complaints in enteralgia and also render the return to the normal condition more difficult, for the following reasons. If the tonic contractions of the longitudinal and circular muscular layers last for some time, the sensory intestinal nerves are to some extent compressed. Since the contractions also hinder the passage of the chyme, of the feces, and of the intestinal gases, or prevent evacuation, these intestinal contents accumulate in front of the spastically contracted intestinal sections. Thus the sensory nerves of the intestines may be irritated both chemically by the fermenting and decomposing chyme, and mechanically by the stagnating and condensed, hardened feces, and, in places where the intestinal wall is distended, also by intestinal gases. In one section the nerves may be compressed by spasm; in another they are put on the stretch by distention. This combination of pathogenic events constitutes distinctly an intestinal colic, and is not strictly a neurosis. It is evident also that the pains in such colic often diminish considerably or disappear entirely, according to the partial or complete discharge of fecal masses and flatus, either spontaneously or after the use of purges or enemata.

Basal Causes of Intestinal Colic.—The number of abnormal irritants which may cause colic by their effect upon the sensory intestinal nerves is very great. In a portion of the cases, the colic is caused by a faulty diet, whether in regard to the quantity or the quality of the food. If a very great amount of food is ingested, which is very hard to digest, and remains in the stomach longer than usual, and is therefore attacked by fermentation and decomposition, when it passes over into the intestine it may cause colic. The same may be brought about by unwholesome or decayed foods and drinks which have started to ferment, decomposed or unseasoned wine or beer, unripe fruit, etc. Enteralgia has also been often observed after drinking very cold water or iced drinks.

Causes of Colic as Distinct from Enteralgia (see vol. 1, p. 394).— In my work on "Diseases of the Stomach" I have pointed out that in some families peculiar idiosyncrasies exist toward certain foods which upon ingestion may cause gastritis or gastralgia. Similarly, some people get intestinal colic every time they eat certain foods,—such as fish, oysters, crabs, fruits, or certain vegetables,—which are neither harmful nor hard to digest, and which agree splendidly with most persons. In such cases we have to do with an idiosyncrasy of the sensory intestinal nerves against the foods in question, which we can not explain. Some people have an idiosyncrasy against certain purges. For instance, they get an attack of colic after taking a very mild purge, and can yet stand a drastic purge of another character very well.

Another fairly frequent cause of colic is a fecal stagnation and an accumulation of gases in the intestine (wind colic), by which its walls are distended and the sensory nerves strongly irritated. This is the reason why little children who are fed on milk and porridge often suffer from wind colic, because such a food very often causes considerable gaseous formation in the intestine. In new-born children a short retention of meconium in the intestine often suffices to cause colic (meconal colic). This soon disappears if one succeeds in removing the meconium by a little castor oil.

Among other causes of colic we may mention gall-stones, foreign bodies, enteroliths, and intestinal parasites (ascarides when in large knots, tapeworms). Abnormal irritations starting from the blood cause colic much more rarely than when they start from the intestinal mucosa. Thus the colic accompanying uric-acid arthritis which at times immediately precedes, and also often supplants, an attack of gout, may probably be attributed to an irritation of the sensory intestinal nerves by excrementitious or tonic substances, especially salts of uric acid (sodium quadriuate and biurate), originating in the blood; for uric acid as such does not occur in the blood nor body secretions. (See vol. I, p. 651.) Personally I have had three opportunities to become convinced of the actual existence of gouty enteralgia, and a number of French writers assert that the products of gouty metabolism may be demonstrated in the gastric contents and stools during the height of the gouty attack. (Hemmeter, " Diseases of the Stomach," second edition, p. 391.) What the French designate as " lithiase intestinale " (Chevalier, "Lithiase intestinale," " Thèse de Paris," 1898; Dieulafoy, " Études sur l'appendicite," " Presse médicale," 1896 ; " Lithiase intestinale et entérrocôlite sableuse," Clin-

iques de l'Hôtel-Dieu, 1896–97 ; Laboulbène, " Sur le sable intestinal," " Archives générales de médicine," déc., 1879 ; Mathieu et
Richaud, " Deux cas de sable intestinal et d'entérite muco-mem-
braneuse," " Bull. et Mémoires de la Société médicale des Hôpitaux," Paris, 22 mai, 1896 ; Mongour, " Note sur un case de
lithiase intestinale," Société de Biologie, février, 1896 ; Oddo,
" Sable intestinal," Société médicale des Hôpitaux, 1896) is not
always gout, but refers to any form of calculous deposit or concretion found in the bowels.   Possibly the colic which occurs as the
result of chronic lead-poisoning, or of the much rarer copper-pois-
oning, is caused by the fact that the toxic lead and copper salts in
the blood irritate the sensory intestinal nerves.   At present we
have not yet succeeded in explaining the origin of the colic which
often sets in after severe colds of the outer skin, especially that of
the abdomen.   It is usually explained by saying that the blood
flowing in great quantities from the contracted vessels of the skin to
those of the intestines and the other abdominal organs, causing
hyperemia of the intestines, irritates the intestinal nerves.

An enteralgia as a genuine neurosis is a painful condition of the intestinal nerves, not like colic, which is the secondary effect of an
intestinal tetanus, but simply the expression of an exaggerated irritability of the sensory intestinal nerves.   It has become customary
to distinguish a plantar neuralgia (plantaris) from an ischiatic or
sciatic neuralgia.   Similarly, we are justified in distinguishing between a neuralgia involving (a) only portions of the intestinal territory supplied by the splanchnic nerve, and (b) that involving the
entire mesenteric plexus.   These two forms differ only in the extent of the regions involved, and have been described as (a) Neuralgia nervi splanchnici and (b) Neuralgia plexus mesenterici, respectively (Nothnagel).   Lead colic (colica saturnina) may or may not be
associated with tetanic contractions of the intestinal muscularis ; the
abdomen may or may not be concavely retracted.   Accordingly it
may be considered secondary to a muscular tetanus, or, in the absence of this, it may be looked upon as a pure neurosis.

Intestinal colic as just described does not represent a typical sensory neurosis, except in those cases in which it is dependent upon
an increase in the normal excitability of the sensory intestinal nerves,
without any other assignable pathogenic cause.   This is observed

most frequently as a partial symptom or resultant appearance of neurasthenia, hysteria, hypochondria, and tabes. In tabes very violent attacks of colic (intestinal or abdominal crises) often occur, with or without gastric crises, and may distress the patient exceedingly. Nothnagel is of the opinion that the abdominal or intestinal crises are not always pure neuroses, but occasionally associated with muscular enterospasm, either coordinate or reflex, and quotes the classical clinical picture given by Romberg of hyperesthesia of the mesenteric plexus, to prove that this venerable neurologist also confused intestinal colic with enteralgia of a purely neurotic type.

The excitability of the intestinal nerves may also be increased by diseases of the bladder, the uterus, the ovaries, the kidneys, and the liver, and give rise to enteralgia. Malaria also may in rare instances cause intestinal colic.

Symptomatology.—There is no such thing as a typical clinical picture of mesenteric enteralgia as a neurosis pure and simple. When we consider that the abnormal irritants which may cause colic are very numerous; that their intensity and duration may greatly vary; that in those cases where enteralgia is a partial or resultant symptom of hysteria, neurasthenia, tabes, and lead-poisoning the symptoms of these basal diseases may also appear, we can well understand why the clinical appearance of the disease varies so extraordinarily in different cases; why the attacks are of a varying intensity, and their duration longer or shorter. If the enteralgia has been caused by a faulty diet, it usually commences with gastric disturbances, eructation, nausea, vomiting, and anorexia. If we are confronted with stercoral colic, it is usually preceded by obstinate constipation and flatulency, which occasionally alternates with diarrhea. If the enteralgia is the result of a chronic lead-poisoning, we can detect traces of lead on the gums, oliguria, and sometimes albuminuria; the pulse is hard and retarded. Paralysis is usually absent at this stage.

The main symptom of enteralgia is the intestinal pain, which entirely dominates the clinical picture of the disease in the more severe cases. It is very seldom that it appears suddenly and in all its intensity. Usually it is of moderate intensity at first and then gradually increases in strength. The pains often have a griping character, but are also frequently described as cutting, boring, and stabbing. Sometimes the patients feel as if the intestine were seized and pulled about at one or more places by tongs or they describe their feeling as a twisting of the bowel. In the majority of cases the patients usually locate the pain in the umbilical region. However, it often radiates thence toward the back, the loins, upward, toward the thighs, and also into the testicles. In those cases where the pain often changes its location, it is usually accompanied by palpable peristalsis, which causes loud rattling and rumbling noises. In the slighter cases the pain usually is endurable and lasts but a short time; in the more severe cases, however, it may reach such an intensity that delicate patients may faint as a result of it. The pale countenance has a suffering look, cold sweat is on the forehead, and the extremities are as cold as in collapse. In many cases the pains are alleviated by external pressure. On this account the patients usually press their hands or some firm substance against their abdomen. During the height of the attack they usually take a bent-up lateral position, sometimes the ventral position. If, however, the entire intestine, and consequently also the abdomen, is excessively distended by gases, then even gentle pressure is sufficient to increase the pains considerably, so the physician may begin to suspect the presence of peritonitis. If the attack ceases, the pain gradually decreases. If it be a case of secondary colic, and not of primary enteralgia, the pain decreases rapidly when the accumulated fecal masses and gases ·are removed spontaneously or by the use of purges or enemata.

In intestinal colic, spastic contractions of the intestines are hardly ever absent if the pains are very violent. If these contractions extend over a large portion of the intestines, as is the case more especially in lead colic, the abdomen presents a boat-shaped depression. The abdominal walls are very tense, and often as hard as a board, because the abdominal muscles are usually affected by the cramp. If the spastic contractions of the muscularis are restricted to single sections of the intestines, then this depression is absent. Indeed, the abdomen may be asymmetrically bulged out at those places where intestinal loops are distended by gases and stagnating feces. In stercoral colic and wind colic the abdomen is usually symmetrically and meteorically distended.

In colic the stools are usually retained; sometimes there is also a retention of gases. If flatus afterward passes off in large quantities, the pains usually cease for a short time; indeed, they may cease altogether, especially in the so-called wind colic. Just as the intensity, so also the duration of colic attacks is subject to very great variations. If the abnormal irritation which caused the enteralgia has excited the sensory intestinal nerves only temporarily, the pain may last but a short time (sometimes only minutes), and there may be only the one attack. If, however, the excitant effect of these strong irritants upon the sensory intestinal nerves is repeated at longer or shorter intervals, and if the excessive increase in their excitability lasts for some time, then the patients are often tortured for hours by violent pains, and the paroxysms recur after longer or shorter intervals.

Besides the previously mentioned symptoms, the following are also found in enteralgia: Asthmatic complaints, palpitation of the heart, feelings of oppression, tenderness, strangury, singultus, and vomiting; priapisms and emissions, which probably are caused reflexly, occur more rarely. When the paroxysm is at its height, the testicles may be drawn upward, and the levator ani muscle may be spasmodically contracted. Even crural cramps and general convulsions have been observed repeatedly during colic. The enteralgia which is dependent upon hysteria is sometimes accompanied by a hyperesthesia of the abdominal walls.

Diagnosis.—The symptomatology of enteralgia and colic is very characteristic, and the disease may usually be diagnosed with certainty. But the clinical distinction between primary enteralgia, the neurosis pure and simple, and secondary (enteralgic) colic in the sense of Nothnagel, is not always easy. Fortunately this differential diagnosis is not very essential to correct treatment, as the therapy of both conditions is much the same. The nervous (or neuralgic) nature of the disease is usually characterized sufficiently well in most cases by the sudden commencement, by its paroxysmal occurrence, and by its cessation; by the presence of other nervous symptoms, and also by the etiology. In secondary enteralgia, which is the result of anatomical diseases of the intestine (inflammation, ulceration), the pain often increases under pressure exerted upon the abdominal wall. These diseases also cause diarrhea more frequently than constipation, and in some cases pathological additions (blood, mucus, more rarely pus) may be discovered in the dejections by means of a repeated, thorough examination. (See chapter on Examination of Feces.)   A careful previous history and record of present examination, which must be extended to the evacuations (gall-stones, fragments of enteroliths, intestinal parasites), are necessary for the determination of the causes of colic in the various individual cases.

There are other diseases which cause pains in the abdomen, and which might therefore be mistaken for enteralgia.   They are rheumatism of the abdominal muscularis, lumbar neuralgia radiating to the abdomen, hyperesthesia of the abdominal walls, appendicitis, the obstructions, peritonitis, gall-stone colic, and nephrolithic colic. Usually, however, they may be differentiated from purely neurotic enteralgia without difficulty.

Rheumatism of the Abdominal Muscles.—The pain caused by this rheumatism often changes its seat.   It may be located by the patients themselves as being in the abdominal walls, not within the abdomen. It usually lasts longer than the pain dependent upon colic, but does not occur in paroxysms, and has no distinct alternating alleviations and exacerbations.   It increases under a moderate pressure upon the abdominal walls, and still more so at the contractions of the abdominal muscularis during defecation.   When the patient is quiet and in the dorsal position, and the tension of the abdominal walls is relaxed, it decreases.   The evacuations in rheumatism of the abdomen are hindered just as in enteralgia.   This is due to the fact that the patients often suppress all desire for an evacuation as long as possible, for fear of increasing the pain.   The pains in rheumatism are often alleviated or even removed by using anti-rheumatic remedies which are without any effects in colic,—such as salol and sodium salicylate,—and also by the application of faradic or voltaic currents upon the abdominal walls.   This is especially true if the rheumatism has existed only for a very short time.   There is, however, a form of enteralgia which occurs in rheumatic subjects and is amenable to the same treatment as the joint or muscular affection.   Here, we naturally presume that the intestinal pain, which is relieved by salicylate of sodium, is caused by the same abnormal conditions, whatever they may be, which cause the general rheumatism.

Lumbo-abdominal Neuralgia.—Here the pains are located on the surface (of the body), and are confined to a very sensitive intercostal region. They often radiate toward the seat, the hypogastrium, and the genitals. They may often be ameliorated or even destroyed by anti-neuralgic remedies such as antipyrin, antifebrin, or sodium salicylate. The recognition of this neuralgia is also rendered easier by detection of so-called neuralgic or pain spots—small circumscribed areas which are extremely sensitive to the slightest pressure.

Hyperesthesia of the Abdominal Walls.—This usually is a partial symptom of hysteria and neurasthenia, and the pains dependent upon it are usually accompanied by other symptoms of the basal disease. The superficially localized pains are greatly intensified by a very slight touch on the abdominal walls, and also by the raising of a fold of the skin; and very often they decrease rapidly after the application of faradic and galvanic currents.

Peritonitis.—This almost invariably causes fever, which is absent in enteralgia. The pain extends over the entire abdomen, continues for a long time, and is intensified by pressure. Marked meteorism is usually present, whereas in enteralgia it is observed in but very few cases, and these are not enteralgias really, but secondary colics. In peritonitis one can often detect a dullness by percussion, due to exudation in the lower parts of the abdomen.

If enteralgia is complicated with hyperesthesia of the abdominal walls, and great meteorism is present at the same time, it may readily be confounded with peritonitis. In such a case we are guided, however, by the usually abnormally high temperature in peritonitis, the leukocytosis, and by the fact that deep pressure does not produce more pain than superficial pressure, and also that the raising of a fold of the skin causes pain, which is not the fact in peritonitis.

Biliary and Nephrolithic Colic.—The differentiation of these conditions from enteralgia should present no difficulty if thorough examination is made. In biliary colic (cholelithiasis) the pains are most severe over the hepatic region ; and, besides, their recognition is made easier by other characteristic symptoms. In nephrolithic colic repeated urinalysis will eventually reveal the nature of the trouble.

Prognosis.—The prognosis of enteralgia is almost always favorable. Even in the more severe cases, where it may be a very troublesome and painful disease, accompanied by frequent relapses, it usually ends in a complete cure. In a case of secondary colic described by Oppolzer, death resulted from a break in the intestines caused by enormous meteorism ; in another case, reported by Wertheimer, death occurred during convulsions. These cases are, however, very exceptional.

Therapeutics.—If the patients complain of very violent pains, it is advisable to start the treatment by giving a sufficiently large dose of opium by the mouth (Tr. opii simplic., 15–20 drops ; Opii puri, gr. ½—0.03–0.05 gm.), or to make subcutaneous morphin injections (morph. sulphat. gr. ¼). These narcotics should also be prescribed when a stercoral colic is present, or a colic due to intestinal indigestion, accompanied by spastic contractions of the intestinal muscularis. For if purges or enemata are at once administered in such cases, instead of these narcotics, in order to facilitate the passage of the accumulated feces and gases, or of the chyme which has begun to decompose and ferment, they usually fail to attain the desired result by reason of the spastic contractions of the intestinal muscularis ; often, indeed, they increase the existing distress. If, however, the narcotics have quieted the spasm of the intestines, very often a copious evacuation occurs spontaneously in my experience. After the pain has been relieved this end may also be attained by giving a mild purge (rhubarb preparations, castor oil), so that it is not at all necessary to give a drastic purge which may cause another attack of the colic. Hot poultices by day, Priessnitz poultices at night, and hot baths, with subsequent sweating superinduced also by several cups of camomile tea, may also have very good results if the colic appeared in conjunction with a very severe cold. During severe attacks of colic the patient may have only small amounts of easily digestible fluid or pulpy food, so that a greater burdening and irritation of the intestines may be avoided. If the disease is very obstinate and frequently recurs, a course of electrical treatment is to be recommended. One electrode is inserted into the rectum, the other is placed upon the abdominal wall. Both currents are recommended, but I give preference to the galvanic current (25 milliamperes) for the relief of pain. Massage has also given very good results, espe-

cially in those cases where the enteralgia was caused by coprostasis,
and where a tendency toward constipation remained even after the
coprostasis had been removed.   If the secondary colic is due to an
irritation of the intestines caused by parasites (tenias, ascarides), one
must administer the anthelmintic remedies, as specified in the next
chapter.   If we are confronted with a secondary colic which may
be traced back to hysteria, neurasthenia, etc., this fundamental
disease, of course, must also receive due consideration in the
treatment.

Neuralgia Hypogastrica (Romberg).

If the enteralgia restricts itself to the lowest section of the intestines (rectum), it is called neuralgia hypogastrica.   It is characterized by disagreeable, sometimes even very painful sensations in the
hypogastric region and about the loins.   These sensations are
combined with a violent tenesmus in the rectum and bladder,
and in female patients these straining sensations are felt also in the
uterus and the vagina.   If the sympathetic nerve-fibers of the hemorrhoidal plexus, which supply the lower portion of the rectum, are
also affected, as is often the case, then the patients complain of
proctalgia and coxalgia, and also of pains in the perineum and the
upper part of the thighs.

Hypogastric neuralgia is especially common in people suffering
from hemorrhoids (hemorrhoidal colics), and in neurasthenic
women, and especially those afflicted with uterine diseases.   A
slight form of this neuralgia frequently occurs in tabes also.   In
such cases the patients have a sensation as if a solid wedge were
firmly stuck into their anus and in the lower part of the rectum.

Therapeutics. — This is exactly the same as in enteralgia and
intestinal colic. The rectum and genito-urinary apparatus should be
thoroughly examined. If the neuralgia is the result of hemorrhoids,
irritation of the bladder, or diseases of the uterus, the fundamental
disease must naturally be considered and treated first of all.   If
the digital examination shows that hemorrhoidal veins are present
which are congested to bursting, then local abstraction of blood
(application of leeches to the anus), hot baths, and more especially
numerous hot sitz-baths, are recommended.   If the pains are
very violent, opium suppositories or opium and starch enemata are

to be administered. The food must be non-irritating and easily digested. Constipation must be guarded against, and the evacuations kept at a soft consistency.

SECRETORY INTESTINAL NEUROSES.

Introduction.—Physiological investigation has made it quite certain that the intestine possesses secretory nerves just as well as the stomach. The correctness of this assumption is supported especially by the fact, which has repeatedly been observed, that the activity of the glands, not only of the small intestine (see preparatory secretion of duodenum, vol. 1, p. 53), but also of the large intestine, which is far removed from the stomach, begins at a time when none of the contents of the stomach have passed over into the intestine; or, in other words, as soon as the food has been introduced into the stomach. According to Fleischer, this would indicate that the secretory nerves of the intestine are excited reflexly from the stomach.

Up to the present time we have not succeeded in discovering these secretory nerves and in ascertaining their properties. Besides this, we can not determine with certainty the existence of disturbances in the secretory functions of the intestines if they do not reach any great intensity. It is not surprising, therefore, that the secretory neuroses of the intestines have received no attention at all until very recently. Trousseau, to be sure, suggested their existence. All this has been changed since Leube and Dieulafoy ("Entérocôlite glaireuse ou sableuse," Cliniques de l'Hôtel-Dieu, 1896 and 1897), in more recent times, have expressed their opinion that a disease called diarrhea tubularis, or membranous enteritis or colitis (see vol. 1, p. 483), which has been known for a long time, but which previously was indistinct as to its etiology, was in the great majority of cases to be considered as a secretory neurosis. This statement caused the attention of the clinicians and physicians to be directed to the secretory neuroses of the intestines. Nothnagel twelve years ago published valuable observations concerning the disease which previously had been called diarrhea tubularis, but which later on received the name of enteritis membranacea, or membranous enteritis. He was the first one to represent the opinion, which was contrary to the views of most of the authors, that there is no inflammatory affection present in the great majority of the cases in spite of the excessive secretion of mucus. On this account he has selected the very appropriate name " mucous colic," or "colica mucosa," for it. In the remaining much rarer cases, where the alterations produced by the disease are dependent upon a peculiar acute inflammation of the intestinal mucosa, he has retained the former name of "enteritis membranacea."

In a separate chapter I have already given the clinical picture, etiology, and pathology of both these conditions, as they do not by right belong under the secretory intestinal neuroses, but under the anatomical diseases of the intestines ; because even in those types which occur in neurotic subjects, the evidences for assuming that they are neuroses are not satisfactory ; they are so stated upon empirical, not experimental or histologic, grounds. All that can be said is that certain types of membranous enteritis or colitis are not due to the histological pathology of acute or chronic inflammation ; but saying this much does not necessarily place them in the class of neuroses. We must rather confess that the etiology and pathological physiology of these types are not understood so far.

Intestinal neurasthenia has been treated in the chapter on Intestinal Indigestion and Dystrypsia.

Nervous diarrhea has been considered in the chapter on Diarrhea (vol. 1, p. 352), and **nervous flatulence** on page 401, volume 1.

LITERATURE ON INTESTINAL NEUROSES.

1. Anacker, "Das Purgativ Oidtmann," "Deutsch. med. Wochenschr.," 1887, S. 823. (A criticism of a proprietary rectal purgative, the active ingredient of which is glycerin.)

2. Boas, J., "Deutsch. med. Wochenschr.," 1893, No. 41.

3. Brunton and Cash, "St. Barthol. Hosp. Report," 1887.

4. Cruveilhier, "Anat. path. gen.," t. II.

5. Da Costa, J. M., "Membranous Enteritis," "Amer. Jour. of the Med. Sci.," 1871, p. 321.

6. Doumer, E., et Musin, "Annales d'Electro-biologie," 1898, p. 722.

7. Dubois, "Gastro-intestinal Troubles in Neurasthenia" ("Des troubles gastro-intestinaux du nervosisme "), "Revue de Med.," Paris, July 10, 1900.

8. Dunin "Ueber habituelle Stuhlverstopfung, deren Ursachen und Behandlung," "Berlin. Klinik," 1891, H. 34.

9. Edwards, "Amer. Jour. of the Med. Sci.," April, 1888, p. 329.

10. Einhorn, Max, "Membranous Enteritis," "Med. Record," January 28, 1899.

11. Ewald, C. A., "Membranous or Mucous Enteritis," "Twentieth Century Practice," vol. IX, p. 265.

12. Fischel, F., "Prag. med. Wochenschr.," 1891.

12, a. Federn, "Ueber partielle Darmatonie," Wiener Klinik, 1891; also "Blutdruck u. Darmatonie," Wien, 1894; also "Ueber Darmatonie," "Wien. med. Presse," 1895, No. 25–28.

13. Flatau, "Berlin. klin. Wochenschr.," 1891, S. 231.

14. Fleischer, R., "Krankheiten des Darms," Wiesbaden, 1896.

15. Gant, Samuel G., "Neuralgia of the Rectum," "Kansas City Med. Index-Lancet," December, 1899.

16. Good, Mason, "The Study of Medicine," cl. I, ord. L, species 7, Philadelphia, 1825, vol. I, p. 162.

17. Hackel, Jeannot, "Deutsch. med. Wochenschr.," "Hydrotherap. of Chronic Obstip.," January 5, 1899, T. I.

18. Henrot, "Des Pseudo-étranglements," Paris, 1865.

19. Illoway, "Constipation in Adults and Children," New York, 1897.

20. Kahn, A., "Centralbl. f. Chir. u. orthopädische Mechanik," Berlin, 1889, Bd. v, S. 4.

21. Kittagawa, P., "Beiträge zur Kenntniss der Enteritis membranacea," "Zeitschr. f. klin. Med.," 1891.

22. Klemperer, "Therapie der Gegenwart," 1899, S. 48.

23. Laboulbene, "Recherches sur les affections pseudomembraneuses," 1861.

24. Leichtenstern, "Verengerungen, Verschliessungen, und Lageveränderungen des Darms," von Ziemssen's "Handbuch der speciellen Pathologie und Therapie," Leipzig, 1878, Bd. VII, 2. Hälfte.

25. Lemazurier, "Arch. gen. de med.," vol. I.

26. Leube, "Ueber Darmschwindel," "Deutsch. Arch. f. klin. Med.," Bd. XXXVI, 1885.

27. Leubuscher, "Centralbl. f. klin. Med.," 1887, No. 25.

28 Levi, "Gazette med.," 1839.

29. Leyden, E., "Verhandl. d. Vereins f. innere med. in Berlin," "Deutsch. med. Wochenschr.," 1882, No. 16 u. 17.

30. Massloff, "Untersuchungen aus dem physiologischen Institut zu Heidelberg," Bd II.

31. Mendelson, Walter, "Mucous Colitis a Functional Neurosis," "Med. Record," January 30, 1897.

32. Moreau, "Centralbl. f. d. med. Wissensch," 1868, No. 14.

33. Noorden, C. von, "Ueber die Behandlung der Colica mucosa," "Zeitschr. f. praktische Aerzte," 1898, No. I.

34. Nothnagel, "Colica mucosa," "Beitr. zur Physiologie und Pathologie des Darms," 1884, 12. Kapitel.

35. Oppolzer, "Wien. med. Wochenschr.," 1867.

36. Pariser, "Deutsch. med. Wochenschr.," 1893, No. 41.

37. Peyer, A., "Die nervösen Affectionen des Darms bei der Neurasthenie des männlichen Geschlechts," Wien. Klinik, 1893, H. I.

38. Romberg, "Lehrbuch der Nerven-Krankheiten," Berlin.

39. Rose, A., "New-Yorker med. Monatsschr.," January, 1893.

40. Rosenheim, Th., "Krankheiten des Darms," 1893, S. 513.

41. Rothmann, Max, "Ueber Enteritis membranacea," "Deutsch. med. Wochenschr.," 1893, p. 999.

42. Ruedi, Carl, "On Indications and Contraindications of High Altitudes in Phthisis," "The Climatologist," July, 1892.

43. Sahli, "Deutsch. med. Wochenschr.," 1897, No. 1.

44. Senator, "Hydrothionaemie und Selbstinfection durch abnorme Verdauungsvorgänge," "Berlin. klin. Wochenschr.," 1868, No. 24.

45. Siredey, J., "Note pour servir a l'étude des concretions muqueuses membraniformes de l'intestin," "Union méd.," Nos. 7–9, 1869.

46. Stewart, Chas. E., "Chronic Constipation and Sympathetic Nervous System," "Jour., Amer. Med. Assoc.," May 21, 1900.

47. Troussard, "Crises of Enteralgia in Mucomembranous Enteritis," "Gazette Hebdomadaire," July 22, 1900.

48. Wallace, "St. Barthol. Hosp. Report," 1888.

49. Wertheimer, "Deutsch. Arch. f. klin. Med.," 1866, Bd. 1.

50. Whitehead, W., "Mucous Disease," "Brit. Med. Jour.," February 11, 1871, p. 141.

CHAPTER XI.

PARASITES OF THE INTESTINAL CANAL.

Introduction.

The consideration of the parasites of the intestinal canal embraces the study of numerous organisms occurring in conditions of health and disease, in animals and in human beings. When existing in the intestinal tracts of individuals, they live at the expense of their host. There are two great varieties: (*a*) those belonging to the animal, and (*b*) those that are to be classed as belonging to the vegetable kingdom.

Besides these animal and vegetable parasites, there are also found in the intestines, or in the evacuations of both healthy and sick persons, various kinds of those organisms which are by some authors classed as transitional forms between plants and animals, and have therefore been named protozoa or protists (Häckel).* The vegetable intestinal parasites, as far as they are of practical interest to the physician, have been considered to a certain extent in the study of infectious intestinal diseases. A large number of the better known parasites which are now classed with the plants have already been described by Dr. Wm. Royal Stokes, in the section on Bacteria of the Intestine (vol. I, p. 135).

Of the animal parasites I shall describe only those occurring more frequently. The detailed discussion of those parasites which are very rarely observed can be all the more omitted since they cause the same disease symptoms as the more common forms, and as a general rule are also cured by the same means.

According to Leukart, there are more than fifty varieties of animal parasites which inhabit the human intestinal canal. In some countries and regions—that, for instance, in Greifswald and its vicinity—almost 50 per cent. of the inhabitants have parasites in their intestines (Heisig), and in Abyssinia persons without intestinal parasites are the exception; yet in other districts they are found

---

* With the exception possibly of a few ameboid forms, all intestinal parasites of man belong to the animal kingdom.

much more rarely.   In Baltimore intestinal parasites are comparatively rare, in my experience.   Wherever compulsory meat and food
inspection has become a law, parasitical diseases of the intestines have
decreased considerably.   The eggs (embryos) and youthful forms
of the animal parasites reach the intestines principally through food
and drink, and they may, under favorable conditions, develop into
mature specimens.   The principal etiologic factor in the transmission of the tapeworm (belonging to the class of cestodes) which is
found in the human intestine or in the evacuations (proglottides) is the
consumption of the flesh of those animals—swine, beeves, fish (especially, pike)—which contain the youthful forms of tapeworms (cysticerci, or bladder-worms).   Animal parasites may, however, reach the
intestinal canal with vegetable foods, with drinking-water, but very
rarely with the air.   The parasites and their eggs are killed or so
weakened by the long-continued action of high temperatures during the preparation of the food that they do not develop further
during their stay in the stomach and intestines ; it is therefore easily
understood why they are most frequently found in persons who
consume the flesh of the aforesaid animals raw, slightly smoked, or
half-cooked.   The greater the care for sanitary and hygienic conditions in the kitchen, in the preparation of the food, and in keeping
the cooking utensils and the dishes, and most especially the hands,
clean,—the less the danger of transmission of parasites (in the food) ;
whereas this transmission is facilitated by uncleanliness in the kitchen
and in the care of the body.   From the latter reason those persons
who come in close contact with agricultural animals and their excrement as a part of their occupation are in considerable danger if
they take their meals without having washed their hands, or having
done so but superficially.   The hands and fingers should be washed
and brushed thoroughly immediately before sitting down at the table.
This is a habit that physicians should practice.   There is no doubt
that the parasites settle and develop more easily in the intestines of
some persons than in others.   This was one of the foundations of
the old hypothesis of a *parasite* or *worm diathesis*.   The quicker
the contents of the stomach are discharged and the chyme and
feces transported downward and out, the less favorable are the
conditions for the settling, development, and increase of parasites in
the intestines.   The contrary is true in the case of a longer stagnation

conditions for the settling, development, and increase of parasites in the intestines. The contrary is true in the case of a longer stagnation of the ingesta in the stomach, and also of the chyme and feces in the intestines as a result of a diminished peristalsis of both organs. To be sure, some individual parasites (see later on protozoa) seem to increase more rapidly in acute and chronic enteritis accompanied with diarrhea than in the normal intestine, in spite of the greatly increased peristalsis. This may probably be explained by the fact that the powers of locomotion and of taking up nourishment are increased for the parasites by the greater amount of water contained in the intestines. In five cases of infection with *Tænia saginata*, all of which occurred among the employees of a butchering establishment, a striking and sudden constipation was the very first symptom the patients could recall. This suggested to me that the infected meat possibly contained a toxic product of this parasite which caused a transient paralysis of the intestinal peristalsis. These five patients all presented themselves within one month, but it was impossible to trace the meat which had caused the ingestion of the ova or cysticerci, and its effect on animals could not be tested.

In children certain nematodes (*Ascaris lumbricoides, Oxyuris vermicularis*) are most often observed; in adults tapeworms are more frequently noticed. This difference is probably conditioned principally by the difference in the diet. The examination of the evacuations, looking for large, macroscopically visible parasites, proglottides, and eggs, the detection of which is absolutely necessary for their diagnosis and differentiation, is best carried out by placing the evacuations on a hair or thin sieve (with fine holes) and gently letting water wash through (Boas stool-sieve). See chapter on Examination of the Feces, by Dr. Harry Adler.

PROTOZOA.

In the chapter on Dysentery (vol. I, p. 524) and in the chapter on Intestinal Bacteria (vol. I, p. 191) the pathogenic rôle and biology of the protozoa have already been partially considered. Numerous observations have been made which show that certain species of protozoa may occur in healthy persons without causing the least discomfort or complaint (Kartulis, Quincke, Nothnagel, Kruse, Pasquale). Parasites of this class, however, are found in great numbers in the evacuations of all diseases of the intestines accompanied by diarrhea, especially those caused by enteric fever, dysentery, cholera, and tuberculosis, but also in noninfectious acute and chronic enteritis. On this account it has been repeatedly maintained that the protozoa in question, if they increase very much, may cause diarrhea. Since, however, they are found in the intestines of perfectly healthy persons without causing any disturbances, one can not exclude the possibility that this great increase in the protozoa in the excreta is not the cause, but the effect, of the diarrhea, and that they find a more favorable soil in the intestine during diarrhea (possibly as a result of the increased amount of water and soluble nutriment). The observation that the protozoa disappeared simultaneously with the diarrhea is not a positive proof for the correctness of the assumption that they caused diarrhea, since with the cessation of the latter the more favorable conditions for their increase were lacking. If, however, the statement be confirmed in the future, that in those cases of diarrhea in which large numbers of protozoa can be detected in the excreta the diarrhea ceases simultaneously with the destruction of the protozoa by means of repeated irrigations with an aqueous solution of quinin (mur.), which is a strong poison for all lower organisms, then this assumption of an etiological relation would gain very much in probability. Quincke ("Berlin. klin. Wochenschr.," November 20, 1899) states that the pathogenic protozoa found in the intestinal tract are *Trichomonas intestinalis, Cercomonas hominis, Lamblia intestinalis* (formerly known under the older names *Megastoma enterica* and *Cercomonas intestinalis*), *Coccidia, Balantidium coli*, and *Amœba coli*. He reports one case in which the coccidia seemed to produce an enteritis, one in which an ameba was found, one in which a peculiar parasite (not exactly an ameba, perhaps a coccidium) was the cause of a chronic recurring diarrhea, and two other cases in which the symptoms had suggested tuberculosis of the lung and intestine, but in which at autopsy ulceration of the bowel was found with amebæ at the bottom of the ulcers. The clinical symptoms of protozoan enteritis are least characteristic in cases of infection with the flagellates occupying the small intestine. There is either a mild, chronic diarrhea, or only a disposition thereto. In the case of *Balantidium* and *Amœba coli* the symptoms referable to the large intestine are much more marked and may resemble those of dysentery. The evacuations are mushy and thin, containing pus and blood; the movements often occur in groups, especially toward morning, and are accompanied by tenesmus and preceded by tormina and borborygmi. In the beginning these parasites produce only a simple catarrh; later the balantidium and the ameba may bring on ulceration. Frequently in cases of ulceration the symptoms resemble those of tuberculosis of the intestines. Death in ulcerative colitis is dependent upon exhaustion from insufficient food assimilation, absorption of the putrefactive products, and, finally, upon septic infection. At times the ulcers lead to purulent peritonitis by continuity or perforation. It is not always possible to find the cause of the ulcers, especially in the case of the balantidium. The ameba is usually found at the bottom of the ulcer. Two cases of extensive colon ulceration in which the genesis was unknown are described by Quincke. They may both have been due to protozoa. As to the source of the protozoa and their mode of introduction, not much is known. The balantidium is found in the hog, and may be transmitted from it to man. Flagellates are found in hogs, sheep, mice, rats, rabbits, and cats. Coccidia are found in the liver of rabbits and in the intestinal epithelium of cattle, dogs, cats, and sheep. "*Amœba coli felis*" is found in cats; perhaps also in dogs. As to the source of the so-called "*Amœba coli mitis*," nothing is known; the drinking-water may have something to do with conveying the ameba. The *treatment* consists in removing the parasites, which, when they are in the small intestine, is accomplished by the administration of castor oil and calomel. In the large intestine irrigation must be used in addition. Calomel should be employed for one or two weeks in increasing doses; it is useful against all of the protozoa. But in infection with *Lamblia intestinalis* large doses of calomel have failed; this parasite is among the most difficult to get rid of. Quinin, in clysters or internally, is used against the balantidium. The flagellates are removed most easily; next, the balantidium; and amebic infection is the most resistant to treatment. The stools do not present anything characteristic, except that in chronic amebic cases they are thin, gelatinous, with a very slightly fecal odor, and have a strongly alkaline reaction (see Amebic Dysentery). The stools should be examined immediately after they are passed; and until the examination they should be kept warm in an incubator or by being covered. Sometimes it is advisable to introduce a thick glass rod into the rectum in order to get a little of its contents for examination. When the stool is not fluid enough, the microscopic preparation should be diluted with saline solution. The balantidium is most easily recognized on account of its size and mobility. The flagellates may also be recognized, but sometimes they are overlooked, on account of their transparency, pallor, and smallness. The ameba is sometimes confounded with the degenerated epithelial cells. Encysted forms and coccidia are least characteristic, but strike the attention by their number and uniformity; at times also by a peculiar greenish shine. They may be mistaken for nematode eggs perhaps. Staining scarcely helps the recognition of the protozoa; at least attempts to stain cover-slip preparations by Mallory's method (" Journ. Experim. Med.," vol. II, p. 530) proved unsuccessful. When the protozoa are to be stained in tissues, this serves admirably.

Protozoa soon become motionless in the excreted feces, and, assuming spherical forms, avoid detection. It is also advisable to look for small particles of mucus in the diarrheic evacuations, and to examine these, because protozoa are often contained in them in large quantities. If an admixture of mucus is wanting in the evacuations, mucus may be taken out of the rectum by means of a spatula or glass rod, and this examined microscopically.

Protozoa are unicellular organisms of such small size that single specimens can be detected with certainty only by the microscope. The body of the cell consists of contractile protoplasm, in which one or more nuclei may be discovered, and occasionally one or more contractile vacuoles. Their propagation or increase is carried out chiefly by fusion or budding. Sporulation, however, has been reported for many protozoa, and we are hardly in a position to deny it for the forms parasitic in man. For their locomotion they use (in the case of rhizopods) pseudopodia, which are protrusions or continuations of the protoplasms of the cell, capable of changing their shape readily, and which are formed as required and then retracted; or the organisms may have persisting flagella, cilia, or also continuations, which make the seizure and absorption of undissolved food-stuffs possible. The various species and kinds are distinguished by pseudopodia, or by the permanent cilia, flagella, or other protoplasmic continuations. In some, a firm protective shell is secreted by the protoplasm ; and still others possess a mouth opening (infusoria). The more important of the class of rhizopods that have been found in the human intestines or evacuations are monadines and ameba ; and of the class of infusoria, *Lamblia intestinalis,* *Trichomonas intestinalis* and *Trichomonas vaginalis*, and *Balantidium coli.*

A number of these flagellate infusoria are classed by C. Claus (English translation by Sedgewick, vol. 1, p. 193) among the monadines.

Rhizopods.

Ameba.—*Amœba coli.*—This protozoon has been fully described in the article on Endemic Dysentery. It was first described by

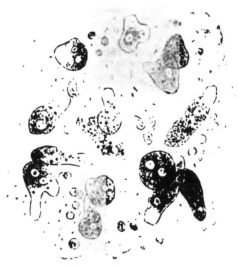

FIG. 12.—AMŒBA COLI.

Lösch, and found in the evacuations of a Russian peasant suffering from dysentery and caseous pneumonia. This organism was present in enormous numbers (seventy amebæ in one visual field when magnified 500 times). During rest it assumes a spherical, granular form, of 0.02 to 0.035 mm. diameter, but often changes its shape when moving. Besides a nucleus with nucleolus, bright vacuoles may be detected within it, the number of which varies between two and eight. At first clear pseudopodia free from granules serve for locomotion, which later on are filled with granular protoplasm. This parasite was communicated to dogs by Lösch, and to cats by Kovacz, Quincke, and Boas, the injection into the intestines generally producing dysentery. It was also occasionally detected in the evacuations in the case of tuberculous intestinal diseases (Lambl). Further investigations have shown that this parasite almost always occurs in the evacuations of endemic dysentery, as it occurs frequently in Egypt (Kartulis) and in many tropical countries. It is therefore assumed that *Amœba coli* is the cause of this disease (amebic dysentery), especially since it was also found in abscesses of the liver, which complicate this disease. Other kinds of amebæ which do not cause any disturbances also occur in the intestines (Quincke, Boas). *Amœba coli* is killed by quinin and tannin injections.

Infusoria.

1. **Cercomonas intestinalis (Lamblia intestinalis; Lambl, 1875).**—This parasite is pear-shaped. At its rear end it has a rigid

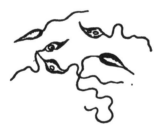

FIG. 13.—CERCOMONAS INTESTINALIS.—(*According to Davaine.*)

tip (tail process); at its forward end a long, quickly vibrating flagellum which serves as a means of locomotion. It is 0.008–0.01 mm. long (Davaine). It was first found by Lambl in the gelatinous, slimy evacuations of children. Later it was found by Davaine, Marchand, and Zunker in the evacuations of typhoid fever and cholera, and also in diarrhea, which was not due to these infections. Zunker also detected it once in sordes.

Lambl's form is now *Lamblia intestinalis* and distinct from

Davaine's species. There is considerable confusion in the medical and zoologic articles, and it is not always easy to recognize the species a man is dealing with. As a rule, however, the following species of infusoria are acknowledged: *Plagiomonas urinarius* (Künstler, 1883); *Trichomonas vaginalis*, Donné, 1837; *Trichomonas hominis* (Davaine, 1854) [*Cercomonas hominis*, Davaine, 1854; *Cercomonas intestinalis*, Lambl, 1875, but not same as Lambl, 1859, see below; *Trichimonas intestinalis*, Leukart, 1879; *Monocercomonas s. Cimænomonas hominis*, Grassi, 1882, 1888]; *Lamblia intestinalis* (Lambl, 1859); [this organism has been described under the following names and by the investigators mentioned: *Cercomonas intestinalis*, Lambl, 1859, but not 1875, see

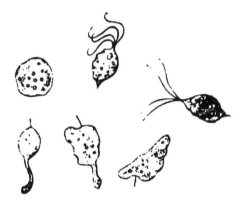

FIG. 14.—CERCOMONAS COLI HOMINIS.—(*According to May.*)

above; *Hexamita duodenalis*, Davaine, 1875; *Dimorphus muris*, Grassi, 1879; *Megastoma entericum*, Grassi, 1881; *Megastoma intestinale* (Lambl, 1859), R. Blanchard, 1885; *Lamblia intestinalis* (Lambl, 1859), R. Blanchard, 1888; *"Dimorpha muris Grassi"* of Senn, 1900].

If these parasites are present in the evacuations in large numbers, they cause a cadaverous odor. The pathogenic significance of these tiny animals is not definitely known; it is not even certain whether they are directly causative of the diseases in which they have been found. Cunningham found *Cercomonas intestinalis* in 66 per cent. of cadavers dead from Asiatic cholera. The parasites in the intestines are usually quickly killed by irrigations of a weak tannic acid, quinin, or boric acid solution.   If these are not successful, calomel in doses of 0.1 gram, three times a day, is recommended (Roos).

2. **Cercomonas coli.**—This parasite, about as large as a red blood-corpuscle, contains a nucleus, and differs from the *Cercomonas intestinalis* by the fact that it has four flagella, all quickly vibrating. It was found by May in the evacuations of an herb-gatherer who suffered from carcinoma of the stomach and colitis.   He had probably become infected by frequently drinking water out of puddles.

3. **Trichomonas intestinalis.**—This infusorium, having a length of 0.015 mm. and a breadth of 0.015 mm., is shaped like an almond kernel.   The ciliary edge, which is on the front part of the body, is in rapid motion ; the rear end has a tail process.   Leyden and Zunker found it in acute and chronic diarrhea ; Marchand

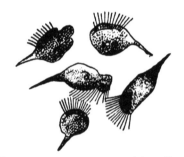

FIG. 15.—TRICHOMONAS INTESTINALIS.—(*According to Zunker.*)

was the first to discover it in the evacuations of typhoid in 1875, and Steinberg in sordes of the teeth.   It can be successfully eradicated by the same means as recommended for the cercomonas.

4. **Lamblia intestinalis (Lambl, 1859), or Megastoma entericum.**—This parasite is also pear-shaped, having a length of 0.015 to 0.018 mm.   It is distinguished by two tail threads, six long flagella, four pairs in all, and two cavities resembling suction cups. Grassi discovered it in diarrheic evacuations in considerable numbers, and proved that it has its abode principally in the upper parts of the small intestine.   Moritz and Hölzl have often found it in healthy persons.   It seems, however, to find a more favorable fostering soil in the diseased intestine, increasing more rapidly there, but not itself causing any great disturbances.   The

organism presents a concave depression on one side of the anterior surface of the body. These are the suction cups by means of which it attaches itself to the epithelial cells (see Fig. 16). Their exact pathogenicity is doubtful.

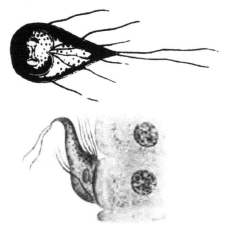

FIG. 16.—MEGASTOMA ENTERICUM.—(*According to Grassi and Schewiakoff.*)

5. Balantidium coli.—This creature is 0.07–0.1 mm. long, has an ovoid shape, and on its circumference has a connected wreath of fine ciliary hairs. The granular center is surrounded by a bright cortical layer, and contains two contractile vacuoles besides the nucleus, and sometimes also red and white blood-corpuscles,

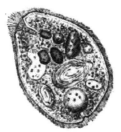

FIG. 17.—BALANTIDIUM COLI.—(*According to Malmsten.*)

besides particles of food (remains of plants). When it occurs in excessively large numbers in the intestines, it has been reported as causing a mucous diarrhea. The parasite was first discovered in man by Malmsten in 1856, in diarrheic evacuations; since then numerous investigators—Edgren, Ekekrantz, Graziadei, Henschen and Waldenström, Orthmann, Perroncito, Roos, Stieda, Windblath, and Wising—have given the results of their observations.   But it is probable that Leuwenhoeck, the inventor of the microscope, really first saw them in his own stools, during a prolonged diarrhea.   These studies show that this parasite is found principally in Sweden, Norway, the Russian Baltic provinces, and in Italy.   In France and England it is not found at all, and in Germany but rarely.   It is always found in the large intestine of swine (Leukart).   Henschen and Waldenström state that the infusion of warm water (37° C.), containing 50.0 vinegar and 5.0 tannic acid to 1 liter of water, kills these parasites and stops the diarrhea.   Quinin clysters (Orthmann), naphthalin (Edgren), and calomel (Roos) have also been used with good effect.

ANIMAL PARASITES (HELMINTHIASIS).

Cestodes (Tapeworm).

. Of the tapeworms found in the human intestinal canal and belonging to the class of cestodes, only three are of practical importance— these are, the *Tænia solium*, the *Tænia saginata* (*mediocanellata*), and the *Dibothriocephalus latus*.   As these three species cause almost the same symptoms, and since the same means are used for their destruction, it is expedient to treat them together in order to avoid repetition, after having discussed the natural history of the several kinds.   The tapeworm infection was known to the Egyptians and ancient Hindus, and it is probable that the forbidding of certain meats in the Mosaic laws was based upon a knowledge of these parasites.

Tænia solium (Armed Tapeworm).—The shape of the tapeworm designated *Tænia solium* (from ταινία, "a band or ribbon"), which usually in its developed state has a length of 2 to 3½ meters, and especially the shape of its head (scolex), is so characteristic that it may be distinguished from the other tapeworms without difficulty.   The determination can be made with greater certainty when the head or segments are slightly magnified (fifty times).   The *Tænia solium* is white, and consists of a head, a thin neck, which is from 0.5 to 2 cm. long and is not jointed, and the body.   The latter is composed of numerous (up to 850) distinctly defined sections (proglottides),

which are at first very short and narrow, but which gradually increase in length and still more in breadth as the distance from the head increases, until finally, about a meter from the head, they are nearly square.   Thereafter they gradually become narrower again, so that the last (80 to 100) mature sections are like pumpkin seeds, about 9 or 10 mm. long and 4 to 7 mm. broad.

The knot-like head, which is known as the scolex (from σκώληξ, " a worm "), is roundish and of the size of a pin-head (1.3 mm. in diameter).   In its upper part it is colored gray or black.   It has four movable suction discs, which can be advanced or retracted, and are often stretched so far that they are connected with the head by a thin stem only.   The rostellum, a disc-shaped or truncated cone-like projection, is on the top of the scolex.   It is surrounded by an outer wreath of small hooks, and an inner one of larger hooks (altogether, about twenty to thirty).   By means of the suction discs and the rostellum, the scolex can get a firm hold on the mucous membrane; this attachment usually occurs in the upper third of the ileum, whereas the other end reaches almost to the ileocecal valve, so that the neck is often broken off before the head lets loose.   In spite of the circle of hooks, the *Tænia solium* can not cause such pathological changes in the intestinal mucous membrane as erosions, ulcers, or bleedings, as was formerly assumed.   Still less can it pierce the wall of the intestine, if intact.   New sections are constantly being formed, starting from the head.   These are forced downward by those sections which are formed still later.   The head, when remaining behind alone, may live and is capable of regenerating the entire parasite.   Only the last (80 to 100) proglottides are mature, and they possess both male and female sexual organs (hermaphroditism).   In the middle of the segments lies the matrix (uterus), which consists of a central canal with eight to ten branch canals extending out like a tree.   (See Fig. 22, p. 558.)   On one side (sometimes the left, sometimes the right), somewhat below the middle of the segment, is the sexual pore, through which the eggs do not pass, however.   In the upper part of the proglottides are the male sexual organs, consisting of bright little testicles.   In the fertilized uterus the round or oval eggs are developed (0.036 mm. long, 0.03 mm. wide), which are surrounded by a fairly thick, coarse, radially striped shell.   These eggs, even while they are still in the uterus,

usually show a scolex with six hooks.   After a shorter or longer
period of time, one or more proglottides are forced off; longer sections of the tapeworm may be detached, however, having a length of a
meter or more, and pass off with the stools.   It has been noted that
after parts of the tapeworm have been absent in the evacuations for a
long time, they again make their appearance, occurring off and on for
days.   This is due to the fact that the development of the tapeworm
up to that stage in which the mature segments are formed requires a
longer period of time (three to four months).   Sometimes the entire

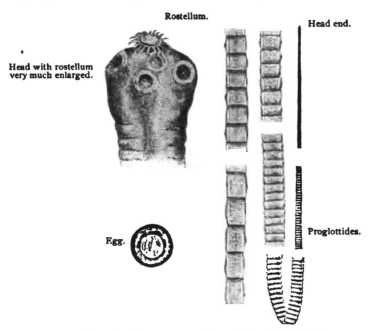

FIG. 18.—TÆNIA SOLIUM.—(*From Author's Collection.*)

tapeworm, head and all, is passed off with the feces.   This has been
repeatedly observed in children and adults after the use of laxative
drinking-cures and strong aperients, after the consumption of food
which is disagreeable or harmful to the tapeworm, and also in the
case of intestinal diseases, especially enteric and typhoid fever.   The
parasite itself may become diseased, as is proved by the malformation
of the individual segments, and thus its expulsion may result. Although as a rule the passage of the proglottides and the emitted eggs
is by means of the stools, yet the former may, although exceptionally,

be vomited, such cases having been reported by Berenger-Férand and Martel. In one case a piece of tapeworm 2 meters in length was vomited; in another a piece of tapeworm more than half a meter in length passed out through the mouth, while long chains of proglottides passed off through the anus. Besides this, the proglottides may leave the body through other channels, if abnormal communications, such as fistulas, exist. Thus, Dacbon and Bundach reported a case of fistula of the intestine and bladder in which they observed proglottides pass through the urethra. They have also been found in abscess cavities. Küchenmeister and von Siebold observed proglottides pass out through an abscess near the umbilicus. In most cases only one tapeworm is found. Repeatedly, however, 10 or even 20 specimens of younger or older teniæ, and at the same time a greater or less number of trunkless heads, have been driven out by one tapeworm cure (Berenger-Férand, Laker, Kleefeld). It is rare that two different kinds of tapeworms occur together; more frequently oxyures and ascarides, and other animal parasites, are found in the human intestine together with the teniæ. Up to the present time the *Tænia solium* has been found only in human beings. Attempts to transplant it to animals have failed.

If the eggs of *Tænia solium* reach the human stomach, the larval stage, *Cysticercus cellulosæ*, develops (this is not the case with *Tænia saginata*).

The disease is acquired by eating the infected meat of the intermediate host —"Zwischenwirth"—rather than by the ingestion of undeveloped ova. For the further development of the tapeworm embryo, its stay in another animal (intermediate host or carrier) is necessary. For the *Tænia solium* this intermediate host is usually the hog. If tapeworm eggs or mature proglottides get into the stomach of hogs that have eaten offal or garbage infected with feces containing tapeworm segments or eggs, and if the capsule of the eggs be cast off, the embryos are liberated. They at once commence their journeys, pierce the wall of the stomach or intestines, and reach the various organs of the body, especially the muscles, being carried there by the circulation of the blood, or traveling there independently. Here they develop, after they have lost their hooks (in the course of two or three months), into bladder or cyst worms (hydatids), or into cysticerci. They retain their vitality three to six years, then die and ossify. In the hog they are generally found in the intermuscular connective tissue as egg-shaped yellow cysts, having their greatest diameter 0.8 to 1.0 mm. long. These cysts have in their middle a bright nucleus which corresponds to the place of the so-called head cone. They may easily be detected with the unaided eye. Besides in the swine, they are reported to have been found also, although much more rarely, in dogs, rats, bears, deer, and monkeys, and, according to some investigators, in sheep.

The head of the future tapeworm is then developed in an invagination of the cyst wall and the complete organism thus formed constitutes the *cysticercus*, or bladder-worm. If the animal is not slaughtered, the cyst and contents will eventually degenerate and die, the cyst undergoing calcification. If the meat of the animal is eaten before the cyst undergoes calcification, the cyst of connective tissue around the hydatid is digested away, the head and neck of the parasite remain uninjured, and passing into the intestines of the human being, there attaches itself by means of its suckers and forms segments by transverse division.

Cysticerci, or bladder-worms, have been observed also in human beings in a great number of cases. If ripe tapeworm eggs get into the stomach by means of antiperistaltic intestinal movements, during vomiting or per os (soiling of the fingers with feces containing eggs), the embryos may also pass into the various organs (brain, eyes, skin, etc.), and are there encysted.

As to the longevity of the *Tænia solium*, it has often been observed that persons have had them ten to fifteen years or more. The *Tænia solium* is especially widespread in middle and northwest Germany. Orthodox Jews, and also those Orientals who do not eat pork on account of their religious tenets, are free from them. In those countries where compulsory meat inspection has been introduced, and especially in the cities where abattoir laws exist, the *Tænia solium* has become much rarer in recent years.

Tænia saginata (mediocanellata, Küchenmeister); Fat, Unarmed Tapeworm.—The *Tænia saginata* is very different from the *Tænia solium*, both in shape and appearance. It attains a length of 6 meters. The segments are thicker, stouter, and broader than those of the *Tænia solium*, and correspondingly also more opaque. The head is 2.5 mm. broad, and is sometimes without

pigment, sometimes colored more or less black. It has four powerful suction discs around which there are usually collected large
amounts of black pigment. A rostellum with its wreath of hooks
is wanting, and in place of it is found a smaller frontal suction disc
in the middle of the others.

The neck is very short, sometimes hardly noticeable, and consequently the segmentation of the tapeworm commences much fur-

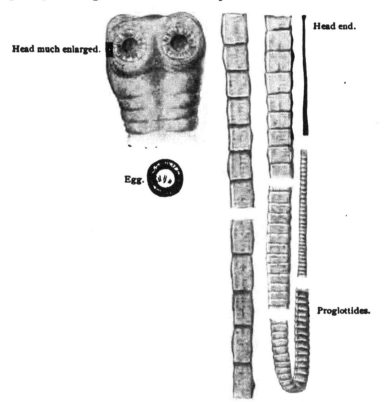

Head much enlarged.

Egg.

Head end.

Proglottides.

FIG. 19.—TÆNIA SAGINATA.—(*From Author's Collection.*)

ther up. The proglottides are mature from about the six hundredth
segment on. These segments are 16 to 20 mm. long, 5 to 7 mm.
broad, and shaped like pumpkin seeds. The side canals of the
uterus are much more numerous than those of the *Tænia solium*
(twenty-six to thirty), and have no arbor-like appearance (not branch-
ing like a tree), but are divided like a fork. (See Figs. 21 and
22.) The sexual opening is sometimes on the right side, sometimes

on the left (not alternating, however), and somewhat below the middle of each section.   The oval eggs are but slightly larger than those of the *Tænia solium*,—0.039 mm. long, 0.035 mm. wide,— and their shells are slightly thicker and brighter.

The infection of human beings is always caused by the consumption of raw beef which contains the youthful forms of *Tænia saginata*, its cysticercus.   These are found in the muscles, the heart, and the brain of the beeves.   Besides the beef, the cysticercus of the *Tænia saginata* has been found hitherto in the giraffe and several other animals ; never in human beings, however.

The *Tænia saginata* is spread all over the inhabited earth.   This is explained by the great consumption of raw beef.   In southern Germany, France, and this country it is oftener observed than the *Tænia solium*.

Dibothriocephalus latus (Grubenkopf), Broad Tapeworm. —In length the *Dibothriocephalus latus* surpasses both of the other tapeworms, being found at times 8 meters long.   Its head is only 2 mm. long, and 1 mm. broad.   It has the shape of a flattened club or almond, and has on both sides a deep, cleft-shaped suction disc, which reaches almost to the neck.   It has no circle of hooks.   The neck, which is as thin as a thread (3 to 5 mm. long), comes after the head. The shape of the segments, the number of which may reach 4000, varies considerably.   Up to about the last 600 mature segments, they are about three or four times as broad as long (10 to 15 mm. : 3 to 4 mm.).   The mature segments, however, have more of a square shape (5 mm.).   Their breadth, however, may increase as they descend.   In the uppermost of the mature segments the uterus is a fairly straight canal ; in the lower ones it is arranged like a rosette (intertwining).   The sexual opening is found not on the side, but in the middle of the segment, and always on the same side. The color of the *Dibothriocephalus latus* is a faint bluish-gray.

The oval egg (0.07 mm. long, 0.045 mm. wide) possesses a slightly brownish hull.   At one end, which is usually referred to as its front end, a sharply defined lid or cup may be observed.   The dibothriocephalus, which has also been observed in dogs, vegetates in the smaller intestine of the human being, just as the other tapeworms.

The intermediate host, or the bearer of the youthful forms of the

Dibothriocephalus latus, of its pleocercoid, as has been determined especially by the observations of Küchenmeister, Braun, Parona, Lonnberg, Zschokke, and others, are pike, burbot, barbel, trout, salmon, perch of certain lakes. The flesh of these fish, if consumed raw or partially cooked, may transmit the parasite. For this reason

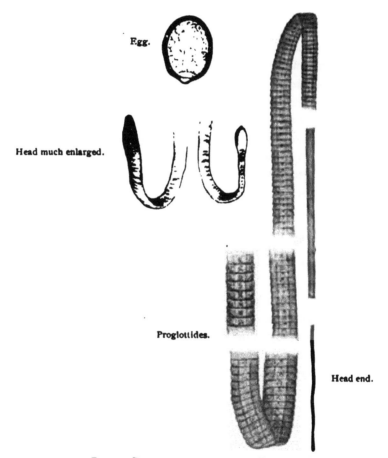

FIG. 20.—DIBOTHRIOCEPHALUS LATUS, HEAD AND EGG.

the dibothriocephalus is especially common in those regions where the consumption of these fish is very great; that is, in northwestern Russia, Poland, the eastern part of Prussia, Pomerania, Finland, Sweden, Norway, Holland, Belgium, in the western part of Switzerland, and the adjacent French districts. It has also been repeatedly observed in the neighborhood of Lake Starnberg near Munich (Bollinger).

The hypothesis has been advanced by Zaesslein that the consumption of green salad growing in trenches irrigated with the water of the western Swiss lakes, where the fish frequently contain the larvæ of the *Dibothriocephalus latus*, may transmit the parasite. He assumes that when the plants are moistened with this water, they retain the pleocercoid and tapeworm eggs. This assumption is biologically impossible.

Besides the tapeworms just discussed,—*Tænia solium, Tænia saginata, Dibothriocephalus latus,*—the following kinds have been found in the human intestines in isolated cases: *Tænia confusa, Tænia Africana, Dipylidium canium, Hymenolepis murina, Hymenolepis diminuta, Davainea madagascariensis, Dibothriocephalus cordatus, Diplogonoporus grandis, Ligula mansoni.* These may, however, be left undiscussed, both because they occur but rarely, and also because they cause the same disease symptoms, and their treatment is identical with the former.

Symptomatology.—Although experience shows that many persons may have one or even more tapeworms for a long time without experiencing any discomfort on their account, but rather enjoy perfect well-being, and only notice that they have a tapeworm when they see proglottides in the evacuations, nevertheless a host of the most varied symptoms has in recent times been attributed to "tapeworms," both by laymen and physicians. There is hardly a symptom for which a " tapeworm " has not been made responsible. Neurasthenics, hypochondriacs, and persons suffering from hysteria often firmly believe that they have a tapeworm, though they have never seen parts of one pass away, and refer their nervous complaints to it; indeed, they sometimes imagine they can distinctly feel the movements of the worm in their body. In a number of cases of "neurasthenia intestinalis" which occurred in my practice lately the patients had been dosed with male-fern and chloroform for no other reason than this. They had said they could feel the undulatory movements of the worm. In neurasthenics this assertion should go for naught. It has hitherto not been accepted for a certainty that the movements of teniæ can be felt. In an experimental infection of himself with *Tænia saginata*, Dr. C. M. Stiles believed, however, that he could distinctly feel these movements. Although it can not be denied that the presence of one or more tapeworms in the intestines can cause not only digestive disturbances in the stomach and intestines, and complaints dependent upon these organs, but also many nervous anomalies, which may arise reflexly, nevertheless one should be very conservative in judging the subjective symptoms mentioned by the persons suffering from tapeworm, especially the nervous symptoms. One can only assume a causal relation between them and the tapeworm, if they cease soon after the expulsion of the latter. Probably the nervous anomalies are usually the results of the digestive disturbances caused by the tapeworm. The following are the usual symptoms observed in people suffering from such a parasite :

Loss of appetite, which may alternate with great, almost insatiable hunger ; eructation ; nausea ; vomiting ; disagreeable sensations of pressure in the abdomen, which are more rarely confined to a certain region (epigastrium), but oftener change their locality, and in many patients are aggravated to violent colic-like pains. The latter, as well as the dyspeptic complaints, frequently set in soon after the consumption of certain foods,—herring, onion, garlic, and sour foods,—or increase after the ingestion of these foods, while, on the contrary, they are ameliorated by the use of milk, eggs, and oily food-stuffs. There may be constipation, diarrhea, and sometimes constipation alternates with diarrhea. In the records of 60 cases in which I could find any reference to the state of the bowels there was constipation in 38, diarrhea in 12, and an alternation of the two conditions in 10 cases. The vitality and movement of a healthy tapeworm when it is contained in its normal environment —the warm intestines of the human host—are not clearly understood, since practitioners of medicine generally see the parasite only in a dazed or dead condition. If a tapeworm that has been expelled dazed but still alive is placed in a basin of lukewarm water, it will soon recover, and then one can observe a wonderful peristalsis of the segmented body. The undulatory movements are quite forcible, the neck is capable of strong flexion and extension, and there is an energetic action of the suction discs. Such movements must exert an intense irritation upon the intestinal mucosa of the infected host.

The ring of hooks of *Tænia solium* enables this parasite to bore deeply into the mucosa. The hooks are composed of chitin, and it has been recorded that they penetrated through the glands of Lieberkühn (Zürn), undoubtedly constituting a serious traumatic condition.

The nervous symptoms to be noted are headache, vertigo, fainting spells, convulsions, delirium, mania, epilepsy, chorea, difference in size of pupils, myosis (Denti), disturbances in sight and hearing, paresthesia in the limbs, singultus, and pruritus. Davaine has called attention to the fact that single nervous disease symptoms—epileptic attacks, spasmodic contractions of the muscles of the neck and of the extremities—ceased after the expulsion of the parasite, and thus were dependent upon them. Dr. Chas. W. Stiles reported an experimental infection of himself with *Tænia saginata* (Bulletin No. 19, U. S. Dept. Agriculture, " The Inspection of Meats for Animal Parasites," p. 87). He describes the most constant symptom—a sensation similar to that which one experiences in the rapid descent of an elevator; it occurred frequently, especially when walking.

Very often patients suffering with tapeworm present symptoms of a severe, gradually increasing anemia, which can not be differentiated from a progressive pernicious anemia, arising from other causes, since the conditions of the blood are the same. Although the patients at first consume abundant food—indeed, sometimes much more than usual—as a result of extreme hunger, the bodily weight rapidly decreases and general nutrition suffers greatly. Later on the patients complain of dyspnea and palpitation of the heart; lack of appetite, diarrhea, and fever may develop. Finally the patients become so weakened that they can no longer walk about, and have to go to bed. If they arise suddenly, fainting spells, flashes before the eyes, and also rumbling in the ears (anemia of the brain) are complained of. Hemorrhages from the mucous membrane and from the retina have been reported by F. Müller. The investigations of Botkin, F. A. Hoffman, Lichtheim, Reyer, Runeberg, Schapiro, and Schaumann have made it probable that in certain forms of anemia an infection with *Dibothriocephalus latus* is the cause. When the parasite is expelled the anemia decreases. A satisfactory explanation for the manner in which the anemia is produced is at present lacking. Albu and Bouchard trace it to the absorption of toxic substances from the intestines.

Diagnosis.—The presence of any one of these forms of tapeworms in the intestines can be determined with certainty only by means of thorough and oft-repeated examinations of the evacuations, and by the detection of segments or eggs of parasites. The statements of the patients themselves can not be relied upon alone, since they have often mistaken remnants of food, sinews, skins, clotted milk, etc., for tapeworm segments. If the suspicion is present that a patient has a tapeworm, and if no proglottides have passed off for a long time in the evacuations, it is advisable to prescribe mild laxatives, tapeworm remedies (in small doses), or the consumption of herrings, onions, or garlic, since the expulsion of single proglottides often follows the use of these means ; this at least has been my experience. The following remedies are available for this purpose :

For children, two or three teaspoonfuls of the compound infusion of senna, or the syrup of senna and manna.

For adults, the following :

> R. Ext. filic. mar. æth., ... 1.0 (or gr. xv)
> Syr. mannæ, ... 50.0 (about ℥ iss).
> M. Sig.—Two or three teaspoonfuls in the morning.

Occasionally a tablespoonful of castor oil will suffice.

If tapeworm segments have passed off with the evacuations, one can easily determine with the aid of the microscope to which class they belong, since the form of the segments, and especially that of the uterus, differs essentially in the three species.

Differential Diagnosis.—As the *Dibothriocephalus latus* and the other species mentioned on page 554 are rare inhabitants of the human intestine, the essential aim of a differential diagnosis in our country would be to distinguish between the *Tænia saginata* (the beef-measle tapeworm) and the *Tænia solium* (the pork-measle tapeworm). A distinction between the two is somewhat facilitated by a close inquiry into the nature of the patient's meat diet. If he has eaten no pork, it is, of course, not probable that he is infected with the *Tænia solium.* If he has eaten no beef, it is not probable that he is infected with the *Tænia saginata.* In certain districts where the inhabitants feed largely upon fish, the possibility of *Dibothrio-*

cephalus latus infection should be considered. Human beings are subject to infection with ten different species of tapeworms, but for practical purposes the differentiation of the forms specially mentioned will suffice. A distinction can be made by an examination of the segments of the tapeworms, or of the eggs and the head, if this can be found. The segments are sometimes found in the bed or clothes of the patient when they wander out of the rectum of their own accord. If several segments are joined together, the

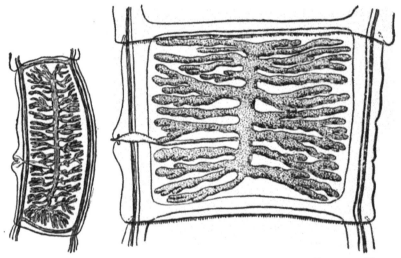

FIG. 21.—GRAVID SEGMENT OF BEEF-MEASLE TAPEWORM (TÆNIA SAGINATA), SHOWING LATERAL BRANCHES OF THE UTERUS, ENLARGED (ORIGINAL).—(*After Chas. W. Stiles, United States Department of Agriculture, Bureau of Animal Industry, Bulletin No. 19.*)

FIG. 22.—GRAVID SEGMENT OF PORK-MEASLE TAPEWORM (TÆNIA SOLIUM), SHOWING THE LATERAL BRANCHES OF THE UTERUS, ENLARGED (ORIGINAL).—(*After Chas. W. Stiles, United States Department of Agriculture, Bureau of Animal Industry*).

parasite is generally of the armed species; viz., the *Tænia solium*, or pork-measle tapeworm. If every portion of the detached parasite consists of a single segment, it is generally the unarmed species, or *Tænia saginata*, or beef-measle tapeworm. In examining the segments passed, the form of the uterus should be especially noticed. The segment can be mounted in glycerin, and placed between two thin glass slides, and examined under a lens, or even with the unaided eye. When held up to the light, one can readily discern and count the lateral branches of the uterus. If there are from 17 to 30 branches on each side of the main trunk, we are dealing with the unarmed tapeworm, *Tænia saginata* (beef-measle). (See Fig. 21.) But if there are only 7 to 10 branches on each side, it is a segment from the armed tapeworm, *Tænia solium*. (See Fig. 22.) The head, if it can be found, should be examined by the microscope. If the hooks are absent, it is the unarmed tapeworm. If there are two rows of hooks present, it is the armed tapeworm, or *Tænia solium*. Fortunately infections with the armed tapeworm are rarer in this country than those with the unarmed, for *Tænia solium* invades the tissues of man, and in its larval state it may develop in the muscles, the eyes, and other portions of the body. Whilst at Strümpell's clinic at the University of Erlangen, in 1896, I had occasion to study a young girl, twenty years of age, who died suddenly in convulsions, and who had never before in her life been sick. The autopsy was performed by Hauser. Nothing abnormal could be found in any of the organs of the body, which was that of a strong, vigorous individual; but in the left lateral ventricle was found a cysticercus of *Tænia solium*. The unarmed tapeworm, *Tænia saginata*, develops only on the intestine, and its larval form is unable to develop in man.

The importance of recognizing which species of tapeworm an individual is infected with has also an important bearing for prophylaxis with regard to the infection of cattle, if the individual live in the country. In case the excrement be passed in or in some way reach the fields where cattle feed, he may infect them should he carry the *Tænia saginata*; but he can only infect hogs if he carry the *Tænia solium*. If there is the least ground to suspect an infection with any tapeworm, it is wisest to disinfect the feces with quicklime until there is assurance that the worm has been effectually destroyed.

If a very great number of tapeworm segments pass off in a short period of time, it signifies that several tapeworms are present in the intestines. Since tapeworms of several kinds may be present in the intestines, a microscopic examination of all the proglottides contained in the evacuations is sometimes necessary if the recognition of the species is desired. Leichtenstern has called attention to the fact that if animal parasites (worms), and especially the *Tænia*

saginata, be present, the evacuations are often full of Charcot-Neu-
mann-Leyden crystals ; thus the detection of the latter is also of
use for the diagnosis of tapeworms.

Prognosis.—In general the prognosis is favorable.   In many
cases the parasites are completely expelled by the use of efficacious
tapeworm remedies.   In others, however, the cure has to be repeated twice or even three times.   Patients having a *Tænia solium*
in their intestines are further exposed to the danger that the tapeworm eggs may get into the stomach, either from the intestines or
per os.   Here they may later develop into cysticerci, which are
much more dangerous parasites than the *Strobila.* *   If the diagnosis
of a *Tænia solium* is certain, the tapeworm must be expelled as soon
as possible.   In the case of *Tænia saginata* or *Dibothriocephalus latus,*
an infection with the cysticerci of the same is not to be feared, since
they have never yet been found in human beings.   It is for this
reason that a recognition of the species should be aimed at.

Therapeutics.—Prophylaxis plays a very important rôle in these
parasite invasions.   This is evident from the fact that in those countries where obligatory meat inspection has been introduced, and
especially in those cities where slaughter-house laws exist, by means
of which a thorough control of the meat of slaughtered animals is
made possible, the *Tænia solium,* and also the *Tænia saginata* (more
especially the former), has become a rare human parasite.   This is
my experience in Baltimore, where *Tænia solium* is rare.   In the
larger hospitals of Berlin not one such parasite is seen in an entire
year.   Prophylaxis is rendered easier by the fact that the larvæ of
the three tapeworms are plainly visible to the naked eye, and still
more so when the meat is examined by a lens, and can be recognized not only by physicians and veterinary surgeons, but also by
intelligent laymen.   The detection of the cysticerci is most difficult
in beef, on account of the great amount of the meat.   It is, however, usually possible for a trained meat inspector to find them if
present.   The prophylactic measures should, however, not be restricted to an inspection of the meat of slaughtered animals.   Both
farmers and cattle-raisers should see that their cattle and hogs get
no food or drinking-water that is contaminated with human excre-

---

* This is a name given to the tapeworm as a whole.

ment. They should also keep their stables as clean as possible. Since, however, the former can not be entirely avoided in the country, because human excrement is often deposited in the grass and on the pastures, as well as on the edge of ditches, from which the cattle later on drink, and since a thorough inspection of the flesh of slaughtered cattle can not be enforced, individuals can guard themselves against tapeworms only by eating nothing but thoroughly boiled and roasted pork, beef, and fish. In beef the chief dangerous parts are the tongue, masseters, and the heart. Even beefsteak should be well cooked. In our country "*interstate*" meat is inspected by the Government.

Medicinal Treatment.—*Tapeworm Cures.*—The treatment for the expulsion of tapeworm must be executed in a systematic manner. Since the expulsion of the tapeworm, which may be obtained both by dietetic and medicinal means, and also by aperients, may weaken the patient very much, though only temporarily, it should not be carried out, or only with the greatest precautions, in very old persons, in weak small children, in consumptives, in cases of gastric ulcer, of ulcers of the intestines, after great losses of blood, and during pregnancy. The treatment is also more critical to undergo during the menstrual period. The tapeworm cure is composed of three stages :

1. The preparatory or preliminary treatment, the object of which is to empty the intestines before the expulsion, and thus create favorable conditions for the prompt evacuation ; and, on the other hand, to irritate and sicken the tapeworm and to make its stay in the intestine as unpleasant as possible by the ingestion of various foods that create a disagreeable environment for him.

2. The Cure Itself.—In this stage the parasite is rendered unconscious by means of anthelmintics, and thus forced to loosen its hold on the mucous membrane, to which it has attached itself. The transportation downward by means of the peristaltic intestinal movements is rendered possible by the teniafuge.

3. The mechanical removal of the parasites, if this be necessary, by means of aperients, enemata, or colon irrigations.

Preparatory Treatment.—For a few days, or at least twenty-four hours, before the actual cure the patient receives only liquid, easily digested food—milk, bouillon, raw eggs. Mild aperients are also to be given, several times a day, such as castor oil (one table-spoonful two or three times daily, preferably in soft gelatin capsules —Parke, Davis & Co.), compound licorice powder, powdered rhubarb, infusion of rhubarb, and mineral waters,—Saratoga, Congress or Hathorn, Hunyadi Jànos, or Rubinat-Condal,—in order to attain thin and fluid evacuations. The evening before the cure, the patient should eat a considerable quantity of very salty herring salad, which must contain onions, garlic, pieces of potato, red whortleberries, and kernel fruits. (Häring-Salat—German recipe; see "Universal Lexikon der Kochkunst," Bd. 1, S. 437.)

Expulsion Cure.—*Tapeworm Remedies.*—Of the latter, only the most important will be mentioned. These will be fully sufficient for the practitioner, and their efficiency has often been tested by the writer.

1. The *extract of male-fern* has proved most reliable in my experiments. But the practitioner must assure himself that the drug is pure and fresh. Failures, as a rule, are due to a decomposed extract. The numerous observations of Liebermeister show that splendid results were attained with this in the case of *Tænia saginata* even without any preparatory treatment. Mosler and Peiper recommend the following administration of male-fern:

R. Ethereal extract of male-fern, ... 7.5–10 gm. (ʒij–ʒiiss)
Simple syrup, ... 40 gm. (fʒx).
M. Entire dose to be taken within ten minutes.

The larger dose is given when the diagnosis of *Tænia solium* has been established. Other eligible forms are the following:

R. Root of male-fern, ... 15.0 to 20.0 (ʒiij, gr. xlv)
White sugar, ... 5.0 (ʒj, gr. xv)
Sugar well flavored with lemon juice or oil, . 1.5 (gr. xxij).
M. To be taken in two equal doses.

R. Root of male-fern,
Ethereal extract of male-fern, ... aa 2.0 gm. (gr. xxx).
M. Sig.—Make into twenty pills. Take ten pills in the morning and evening.

A number of clinicians (Caglioni, Giaccone, Perroncito, Schönbaechler) used much larger doses than the above—as much as 20 to 30 grains of the extract—without observing the slightest unpleasant side-effects. On the other hand, Eich has collected twenty-

our cases in which the extract of male-fern produced serious phenomena of intoxication, and in one case even death. It will in all
cases, therefore, be safe not to give more than 10 grams of the extract to adults; to children, according to the age and state of constitutional vigor, from 1 to 4 grams. There can be no doubt that
the administration of castor oil together with the extract of filix mas
increases the liability of intoxication. The practitioner must reckon
with the possibility of provoking an amaurosis or other severe disturbance of health as a result of this teniafuge. I have had occasion to observe three cases of intense jaundice (icterus) after large
doses of male-fern extract given by tapeworm quacks. The medico-
legal aspects of such unintentional complications have been considered by Leichtenstern, who advises the following precautions:
(1) The maximum dose of 10 grams should never be exceeded;
(2) extract of male-fern should never be given on two consecutive
days; and (3) never on an empty stomach, but only after a meal
(breakfast). The administration of a laxative simultaneously with
the male-fern is irrational, because it drives the teniafuge past the
parasite too rapidly. Castor oil, calomel, jalap, or senna should not
be given until two hours after the tapeworm remedy.

Flores kousso: These contain as their efficacious component the
" *Koussin* " (Bedall).

Bark of the root of the *pomegranate tree (cortex. rad. granati):*
This was used in ancient times as a tapeworm remedy.

All these tapeworm remedies are best taken in the morning on
an empty stomach. Patients who vomit easily should take the
remedy after a cup of very sweet black coffee (also with some
brandy). The effective quantity should preferably be taken in
two doses with an interval of half an hour. Whilst under this
treatment and after it, the patient should stay in bed, because
nausea, vomiting, and fainting spells are most easily prevented by a
recumbent position. If the patient vomits very easily after taking
evil-tasting medicines (with the exception of kamala all the anthelmintics taste very bad, and such correctives as honey, lemon juice,
rum, or red wine disguise the taste but very little), it is sometimes
advised to introduce them into the stomach with the stomach-tube.
This procedure I have never found it necessary to resort to. The
failures which are observed fairly often in tapeworm cures may very

probably be traced to the fact that the amount of effective matter contained in the plants in question may vary both with the age of the plant and the locality of its growth, and that this amount decreases as a result of decomposition if the preparations are stored for some time. It is very important for the practitioner to assure himself that all tapeworm remedies are perfectly fresh, otherwise his efforts may be futile.

1. *Ethereal extract of male-fern* (extractum filicis maris æthereum) (dose 8 to 10 grams—ʒiss to ʒiiss): The same can be prescribed either in gelatin capsules (2.0 grams, or 20 to 30 grains, per dose) or in the form of pills (℞. Felic. maris, 4.0 grams (ʒj); make 30 pills; 15 pills twice daily).

2. *Blossoms of kousso* (*Flores kousso*): Dose about 20 to 25 grams (ʒv to ʒviiss). This is best introduced in the form of compressed tablets (1 to 2 per tablet), also in two portions.

3. *Bark of fresh pomegranate roots* is to be prescribed as a macerated decoction. Bark of pomegranate root (cort. radicis granati), 50 grams (also more); macerate for twenty-four hours with 500 c.c. water, then evaporate down to 250 c.c.; add syrup of orange peel, 30 grams. To be taken in two parts.

The oily alkaloid separated from pomegranate bark, known as *"pelletierin,"* after the chemist Bertrand Pelletier, who first isolated it, is most efficaciously employed in the form of the tannate. The dose is from 5 to 15 grains in 1 ounce of water, followed by half an ounce of castor oil. It is an effective teniafuge if it can be procured in a fresh and reliable form. Unfortunately the preparations brought into commerce under the name of pelletierin tannate vary greatly in their teniafuge power and toxicity. Doses of 0.04 to 0.5 gram (5 to 8 grains) have been known to cause faintness, formication, disturbances of vision, and cramps in the legs in human beings. My experience with this alkaloid is limited to five cases of *Tænia saginata*, all of which were expelled completely without any ill effects. It is an expensive teniafuge.

4. Kamala: Dose, 10 to 15 grams (ʒiiss to ʒiiiss). This is to be introduced in sweetened coffee or tea, or as an electuary. In two equal portions.

If the anthelmintic has been well borne and the tapeworm has not passed off within two hours after the taking of the medicine, it must be expelled by the use of aperients. For instance, a table-spoonful of castor oil every four hours, either in emulsion or gelatin capsules; calomel (0.2) with pulverized jalap (0.5 to 1.0), two or three times in twelve hours; mineral waters; infusion of rhubarb or senna, 10 : 150, by the tablespoonful; effervescent citrate of magnesia, one pint. The most reliable or expeditious way of hastening an already dazed tapeworm outward is by large colon irrigations of 1 or 1½ quarts of warm water. If a portion of the tapeworm has already protruded at the anus, one should never pull at the extruding piece, since the portion might easily tear off and thus hazard the success of the cure. Instead of the infusion of water, Eichhorst recommends injecting a decoction of the roots of ferns (decoct. rhizom. filicis, 50 : 500) into the rectum. If the head has passed off, the desired end is obtained. If the head can not be found, it is not always certain that the treatment was unsuccessful ; but as there is doubt concerning the complete expulsion, the patient should be impressed with the expediency of presenting himself in three or four months for supervision, and if need be, examination of the evacuations. If proglottides again pass off after three or four months, the treatment has to be repeated. If this is not the case, the tapeworm is destroyed. A light diet is advisable for a few days after the cure, because the intestines are very often highly irritated as a result of the treatment. In susceptible cases ascites or chronic intestinal catarrh may sometimes supervene.

With the remaining drugs recommended as teniafuges I have only a limited personal experience. They are : Cocoanut (the milk and entire nut should be consumed within an hour); salol, gr. xl, in capsules ; naphthalin, gr. x to xxx, in capsules. But I have had four satisfactory results with benzin. The patients received ½ ounce of castor oil and an enema of 1 quart warm water containing 15 grains of benzin. Three hours later the following mixture was given :

R. Benzin, c. p., ... 6 gm. (ℨiss)
    Mucilage of acacia,
    Licorice syrup, ... aa 30 gm. (about ℨj)
    Peppermint water, ... 120 c.c.
One tablespoonful every hour.

Trematodes (Flukeworms).

The trematode worms which are important clinically—that is, those which have so far been discovered as being parasitic in man— are the following: *Monostomulum lentis, Agamodistomum ophthalmobium, Fasciola hepatica, Fasciolopsis Buskii, Paragonimus Westermanii, Dicrocælium lanceatum, Opisthorchis felineus, O. sinensis, Heterophyes heterophyes, Schistosoma hæmatobium, Amphistoma hominis.*

The names used in older works, like Mosler and Peiper's "Thierische Parasiten" (Nothnagel's "Spec. Path. u. Ther.," Bd. VI), Fleischer's "Magen- und Darmkrankheiten," J. Ch. Huber's comprehensive work, "Bibliographie der klinischen Helminthologie," and various publications of Leichtenstern (vol. IV of Penzoldt and Stintzing's "Handbuch d. spec. Therapie innerer Krankheiten"), are:

MODERN NAME.	OLD NAME.
Monostomulum lentis.	*Unknown.*
Agamodistomum ophthalmobium.	*Distoma ophthalmobium.*
Fasciola hepatica.	*Distoma hepatica.*
Fasciolopsis Buskii.	*Distoma crassum.*
Paragonimus Westermanii.	*Distoma pulmonale.*
Dicrocælium lanceatum.	*Distoma lanceolatim.*
Opisthorchis felineus.	*Unknown.*
Opisthorchis sinensis.	*Distoma sinense.*
Heterophyes heterophyes.	*Distoma heterophyes.*
Schistosoma hæmatobium.	*Distoma hæmatobium.*
Amphistoma hominis.	*Unknown.*
Distoma conjunctum.	*Distoma conjunctum.*

The *Paragonimus Westermanii*, or lung fluke, has become of interest to us because it has been established that it is the cause of parasitic hemoptysis, common in Asia, and has already been introduced into this country by returning troops. According to a report from the United States Department of Agriculture, entitled "Notes on Parasites," No. 50 to 52, by Chas. Wardell Stiles, Ph.D., and Albert Hassall (p. 592), the eggs of the paragonimus have been found in the mediastinum, diaphragm, mesentery, and in the walls of the intestine. Cysts of paragonimus eggs have been found in the mesentery and great omentum, but it is claimed they have not produced any notable symptoms when present only in this locality. For a closer description of this parasite, as well as for a review of the medical literature of pulmonary infection by it, reference must be had to the article from the United States Bureau of Animal Industry (*l. c.*).

The *Opisthorchis sinensis*, or *Distoma sinense*, is the cause of a common liver disease in Asia, and it is conceivable that it may be imported to this country by some of our troops who have been engaged in China.

The *Opisthorchis felineus* (or the *Opisthorchis tenuicollis*) is the cause of a liver disease to which the Russian troops are subject. These diseases may be brought to the United States by our returning troops, and they cannot be diagnosed except by recognizing the eggs of these worms in microscopic examination of the feces. These forms, as well as the *Amphistoma hominis*, are fortunately so extremely rare in our country that I have no personal experience with the clinical aspect of their infections.

The *Fasciola hepatica*, or *Distoma hepatica*, is a trematode which has been repeatedly found parasitic in the human intestine, bileducts, and liver. Virchow found two distomas in the liver of a patient who showed no special symptoms during life. There were no signs of any dilation or other changes in the bile-ducts. Carter, Wyss, and Lambl have reported similar findings without anatomical changes. According to Baelz (" Berliner klin. Wochenschr.," 1883, p. 234), distomatosis can be recognized with certainty during life by the presence of characteristic eggs in the feces.

The proper course to pursue is for the physician to send any eggs which he may find in the feces of patients returning from China and the Philippine Islands, or other tropical countries, to an experienced zoologist.

The cases described by Baelz showed marked cyst-like dilations of the bile-ducts which contained hundreds of small red worms. The cysts varied from the size of a hazelnut to that of a walnut. Some of the *Fasciolæ hepaticæ* were found free in the bile-ducts, and others in the duodenum. The liver tissue in the environment of these cysts was atrophic. Pallas and Fortassin found them in the biliary passages of female cadavers, but there were no changes in the liver in either case. Brera found this parasite

in the liver of a scorbutic and anasarcous man.   The liver was
hard and enlarged and its glandular substance filled with distomæ.
It seems that pathological changes are not caused unless the parasites are very abundant.   Chronic induration and stenosis about
the bile-ducts with persistent icterus were caused by this parasite
in the cases reported by Biermer (" Schweiz Zeitschr. f. Heilk.,"
1863, Bd. II) and Bostroem (" Deutsch Arch. f. klin. Med.," Bd.
xxx, p. 557).

The **treatment of distomatosis**, trematode infection of the
human intestine, consists in the administration of purgatives in conjunction with anthelmintics, in the same manner as has been
described in the paragraph on oxyuris.   If the trematodes have
become localized in the bile-ducts and liver, the treatment becomes
difficult.   It is suggested that medicines directed toward increasing
the secretion of bile might effect a discharge of the invading
Fasciola hepatica.   Whether this can be accomplished or not is a
problem for future experimental therapeutics.

The treatment for expulsion of the trematodes is the same as for
the cestodes.

Roundworm (Nematodes).

Ascaris lumbricoides (the Long Roundworm).—The long
roundworm designated as the *Ascaris lumbricoides* is of great clinical
importance, because it is frequently found in the intestines and evacuations of human beings, much oftener probably than the other animal parasites.   It is easy to recognize and can not be overlooked
in the stools.   The color may be a whitish-yellow, reddish, or
brownish tint, the shape cylindrical, like that of an earthworm ; the
size is considerable.   The male ascaris is slender, and often has the
tail rolled in toward the ventral side.   It may attain a length of 20
to 25 cm.   The female is thicker, and may attain a length of 30 to
40 cm., and is 6 mm. in thickness.   At the tail end of the male is
the cloaca from which the slender, slightly curved chitinous spicules
(copulative organs) project.   In both sexes the roundish button-
shaped head has three cone-shaped lips with tactile papillæ, and
fine teeth, numbering about 200.   Both male and female have,
besides the numerous cross-striations, four longitudinal lines running from head to tail, one of a faint white color, on both the ventral

and the dorsal aspect, and one of a more brownish tint laterally between these. The female has two long stretched uteri. The sexual opening is on the abdominal line, at the joining of the first and second thirds of the body. The fecundity of *Ascaris lumbri-*

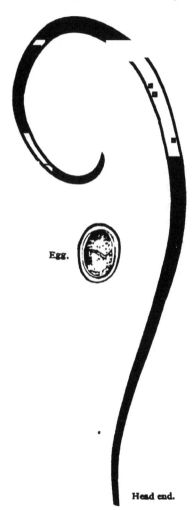

Egg.

Head end.

FIG. 23.—ASCARIS LUMBRICOIDES.

coides is something enormous. The number of eggs in the sexual organs of a pregnant female is given by Leuckart and Eschericht as about 60,000,000.

The oval eggs, which attain a length of about 0.05 to 0.075 mm.,

are surrounded with a coarse dark shell, having an outer albumi-
nous covering which shows hilly protuberances and is often colored
yellowish-brown or green by the bile coloring-matter.   The seat of
the parasite is in the small intestine.   To be sure, it occasionally
gets into the larger intestine, even into the stomach and into other
cavities of the body, but in these places it usually remains alive but
a few days.   Hippocrates was acquainted with the tendency of
ascarides to migrate in order to reach the exterior.   In one of my
patients, a youth aged nineteen, emesis brought out 11 ascarides.
Another patient, a young lady aged twenty-six, reported that two
such worms crawled out through her nose during sleep.   In both
cases treatment caused evacuation of ascarides from the bowels.

Etiology.—As the ascaris, according to Grassi, Lutz, and Leuckart requires no intermediate host, the only mode of transmission
is by ingestion of the embryos of the *Ascaris lumbricoides*, which
may enter the body with vegetables, fruits, and drinking-water.   The
embryo must enter; if the ovic cell enters, it will not develop.
Mosler has proved the presence of the eggs in drinking-water.
Lutz (*l. c.*) attributes the failure of experiments attempting the infection of human beings with ova of the ascaris to the maceration
and destruction of the outer mulberry-like envelop, and consequent
exposure of the young embryos to the digestive juices.   The
rough outer envelop of the ova, if intact, is capable of resisting the
action of digestive juices.   Since a species of *Ascaris lumbricoides* is
also found in hogs and beeves, it was suggested by Fleischer that
the parasite may be further propagated by these animals.   But the
ascaris found in hogs and beeves represents an entirely different
species and hence can have no influence in spreading the human
infection.   Its development and growth seem to proceed very rapidly, since young specimens are found very rarely.   The transmission of the ascarides is favored by lack of cleanliness.   This explains why they are so often found in the insane.   *Ascaris lumbricoides* is found in all ages and both sexes; but, according to Zenker,
it occurs more frequently in females and in children.   Nothing
definite is known concerning the duration of life of the worm.

Symptomatology.—Although disease symptoms may be entirely
wanting when several or even numerous ascarides are in the intestines, yet in many other cases they cause about the same symptoms

as tapeworms—that is, disturbances of both local and general nature. It is important to recognize the nervous anomalies arising reflexly and attributed to ascarides; the explanation of these nervous disturbances is the same as of those found in patients having tapeworms. We can assume a direct dependence of these disturbances on the presence of the worms in the intestine only when these disturbances cease after the expulsion of the worms and again commence if they should develop again.

Ascaris lumbricoides possesses a strong, odoriferous principle, which continues to be perceptible after the worm has been carefully washed. The substance to which this odor is due may, according to Huber ("Twentieth Century Practice of Medicine," vol. III, p. 583), cause urticaria in patients having a predisposition to this eruption. It is conceivable that some of the so-called nervous symptoms may be due to the absorption of this ascaris toxin. It is, however, often observed that these nervous disturbances continue with the same or but slightly diminished intensity after the expulsion of the parasites. In other cases, however, they disappear at once.

The local disturbances observed in ascarides are loss of appetite, bad taste in the mouth, salivation, extreme hunger, offensive breath, eructation, nausea, sensibility of the stomach to pressure, and colic-like pains, especially in the region of the navel, constipation, and also diarrhea.

The general condition and the nutrition sometimes suffer very much, especially in children if they are hosts to a large number of roundworms. The face becomes pale and yellow, as in the case of very sick persons; the eyes lie deep in the sockets and have dark rings about them; the face shows suffering, and the patients lose weight.

The nervous symptoms may be prominent and persistent: tickling sensations in the nose, difference in the size of the pupils, fainting spells, vertigo, flashes before the eyes, cramps, chorea, epilepsy, disturbances in sight and hearing, paralysis, neuralgia, asthma, singultus. Indeed, Henoch has observed ecstatic conditions accompanied with great unrest and occurring every evening in a boy twelve years old. Before these attacks he would complain of violent pains in the region of the descending colon. After the expulsion of large ascarides they suddenly ceased.

If ascarides pass over into the colon, they are passed off with the evacuations.   If the stomach is invaded by ascarides, disagreeable sensations of nausea and pain are produced, which quickly cease as soon as the parasites are expelled by vomiting.

Unpleasant, and indeed very serious, results may, on the contrary, be caused by the passage of ascarides into other organs and parts of organs, and especially by their tendency to slip into narrow channels and obstruct them.   If a large roundworm gets into the upper part of the esophagus and thence into the larynx, it may quickly result in death by suffocation.   If the worm is breathed into the deeper air-passages from the larynx, the dyspnea, to be sure, decreases, but the occurrence of traumatic inflammation of the lungs or of a lung abscess is to be feared.   In isolated cases roundworms have also been found in the nose and in the lacrymal duct. In a case in my own practice the first intimation of the real cause of an apparent gastritis in a young girl, aged twenty years, was the expulsion through the nose of an ascaris after a violent fit of sneezing.   The stomach-tube had brought out no worm previous to this.   Proper treatment caused the evacuation of eleven ascarides in the feces.   A singular case has been reported by Bruneau.   A girl was seized with violent convulsions during mass.   After a roundworm had been taken out of the external ear-passage, these ceased.   The worm had started from the mouth through the Eustachian tube, to the inner (or middle) ear, and thence had reached the external ear-passage through a pre-existing perforation in the tympanum of the ear. ·

If large-sized ascarides slip into the pancreatic, or, what is more frequent, into the common gall-duct, the secretion of the pancreatic juice into the intestine ceases.   In the second case the patients often succumb to a fatal jaundice.   If little ascarides get into the gall-bladder and die there, they may, just as any other foreign body, favor the formation of gall-stones.   If they get into the bile-passages of the liver, they may first cause an ulceration of the mucous membrane of the bile-ducts and finally the formation of abscesses in the surrounding hepatic tissue.

When abnormal communications have been formed between the intestine on the one side and the peritoneal cavity, the bladder, the uterus, the pleura, and the pericardial cavity on the other, as a result of perforation, of follicular, tuberculous, or other kinds of intestinal ulcers, or as a result of the breaking through of perityphlitic and other abscesses, ascarides may get into the peritoneal cavity, and the other cavities mentioned above, and leave the body through the urethra or the vagina. Roundworms have also been found fairly often in peritonitic abscesses communicating with the intestine. These are usually caused by the compression or incarceration of an umbilical hernia (especially in children) or of an inguinal hernia (especially in adults); they are also caused by perforating intestinal ulcers. The old designation "worm-abscess" proves that in former times it was thought that the ascarides caused the compression and inflammation. It is, however, highly improbable and entirely unproved that the roundworms may cause an ulcerating inflammation or perforation of the intact intestinal wall, with consequent suppuration. They may at most help to increase an already existing inflammation, especially a perityphlitis, acting as an irritant, just as any other foreign body would. Heller denies that anatomical changes in the mucous membrane may result from the presence of ascarides in the intestines. F. Mosler ("Thierische Parasiten," von Mosler u. Peiper, Nothnagel's "Spec. Path. u. Ther.," Bd. vi, S. 196) gives the statistics of cases where small erosions and enteritis were caused by the ascarides. Huber (*l. c.*) defends the idea that the ascarides secrete a strong chemically irritating toxin. While he was engaged in studying the lumbricoid worms, he noticed that an irritating itching occurred on his own head and neck; that large lumps appeared on his neck and smaller ones on his forehead. His right ear became swollen; the ear-passage discharged profusely for an hour; there was a continuous throbbing in his head, starting from the right ear. Besides these there was catarrh of the conjunctivæ, accompanied by violent itching, which increased to chemosis on the right side, and itching of the hands. Miram has twice observed similar symptoms in his own case, while examining *Ascaris equorum.*

In many cases only single specimens of *Ascaris lumbricoides* exist in the intestine. They may, however, be present in the intestine in enormous quantities, especially in children. In the case of a twelve-year-old boy, observed by Fauconneau-Dufresne, over 5000 roundworms passed off in a period of two to three months, and on one occasion 103 specimens were vomited.

It was formerly positively denied that ascarides, even if present in great numbers, could cause obstruction of the intestine. Recent observations, however, show that they may completely obstruct the intestine, not only temporarily, but even for a longer period of time. This is shown by an interesting case, described by Stepp, in which roundworms caused fatal ileus in a child four years old. Dr. Basil M. Taylor described a case of intestinal obstruction (" Am. Journ. Obstet.," June, 1899) in a boy four years old due to a mass of ascarides and necessitating operation. The child died three days after the laparotomy. Dr. Donald R. McCrae has reported a case where lumbricoids were the cause of obstructing the small intestine (" Lancet," Sept. 16, 1899). My personal opinion is that obstruction caused by conglomeration of lumbricoids is undoubtedly possible, for the parasites have a way of intertwining in the bowel of the living host, and must act as an obturating mass, both mechanically and reflexly.

Diagnosis.—This is easy, if ascarides are found in the matter excreted or vomited, or if the eggs of the ascarides, which may easily be recognized by their shell and covering of albumin, can be detected in the evacuations. Eichhorst states that the latter are often found in the bits of excrement sticking to the anus. Charcot crystals are found but seldom in the evacuations in the case of ascarides.

Prognosis.—In general the prognosis is favorable, since the previously mentioned serious results are rare in comparison with the frequent occurrence of ascarides. It is better, however, to prevent these entirely and to expel the ascarides as soon as their presence is discovered.

Therapeutics.—*Preventatives.*—Bodily cleanliness and cleanliness in the kitchen (careful cleansing of vegetables and fruits), and avoiding the use of water from springs or wells too near to the privies, are fundamental rules. Whenever there is the least suspicion of impure water, it should be sterilized prior to drinking, if better water can not be secured. This at least renders the transmission of ascarides to human beings more difficult; uncleanliness, on the contrary, facilitates it. This is proved by the fact that the parasites are found much more rarely in civilized peoples, and in the adults of the higher classes, while they are much more widespread in uncivilized nations, in uncleanly insane, and also in children . whom the habit of cleanliness is not developed, and who often infect their mouths with their fingers which may be contaminated with earth possibly containing ascaris eggs.

For expelling the ascarides, santonin, which has completely displaced the formerly used *Flores cinœ* (the mother-plant of the santonin), is recognized to be the best remedy. It does not, according to Schroeder's observations, kill the roundworms, but renders their stay in the small intestine so unpleasant that they go into the large intestine and then easily pass off with the evacuations. Since santonin, if repeatedly taken in large doses, may cause the symptoms of intoxication, urticaria, vomiting, yellow vision, convulsions, and delirium, it is advisable to give an aperient a few hours later,—calomel, castor oil, pulv. liquor. comp., effervescent citrate of magnesia, etc.,—so that the santonin may be removed from the intestines after it has done its work. In children, santonin is to be prescribed in doses of 0.02 to 0.05 gram, or ⅓ to 1 grain, three times daily, as a powder or in the form of troches. Santonin may be given in combination with calomel thus :

> ℞. Calomel, ... gr. j to gr. ij
> Santonin, ... gr. ⅓.
> M. SIG.—One powder three times daily.

Wormseed or chenopodium in doses of grains xx to xxx is an effective remedy. The oil of chenopodium, dose 5 to 10 drops, acts similarly. Thymol in doses of ½ to 2 grams (grains viiss to xxx) is effective for the expulsion of ascarides. But the practitioner will rarely require anything more than santonin.

Oxyuris vermicularis (Seatworm, Pinworm).

This is a small white filiform or thread-shaped parasite. The male is 5 mm. long, 0.2 mm. thick; the female is 12 mm. long, and 0.5 to 0.6 mm. thick. The head of both male and female is a small knob; the mouth is surrounded by three lips. The blunt tail end of the male is rolled in toward the ventral side; that of the female is drawn out like a bodkin. The eggs have a length of 0.05 mm., with a breadth of 0.025 mm. They are oval-shaped, but bulge out more on one side than on the other. The contents of the unfertilized and undeveloped egg, consisting of large granules, have a nucleus with a nucleolus inside the latter, and are surrounded by a shell possessing several layers.

The developed eggs contain embryos; they are not discharged from the pregnant females whilst they are in the human intestine. The oxyuris eggs are not discharged until after this parasite leaves the intestines of the host. Hence the feces very rarely show oxyuris eggs, even when the seatworms are present in the bowel. In rare instances, dead female oxyures may abort (Leichtenstern) just as they die, and then eggs may be observed in the feces. It is not necessary to look for eggs in attempting the diagnosis. In this infection the oxyuris itself is, as a rule, found in the feces.

This parasite at first stays in the small intestine. Later on it goes into the large intestine, and especially into the cecum. The pregnant

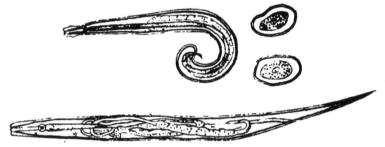

FIG. 24.—OXYURIS VERMICULARIS.
The eggs above represent the undeveloped form.

females go to the lower part of the large intestine and to the rectum, and do not deposit their eggs until they leave the latter.

Infection with oxyuris always occurs by ingestion of ripe ova of the parasite, which on reaching the stomach are deprived of their shell by the gastric juice—at least so it is presumed. I have not been able to find any report in the literature of the subject whether oxyuris eggs can really be digested, or rather whether the shell can be digested in human gastric juice or not.

The liberated embryos settle in the small intestine. After some time the cohabitation of the developed parasites takes place here. Then they spread over the entire large and small intestines. The pregnant females seem to prefer settling in the cecum. If their ovaries are full of eggs, they proceed to the lower part of the large intestine and to the rectum and deposit their eggs there.

Since oxyures and eggs are often found on the mucous membrane of the anus and in its immediate neighborhood, and since the patients, especially at night, just before and during sleep, are often forced to scratch these places with their fingers on account of great itching, the fingers as a result are very easily infected with oxyuris eggs. If live female oxyures are in the vicinity of the anus, children may crush the females and thus infect their hands. Oxyuris eggs are rarely found in the feces. Zenker has repeatedly detected the eggs under the finger-nails and at the base of the nails. These eggs may get into the mouth and thence into the stomach, in the morning before the hands are washed.

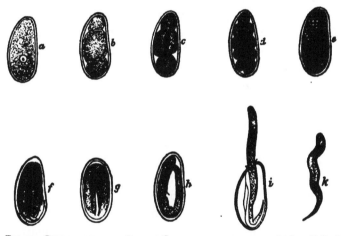

FIG. 25.—DEVELOPMENT OF OVA OF OXYURIS VERMICULARIS.—(*After Heller.*)
a to *e*, Segmentation of the yolk. *f*, Ovum, showing embryo of tadpole shape (lateral view). *g*, Same embryo as *f* in abdominal view. *h*, Ovum containing worm-shaped embryo. *i*, Embryo escaping from the shell. *k*, Free-moving embryo.

Although the duration of life of the parasite is but short, and large numbers of worms are removed daily in the evacuations, yet in many cases (especially children) apparently their number does not diminish. This is because new mature eggs are always being brought into the stomach and intestines as a result of self-infection, and their embryos develop here very quickly. The worms may also be spread by uncleanly bakers, waiters, and fruit-dealers, if their hands are infected with eggs, and the parasites deposited on bread, fruit, and vegetables, as well as other food-stuffs, thus contributing to the propagation of the parasite.

Curious discrepancies occur, in various special works on human intestinal parasites, concerning the deposit of the ova of oxyuris and the method of their dissemination. Thus, R. Fleischer ("Spez. Pathol. u. Therapie d. Magen u. Darmkrankheiten," S. 1380) and Mosler and Peiper ("Thierische Parasiten," S. 227) state that the oxyures deposit their ova in the colon and rectum so abundantly that the mucosa is covered like a fur (Fleischer). Furthermore, that the feces contain enormous numbers of ova which may become dried in the sun and be disseminated by the wind, insects, flies, etc. (Mosler and Peiper). These errors have been copied from text-book to text-book.

The truth is that the pregnant females practically never deposit their ova as long as they live within the human intestine. Emigration of the oxyuris is the first act of propagation, and the discharge of the eggs is associated with the death of the mother worm. The sexual fertilization of the females takes place in the small intestine. After this the migration begins at once, and the pregnant females tarry for a time either in the cecum or in the rectum. This delay varies according to the degree of maturity of the eggs. When they are ripe, the female leaves the rectum.

Drying of the eggs so that they could be carried by the wind would, in the opinion of Dr. Chas. Wardell Stiles, probably kill them. The temporary sojourn of pregnant females in the rectum and colon gives us a valuable therapeutic hint—namely, the use of colon and rectal irrigation with quinin, gr. xv to 1 quart of warm water, or of benzin, grams 1.2 to one quart warm water, or of one quart of quassia infusion, after these parasites have been driven down from the small intestines by santonin.

Fleischer (*l. c.*, p. 1381) asserts that oxyures are not transmitted by drinking-water, and there are other authors who assert that water infection does not play a great rôle. However, this question has as yet not been satisfactorily investigated, and to be on the safe side it will be wise to boil the drinking-water in families where oxyuris infections exist.

Oxyures are found all over the globe. They are most frequently found in children. Heller reported a case of oxyuris infection in a child five weeks old. Women, however, often suffer from them, but they are most frequent in the uncleanly insane. There are few human beings who at one period or another of their life have not been hosts of this parasite.

Symptomatology.—The oxyures present in the small intestine and in the upper part of the large intestine do not cause any distinct disease symptoms. If the oxyures are present in great numbers, marked irritation of the mucosa results, which often ends in catarrhal inflammation, and causes diarrhea (diarrhœa verminosa). In this case oxyures, together with large quantities of mucus, may be found in the evacuations. The usual, indeed almost the regular, symptom is a severe itching in the anus and its neighborhood. This is a result of the irritation of the mucous membrane by the parasites, and usually starts at night in bed, or increases considerably at this time, because the oxyures, probably as a result of the warmth of the bed, and of quiet, proceed partly toward the anus and the outside. On this account oxyures are often found on the bed-sheet in the morning. This itching may be so violent and persistent that it may prevent the patient from sleeping, and may even increase to violent pain and tenesmus. If the skin of the perineum is moistened with vaginal secretion, oxyures may pass from the neighborhood of the anus into the vulva. This is not possible if the skin is dry. The oxyures are doubtless more frequently carried into the vagina by scratching with hands infected with the eggs pressed out of dead female oxyures. Here the oxyures cause hyperemia, increased secretion of mucus, and sometimes also hyperesthesia and leucorrhea. Nymphomaniac conditions, masturbation, erections, pollutions, prostatorrhea, and spermatorrhea may be caused by the itching irritation of the vulva, testes, penis, and rectum. The oxyures get under the prepuce more rarely (itching irritation, balanitis, balanoposthitis). In severe cases an itching (nervous) of the skin may also appear at other places in the body. The remaining symptoms correspond with those observed in the case of ascarides. Two cases of intractable pruritus vulvæ in my practice were traced to oxyures, and this very annoying symptom was cured by santonin treatment and vaginal irrigations with infusion of quassia to remove possible oxyures in the genital passage.

Diagnosis.—This can be easily and certainly made, since oxyures, which usually are in quick motion, are always found in the evacuation in this infection, and at times the eggs can be found in the neighborhood of the anus; their presence there being caused by the scratching of the patient, during which pregnant and emigrated females are mashed and killed. Charcot-Leyden crystals are found but seldom in the feces in these cases.

Prognosis.—This is favorable, for even if the disease may be persistent as a result of frequently repeated self-infections, it may nevertheless be absolutely cured by rational therapeutics and by cleanliness.

Therapeutics.—Just as in the case of ascarides, santonin usually renders valuable service in driving out these parasites from the small intestine into the larger. (See Treatment of Roundworms.)

The following formula of Mosler is one which I have prescribed with uniformly good results, particularly in children:

    ℞. Santonin, ... 0.2
        Olei ricini,
        Syr. rubi idæi, ... āā 50.0
        Chloroform, ... 1.0.
    M. Sig.—One to two tablespoonfuls in the evening.

Benzin given internally as described in the section on the treatment of tapeworms, and also when used in the form of colon irrigations (20 drops to a pint of warm water), has in my experience proved efficacious in three cases. Aperients are required simultaneously.

It is also advisable to rinse out the large intestine frequently with water to which thymol, salicylic acid, quinia, soap-water, and, in very obstinate cases, boric acid has been added. Infusions of quassia and of garlic as enemata are highly recommended. If the neighborhood of the anus itches very much, it is to be anointed with gray ointment (hydrarg. ciner.), which also prevents the passing over of the oxyures into the vulva. It is sometimes very difficult to rid children completely of them, and several attempts are always necessary for a satisfactory result. Some cases require daily irrigation treatment and weekly doses of santonin for a month or more.

Trichotrachelidæ (Leuckart) (Whipworm). Trichuris trichiura (old name, Trichocephalus dispar).

This parasite was first observed and described by Morgagni. The designation whipworm is well merited, since it really has the shape of a whip, the handle of which is formed by the thick tail end, the thong by the head extremity, which is elongated and thin, resembling a hair. The tail end of the male is rolled in, not toward the ventral side, as in the case of *Ascaris lumbricoides* and *Oxyuris vermicularis*, but toward the dorsal side. The male has a length of 40 mm., the female 45 to 50 mm. The vulva in the female is at the beginning of the lower part of the body ; in the male the cloaca is at the end of the body, and a spicule projects from it. The eggs are oval, 0.05 mm. long, colored brownish, have small shining knobs at both poles, and may thus be easily distinguished from other eggs.

The whipworm has its usual habitation in the cecum, very rarely lower down in the colon. It has been asserted by Klebs and

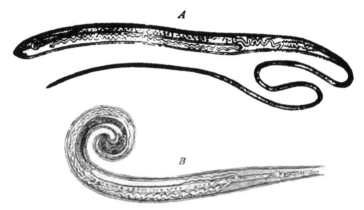

FIG. 26.—TRICHURIS TRICHIURA (OLD NAME, TRICHOCEPHALUS DISPAR).
A. The organism with the elongated whip-like thread is the female parasite. *B.* The shorter form is the male parasite. The elongated whip is not the tail, for the tip end of it represents the head.

Heller that the parasite encircles and grasps projecting bits of mucosa and thus holds on to it by its narrow whip-like head end. But Leuckart, Küchenmeister, Mosler, and Peiper have observed that this long thin head end is actually embedded under the mucosa beneath the epithelium.

Etiology.—The embryos of the whipworm do not need an intermediate host for their development. They get into the stomach probably in the drinking-water or with vegetable food (fruit or vegetables). The whipworm requires no intermediate host for its life history (Leuckart), and its eggs require from four to six months, even one year, for development of the embryo (Davaine-Leuckart) within the egg.   After maturity and escape of the embryo from the egg it requires four to five weeks to reach full growth in the human intestine.   They then migrate to the cecum, where they usually remain.   Moosbrugger reported a case of whipworm infection in a little boy which ended fatally.   It had been brought on by the ingestion of garden earth, which contained the eggs of this parasite, as was later determined.

Symptomatology.—Single specimens of the parasite do not cause any disease symptoms.   If larger numbers occur in the colon, diarrhea and nervous symptoms may appear.   Pascal, Valleix, and Barth report cases that died under manifestations of severe cerebral symptoms ; at autopsy the brain and meninges were found normal, but enormous numbers of trichocephalides were found in the intestines (see Pascal, " Bull. Soc. Méd.," No. 3, p. 59 ; also Valleix, " Guide du Médicin praticien," VI, p. 98).   Burkhardt (" Deutsche med. Wochenschr.," 1880, No. 34) reports a case of intractable diarrhea and emaciation extending over a period of nine months and finally eventuating in icterus which was due to intestinal infection with this parasite.   The case eventually recovered.

Diagnosis.—If the parasites or their eggs are found in the feces, the diagnosis is easy.   The eggs have the shape of minute almonds, but more symmetrical.   Charcot crystals are also often found.

Therapeutics.—The manner in which this parasite penetrates under the mucosa, and its frequent envelopment in masses of mucus, render the complete eradication difficult at times.   The treatment requires time and patience.   The best results are obtained from benzene irrigation of the colon ($3j$ benzene to one quart warm water) ; at the same time benzene is given internally.   Extract of male-fern is recommendable, employed in the same manner as advised under paragraph on tapeworms.   Rosenheim recommends thymol (2.0), to be given several times a day.

Trichinella spiralis.   Trichina spiralis Owen, 1835 ; Trichinella spiralis (Owen) Railliet.   Trichinosis.

The infection with this parasite occurs by the ingestion of meat, particularly pork, containing the trichinella.   There are three stages of the disease : (1) The intestinal, (2) the migration, and (3) the encapsulation stage.   It appears that this parasite was first observed in 1832 by Hilton, prosector at Guy's Hospital, London. He did not recognize the true character of the minute worm, but described countless small, calcareous concretions which he mistook for " gargols." James Paget, in 1835, first discovered the round-worm contained in the capsules. The fine, hair-like and curled-up parasite was more closely described by Owen, and defined as *Trichina spiralis*.

The credit of having methodically studied and clearly set forth the histogenetic relations of trichinosis and the rôle played in the pathogenesis by the trichinella is due to Zenker ("Deutsch. Arch. f. klin. Med.," Bd. 1, 1866). The parasite is found in two forms : (1) The intestinal trichina, which is sexually mature, and (2) the muscle trichina, which is sexually immature.

1. The *intestinal trichinella* is a fine, hair-like worm, narrower at the cephalic end, and possessing a head smaller than the rest of the body. The tail of the male has a bilobed prominence, between the divisions of which the cloaca is placed ; the parasite does not possess any spicule. The female has a blunt rounded tail, the reproductive outlet being situated near the anterior part of the body. The ova are exceedingly small, and are developed inside the body of the maternal worm, the embryos being viviparously produced at the rate of 100 a week after the entrance of the female into the intestine.

2. The *muscle trichinella*, as it is ingested in the infected meat, develops its sexual apparatus after it has entered the intestinal canal of its host. About three to four hours after ingestion of the infected meat the capsules containing the embryos open and the latter rapidly develop. Within two days these muscle larvæ are matured and fecundation of the female takes place. The development of the parasite from the period of the impregnation to the time of sexual maturity is, under favorable conditions, less than three weeks, the various steps of development occurring approximately in the follow-ing periods of time :

(*a*) Maturation of muscle larvæ within two to three days of in-gestion of infected pork.

(*b*) Birth of embryos occurs in seven days more.

(*c*) In about two weeks the young brood has migrated from the intestine of the host into his muscles, where further changes occur ;

namely, the formation of a minute capsule and deposition of lime salts in the capsule and parasite. According to Zenker, cases in which none but encapsulated trichinellæ are found are instances of healed trichinosis.

Symptoms.—The gastro-intestinal symptoms, which appear in from two to three days after the ingestion of the infected meat, consist of anorexia, gastric distention, nausea, vomiting, diarrhea, and colicky pains. The blood examination shows marked eosinophilia.

The symptoms after the penetration into the muscles are fever, nausea, marked myalgic pains, with stiffness and swelling of the muscles, edema of the face, and in some cases insomnia, delirium, and death from marasmus or pneumonia.

Diagnosis of Infection with Trichinella spiralis.—During the first week of this infection the diagnosis can very rarely be established. In fact, the diagnosis always presents difficulties when one is confronted with an isolated case or the first cases of a coming epidemic. The recognition of the trichinosis is easy only in cases that occur during the prevalence of an epidemic of this infection. Aside from the phenomena which are expressions of disturbances of the central nervous organs and peripheral nerves, the delirium, hyperesthesia, and anesthesia of the skin, the distress felt at all muscular movements, even those of chewing and deglutition, the dyspnea in consequence of invasion of the respiratory muscles, mydriasis and painful movability of the eyes, there are peculiar cutaneous edemas which are almost constantly present and are quite characteristic and important, especially when one has limited the diagnosis by exclusion of other possible infections.

The clinical picture that trichinosis presents is really only available for exact diagnosis after the expiration of the first week following the infection. Then we are confronted almost invariably with bronchitis, which may later eventuate into pneumonia, particularly so if the accumulated secretion can not be expelled on account of the insufficiency of the expiratory muscles. If in addition to these nervous and respiratory symptoms we can also observe muscular pains and edemas following an acute gastro-intestinal attack, the practitioner should think of trichinosis, especially if fever is present. The next efforts should be directed to eliminating other possible infections, that may produce similar effects—namely, the exanthematous fevers, typhoid fever, influenza, and malaria. Nephritis and hepatitis will have to be excluded, also cardiac diseases, because these also may lead to edema. Here frequent analyses of the urine are helpful, because these diseases are, as a rule, associated with albuminuria, whereas trichinosis only exceptionally gives rise to albuminuria. If the practitioner has gone through with all these differentiations, he has finally limited his diagnosis to infectious polymyositis or trichinosis. Both of these may present the identical symptoms. An initial edema of the face, and especially of the eyelids, speaks for trichinosis, if these signs are present. *But the only reliable evidences for the diagnosis can be obtained from microscopic examination of the feces, if for intestinal trichinellæ, and of an excised piece of muscle for muscle trichinellæ.*

Unfortunately, examination of the feces is often negative and no trichinella are found, although undoubted trichinosis exists, so that absence of trichinella from the feces does not exclude trichinosis. Even excision of a piece of the biceps or deltoid muscle may show no trichinella. However, this effort of diagnosis is more frequently rewarded by finding the parasite than by examination of the stool. The anamnesis is important if the patient has eaten imperfectly cooked pork ; and if some of the meat of the same pig is obtainable and can be shown to be infected, the diagnosis is naturally beyond a doubt.

Prognosis depends on the amount of infected pork eaten and the degree to which it was contaminated. The statistics of German reports show a variable mortality. Dr. C. W. Stiles reports that his figures of the German total mortality are 5.6 per cent. The fatality depends upon the intensity of the infection. In 108 infections in Weimar, for instance, there were no deaths ; but in an epidemic in Hedersleben there were 30 per cent. of deaths (Mosler and Peiper, *l. c.*, p. 297), so that it is hardly possible to correctly express the mortality in percentages.

Prophylaxis consists in the avoidance of meat food that has not been prepared in such a way as to kill any trichinæ that might exist (by thorough cooking, exclusion of trichinous pork by governmental meat inspection). The objection of the German and French Governments to American pork is logically set forth in Mosler and Peiper's work (*l. c.*, pp. 279 and 280).   They base their statements on the investi-gations of Billings, who in examining meat from 2701 pigs (Boston, 1879) found 154 cases of trichinosis, or one pig in 17.53.   In 1881 Billings found 75 pigs infected with trichinella among 2068 animals examined; this makes a proportion of one in 27.46.   These investi-gations of Billings require confirmation, and it does not appear exact nor logical for German authorities to be guided by them exclusively when the official statistics of the United States Government, based upon thousands of examinations, indicate an average occurrence of trichinosis among hogs in the United States in only 2 per cent. of these animals.

Treatment.—If the infection is recent,—within three to five days,—gastric and colon lavage is indicated to remove the parasites. Emetics and purgatives—ipecac and calomel—are available under these conditions.   After these have acted, antiseptics are indicated to destroy the remaining trichinæ.   The best are: Salol, gr. v, t. i. d.; carbolic acid, gtt. iij, t. i. d., largely diluted; tincture of iodin, betanaphthol, bismuth salicylate, and glycerin.   There are no reme-dies that can influence the embryos in their migration through the muscles.   Merckel and Fiedler recommended large doses of gly-cerin.   One patient who had eaten trichinous sausage took 15 table-spoonfuls in a day and recovered.   But Peiper and Lesshaft were unable to prevent trichina infection in rabbits and pigs by glycerin (Mosler and Peiper, *l. c.*, p. 307).   So I conclude that the glycerin treatment is unreliable.

There can be no doubt, however, that benzene is an effective remedy against trichina.   It should be given both internally and at the same time by colon irrigation.   Inwardly it is given in the fol-lowing form:

> ℞. Benzene, c. p., ...   6.0
>   Mucilag. acac., ... 25.0
>   Succi liquor., ...   8.0
>   Aquæ menth. pip., ... 120.0.
> M. Sig.—Dose, one tablespoonful every two hours.

As a colon irrigation, it should be injected through a high rectal tube in the strength of 4 to 8 grams of benzene to one quart of water.

Santonin, especially when combined with calomel and jalap in form of a powder (santonin, 0.2 ; calomel, jalap, and white sugar, each 0.5 ; make into 6 powders ; give one powder twice daily .

In systemic trichinosis the recovery depends upon the "vis medi-catrix naturæ." But individual symptoms need attention. The muscular pains are best treated by inunctions with hot oil and chloroform, and hot baths; the insomnia by morphin, sometimes chloral and sulfonal, 5 grains of each at one dose; the profuse sweating by quinia, atropin, and sponging. There may be grave cardiac depression, requiring strychnin and digitalis. The diet must be nutritious but easily digestible. Careful attention should be given to the feeding.

Strongylides. Correct name: Uncinaria duodenalis (Dubini, 1843) Railliet, 1885 (Hook-worm).

Synonyms.—*Anchylostoma duodenalis* Dubini, 1843; *Strongylus quadridentatus* Siebold, 1851; *Dochmius anchylostomum* Molin, 1860; *Sclerostoma duodenale* (Dubini, 1843) Cobbold, 1864; *Strongylus duodenalis* (Dubini, 1843) Schneider, 1866; *Dochmius duodenalis* (Dubini, 1843) Leuckart, 1876.

Introductory Remarks.—Infections with uncinaria, or anchylostoma, as it is better known, several decades ago seem to have been common in Italy. It was observed by Dabini in 1838 as widespread in Milan and upper Italy. Later it was observed in Egypt by Bilharz and Pruner. In 1851 Griesinger recognized it as the cause of the so-called Egyptian (tropical) chlorosis. Wucherer, after numerous dissections, completely confirmed Griesinger's views. By him and by Lutz and other investigators the parasite was found in other tropical and subtropical lands. It has been found to occur in Brazil, Peru, Bolivia, Cayenne, Jamaica, Porto Rico, and Cuba, the eastern and western coasts of Africa, India, and Japan. The causal relation between the parasite and severe anemia was also determined by Wucherer and Lutz. Italian investigators, especially Bozzolo, Concato, Grassi, Perroncito, later on showed that the *Uncinaria duodenalis*, or *Anchylostoma duodenale*, not only caused the well-known severe anemia of the Italian tile (brick) makers, but also the so-called tunnel anemia, from which so many persons employed in the construction of the St. Gothard tunnel suffered. Perroncito has since caused numerous examinations of the evacuations of the miners working in the mines of Sardinia, southern France, and Hungary (Kremnitz, Schemnitz) to be made. These miners often suffer from marked anemia, and these investigations were made to determine its cause. They showed that it might also be traced to the presence of hook-worms in the intestines.   Since then every year brought new facts, by which our knowledge of uncinariosis or anchylostomiasis and its dependent symptoms has been enlarged.   Menche and Meyer (1882 and 1883) first detected uncinariosis or anchylostomiasis in Germany in brickyards in the neighborhood of Bonn and Aix-la-Chapelle. Leichtenstern observed it in the neighborhood of Cologne, and he instituted thorough investigations by which the etiology, symptoma-tology, and pathological anatomy of the disease were materially advanced.   Francotte and Masins found it (1884) existing in the coal miners near Lüttich ; van Beneden found it in the coal miners at Monts.   While Müller and Seifert found the parasites in brick-makers near Würzburg, Grawitz found them in four Italian brick-makers employed near Berlin, and Bernheim in a brickmaker near Baden.   Since that, hook-worms have been observed in numerous lands and districts—United States, Germany, Switzerland, Nether-lands, Belgium, France, and Hungary.   According to my experience, there is no doubt that this parasite is being introduced into the United States by Italian and Polish laborers and their families, who at times are found to have uncinaria in their stools.   Anemia due to this condition has been observed among them in certain definite dis-tricts in Baltimore.   Our soldiers are bringing this parasite from Porto Rico (" Phila. Med. Journ.," Mar. 10, 1900, p. 541); also Dr. Bailey K. Ashford, "Ankylostomiasis in Porto Rico," "New York Med. Journ.," April 14, 1900).   A recent report on anchylostomiasis in the United States is by Drs. Herman B. Allyn and M. Behrend in " American Medicine," July 13, 1901, p. 63, to which reference should be had for illustrations and literature.   We may in future expect to see more of this hitherto rare parasite in our country. About fifteen new cases have been diagnosed this summer (1901).*

Natural History of the Uncinaria duodenalis, or Anchy-lostoma duodenale.—This worm, which has a yellow-white or brownish color, has a cylindrical shape.   The length of the female is 10 to 12 mm., at most 18 mm.; that of the male is 6 to 8 mm.,

---

* Dr. John L. Yates has discovered a case of uncinariosis at autopsy at Bay View Asylum, Baltimore.

rarely 10 mm. Many more females than males are found in the human intestine—22 to 24 of the former, 10 of the latter (Leichtenstern); or after longer duration the relation is 6 : 1 (Schulthess). Under high powers a bell-shaped mouth capsule may be seen at the cephalic end. This capsule is provided at its dorsal edge with two small teeth ; at its ventral side with four larger ones, curved inward. Further down it has powerful dagger-shaped strips of chitin, by means of which the parasite pierces the mucous membrane to which it attaches itself. The males are shaped like threads, white in color, and often bent in angles. The females are stretched out, thicker, and colored yellowish-white or brownish (the color being due to the blood with which they are filled). The fecundity of these parasites is something enormous. According to Leichtenstern, one evacuation weighing 233

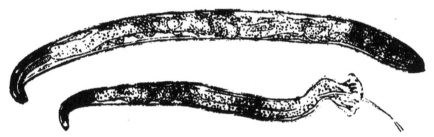

FIG. 27.—UNCINARIA DUODENALIS, OR ANCHYLOSTOMA DUODENALE.—(*From the Author's Clinic.*)
The smaller one is the male parasite.

grams may contain 4,216,930 eggs. These possess a bright shell, while their contents are brownish. They are usually found in the stage of segmentation. They are oval in shape, 0.05 mm. long and 0.025 mm. broad. The further development of the eggs proceeds outside of the intestine only. The number of the parasites in the intestine may vary between 15 and 3000 or more (Grassi). If there is a great number of eggs in the feces, we may infer that there are many female hook-worms in the intestines. The parasites adhere to the intestinal mucosa by suction. They act like cupping glasses, the six teeth and the dagger-shaped formation of chitin at the bottom of the mouth capsule taking the place of knives and executing the preliminary scarification.

The females seem to be much more gluttonous than the males,

and to suck more blood than is requisite for their nourishment. For this nourishment the blood plasma principally is used; most of the red blood-corpuscles leave the intestinal canal of the parasite unutilized and unchanged. Since the severity of the symptoms does not always stand in a fixed relation to the number of the parasites present in the intestines, and since the amount of blood sucked out would scarcely suffice to produce a severe anemia in a relatively short period of time, it is probable that some other injurious influences, as yet unknown, are concurrent with the loss of blood and the digestive disturbances occurring in uncinariosis, or, as it was formerly called, anchylostomiasis. The intestines may be infected simultaneously by *Uncinaria, Strongyloides, Ascaris lumbricoides,* and *Oxyuris vermicularis.*

Lussano ("Contributo allo patogenesi dell' anemia da anchilostomiasi," "Rivista Clinica," 1890, No. 11) has extracted substances from the urine of persons having hook-worms which, if introduced into the circulation of the blood, caused a diminution of the red blood-corpuscles and of the hemoglobin. From this he infers, possibly correctly, that toxic substances are formed in the intestines in the case of uncinariosis, and again absorbed, which tend to damage the normal composition of the blood (see discussion on Uncinariosis in "British Med. Journal," Sept. 1, 1900).

The uncinaria does not live in the duodenum alone, as one might infer from the specific name *"duodenalis."* It is even more frequently found in the jejunum and ileum, and may be entirely lacking in the duodenum.

Etiology.—The origin of new hook-worm epidemics in any district can always be traced to the introduction of the parasite by one or more persons who carry them in their intestines. The transmission to healthy persons occurs by way of the feces of the sick, which almost always contain eggs in greater or less amounts. If the infected patients evacuate the feces charged with the eggs on the open ground, the embryos under favorable conditions may develop into larvæ. If these get into the stomach and the intestine, they may in a short time develop to mature parasites, as the beautiful experiments carried out by Leichtenstern upon human beings prove. He studied more particularly the manner of infection in the brickyards near Cologne and Aachen, where mostly Italians and

Poles work. These, with their families, often had hook-worms in their intestines, and wherever they went the parasite was discovered in other individuals with whom they associated. If the infected laborers deposited their evacuations in the brickyards,—a frequent occurrence,—the clay of which the bricks were made was impregnated with the embryos of the parasites, especially after a rain. As the face and hands of the laborer are usually covered with a thick layer of clay, and since the hands are usually not washed before meals, or but superficially, the larvæ may easily get into the mouth and stomach, and develop further in the intestine. Indeed, Leichtenstern has repeatedly detected clay in the feces of the laborers. Besides, the contagion in the brickyards at Cologne, Aix-la-Chapelle, etc., was often caused by the drinking- or wash-water. This came through wooden pipes which were rendered tight by infected clay, not through impermeable iron pipes, so that eggs could readily get into the water. The water was still more contaminated if it flowed through earth mixed with feces containing eggs before it got into the water pipes.

It has been suggested that the larvæ may also get into the mouth and stomach through the air—an assumption which is based upon von Schopf's interesting experiments. This observer carried on his studies in mines where the miners, in spite of all precautions (washing the hands before meals, sterilizing drinking-water), often suffered from anchylostomiasis. He therefore inferred that the larvæ must in this case get into the mouth from the air. A proof of this assumption was sought in the discovery that numerous anchylostomes or larvæ were found in the intestines of a dog that had been tied at a place where the air forced out from a ventilating shaft passed by. They were also found in the water which was condensed from the aqueous vapor of the air on a glass plate. Dr. Chas. W. Stiles, zoologist to the United States Bureau of Animal Industry, is of the opinion, however, that this is far from proof. The chances for error here are too great. The observation on the dog is worthless until it is shown that all other sources of contamination were excluded and that the larvæ found in this animal were really those of *Uncinaria duodenalis*, for there are two other species that occur in the dog. Drying the embryo to a point that they can be carried by the wind is almost sure death to them.

In winter the cases of uncinariosis or anchylostomiasis in the brick-yards near Cologne, Aix-la-Chapelle, and other cities usually cease, since the eggs are killed by the cold. They usually recommence, however, in the spring and summer, when the Italians and Poles return, for these laborers usually work in mines in more southerly climates during winter.

Symptomatology.—The disease symptoms observed in uncinariosis (anchylostomiasis) may be divided into two groups. To the first belong digestive disturbances in the stomach and intestines, and complaints dependent on these organs. Usually these complaints appear soon after the first infection with the larvæ of the hook-worms. They may, however, continue during the entire duration of the disease, and even increase in intensity. To the second class belong the symptoms of a disease of the blood. In severe cases this appears as a pernicious progressive anemia. These symptoms usually appear a few weeks after the beginning of the disease, and may . reach considerable intensity two months after the infection. The symptoms are dependent not only on the number of parasites in the intestines,—since they may cause severe sickness even if present in only moderate numbers,—but also on the varying power of resistance of the patients and on the degree of the digestive disturbances caused by the parasites. If the number of the female parasites in the intestine is especially large, the anemia increases somewhat more rapidly, as the females suck more blood than the males. Uncinariosis or anchylostomiasis in Porto Rico is sometimes associated with malaria (the malarial parasite occurring in the blood) and dysentery. Charcot-Leyden crystals are a constant element in the evacuations.

Local Disturbances (Digestive Organs).—Disagreeable sensations of oppression and fullness in the gastric region, especially in the epigastrium, which may increase to pain, loss of appetite, sour eructation, nausea, and vomiting, are the first consequences of uncinariosis or anchylostomiasis. Meteorism and constipation often occur simultaneously. Diarrhea seldom occurs by itself, but often alternates with constipation. At this stage all symptoms of an anemia dependent upon uncinariosis or anchylostomiasis are wanting.

Symptoms of Anemia.—These are observed a few weeks after the infection. The color of the face and of the visible mucous membranes becomes pale, and especially the lips, the conjunctivæ, and the sclerotics show great pallor. To this are added a decrease of strength, loss of breath at least during bodily movement and exertion, when the patient easily gets into perspiration, experiences palpitation of the heart, flashes before the eyes, rumbling in the ears, fainting spells, chilly sensations, and weariness.

The pulse is at first soft, but quite strong ; later it becomes weak and rapid. In some cases fever sets in, especially during the evening. Besides a dilation of the right, or occasionally of the left, ventricle, systolic anemic noises at the heart and in the larger arteries are always to be detected. One can also hear strong pulsations over the carotid veins, and also bellowing murmurs over the jugular and crural veins. The voice is often hoarse. Auscultation and percussion give evidence that the condition of the lungs is either normal or a slight bronchial catarrh exists. Uncinariosis or anchylostomiasis may predispose to or hasten pulmonary tuberculosis. As the disease advances, the functional disturbances of the digestive organs increase. The appetite ceases entirely. Sometimes, however, intense hunger and abnormal desires toward entirely indigestible matters are manifested,—earth, clay, lime (geophagy, allotriophagy), —especially in patients in tropical countries, and among these more especially the children. Duprey (" Lancet," Oct. 27, 1900) believes that dirt eating is the cause, but in my experience it was also frequently a result, and did not exist before the pronounced anemia. The tongue is coated, the taste is pasty, sometimes there is a strong *fœtor ex ore*. Muco-serous masses are vomited fairly often, and these are said to occasionally contain hook-worms. In some patients the feeling of tension in the upper part of the abdomen and nausea never disappear entirely. Usually persistent constipation exists. In the later stage of the disease diarrhea often occurs. In two soldiers that had been to Porto Rico I observed typical dysentery, the evacuations containing very large numbers of the ova of uncinaria. If the evacuations are scanty, they are also colored dark brown or black. The large admixtures of blood, which are often observed in the tropics, are hardly ever noted in the United States and Europe. Microscopic examination, however, shows red blood-corpuscles in the evacuations fairly often. This can be explained by the habits of the parasite and the formidable cutting apparatus in its mouth. The evacuations are also rich in undigested food particles (muscle-fibers, starch particles), and in a thorough microscopic examination Charcot crystals are always found (Bäumler, Leichtenstern, Perroncito), just as in the case of the other intestinal parasites. Since these crystals are often contained in considerable numbers in the mucus of the evacuations, the mucous particles must be especially examined microscopically. If they are wanting, it is advisable to prescribe a moderate dose of calomel, so that the increased peristalsis may cause the mucus adhering to the mucous membrane to pass out. If Charcot-Leyden crystals are still found in the feces after the treatment for expelling the parasites, it is an indication that there are still parasites remaining in the intestines (Leichtenstern).

Although hook-worm eggs are usually found in the evacuations, the parasites themselves do not appear or are found only in isolated cases so long as no anthelmintic has been administered (Pistori-Parona). There are cases of typical uncinariosis or anchylostomiasis in which neither the parasite nor ova can be found in the stools for a long time. The reason for this negative result may be that very few parasites are present, and these firmly attached. Besides the ova of uncinaria, the eggs of oxyures, ascarides, and whipworms are often found in the feces simultaneously. If antiparasitic remedies are given, hook-worms and also specimens of *Strongyloides intestinalis*, oxyures, roundworms, and whipworms are found in the evacuations. The urine, which is usually plentiful, ordinarily contains much indican and sometimes also albumin in small amounts. Hemorrhages into the retina, which are sometimes observed in progressive pernicious anemia due to other causes, are usually lacking, but they do occur in rare cases of uncinariosis (Grassi).

Condition of the Blood.—This is of great practical importance, especially for diagnosis. The blood flowing from a needle puncture in the finger is very pale, serous, more rarely of a grayish-red color (Masius and Francotte). In severe cases the number of the red blood-corpuscles is very much reduced (according to Leichtenstern, to one-third; according to Stahl, to one-sixth). The hemoglobin of the blood is correspondingly diminished (according to Leichtenstern, to one-sixth of the normal blood). The number of the white blood-corpuscles was moderately increased (leukocytosis) in both of my cases (14,000 and 15,000); sometimes it is increased so much that the condition of the blood coincides with that of leukemic patients. Giles ("Brit. Med. Journ.," Sept. 1, 1900) reports that in Assam the leukocytes were decreased; he states that the hemoglobin was 11.5 per cent., the red corpuscles 1,145,000, the white corpuscles 5338. In the case reported by Allyn and Behrend (*l. c.*) the red blood-cells numbered 1,220,000 and the white blood-cells 8650 on the first count. Poikilocytes and microcytes are found in the blood some-what more rarely than in the case of progressive pernicious anemia. The eosinophilic cells, however, are always present in larger numbers (Leichtenstern). Besides these, gigantoblasts, nucleated red blood-corpuscles, and white blood-corpuscles containing fat particles (marrow cells) are found in the blood fairly often in the case of anchylostomiasis. The disease may cause death in a few weeks in especially acute cases if not treated; it usually lasts for many months and even years, even with good treatment. Since the life of the parasites in the intestines lasts at most eight years, the disease may heal of itself if a new infection is avoided. This self-limited ter-mination, however, occurs very rarely, especially in patients belong-ing to the lower classes. The disease oftener goes into the third stage, which is characterized by marasmus and severe complications. In this stage the patients grow weaker and weaker, so that finally they can no longer leave their beds. Edema, effusions into the serous cavities, albuminuria, nephritis, wasting of the muscles, and great dyspnea set in, accompanied by hemorrhages in the mucous membrane, the brain, the kidneys, and also by enlargement of the spleen and the liver. Sometimes the patients complain of pains in their bones, which are probably caused by changes in the marrow (as in the case of leukemia), and also of violent headache, hyper-esthesia, paresthesia, and rumbling noises in the ears. Delirium and muscular cramps may also appear, with increasing apathy and weakness, terminating in marasmus.

Pathological Anatomy.—The anatomical changes correspond almost entirely to those observed in progressive anemia. Besides the advanced anemia of all organs, one can detect a pronounced fatty degeneration in all the glandular organs, especially in the gland cells of the stomach, the intestines, the pancreas, and the liver. It may also be noted in the kidney and the heart-muscle.

Hemorrhages of the meninges, of the dura, of the medullary substance of the brain, and also changes in the marrow of the bones
like those occurring in medullary leukemia, have been found.   In a
few cases amyloid degenerations of the liver, the kidneys, the spleen,
the stomach, and the intestines have been observed (Leichtenstern).
The small intestine contains bloody mucus, and here and there
clotted blood.   Very often the intestinal mucosa is in a state of
intense enteritis.   At those places where the worms have attached
themselves, numerous ecchymoses and bloody infiltrations can
always be detected.   If the autopsy be made soon after death,
numerous live and moving parasites may be found in the intestine,
attached to the mucous membrane, while others that have become
detached from the mucous membrane are already dead.

Diagnosis.—The recognition of uncinariosis or anchylostomiasis
and its differentiation from a progressive pernicious anemia arising
from other causes, and also from cancerous cachexia, are facilitated
by the discovery of the eggs of the hook-worms and of Charcot-
Leyden crystals in the evacuations.   A thorough microscopic examination of the feces is therefore absolutely necessary in all cases
where there is any suspicion of these parasites.   The diagnosis is
made still more certain if the parasites themselves are found in the
evacuations, and it is therefore advisable to administer an aperient
and an anthelmintic, that their passage outward may be facilitated.
If the anamnesis shows that the patient has lived in a region in
which uncinariosis or anchylostomiasis occurs endemically, if he is
a brickmaker or miner, the detection of eggs alone constitutes a
positive diagnosis.   The presence of Charcot-Leyden crystals is, of
course, confirmatory.   If the evacuations still contain the above
crystals after the expulsion treatment, it means that some parasites
have remained in the intestines.   After several weeks have elapsed
during which no eggs or crystals have been found in the evacuations
we can assume a complete cure.

Prognosis.—Uncinariosis or anchylostomiasis is a severe and dangerous disease, which may, if let alone, cause death in a period of time
varying from a few weeks to several months.   Authentic reports of
spontaneous cures have not come to my notice.   The prognosis is
favorable if the expulsion be carried out in time.   Indeed, patients in
whom the anemia has already reached an advanced stage may rap-

idly recover if the parasites be expelled. If the removal of the parasite is incomplete, there is first an improvement, and then the anemia increases again, rendering a new expulsion treatment necessary. Even in those cases where the disease has entered the third stage, it may in some cases yet be cured if the treatment is rational and if no incurable complications have set in. If the latter is the case, the prognosis of course is unfavorable.

Therapeutics. — *Prophylaxis.* — Those persons suffering from uncinariosis or anchylostomiasis must be separated from healthy persons and those suffering from other diseases in order to prevent transference of the infection. The evacuations are to be either burned, disinfected, or covered with boiling water. Corrosive sublimate solution (1 : 1000) or carbolic acid or formaldehyd solutions are also effective. In the absence of these an abundance of chlorid of lime should be used, or the evacuations should be burnt, and the tools used in handling them (shovels) held in the fire. The owners of brickyards should be compelled to construct a sufficient number of tight privies, which should be frequently disinfected, and in the construction of which care should be taken to prevent contamination of the neighboring soil with the feces. The water must not be carried in wooden but in iron pipes. Pure drinking-water should also be provided in mines, and both brickmakers and miners should be admonished to wash and brush their hands thoroughly and to clean their finger-nails before eating.

Medicinal Treatment.—If one wishes to expel the hook-worms, experience shows that the ethereal extract of male-fern and thymol render equally good service. Extract of male-fern may be given in large doses, according to Perroncito (10 to 30 grains at a time), or in repeated smaller doses (2 to 4 grains daily on an empty stomach), according to Parona. (See the paragraph on treatment of tapeworms.) The evening before the patient takes two tablespoonfuls of castor oil, or a pint of the effervescent citrate of magnesia, and the next morning the anthelmintic remedy, either on an empty stomach or after drinking a small cup of black coffee. The patient is to take the drug in bed, on account of the nauseating and sometimes debilitating effect. The parasites are poisoned by the remedy, release their hold on the mucous membrane, and are carried out with the feces. According to the results of the examination of the evacuations, the administration of this remedy can be omitted or is to be repeated. At first usually the females pass off, and later on the males. If more males than females are found in the evacuations, it is a proof that the cure so far has been a success. After the administration of the extract of male-fern, other aperients are also to be prescribed to remove both the parasites and the remedy from the intestines. If the administration is repeated, we must not forget that it may cause intoxication phenomena, vertigo, double vision, and albuminuria. If no more eggs and Charcot-Leyden crystals can be discovered in the stools two or three weeks after the treatment, the cure is complete. If, on the contrary, new eggs are found, the treatment must be repeated.

Besides the extract of male-fern, Bozzolo and Graciolo also advise the use of thymol in daily increasing doses (2.0 to 10.0). In the use of this remedy great care is required; Mosler and Peiper caution against it and Leichtenstern observed a fatal collapse in a patient after the administration of 6 grams. The autopsy, however, showed a fatty degeneration of the heart (" Deutsch. med. Wochenschr.," 1887). Thymol is to be given in gelatin capsules, together with coffee or bouillon, and later on an aperient must be prescribed, *but alcohol in any form must be avoided.* It is a constant preparation, whilst extract of male-fern varies greatly in pharmaceutic efficacy. Thymol is decidedly the cheaper drug of the two. Failures to expel the anchylostoma occur under both remedies, but they are rare exceptions. Santonin and pomegranate have also been employed for this purpose, but they possess no special advantages.

The ova of the hook-worms are so characteristic that they can scarcely be confounded with those of other parasites. They might possibly be mistaken for oxyuris eggs, but these always contain embryos. The eggs of oxyuris on treatment with dilute acetic acid exhibit a separation of the external layer of the chorion, raising it from the inner layer like a blister. This does not occur with the eggs of uncinaria.

After the destruction of the parasites, good nourishment and iron preparations are to be prescribed if the anemia does not quickly improve. This is a most important part of the after-treatment. The form of iron must necessarily vary with the special indications and requirements in each case. The organic forms of iron do not, in my experience, accomplish better results than the Blaud pill or the ferric chlorid. The iron administered does not become absorbed into the blood; it benefits by protecting the iron in the nucleo-albumins of the food from becoming converted into sulphids (Hemmeter, "Phila. Med. Jour.," vol. v, p. 168; "Absorption of Iron from the Gastro-intestinal Tract," etc.). In very rare cases the gastric mucosa is so sensitive after an attack of uncinariosis or anchylostomiasis that these forms of iron may disagree. In those cases a trial should be made with ferratin if iron is indicated.

Strongyloides intestinalis.

Synonyms: *Anguillula intestinalis* Bavay, 1877; *Anguillula stercoralis* Bavay, 1877; *Rhabditis stercoralis* (Bavay, 1877); *Leptodera intestinalis* (Bavay) Cobbold, 1879; *Leptodera stercoralis* (Bavay) Cobbold, 1879; *Pseudorhabditis stercoralis* (Bavay) Perroncito, 1881; *Rhabdonema strongyloides* Leuckart, 1883; *Strongyloides intestinalis* (Bavay) Grassi, 1879; *Rhabdonema intestinale* (Bavay) R. Blanchard, 1885.

This parasite was first discovered in the evacuations of soldiers affected with the so-called Cochin-China diarrhea, by Normand, in 1876. Bavay studied the worm more carefully (1876) and described it under the name of *"Anguillula stercoralis"* asserting that it differed but little from a worm which occurred in the earth, and known as the *Rhabditis terricola* Dujardin, genus *Leptodera* Schneider. There can be no doubt from the scholarly description given by William Sydney Thayer ("Journ. of Experimental Med.," vol. VI, p. 75, "On the Occurrence of Strongyloides in the United States") that infection with this parasite occurs in this country. I refer to this article for a full description of the biology of this organism, and the clinical features manifesting themselves when it affects the human intestinal canal; also for a very full bibliography on this subject. Dr. Richard P. Strong, who is now Director of the United States Army Pathological Laboratory at Manila, has also given an excellent account of a case of infection with this worm, which is, however, embodied in the report by W. S. Thayer. (See Richard P. Strong, "Cases of Infection with *Strongyloides intestinalis*, First Recorded Occurrence in North America," "Johns Hopkins Hospital Reports," vol. x, 1901, p. 91; Strong has reported, further, cases and studies carried on in the Philippine Islands in "Circulars on Tropical Diseases," Chief Surgeon's Office, Manila, P. I., Feb., 1901.) These worms, when observed in the evacuations of patients, are extremely active, about 0.3 mm. long, and 0.022 wide. They

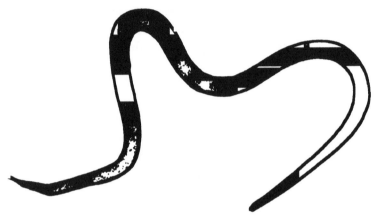

FIG. 28.—ADULT STRONGYLOIDES INTESTINALIS (PARASITIC FORM).—(*After Richard P. Strong, Johns Hopkins Hospital Reports*, vol. x, Plate II.)

are generally found intimately mixed with fecal matter, swimming forward and backward with eel-like motions. These are the larvæ which later on develop into sexually mature forms. In the larvæ the esophagus can be seen within the body of the worm; it is dilated at two places. The sexual apparatus, which is rudimentary in the larva, can be recognized as an oval, glistening body, on the anal

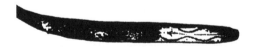

FIG. 29.—RHABDITIFORM EMBRYO OF ADULT FIG. 28. – (*After Richard P. Strong, Johns Hopkins Hospital Reports*, vol. x, Plate II.)

side, between the intestine and the body surface. Sexually mature forms are never found in the fresh or recent dejection. The esophagus, as already stated, shows two distinct expansions. In the expansion nearest to the intestine, three conical, chitinous teeth are recognizable, which are placed in the form of a Y. The intestinal canal proceeds from the esophagus, extends through the worm, and ends in a papilla situated on the right side of the animal, just above the base of the tail.

When fecal masses containing embryos of *Strongyloides intestinalis* are placed in an incubator, at 30° to 35° C., and allowed to remain there for thirty hours, the rhabditis embryos are developed into fully formed male and female rhabdites. · The transition into the sexually

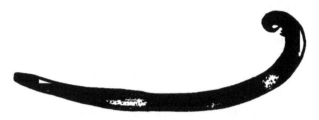

FIG. 30.—ADULT MALE OF FREE-LIVING GENERATION.—(*After Richard P. Strong, Johns Hopkins Hospital Reports*, vol. x, Plate II.)

mature forms occurs by a process of molting, which may start after twenty-four hours. The males may then grow to a length of 0.7 mm., and a thickness of 0.04 mm.; the females may grow to 1.2 mm. in length, and 0.075 mm. in thickness. The characteristic shape of the esophagus is now much more distinct than it was in the larvæ. The head end is rounded, and near the mouth

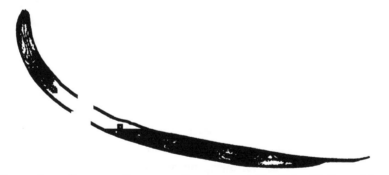

FIG. 31.—ADULT FEMALE OF FREE-LIVING GENERATION.—(*After Richard P. Strong, Johns Hopkins Hospital Reports*, vol. x, Plate II.)

orifice there are four ˙small cuticular openings, which are tactile papillæ. The larger female has a sharp and conical tail ending, but in the smaller male the tail ending is curved in and grows narrower more abruptly than in the female. The vulva of the female lies somewhat below the middle of the body, and in it terminate both uteri.   In close proximity to the anal opening, in the male, there are two thin spicules, representing the copulatory organ.   The spicules are slightly curved and cone-shaped.   The sexual opening in the female is situated about the middle of the body.   The uterus contains a number of eggs, some of which permit of recognition of the young embryo.   Soon after the development of the sexually mature stage fecundation takes place with the passage of the eggs into the uterus.   The eggs are ellipsoidal in form, 0.07 mm. long, and 0.045 mm. broad.   They are deposited at a stage of advanced segmentation; sometimes the escape of the embryos occurs in the uterus.   The embryos of the second generation are very similar to the former embryos, those of the first generation.   A further interesting metamorphosis occurs when these embryos of the second generation are transformed into worms, which represent the youthful strongyloides.

Then the esophagus loses its characteristic bulbous and club shape, and becomes a uniform cylindrical tube, extending to the middle of the body, beyond which it is not recognizable.   The tooth apparatus is lost, the tail end is converted into a slender process, gradually becoming smaller, ending not pointedly, but bluntly.   The sexual apparatus also disappears.   This transformation into the adult *Strongyloides intestinalis* occurs in about thirty to thirty-six hours.   On the fifth day of the culture the filaria-like larvæ of this phase are already present in large numbers, and after eight days they are present exclusively, for at that time the sexually mature rhabditiform types have perished.   The filaria-form larvæ of the adult strongyloid form do not undergo any further changes.   It seems that they are not equipped for any extensive free life, though by some investigators it has been suggested that such a life, of this phase of the parasite, may possibly occur in other hosts.

We have, then, the following phases of metamorphosis : (1) Adult parthenogenetic strongyloid forms produce the ova, either in the stage of segmentation or with embryo already forming within the uterus ; (2) the ova develop into rhabditiform embryos ; (3) sexual maturity by molting ; (4) conjugation and fecundation ; (5) embryos of the second generation ; (6) transformation into the large strongyloid form.   These larvæ undergo no further changes outside the body of the host.

The alternation of free and of parasitic generations, which was first studied by Leuckart, in a (frog) nematode known as *Ascaris nigrovenosa* (= *Rhabdonema nigrovenosum*), has been designated by this investigator as "*heterogonia*." Ercolavi designates it "*Dimorphobiosis*." If deductions are to be made from the studies of Leuckart with this parasite, we must look for the sexually mature condition of the filaria-form larvæ of *Strongyloides intestinalis* in the original host, the human being. According to Grassi, Segrè, and Leichtenstern, the rhabditiform larvæ are usually transformed directly into the filaria-form, and the sexually mature free-living intermediate generation ("Zwischengeneration") is the exception. It is not known whether these parasites are true hermaphrodites or whether they are parthenogenetic ("parthenogenesis" meaning the virginal reproduction, in which the whole development of the embryo is effected without the aid of fecundation). Leuckart believes that the worms are hermaphrodites, but Grassi and Calandruccio conceive the reproduction to be parthenogenetic.

Symptoms of the Infection of Human Intestinal Canal.— Grassi, Seifert, and Parona conclude from their observations that the presence of millions of these parasites in the human intestinal canal does not cause specific morbid symptoms. Leichtenstern ("Ueber Anguillula intestinalis," "Deutsch. med. Wochenschr.," 1898, xxiv, p. 118) has also observed large numbers of rhabditiform embryos of strongyloides in the stools of the same individuals for years. They were constantly present, and the persons infected appeared in normal condition. He concedes that the presence of such enormous numbers of these parasites may increase an already existing diarrhea, but believes that the diarrhea must be due to some other primary cause. This view was previously expressed by Calmette ("Archiv de Méd. Nav.," 1893, LX, pp. 207, 261, and 335). R. P. Strong (*l. c.*), from a microscopic study of sections from two fatal cases in Manila, and from observations made on five clinical cases, does not regard the parasite as harmless; but, on the other hand, he does not consider it particularly dangerous. He believes that it is capable of setting up an enteritis, expressing itself in an intermittent diarrhea. In the plates accompanying Dr. Strong's article ("Johns Hopkins Hospital Reports," vol. x) the embryos are shown beneath the epithelium of the villi, and in figure 7, of Plate III, the embryos are shown lying within the walls of the crypts of Lieberkühn; and in a note appended to the article Dr. Strong announces that monkeys have been successfully infected by feeding them the embryos of *Strongyloides intestinalis* through a stomach-tube. The animals suffered from diarrhea, and their stools contained large numbers of the ova of strongyloides, containing unhatched embryos.

In the feces of human beings infected with this worm Strong could find no ova, and Thayer could find only two eggs in the examination of a great many stools from his three cases. So much is evident: the diagnosis of this infection in the human being can practically not be made by the discovery of the eggs in the feces. We will have to look for rhabditiform embryos. Nor was Strong ever able to find the adult female strongyloid form in the feces. As the *Strongyloides intestinalis* frequently occurs simultaneously in the human intestinal canal with the *Uncinaria duodenalis*, a distinction between the two becomes necessary, and can be facilitated from the description of the *Uncinaria* already given. In severe infections with this latter parasite (uncinariosis) the eggs are always very numerous in the stools.

Treatment.—Strong asserts that the mild forms yield to the treatment of thymol in the same doses as recommended for the *Uncinaria duodenalis*. Thayer's cases were treated with bismuth subnitrate, rest in bed, and diet. Thymol was also given on several occasions in two doses of 30 grains taken with an hour's interval, and in one case fluid extract of male-fern, but neither eggs nor mother worms were found in the stools. The diarrhea, if present, should be treated like any other diarrhea of infectious origin (see vol. I, p. 352, "Entozoic Diarrhea"). Tannigen, bismuth subgallate, and opium may become necessary. Tonic treatment by strychnin, iron, and quinin, appears to be useful.

The conclusions of Dr. Richard P. Strong, and those of Dr. Wm. S. Thayer, with regard to the biology of the strongyloides, have been confirmed by Dr. Chas. Wardell Stiles, of the United States Bureau of Animal Industry, Department of Agriculture. Literature concerning this parasite will be found in the report by Dr. W. S. Thayer (*l. c.*), which embodies the first three cases that have been observed in this country.

It is not considered necessary to append the literature on intestinal parasites. It is very satisfactorily compiled in the "Index-Catalogue of the Surgeon General's Library" and "Bibliography of Medical and Veterinary Zoology," by Stiles and Hassall, now being published by the United States Bureau of Animal Industry, and in the treatise on "Animal Parasites" by Mosler and Peiper, in Nothnagel's "Spec. Path. u. Ther.," Bd. vi; also in J. Ch. Huber's comprehensive work, "Bibliographie der klinischen Helminthologie," and various publications of Leichtenstern, especially in volume iv of Penzoldt and Stintzing's "Handbuch d. speciellen Therapie innerer Krankheiten."

CHAPTER XII.

DISEASES OF THE RECTUM.

By Thos. Chas. Martin, Ph.D., M.D.,

Professor of Proctology in the Cleveland College of Physicians and Surgeons; Proctologist to
the Cleveland General Hospital; President of the American
Proctologic Society, etc.

The pathology and etiology of rectal diseases are essentially the same as those of the abnormalities as they occur in other parts of the intestine. The reader is referred to previous chapters (vol. 1) for questions of physiological or pathological interest; accordingly, this chapter will be devoted more especially to diagnosis and treatment of rectal diseases.

Examination of the Rectum.

Elevation of the patient's hips is an essential to the proper examination of the rectum. Without instruments the physician who has acquired some degree of skill in the use of his fingers may achieve a complete ocular inspection of the rectum by the following method: The patient should be anesthetized as he lies on his back. When the anesthesia is complete he should be turned to the Sims posture; his left arm, however, should be drawn forward beneath him and across his chest. His thighs should be drawn toward his chin until they are at an angle of about 95° with his trunk. The physician should now lean himself against the patient's knees, pass his right arm under the patient's hips, and lift the trunk toward him. At the same time, with his left hand clasping the patient's right foot, the physician should steady the patient's right thigh. The patient now resting on his left shoulder and knees may be easily supported by the assistant who at the same time manages the anesthetic. The physician should now point his index-fingers as shown in figures 32 and 33, and after well lubricating them bury them in the anus to the depth of his knuckles. Now he should forcibly separate his fingers in the direction of the ischial tuberosities. This manipulation opens the anus and permits an inrush of air to the rectum, which inflates this organ to such a degree that the mucosa may be seen smoothly lining the rectum to the depth of 6 to 8 inches (15.24 to 20.32 cm.) if the rectal valves do not obstruct the view. The transverse diameter may be from 2 to 4 inches (5.08 to 10.16 cm.). Under certain conditions the rectum will not inflate. The absence of in-

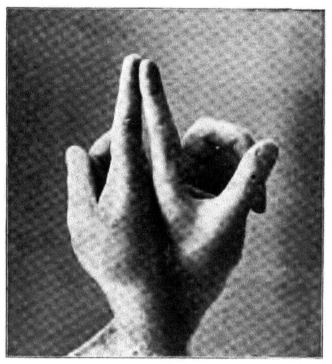

FIG. 32.—THE POSITION OF THE HANDS FOR NONINSTRUMENTAL PROCTOSCOPY.

flation instead of being regarded as evidence of the inutility of this method of examination, should be regarded as a sign of one or the other of the following several conditions: namely, acute rectitis with edema; far-advanced hypertrophic rectitis; a close tubular stricture of rectum; malignant growth or extrarectal and intrapelvic disease which limits the expansion of the rectum; invagination of the sigmoid into the rectum or the rectum into itself; gaseous distention of a part of the bowel above the rectum; accumulations of intra-abdominal fat; peristalsis or spasm of the circular muscular fibers of the rectum; or it may be the result of the patient's voluntary resistance. All of which may be easily differentiated by a method which presently will be described. If this method of examination is practised by the physician, he will be able to discover at a glance most of the diseases to which this organ is subject; it

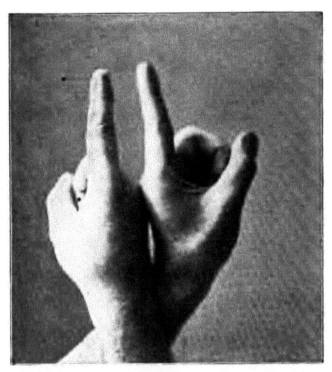

FIG. 33.—THE POSITION OF THE FINGERS AFTER THEIR INTRODUCTION INTO THE ANUS.
Figures 32 and 33 have been previously used in the " Journal of the American Medical Association " and in the " Philadelphia Medical Journal."

does not, however, permit him to accomplish more than the diagnosis of the disease.

Certain instruments and appliances are required for a perfect and painless inspection of the rectum. The chair and the instruments which I have designed for this examination are shown in the illustrations, figures 34, 35, 36, and 37. The following method of examination requires neither local nor general anesthesia, for the reason that it is painless and, as the rectum is normally empty, neither physics nor enemata are required for the patient's preparation. Such measures may be useful in the preparation of the patient for local treatment after diagnosis is made, but if they be not employed the condition in which one then finds the rectum may have an obvious diagnostic significance; for example, the presence and location of pus or blood in the rectum may signify the location of the lesion

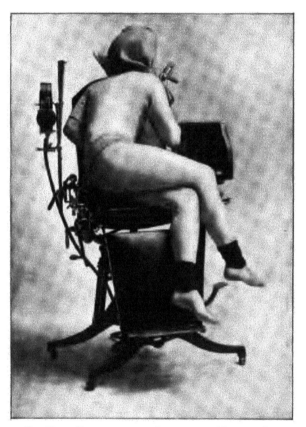

FIG. 34.—THE FIRST POSITION OF THE PATIENT FOR MARTIN'S PROCTOSCOPY.

in which they have their origin. The presence of feces in the case of obstipation may help to determine the location of the obstructing rectal valve.

The patient should be required to sit on the operating chair with his right knee crossed over his left. His knees should be lifted to touch the knee-piece which is attached to the left arm of the chair.

The patient's left arm should be folded at his side and his elbow drawn a little behind him and his right arm folded across his chest in such a way that his hand shall rest upon the small pillow beneath

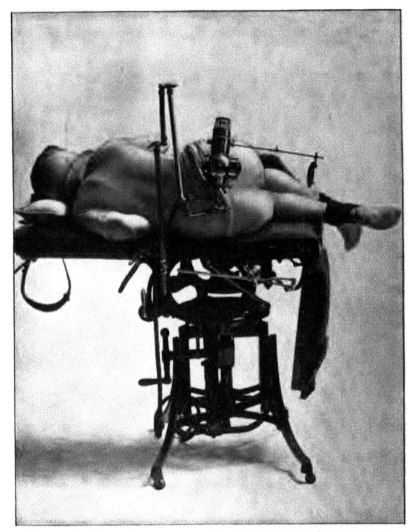

FIG. 35.—THE SECOND POSITION OF THE PATIENT, ILLUMINATION APPARATUS, ETC.

his left cheek (Fig. 34). The physician should now carry the back of the chair from the upright to the horizontal position. It may then be observed that the patient lies comfortably in the Sims posture. The illumination apparatus should now be carried forward as shown in figure 35. After a careful ocular inspection has been made of the ischiorectal region and anal verge, these parts should

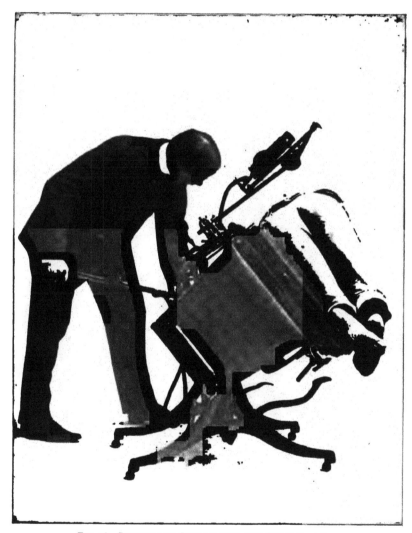

FIG. 36.—PUTTING THE PATIENT INTO THE THIRD POSITION.

be subjected to a careful palpation and then the interior of the fixed or anal rectum should be examined with the finger. Before the physician proceeds to a specular examination he should palpate the pelvic floor between the inserted finger and that of the free hand.

The introduction of an instrument into the rectum may be much

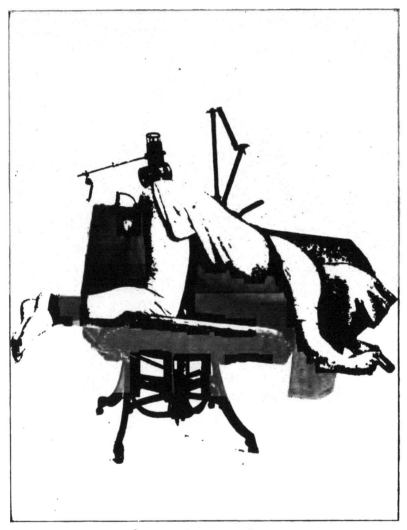

FIG. 37.—MARTIN'S POSTURE FOR PROCTOSCOPY.
Figures 34, 35, 36, and 37 have been previously used in the "American Gynæcological and Obstetrical Journal" and in the "Philadelphia Medical Journal."

facilitated by thoroughly lubricating it and placing its end .against the external sphincter and requiring the patient to bear down.

Bearing down depresses and thins the pelvic floor, relaxes the levator ani, expands the external sphincter, and presses the relaxing internal sphincter over and upon the proctoscope (Fig. 38). A tight or spasmodically contracted sphincter may thus be entered without difficulty and without provoking pain. The obturator (Fig. 39) should now be withdrawn and the inspection of the anus made. This inspection should be made coincident with a very slow withdrawal of the anoscope, as suggested by H. A. Kelly.

The examination of the movable inflatable rectum, which is the portion that is above the pelvic floor, requires that the patient shall be turned into a posture which is equivalent to the knee-chest posture.

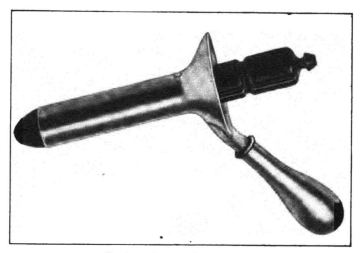

FIG. 38.—MARTIN'S PROCTOSCOPE.

This is achieved by placing upon the patient's right shoulder a suspender which is attached to the chair and by tilting the chair to Martin's posture, which is shown in figure 37. The foot-board of the chair should now be lowered to afford an easier access to the patient. The protoscope should be introduced by the manœuver previously described till its end shall have passed the levator ani muscle, at which time its point must be directed backward and upward into the hollow of the sacrum. The withdrawal of the obturator is followed by spontaneous inflation of the rectum. The physician should now observe the degree of rectal distention, the color of the mucosa, the situation and number of the rectal valves, their propinquity to one another when passive, and the degree of resistance to the test-hook (Fig. 40). He should also observe the character of the contents of the rectum, if there be any. The rectum may present to the eye of an imaginative observer the appearance of a chain of urinary bladders, communicating one with another by means of irregular elliptical openings set at varying axes, and bounded by the nonparallel borders of the rectal valves. In the normal rectum the air pressure smooths the mucous membrane evenly over the entire surface of the gut, as may be observed in the photographic illustrations. The normal mucous membrane of the rectum appears at first wet and of a shining pinkish-gray. When the examination is completed the proctoscope should be withdrawn, the gas-fixture secured in its original position, the chair's lever extended, then manipulated to carry the chair back to the horizontal, and then the chair-back should be lifted to the upright position. In this manner the patient is carried from a sitting posture to one equivalent to the knee-chest pos-

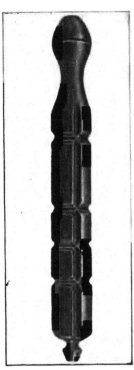

FIG. 39.—THE OBTURATOR FOR ANOSCOPES AND PROCTOSCOPES.

FIG. 40.—MARTIN'S TEST-HOOK.

ture, and painlessly a complete inspection is made of the anus and rectum, and the patient carried back to the sitting attitude.

RECTITIS OR PROCTITIS.

The several **varieties** of inflammation of the rectum are the catarrhal, dysenteric, gonorrheal, syphilitic, and diphtheritic. The first may be acute or chronic, but more often is seen in the chronic variety. Dysenteric inflammation of the rectum has, of course, the same pathology as that which affects the higher portions of the intestine, and is discussed more fully in volume I, pages 515 to 591.

The more common **causes** of inflammation of the rectum are trauma, infection, and impaired circulation of the rectum due to the presence of disease of other organs. Residual hardened feces may under the efforts of defecation be driven so forcibly against the rectal mucosa as to abrade the surface; the presence of foreign bodies which may have descended with the feces from above or may have been introduced through the anus may likewise injure the rectum and initiate an infection which may be followed by local or general proctitis. The presence of a pelvic tumor or the existence of a low grade of peritonitis or any disease of any contiguous organ or tissue which obstructs the circulation of the rectum may cause a chronic rectitis or may be the source of an acute infection of the rectum. So, also, may a rectitis have its origin in a disease at the anus. In the chapter on Sigmoiditis, Professor Hemmeter has described a form of dysentery in which the original infection takes place at the anus, and spreads thence to the rectum and sigmoid (see vol. I, p. 509). Among the commoner causes of proctica or rectitis are displacements of the uterus or adnexa in women, hypertrophied prostate in men, enteroptosis, pelvic abscess, ischiorectal abscess, hemorrhoids, fissure, fistula, prolapse of the rectum; the presence of a tumor at the anus or in the rectum; and neglect or inability to properly empty the rectum of feces. Rectitis rarely follows operation upon the rectum or anus in spite of the fact that it is of all fields the most exposed to the sources of infection. Gonorrheal rectitis is a rare infection, and is even rarer in men than in women for the obvious reasons that in women the usual seat of gonorrhea is in closer communication with the rectum. I have seen one case of gonorrheal rectitis acquired by the patient's using for enemata a syringe previously used by a subject of gonorrheal vaginitis. In all, I have seen but five cases of gonorrheal rectitis in which the diagnosis was confirmed by the discovery of the gonococci, and though the disease was encountered in both the acute and chronic forms, it yielded readily to the treatment presently to be described. Syphilitic rectitis develops insidiously, is of the interstitial variety, and is rarely an independent manifestation of the infection. Exposure to cold is a more frequent initial factor to rectitis. Any circumstance or condition which may drive the blood from the surface or from the extremities to the abdominal viscera may be responsible for an inflammation of the rectum. The abuse of purgatives, with the exception, perhaps, of the salines, is the most common of all causes of rectitis.

Rectitis of the simple exudative form usually runs a short course and is not fatal. The epithelial and connective-tissue tunics of the rectum are more or less congested and edematous, and there is more or less infiltration of lymph into the structure of the rectum. An excess of mucus is secreted which may be deposited in the chambers of the rectum in gelatinous masses or may be discharged in such form with the feces. In mild cases there is usually no bleeding from the rectum. In more violent states of inflammation the wall is very much congested, and edematous to a degree which interferes with inflation on proctoscopy. Not only are the glandular and connective-tissue coats of the bowel infiltrated with serum and pus cells, but the muscular and peritoneal coats of the rectum and the contiguous perirectal structures may also be involved. There is an excessive production of pus cells, and areas of necrosis of the mucosa may appear. There is mucopurulent and sanguineous discharge from the rectum. This form of rectitis, if not checked early, is sometimes fatal. On the other hand, the process may be arrested at any stage in its development and the disease become proliferating as well as exudative, and then a chronic hypertrophic rectitis ensues.

The symptoms of rectitis vary with the degree of the lesion and are dependent in their severity upon the extent and intensity of the inflammatory changes. When the rectum alone is involved in the inflammation they are not as severe as when the anal mucosa is simultaneously affected. Rectitis is usually initiated with the symptoms of sacral and lumbar backache, and the sensation of heat and weight in the sacral region, which sensation extends down the thighs in the course of the great sciatic nerve. In the initial stage of the affection there is usually an inordinate desire for defecation, and attempts accomplish only the dejection of mucus, perhaps, also, of a little blood and pus. Obstipation rather than diarrhea characterizes the first few days of the affection. Defecation is not painful excepting when the anal mucosa is involved in the inflammation; if it be, there will follow considerable tenesmus on each attempt at defecation. About the third or fourth day, provided the attack be not of the most mild character, there will follow a short period of diarrhea. Rectitis of the hypertrophic type is essentially of a chronic form and is almost never attended by symptoms of great pain and distress in the beginning. It is of a recurrent character, lasts for a few days, is accompanied by obstipation, and followed by a day or two of mild diarrhea. The condition is alternately exacerbated and ameliorated, until finally the former state attains the ascendency and there is a chronic hypertrophic rectitis and hypertrophy of the rectal valve; succeeding which there follows a greater hypertrophy of the lower rectum and a dilation, thinning, and perhaps atony of the rectum and colon above the most obstructed point. The colon may be thickened. The defecations are attended with great straining, and enemata may bring from the bowel membranous, cord-like, or cast-like deposits of mucus. The symptoms of this more chronic form are now the symptoms of the complications following upon the original rectitis—namely, tenderness and more or less continuous soreness in the region of the sigmoid flexure and colon and gaseous distention of these portions of the bowel. As the gas accumulates the pain increases and becomes colicky in character. There will be occasional onward movements of the gas, and almost immediately following upon such advance of the gas it will be easily discharged from the rectum. Any of the various manifestations of intestinal autointoxication may attend this period of the disease.

The **treatment** of acute rectitis or the severe form of chronic rectitis consists in keeping the patient in bed in the lateral posture with the hips slightly elevated. In the early stages of acute rectitis a bag filled with cold water should be fastened over the sacrum. Hot water is more helpful in the chronic form of the disease.

The patient should be required to take hot sitz-baths twice a day; the diet should consist of eggs, meat, and meat broths. Contrary to the general belief, local treatment need not inflict pain if the proper technic be employed in its administration. The treatment consists in irrigation and in the application of atomized solutions. The best means for irrigation of the rectum is that devised by Dr. Herschell, of London. It consists of a cylindrical tube or proctoscope to the proximal end of which is attached a large-sized rubber hose of sufficient length to reach to a receptacle beneath the patient's bed. A vertical slit occupies the attached end of the hose at a point near the metal tube. Into this slit is inserted

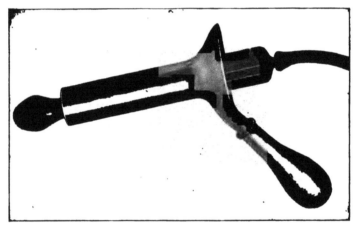

FIG. 41.—A TWO-WAY IRRIGATOR.

an ordinary stomach-tube. The hose fits closely about the stomach-tube and yet not snugly enough to compress the latter. The proximal end of the stomach-tube is connected with the hose of a fountain syringe. This device permits of a ready introduction of the fluid into the rectum and of its more ready escape from the bowel through the metal tube and hose; it also permits of the easy washing away of such fecal matter as may be in the rectum or sigmoid flexure. My own proctoscope and obturator (Fig. 41) also provides a two-way irrigator for the rectum, but is not so serviceable as the device of Dr. Herschell, for the reason that it does not permit of the escape of the fecal matter. The most useful irrigating solutions are bicarbonate of sodium, boric acid, and normal salt solution. After the bowel has been thoroughly irrigated and the solution has been completely evacuated the patient should be put into the knee-chest posture or the Martin posture, and the rectum sprayed with a silver nitrate solution. If the patient be treated in the diarrhea stage, a solution of 5 or 10 grains of nitrate of silver to the ounce of water will be required. If there be obstipation or constipation, a weaker solution should be employed.

HYPERTROPHIC RECTITIS AND STRICTURE OF THE RECTUM.

Often an acute rectitis is followed by the organization of the exudate and consequent thickening of all the coats of the rectum. A slow progressing chronic rectitis may have developed from the acute form, the acute state having been so mild in character as to have escaped the notice of the patient. In either case there results an increase of the fibrous elements. This condition obstructs defecation to such a degree that it robs the rectum of its elasticity or contracts and fixes the rectum (*proctic cirrhosis*). Stricture of the rectum, therefore, in this case is a localized hypertrophic rectitis.

The **causes** of stricture are the same as those of rectitis. However, there are certain exceptions to this statement; these will be discussed in the chapter on Tumors, and have already been considered in chapter xxi, volume i.

The **symptoms** of hypertrophic rectitis are straining at stool for the passage of solid or semisolid feces and the inability to pass other than semisolid or liquid feces. For a long time the patient will have no other symptoms than those of infrequent or difficult defecation. Concerning the various sizes, forms, and shapes of the feces in this condition, I refer to the chapter on Examination of the Feces (vol. i, p. 229), and also that on Enterostenosis. Gradually the difficulties of defecation increase, until finally cathartics and enemata fail to secure the desired result. Before this stage is reached certain complications will have developed. The first of these will be dilation and hyperemia of the colon and sigmoid flexure; in some cases there will be a marked thinning of the bowel, while in others there will be a hypertrophy of the wall. (See Intestinal Obstructions.) To the symptoms previously mentioned there will be added tenderness, a sense of heat, and occasionally pain in the sigmoid flexure, and finally throughout the course of the colon. Flatus will be more or less constant. There · will be discharges of mucus and perhaps of small quantities of pus from the bowel. Membranous shreds or casts consisting of mucus, epithelium, and pus cells may be detected, and the symptoms of intestinal autointoxication may be present in varying degree. The commonest of these are depression of spirits and insomnia. Occasionally the patient may experience for a short period an inexplicable elation, and occasionally, too, instead of insomnia he may experience an uncontrollable drowsiness. He may also grow wholly altered in nature and become insufferably irritable and incapable of concentrating his faculties upon any business in hand. ·

In the chronic form of rectitis the glands of the mucosa gradually become changed in form and there is a tendency for the epithelial cells to lose their columnar shape and become more or less stratified. The muscularis mucosæ becomes fibrous. The muscular tissue will degenerate to fibrous tissue, and there will be a very considerable increase of fibrous tissue in the part of the rectum most involved in the process. An acute rectitis may rapidly build an obstruction in the rectum if it be accompanied by a very considerable infiltration of lymph into the structures of the organ, which, organizing, fixes a portion of the bowel in a state of contraction.

Physiology and Pathology of the Rectal Valves.—The perfect comprehension of hypertrophic rectitis and stricture of the rectum requires a study of the rectal valves, and forces upon the reader a positive conclusion to the moot question of their existence. Mathews, Kelsey, and other recognized authorities deny recognition to these valves, but I hold them to be the key to our knowledge of obstruction of the rectum.* The accompanying illustrations are offered as documentary evidence of the positive existence of the rectal valve (Figs. 42 and 43). The specimens from which the photographs were taken were prepared by a method consisting in fixing the cadaver in the knee-chest posture and pouring melted

---

* For the historic literature on this subject and the protocols of my own anatomical researches the reader is referred to "Obstipation, a Practical Monograph on the Disorders and Diseases of the Rectal Valve," the Philadelphia Medical Publishing Company.

PLATE 12.

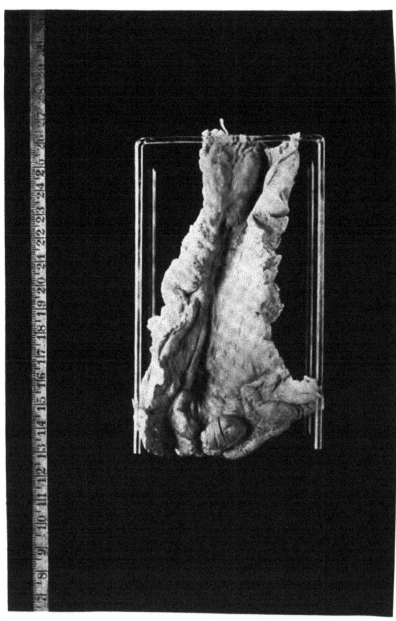

CHRONIC HYPERPLASTIC RECTITIS AND STRICTURE OF THE RECTUM OF LUETIC ORIGIN. A GUMMA HAS TAKEN THE PLACE OF THE ANAL PILASTER.—(*From Professor Hemmeter's Clinic.*)

paraffin into the atmospherically inflated rectum; when the wax had sufficiently hardened the gut was carefully removed, for a few weeks immersed in alcohol, and subsequently dried, varnished, and finally dried and cut into longitudinal, shell-like halves. A comparative study of rectal interiors reveals the fact that the prominence of the rectal valve is increased with the degree of distention of the rectum. The attached border of each valve spans a little more than half the circumference of the rectum, and its free border projects nearly half-way across the diameter of the inflated rectum. Each valvular partition projects at nearly a right angle to the wall

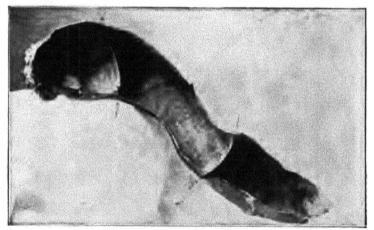

FIG. 42.—INTERIOR VIEW OF THE LEFT HALF OF THE RECTUM OF AN ADULT, PREVIOUSLY FILLED WITH MELTED PARAFFIN.

The subject in the Martin posture. The rectum is distended only to the degree of normal atmospheric inflation. The anus is at the picture's left. The valves are respectively 2½ and 7 inches from the anus.

of the compartment below it and terminates in a sharply defined free border. The free margin of the valve is slightly concave in form and is directed a little obliquely. The number of rectal valves is variable. Some subjects have but two, others have four or more, but 90 per cent. of persons possess three.

The function of the valve is to beneficently retard the descent of the feces.

The degree of obstruction which the valve affords is determined by the depth of the valve from its attached to its free border, by the proportion of fibrous tissue in it and by its propinquity to an adjacent valve.   Figure 44 shows a longitudinal vertical section of a normal rectum.

Hypertrophy of the Rectal Valve.—Hypertrophy of the rectal

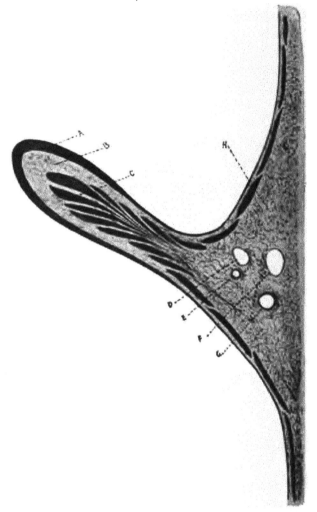

FIG. 43.—A RECTAL VALVE DRAWN AS SEEN UNDER THE MICROSCOPE.
A, Mucous membrane; B, fibrous tissue; C, bundles of circular muscular fibers; D, vein; E, artery; F, vein; G, artery; H, areolar and adipose tissue.

valve constitutes the annular or semilunar stricture of the rectum. Hypertrophy of two valves, or an excessive deposit of fibrous tissue in two or more valves, contraction of the chamber walls between the valves and their fixation constitute what is called tubular stricture of the rectum, and the fact that the valves are the foundation on which strictures are built, and that the valves are situated upon the alternate sides of the rectum, explains the well-known tortuous course of the tubular stricture.

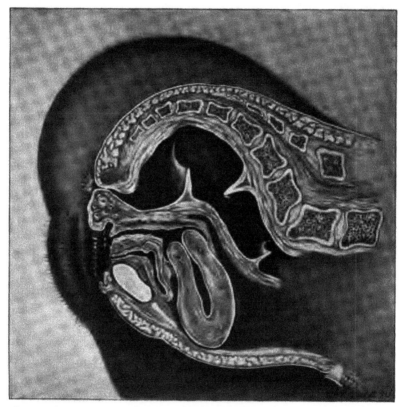

FIG. 44.—A LONGITUDINAL VERTICAL SECTION SHOWING THE POSITION OF THE PELVIC ORGANS IN MARTIN'S POSTURE.
The rectosigmoidal valve-strait is here shown somewhat more contracted than normal.

The **diagnosis** is accomplished by putting the patient into the proper posture for proctoscopy and by the introduction of the proctoscope. The number of valves, the height and thickness of each, and the distance between them, should be determined. If the obstruction be congenital in origin, the valves will not appear thicker than normal, but their free edges will be seen to overlap in such a way that under the pressure of the descending feces the two valves unite to form a temporary diaphragm which prevents the onward progress of the feces.   Each of the valves should now be subjected to the pressure of the test-hook (Figs. 45 and 46).   If any of them be hypertrophic and obstructive, the hook will be lifted and will

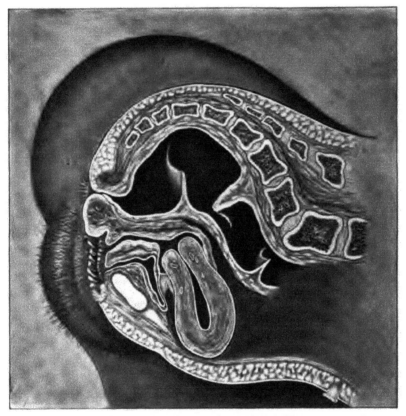

FIG. 45.—A LONGITUDINAL VERTICAL SECTION SHOWING THE POSITION OF THE PELVIC ORGANS IN MARTIN'S POSTURE.
The rectosigmoidal valve-strait is here shown somewhat more contracted than normal. The posterior rectal valve is shown much hypertrophied.

slide over the free margin of the valve without effacing the valve. On the contrary, if the valve be normal, it will be sufficiently elastic to be effaced temporarily without lifting the hook away from the rectal wall.

The **treatment** of hypertrophy of the rectal valves in a case where the obstipation has been recurrent in character and not continuous consists in massage of the valves by means of a rectal sound or a strong forceps guarded with cotton. By means of the proctoscope the massage may be applied with the field directly under the command of the eye of the operator. In addition to the massage, which should be applied daily or weekly, according to the

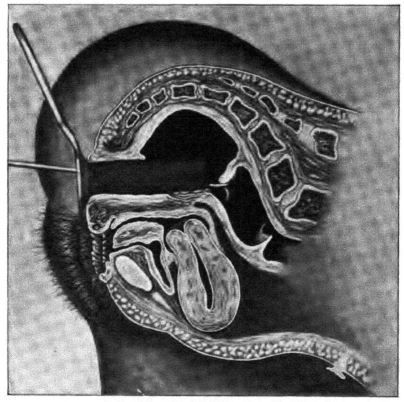

FIG. 46.—SHOWS THE METHOD OF USING THE TEST-HOOK; AN OBSTRUCTING VALVE CAN NOT BE EFFACED UNDER ITS PRESSURE.
The lowest anterior normal rectal valve is shown somewhat effaced under the pressure of the proctoscope.

gravity of the condition, occasionally the rectum should be sprayed with a 0.1 per cent. solution of nitrate of silver. Saline enemata 108° to 130° F. should be employed daily by the patient. After a lapse of a period of about six weeks all treatment should be discontinued and the patient kept under observation that it may be learned how much has been accomplished toward a cure.

Operative Severance of the Rectal Valve.—In cases of congenital propinquity or anatomical coarctation of the valves and of marked hypertrophy, the radical operation of division of the valve is demanded. The technic consists in first measuring off the depth from free to attached border of the valve to be operated, by means of the curved hook. The curved hook (Fig. 47), being bent to three-fourths of a circle, will place its point at least ¼ inch (0.63 cm.) from the wall of the chamber immediately above the valve to which it is applied. The blanched eminence which presents to the eye over the point of the hook as it is drawn toward the operator will indicate the depth to which the valve may be safely cut. The surgically safe part of the valve may also be determined by carrying the end of the proctoscope over the valve's free margin and depressing it till the edge rests on the

FIG. 47.—MARTIN'S CURVED TEST-HOOK.

chamber-wall above and adjacent to the base of the valve. The proctoscope should now be cautiously drawn toward the operator while he carefully maintains it in the same axis, and at the instant it is drawn below the valve this organ will jump across his field of vision. The edge of the proctoscope will point directly to the upper attached margin of the valve. The free border of the valve should now be seized by two tenacula, which should be manipulated in such a way as to draw the margin of the valve taut and an incision made between the two by means of the scalpel (Figs. 48 and 49). The incision should be made by repeated gentle sweeps of the scalpel. If an artery be cut, it should be seized at once by means of the clamp. The use of the scalpel should be interrupted frequently and the bent test-hook applied to determine when the valve's resistance has been overcome. In some rare cases the fibrous tissue in the valve affords such resistance that the scalpel will not sever its fibers. Such cases require tact and experience. The operator should proceed to transfix the *most superficial* portion of the valve by means of the bistoury, and this instrument should then be carried from its position and through the free border of the valve. The wound now being started, the scalpel should be substituted for the bistoury and the incision completed. When the knife has reached the circular muscular fibers, there will suddenly appear a depression at the deep angle of the wound. The wound should not be further deepened. The circular and longitudinal muscular and peritoneal coats of the rectum remain thus uncut. Should the obstruction not yet have been overcome, another incision should be made in some other portion of the valve. Now

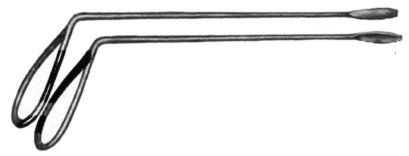

FIG. 48.—MARTIN'S OVER- AND UNDER-VALVOTOMY SCALPELS.
But one knife is necessary if it be provided with a reversible handle.

the wound should be sutured. If an artery should have been cut, the bleeding may be controlled by the clamp. The first suture should be placed in such a position as to effectually prevent the recurrence of the hemorrhage. The first suture for the purpose of coaptating the mucous surfaces of the valve should be placed in the deep angle of the wound. From three to five sutures may be required. The rectum should be tamponed as a preventive measure against secondary hemorrhage. The pledgets should consist of cotton wool, powdered persulphate of iron in limited quantity, and gauze strands. The rectal chamber above the valve operated should be packed tightly, as should also all that portion of the rectum below. Thus, in addition to the sutures, the patient is fortified against secondary hemorrhage by the presence of both mechanical

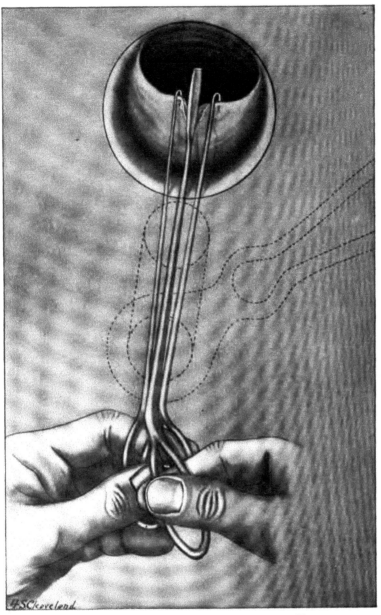

FIG. 49.—ILLUSTRATES THE METHOD OF CUTTING THE VALVE.

and chemical styptics. Should a secondary hemorrhage occur in spite of these precautions, the gauze drains protruding from the anus serve as a diagnostic measure. In the case of hemorrhage the packing should be removed at once and the rectum repacked with a greater quantity of tampons. As the rectum is as insensitive to pain as is the nail's end, neither general nor local anesthesia is required for valvotomy. However, it is wise to administer, hypodermically, a small dose of morphin half an hour prior to the

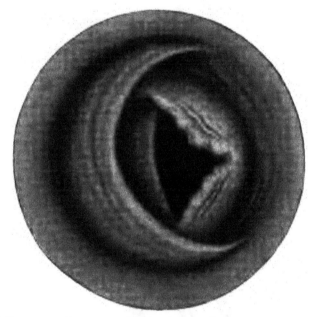

FIG. 50.—A TRANSVERSE VIEW OF THE RECTUM SHOWING TWO NORMAL RECTAL VALVES ON THE LEFT AND THE HEALED OPERATED VALVE ON THE RIGHT.

operation. During the twenty-four hours succeeding the operation it is well to keep the patient under the influence of morphin, that an undue peristalsis may not be provoked by the presence of the tampons. At the expiration of this time the packing should be removed. At the end of forty-eight hours the rectum should be irrigated, and daily thereafter for a fortnight or until the wounds have healed and the congestion subsided. At the expiration of this period the patient should be provided with a liberal diet, from which I prefer to exclude starchy foods. If the diagnosis is correct, the

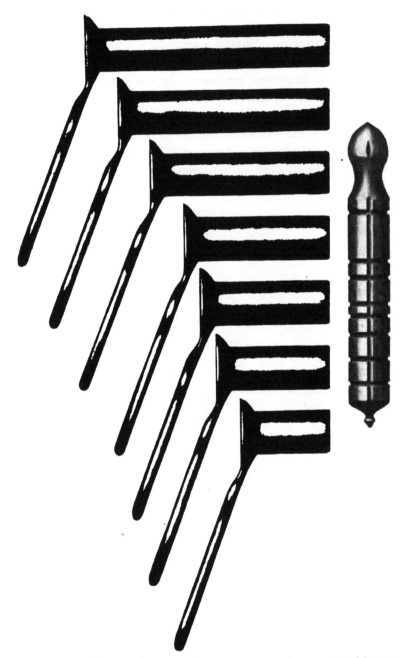

FIG. 51.—A SET OF MARTIN'S GRADUATED PROCTOSCOPES; THE SMALLEST IS 1¼ INCHES IN DIAMETER AND 2 INCHES IN LENGTH.

operation thorough, and there does not exist any obstructing complication, normal defecation will be established (Fig. 50).

Hypertrophic rectitis in that degree which constitutes a tubular stricture of the rectum requires frequent massage by the methods previously described until the chamber walls have become sufficiently elastic to permit that inflation on proctoscopy which renders

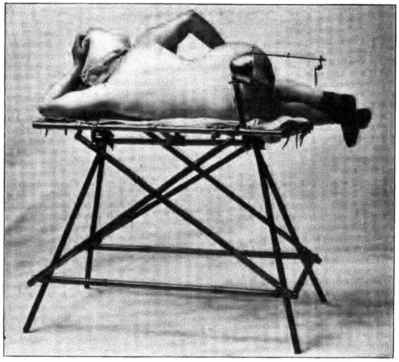

FIG. 52.—THE PATIENT IN SIMS' POSTURE WITH MARTIN'S TABLE AND ILLUMINATION APPARATUS ADJUSTED FOR EXAMINATION AND OPERATION UPON THE ANUS.

the valves accessible for valvotomy. It may require months to achieve this step.

Colostomy and resection of the rectum are unwarranted and outrageous for this condition except when the patient be the subject of complete obstruction. A complete obstruction in such an instance may be due to an invagination of the bowel from above, which, becoming edematous in the grasp of the stricture, may render the case *apparently* hopeless without colostomy. I have relieved such patients by putting them into the proctoscopic posture and making the rectum ischemic by the application of 4 per cent. solution of cocain and massaging the part with cotton-guarded forceps till the invagination reduce itself. However, an invagination should never be permitted to exist longer than twenty-four or twenty-six hours lest adhesion of its peritoneal surfaces render it irreducible. Therefore, internal reduction proving impossible, an attempt should be

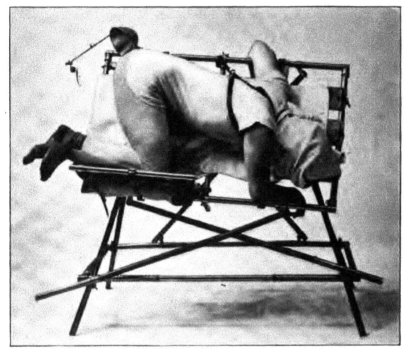

FIG. 53.—THE PATIENT IN MARTIN'S POSTURE WITH TABLE AND ILLUMINATION APPARATUS ADJUSTED FOR EXAMINATION AND OPERATION WITHIN THE RECTUM. THE PASSIVE PATIENT IS SUPPORTED BY THE SHOULDER-SUSPENDER AND KNEE-PIECE.

made through the abdominal route at reduction of the intussusception before colostomy is resorted to. In advanced cases, abdominal or sacral approach and resection of tubular and invaginated obstructions may be necessary, and a temporary colostomy may be the best preliminary step to this.

Obstructions at the anus are built upon the levator ani, the internal sphincter, or the external sphincter muscles or their sheaths, and in a single case all of these organs may be involved. This is especially liable to be the case when the stricture ensues upon an inflammation at the anus, the commonest cause of which is imperfect surgical operation. A stricture situated within the levator ani zone should be cut bilaterally and not posteriorly, which is the conventional method. A bilateral incision cuts across the fibers of the levator ani and is not followed by a recontraction of the lumen, while a posterior linear proctotomy may be immediately followed by coaptation of the wound-edges and a re-establishment of the stricture. The same may be said of a stricture situated in the external sphincter muscle. An external sphincter muscle should not be cut anteriorly, though there is no danger of the re-establishment of the stricture if these structures be cut in the anterior quadrant. On the contrary, incontinence of feces is a probable consequence, for the transversus perinei muscles will prevent the coaptation of the wound's edges and rob the external sphincter of its purchase point. The physician should be very chary of dividing the internal sphincter under any circumstances, for this muscle maintains a state of tonic contraction, and if once divided its function is almost irrevocably impaired. A stricture involving both sphincters and the levator ani should for a long time be subjected to repeated gentle and progressive dilation in the hope that the fibrous tissue may become absorbed. This failing, an obviously qualified prognosis should be made and a posterior linear proctotomy performed, or the stricture completely dissected out and an artificial anus made near the tip of the coccyx.

PERIPROCTITIS.

Inflammation may occur in the cellular tissue about the rectum either above or below the levator ani muscle. When it occurs above the levator ani, it may more properly be termed *pelvic cellulitis*. When it occurs in a situation below the levator ani muscle or anal fascia, it should be termed *ischiorectal cellulitis*. This latter is the most frequent situation of the disease.

The **causes** of periproctitis are the same as those of proctitis and are described in a previous chapter.

The **symptoms** are usually rise of temperature, constipation, more or less feeling of malaise, impaired digestion, and pain and tenderness in the region of the inflammation. Pain is by no means a constant symptom. If the inflammation be deep seated in the cellular tissue, there will be but little pain until the tissue involved, by reason of its swelling, is resisted by the surrounding structures. On the other hand, if the inflammation be situated very near the skin, and particularly if it be situated at the anal verge, between the cutis vera and corrugator cutis ani muscle, the pain will be intense from the beginning.

If the inflammation be in the ischiorectal fossa and deeply situated, there may be no apparent swelling, and the presence of induration may be detectable only by the introduction of the finger into the anus and the palpation of the parts between this finger and the thumb externally placed. If the inflammation be situated superficially, there will be apparent swelling and redness of the area involved. When the periproctitis is situated above the levator ani muscle, the inserted index-finger will usually be able to determine the presence of an induration.

Treatment.—The patient should be required to maintain a state of rest with the body in the horizontal semiprone-semiflexed posture with the hips slightly elevated. In the initial stage the integument of the part should be painted with mentholated collodion, or cold antiseptic and sedative fomentations should be applied. In later stages hot fomentations should be applied. Incision will abort the process, and should be resorted to at once when the question of the presence of suppuration is otherwise unanswerable.

RECTAL AND ANAL ABSCESS.

Abscess in the pelvic floor about the anus often presents the most complex problems. Its perfect comprehension involves a study of the fasciæ of this region.

The symptoms of periproctitis just described may have preceded the suppuration. In many cases, however, the suppuration may have occurred without the previous stages having been noticed by the patient. Pus may be present and there may be no pitting of the part on pressure. The induration about the focus of pus may be so great that a softened spot may not be detectable. Again, pitting and redness may be the only objective signs present in a given case.

When the physician is in doubt whether the condition be one of suppuration or not, the parts should be freely incised lest ultimately fistula ensue.

An abscess situated below the anal fascia and posterior to the transversus perinei muscle points to the skin at a point ½ inch (1.27 cm.) or 1 inch (2.54 cm.) from the sphincter and the same distance from the posterior median raphe, or else it inclines to perforate the anal structures at a point between the external and the internal sphincter. An abscess situated anterior to the transversus perinei muscle and between the superficial and deep layers of the perineal fascia extends in the anterior direction toward the scrotum or labia majora. An abscess situated in the anterior perineum and between the two layers of the triangular ligament tends to perforate the anal structures between the internal and external sphincters, or else tends forward into the membranous urethra. An abscess situated above the levator ani muscle destroys the cellular tissue in the mesorectum, but tends to break into the rectum in the posterior median line at a point immediately above the coccygeolevator muscle.

The **treatment** of anorectal abscess consists in immediate free incision, curetting of the cavity, and packing the wound with antiseptic gauze. This may be done under infiltration anesthesia. If the wound made be undoubtedly larger than the greatest diameter of the cavity, solutions of hydrogen dioxid should be employed in its cleansing; otherwise, other antiseptics must be used. The daily use of sitz-baths is to be enjoined. The wound edges should be opened often enough to insure progresssive healing from the bottom.

FISTULA.

Fistula is an adventitious channel and may open into the bowel or on the body surface, or both. It is a sequel of an abscess. Its walls are lined with granulation or fibrous tissue.

The characteristic **symptoms** are mucopurulent discharge from the rectum or seropurulent discharge from an opening in the adjacent anal surface.

Diagnosis.—With the patient in the Sims' posture manual eversion of the buttocks should be practised at a time when the patient is required to bear down. At this moment ocular inspection of the

field should be made.   Crypts, lacunæ, or other depressions of the
surface should be critically examined by means of the probe's point.
Should the probe enter, the patient should be required to relax the
parts, and a tentative search should be made for the internal orifice of
the fistula.   The probe should be steadied and the patient put into
Martin's posture, which smooths out the intraanal folds of membrane, and the anoscope introduced, and, by means of another probe,
inspection made of the mucous surface of the anus to determine if
there be an internal orifice.   The internal orifice of a fistula discharging internally is usually marked by small granulations or vege-
tations.   If this search fail to discover an internal orifice, a fenestrated conoid speculum, such as Aloe's, should be inserted on its
obturator and the obturator or slide withdrawn.   This instrument
should be introduced with its fenestrum straddling the tissues penetrated by the first probe.   Careful search for an internal orifice
should be repeated.   This failing to discover one, the probe should
be withdrawn and the cavity of the fistula injected at its external orifice
with a sterile solution of milk or peroxid of hydrogen and anoscopy
repeated.   If this manipulation fail to discover an internal orifice,
further search should be abandoned till the time of operation.

Treatment.—The probe should be introduced into the external
orifice of the fistula and the conoid speculum reintroduced and its
fenestrum made to straddle the probe as already described.   The
tissues from the fistula's external orifice, to a point within the anus
as high as the probe's distal end, should be subjected to infiltration
anesthesia.   The probe should be thrust onward through the
mucous membrane and into the lumen of the rectum.   An incision
should be made through both mucous and cutaneous surfaces down
to the probe.   If, on the other hand, the fistula have an internal
and no external opening, the probe should be bent to form a long
hook-end and should be carried through the anoscope or Aloe's
speculum and into the internal orifice.   When it has been made to
pass as deeply toward the cutaneous surface as possible, the anoscope
should be withdrawn and an effort made to draw the probe-hook
deeper through the relaxed tissues and toward the skin.   The probe
should be steadily maintained in this position while the fenestrated
conoid speculum is made to straddle it.   Infiltration anesthesia
should be established and an incision made in the manner already

described. The wound should be packed with antiseptic gauze and cared for as described in a preceding paragraph. The more radical operation, consisting in dissecting out the sac and suturing together the freshened surfaces of the abscess-walls, may be performed under local anesthesia. Simple external fistulas of recent origin may be cured by injection of stimulating fluids and by vigilant general care. In case there be much fibrous tissue about the fistula, it should be subjected to frequent massage. Sitz-baths should precede the massage.

ANAL ULCER OR FISSURE.

As an independent or circumscribed lesion, fissure is seldom observed by the proctologist in the earliest and acute form. When present in the chronic form it has received the names of circumscribed ulceration, ulceration of the pocket of Physic or of the saccule of Horner, painful anal ulcer, anal torment, or fissure in ano.

Salient Symptoms.—Often there is itching at the anus. Pain on defecation or immediately thereafter is characteristic. Intolerably painful anal spasm is often present. The patients seek to avoid defecation and even the escape of flatus. This suppression of gaseous evacuation may lead to tympanites. This disease sometimes affords a multiplicity of reflected symptoms.

Diagnosis.—Anoscopy reveals a narrow gray or red erosion or ulceration lying between the pilasters. Careful and systematic digital eversion of the anal folds at a time when the patient bears down may disclose the lesion. When the probe's point is brought in contact with the fissure, it provokes the characteristic pain or spasm, and the patient usually signifies that the lesion is discovered. Fissures are most commonly posteriorly situated, but may be situated at any point in the anal circumference.

A hypertrophied bit of tissue of a gray color and of about the size of a pinhead is often noticeable at the lower end of the fissure ; this is the thickened wall of the anal pocket—to which Ball has given the name of "sentinel pile." It has been described by von Esmarch as the lower "*edematous polypoid fold.*"

Treatment.—*Prophylaxis.*—As the fissure is most frequently caused by chronic obstipation, this condition must be treated accord-

ing to principles laid down in chapter xv, volume I.   The patients
must be cautioned not to strain or press during defecation.   Boas
(*l. c.*, p. 534) is not in favor of efforts at regular evacuations during
the treatment, but recommends a period of artificial obstipation for
eight days by giving 10 drops tr. opii 3 times daily.   During this
period of rest to the anus, he treats the fissure locally with dry
antiseptic powders, such as airol, xeroform, orthoform, calomel.
The diet consists of soups and gruels.   After eight days he liquefies
the stools by giving castor or olive oil.   He reports 6 cases cured
in eight days, 2 cases cured in three weeks, and 2 in four weeks.
Of 12 cases, only 2 had to be treated operatively.   The ulcer, if
superficial, is to be touched with caustic or the electric cautery.
This treatment is to be repeated at intervals of several days.   It
may be alternated with or substituted by the application of ointment,
stimulating or sedative, according to the requirements of the ulcer.
The following formulas of ointments have been used :

R. Chrysarobin, ... gr. xij
Ext. belladonnæ, ... gr. x
Petrolatum, ... ℥j.
M.

R. Cocain hydrochl., ... gr. ij
Ext. belladonnæ, ... ʒj
Acid. tannic., ... ʒij
Petrolatum, ... ℥j.
M.

Convenient means of applying the ointment is shown in the
obturator-applicator.   This may be done by placing the ointment
in the neck of the instrument, lubricating its distal end with the
ointment, and introducing the anoscope to the necessary depth.
This manœuver places the ointment at a point opposite the diseased
area, where the obturator is to be steadied while the anoscope is
drawn off it.   The anus clasps the applicator around its anointed
neck.   Gentle rotation and withdrawal of the instrument expand
the anus and expose the otherwise infolded and concealed diseased
area and rub into its surface the medicament which the grasping
anus completely strips from the obturator.   Application of the nitrate
of silver solution is efficacious.

The simplest and most effective treatment in that form of fissure which undermines the integument at its inferior end consists in infiltration anesthesia by means of eucain or nirvanin solution and the splitting of the pocket by means of a small scalpel. The hypertrophied tissue should be trimmed away. The ulcer should then be touched with a solution of nitrate of silver, 40 grains to the ounce, and an opium suppository introduced. Subsequently the anus should be dilated twice daily and the wound kept open till perfectly healed. Semidaily immersion of the hips in hot water should be practised. The conventional operation for fissure, which requires general anesthesia, divulsion of the sphincters, and their division by incision, is haphazard surgery, is not uniformly curative, mutilates an important organ, and is hazardous to its functions and in a measure is dangerous to the life of the patient.

ULCERATION OF THE RECTUM.

Pathology and Etiology.—The character of the ulcers which may occur in the rectum and their pathological nature and cause are the same as those of intestinal ulcers, which have been described in a previous chapter (vol. 1, p. 592).

Salient Symptoms.—The feces are sometimes streaked with mucus, with patches of membrane and specks of blood, and there is always more or less purulent material discernible. Pain and soreness are not uniformly present when the disease is situated high up in the rectum, but are invariably present when situated near or at the anus.

Diagnosis.—The ulceration is characterized by the destruction of a circumscribed area of epithelium which is occupied by reddish granulation tissue ; the surface is often seen coated with inspissated mucopus. Ulceration may be accompanied by a more or less diffused chronic rectitis and with general superficial erosion of the mucous membrane. Venereal ulcers present their typical features when situated in this organ. Tubercular ulceration presents a clearly defined border, and is usually surrounded by a pale blue mucous membrane, and the evacuations frequently contain tubercle bacilli. Microscopical examination of scrapings positively determines the character. (See chapter on Intestinal Ulcers, vol. 1, p. 592.)

Treatment.—The ulcer may be stimulated to repair by the application of stimulating lotions, which may be conveniently done by means of the spray or applicator through the proctoscope (Fig. 54).

Because of the humidity of the rectum the actual cautery should not be introduced into this organ, as the consequent rapid evaporation occasions pain. Chancroid ulcers should be coated over with the charcoal and sulphuric acid paste. Enemata of bovinin prove decidedly reparative. Rectal lavage should be employed daily. In

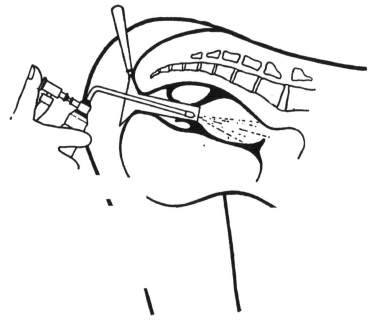

FIG. 54.—SHOWS A METHOD OF SPRAYING THE RECTUM AND SIGMOID FLEXURE.

the section on Intestinal Ulcers, Hemmeter has described the healing of a tubercular rectal ulcer by injections of tuberculin in a subject affected with pulmonary tuberculosis. Petruschky similarly reported healing of tubercular gastric ulcers by tuberculin ("Verhandl. d. XVII. Congress. f. innere Medicin," Karlsbad, 1899, S. 366).

PRURITUS.

Pruritus may be present as a local manifestation of any one of a great variety of constitutional diseases, or it may be a manifestation or a result of any of the diseases within the realms of proctica. Internal hemorrhoids should be suspected as a cause in each case. In persistent cases the feces should be examined for intestinal parasites or their ova. Certain articles of food may cause anal pruritus.

Salient Symptom.—Itching at the anus.

Diagnostic Appearances.—The circumanal skin is often thickened and may be abraded or cracked, or it may appear normal. The anal verge may be perpetually moist with secretion.

Treatment.—The initial cause is to be sought and removed. Mechanical irritation should be stopped. The parts should be painted with a solution of nitrate of silver or with some other astringent lotion. Sedative ointments or powders may be profitably applied. Fomentations are objectionable. Chrysarobin ointment will rapidly remove the hypertrophy of the integument. The patient should be required to practise daily gradual dilation of the anus by means of a conoid or cylindrical anal dilator. Sitz-baths are required daily. If parasites are present, the treatment is that outlined in the chapter devoted to this subject.

ACUTE INFLAMMATION AND PROLAPSE OF THE ANAL MUCOUS MEMBRANE.

Salient Symptoms.—This disease is characterized by intense pain at the anus and consequent prostration of the patient.

Diagnosis.—The anal mucous membrane is observed everted and swollen. The membrane is more prolapsed in the lateral halves than in the anterior and posterior quadrants. The tumor is marked usually by three sulci if the prolapse be bilateral and considerably swollen. There is usually a deep median depression in the mass extending from before backward and in a line continuous with the raphe (Fig. 55). The middle of this line marks the channel of the gut. Near the summit of each lateral mass may be distinguished the linea dentata (Stroud), which in this condition is much exaggerated in depth and dentation. The fitness of Stroud's term is pathologically emphasized. The mucous surface on the rectal side of this line is usually of a deep red color. It is often eroded and is usually covered with a profuse secretion of mucus. The tissues external to this line are yellow-white or they may be of

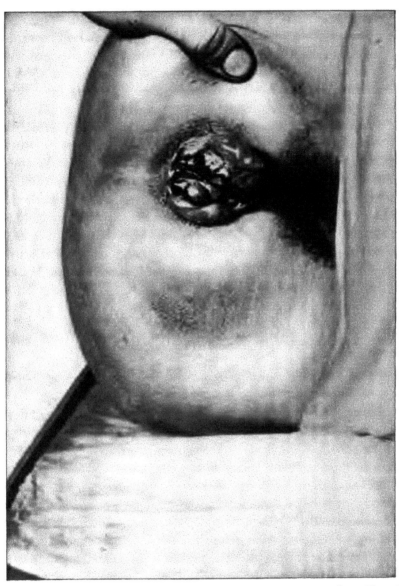

FIG. 55.—SHOWS A PROLAPSE OF CONNECTIVE-TISSUE HEMORRHOIDS AND ANAL MUCOUS MEMBRANE.

a deep purple; the color is dependent upon the degree of edema, venous engorgement, and vascular obstruction.

BIDIGITAL PALPATION OF

Acutely inflamed and prolapsed anal mucous membrane	Prolapsed internal hemorrhoids

REVEALS

Uniform density and elasticity throughout the mass.	Localized induration in one or more parts of the prolapsed mass and irregularity of contour.

Treatment.—Application of astringent and sedative lotions is required. The patient should be kept in the horizontal semiprone-semiflexed posture with the hips slightly elevated. In patients affected with the more aggravated states of prolapse the sphincters should be anesthetized (0.1 per cent. eucain solution) at several points in their circumference to secure their relaxation; the mucous membrane of the mass should be painted with the cocain solution (4 per cent.), and when the parts are sufficiently anesthetized the patient should be put in the knee-chest or Martin posture and the prolapsed parts subjected to taxis and reduced. If this manipulation is not immediately successful, the mass should be vertically incised and depleted, when it may be readily reduced. After reduction of the prolapse the buttocks should be strapped together.

CHRONIC NONINFLAMMATORY PROLAPSE OF THE ANAL MUCOUS MEMBRANE.

Salient Symptoms.—The patient tells of the recurrent character or continuous state of prolapse. There may be itching and proctorrhea.

Diagnosis.—Obvious by inspection. (See preceding section.)

Treatment.—The removal of elliptical portions of the prolapsed mass is demanded and may be done by a method to be described in the section on the treatment of hemorrhoids. If the sphincters be excessively relaxed or contracted, they may be gymnastically developed by the daily introduction of anal dilators, against which the patient should be required to make voluntary slight resistance, or the intrarectal application of electricity may be found useful.

Excision of a circular portion of the prolapsed membrane may be necessary.

NONMALIGNANT ANAL GROWTHS.

Considerations of technic justify that in a practical clinical synopsis the benign growths of this region be classified according to their form and anatomical situation rather than according to their histological character, which has been described in the section on Benign Neoplasms of the Intestines (vol. 1, p. 708). The nonmalignant anal growths are either sessile or pedunculated, and those which are originally sessile, because of the mechanism of this organ, tend to pedunculation. Sessile growths, because of their attachment to a movable structure, are susceptible to being compressed at their bases under the traction of the operator, and, as far as the application of the technic which accomplishes their removal is concerned, will be regarded as pedunculated. The commoner of the benign anal growths are hypertrophied anal pilasters (columns of Morgagni), angiomata of the hemorrhoidal plexuses, fibromata, mucocutaneous hypertrophies, and varices.

Varix of the Anal Pilaster.—A variety of hemorrhoid.

Salient Symptoms.—Steady aching, often referred to the end of the spine, more or less backache, and a great variety of reflected symptoms are ordinarily experienced by the patient.

Diagnosis.—Bimanual eversion of the buttocks may reveal the blue or purple colored projecting varicosity. Anoscopy may reveal a dilated blue or magenta vessel displacing, obliterating, enlarging, or projecting from the pilaster.

Thrombotic Varix.—A form of inflamed pile.

Salient Symptom.—Pain coming suddenly and continuing is characteristic.

Diagnosis.—Bimanual eversion of the buttocks discovers a more or less hemispheroid or columnar mass of tissue projecting from the anal verge. Bidigital examination determines the presence of the organized blood-clot, which is centrally situated in the mass, and the skin is movable over it.

Simple Hypertrophy of the Anal Pilaster.—Connective-tissue pile.

Salient Symptoms.—Anal itching, aching, or occasional pain is significant of this disease. If the mucosa be abraded or necrosed, there may be hemorrhage.

Diagnosis.—Anoscopy reveals an enlarged pilaster whose surface may appear, if not necrosed, somewhat like that of the hypertrophied tonsil which is pitted with lacunæ.

Angioma of the Anal Pilaster or of the Inferior Hemorrhoidal Plexus.—Internal or external hemorrhoid. (See Dilation of Hemorrhoidal Veins, this volume, p. 490.)

Salient Symptoms.—Pain, backache, sciatica, restlessness, and more or less constant sense of fatigue are the common manifestations of this disease. There may be bleeding.

Diagnosis.—The tumor presents in a much aggravated degree the appearance of a hypertrophied anal pilaster, or when the growth is very large all trace of the pilaster may be effaced. The mass (internal hemorrhoid), though it has its attachment at the anal pilaster in the zones of the *linea dentata* and internal sphincter, by reason of the tonic contraction of the latter is projected upward into the levator hollow and into the abdominal rectum, or else is prolapsed externally, dragging with it, sometimes, the anal mucous membrane. Angioma of the inferior hemorrhoidal plexus (external hemorrhoid) presents somewhat different contours and colors. This growth is usually nonpedunculated and is covered with the mucocutaneous integument (Figs. 56 and 57).

Treatment for the Removal of Benign Neoplasms.—In case the nonmalignancy of a growth appear doubtful, under proctoscopy and local anesthesia a section may be taken for microscopic examination. The other benign growths affecting this region present much the same features and clinical phenomena as these just described. The radical treatment aimed at their cure requires their removal, and the technic which is to be proposed, *if executed by trained hands*, in most instances painlessly achieves the desired result without general anesthesia. This technic escapes several of the disadvantages urged against the familiar clamp and cautery operation.

The Clamp (Fig. 58).—This instrument consists of a hollow cone 3¼ inches (8.25 cm.) in length and ¾ inch (1.90 cm.) in diameter at its distal extremity and 1¾ inches (4.44 cm.) in diameter at its proximal end. One quadrant of the cone is fenestrated

(Fig. 59); this is occupied by a movable blade with a serrated edge, which makes contact with the serrated cone edge. The movable blade is sheathed in the cone when the jaws of the clamp are separated.

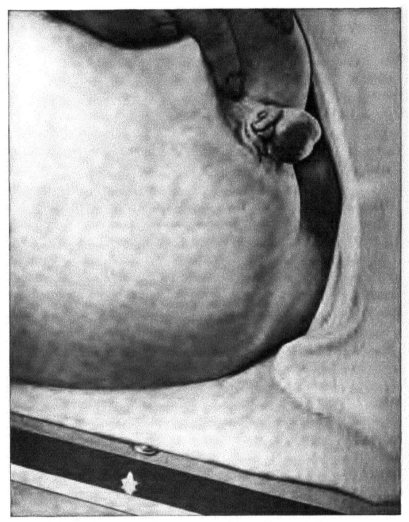

FIG. 56.—SHOWS A PROLAPSE OF CONNECTIVE-TISSUE INTERNAL HEMORRHOID.

The preliminary preparation of the patient consists in daily gradual dilation of the anus by means of Kelly's conic dilator until the anus may be made to open painlessly to the degree necessary

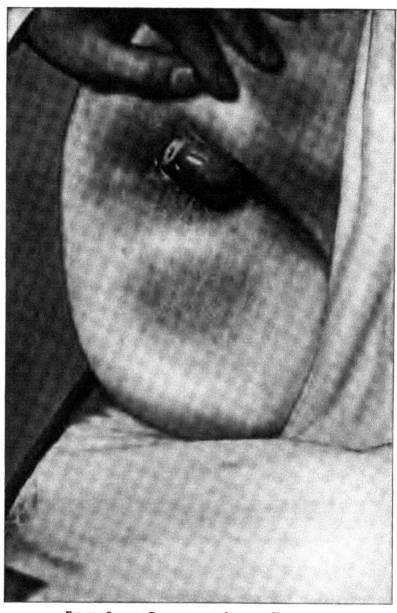

FIG. 57.—SHOWS A PROLAPSE OF AN INTERNAL HEMORRHOID.

for the introduction of the clamp.   Immersion of the patient's hips
in a tub of hot water twice daily will assist in this achievement.

The Technic.—(*A*) The patient should be placed in the horizontal semiprone-semiflexed posture, the upright knee-rest adjusted
to the table, and the light focused on the field of operation.

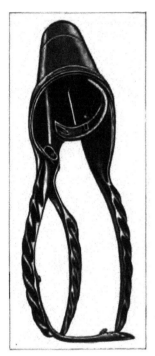

FIG. 58. — MARTIN'S   CONOID
CLAMP FOR THE REMOVAL OF
HEMORRHOIDS UNDER LOCAL .
ANESTHESIA.

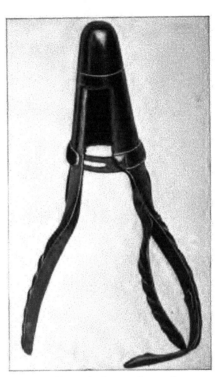

FIG. 59.—MARTIN'S CONOID CLAMP OPENED.

(*B*) The exact situation of the tumor should be determined under
anoscopy.

(*C*) (1) Hypodermic injections of about ten minims of 0.1 per
cent. solution of eucain into the ectal and ental sphincters to secure
their painless dilation are sometimes necessary ; (2) introduction
into the anus of the closed clamp with the blade directed toward or
against the tumor ; (3) separation of the clamp's jaws ; (4) injection
of the eucain solution (*a*) into the membrane covering the now

accessible tumor base, and (*b*) into the connective tissue composing the tumor; (5) clamping the tumor; (6) cutting away the tumor; (7) application of Paquelin's cautery, or of sutures to the pedicle; and (8) (*a*) releasing the pedicle and (*b*) withdrawing the clamp.

Occasionally difficulties may be encountered in an attempt to get an anal polypus through the jaws of the clamp. This may be

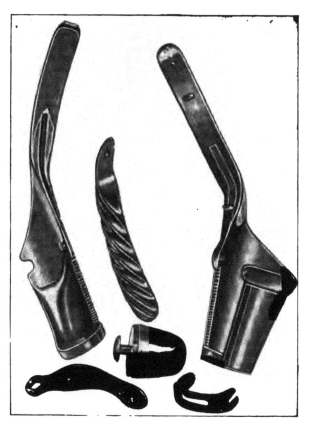

FIG. 60.—THE CLAMP SEPARATED FOR CONVENIENCE IN CLEANSING.

easily accomplished under anoscopy by casting a noose about the polypus. The noose should be drawn taut and the anoscope withdrawn. The tumor is to be held down by traction on the ligature while the clamp is introduced. The operation is then to be performed as described in the preceding paragraph.

Thrombotic inflamed hemorrhoids ordinarily require infiltration anesthesia, incision through the mass, and eversion of the clot. Subsequently, if the tissues be sufficiently hypertrophied and become subject to recurrent attacks of inflammation, the tumor should be removed by means of the technic above described. Inflamed and thrombotic hemorrhoids, if prolapsed, should not be subjected to manipulations designed for the reduction of the prolapse, lest the thrombus be converted into serious or fatal emboli.

Varicose hemorrhoids require the exercise of the greatest precision in placing the hypodermic needle for anesthetization lest the solution be injected directly into the circulation and not into the tissue which it is designed to anesthetize. It is difficult to painlessly remove this lesion. If the operator's technic be in the least degree imperfect, the operation will completely fail.

The clamp effectually blocks the field of operation against the accidental invasion of feces or other intestinal detritus ; the field of operation therefore may be made practically sterile.

By means of this clamp the surgeon experienced in the use of the hypodermic syringe for obtaining local anesthesia may with but trifling discomfort to his patient successfully remove the largest hemorrhoid. Two hundred minims of o. 1 per cent. solution of eucain are sufficient, ordinarily, for the painless removal of tumors of great size. More than three-fourths of the quantity of the solution used may be recovered with the removal of the tumor ; hence the amount of the drug which may enter into the patient's circulation is inappreciable.

This operation, when applied to the largest connective-tissue growths, usually requires of the patient not more than three or four days' restraint from exercise.

The following conditions may contraindicate the use of eucain and the conoid clamp unless the nerve-trunks be attacked. Two or more inflamed internal hemorrhoids and extensive hemorrhoidal varix ; neurasthenic subjects and persons of particular idiosyncrasy to this drug should be put into a state of general anesthesia for operation.

The removal of the nonmalignant growths at the anus by means of the ligature and by the conventional clamp and cautery methods requires that the patient be placed in a state of general anesthesia.

The ligature method requires that the anus be divulsed till the sphincter lies dilated and relaxed. The tumor is seized by means of the volsella, its mucocutaneous surface incised, and the ligature placed and tied. This operation ordinarily entails several days of suffering on the part of the patient. The tumor may be cut away or else it sloughs away and leaves a granulating wound in its stead, which may promptly heal, though it sometimes cicatrizes and establishes a stricture.

ANAL HEMORRHAGE.

Postoperative anal hemorrhage may be effectually controlled as follows: The anoscope should be introduced till its distal end be beyond the levator ani and the obturator removed. A piece of gauze 2 feet (60.96 cm.) square should be folded in lines radiating

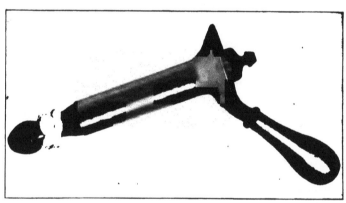

Fig. 61.—The Proctoscope Cotton-wrapped Obturator Prepared for the Control of Hemorrhage.

from its center to its four corners, and into this pouch a small moist sponge or wad of gauze should be placed by means of the forceps and the three carried through the anoscope and above the levator ani. The forceps should be removed and traction placed on the gauze to bring the expanding sponge hard against the distal end of the anoscope and levator ani muscle. That part of the gauze which is within the anoscope should be packed in an orderly manner with strips of gauze and the anoscope withdrawn, leaving the dressings in place. The exposed portions of the gauze pouch should now be packed with pads of gauze and its four corners tied down upon the mass.   Masses of cut gauze should now be padded over this dressing and a T-bandage fixed over all.   After a reasonable time the outer dressings are to be removed, the intra-anal gauze stalk carried through the anoscope, and the anoscope carried deeply into the rectum on the stalk of gauze which serves the purpose of a guide.   The gauze within the pouch may now be removed and irrigation employed to soften the sponge.   Under the grasp of the forceps the sponge may be twisted into a small compass and removed from the rectum through the anoscope.

Ordinarily the following simpler means of arresting hemorrhage is efficacious: Wrap about the neck of the obturator a piece of absorbent cotton (Fig. 61), upon which place a small amount of the persulphate of iron.   Sheathe the obturator, lubricate the anoscope, and introduce it into the anus ; withdraw the anoscope, leaving the cotton-wrapped neck of the obturator within the grasp of the sphincters, where it will be retained.   It may, if necessary, be fixed in its position with tapes.

Anal hemorrhage may be controlled under the pressure of an inserted thumb.   Ice-bags secured to the sacrum by means of the T-bandage are often efficacious in preventing the recurrence of the bleeding.   In all cases the patient's hips should be elevated.

NONMALIGNANT RECTAL GROWTHS.

Nonmalignant rectal growths are sessile or pedunculated, and the sessile growths, because of the mechanism of this organ, tend to pedunculation.   The sessile rectal growths, being situated, like those of the anus, upon a membrane freely movable on an elastic submucosa over the muscular coats of the rectum, may usually be converted by the operator, by a process of lifting the growth and compression of the circumjacent mucous membrane beneath the growth, or by lifting and twisting the tumor, into a surgical pedicle which will facilitate its excision by means of the technic presently to be proposed.   Execution of the technic and the results will improve with the advanced skill, experience, and good judgment.

Salient Symptoms.—Nonmalignant rectal growths present no characteristic symptoms ; the patient may, however, be the subject of occasional attacks of obstipation, diarrhea, hemorrhage, proctorrhea, or of any one or of several of the various manifestations of proctica.

Diagnosis.—Proctoscopy reveals the tumor (Fig. 62).

Treatment.—A silver-wire noose may be thrown about the pedicle, twisted down upon it, the wire's ends cut off and guarded by a compressed shot, and the tumor left to slough off, or it may be cut away, leaving the wire ligature to guard against hemorrhage; subsequently the wire may be removed. A polypus may, how-

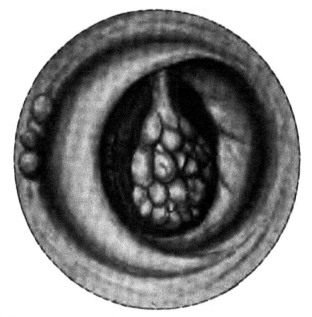

Fig. 62.—A Composite Proctoscopic View of a Rectal Polypus, Papillomas, and a Hypertrophied Rectal Valve.

ever, be more quickly and effectually removed by means of a strong snare (Fig. 63). One provided with a long shaft and with a handle bent at an angle obtuse to the shaft should be introduced through the proctoscope, the tumor base embraced, and the operation finished with a technic similar to that employed by the rhinologist on nasal polypi.

MALIGNANT DISEASE OF THE RECTUM.

Of all portions of the intestine the rectum is most frequently the seat of malignant disease (see statistics compiled by Hemmeter, vol. I, p. 680).   In fact, statistics tend to show that this part of the intestine is as frequently affected as are all other portions of the bowel.   Sarcoma very rarely attacks this organ.   Of the carcinomata, the adenocarcinoma is the commonest form.   The squamous variety is encountered at the anus below the levator ani.   That repetition may be avoided, I am requested to refer the reader to the chapter on the Morbid Anatomy of the Malignant Diseases of the Intestine, by Prof. Hemmeter.   According to this author, 20.22

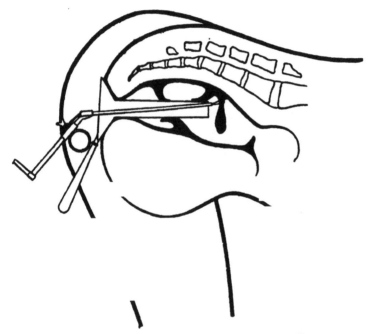

FIG. 63.—A METHOD FOR THE REMOVAL OF A RECTAL POLYPUS.

per cent. of all intestinal cancers are located in the rectum (vol. I, p. 681).

The symptoms which are regarded as characteristic of malignant disease of the rectum usually present themselves or are recognized when the disease is so far advanced as to render its treatment unpromising or else absolutely to forbid surgical intervention. These symptoms are as follows: Diarrhea of a recurrent or chronic character is significant, the defecations being most frequent in the morning.   Even before the tumor sloughs the discharges will contain much mucus, pus, and epithelial cells, and shreds of

PLATE 13.

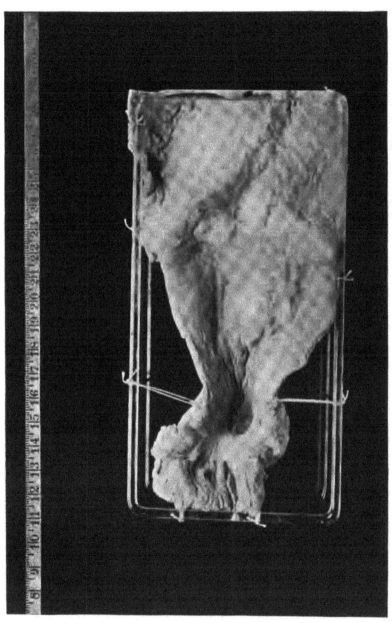

CARCINOMATOUS STRICTURE OF THE RECTUM.

pseudo-membrane. The discharges are characterized by a peculiarly offensive odor, are streaked with blood, and contain blood-clots or bright fresh blood. When necrosis of the growth occurs, masses of necrotic tissue are not infrequently discharged. If the growth be situated in the anal structures, pain is an almost constant symptom, and an excruciating tenesmus is experienced with each defecation, and is often present in intervals of defecation. Sometimes there is an ineffectual straining at stool. The pain is due to the irritation of the exposed tissues, occasioned by contact with the acrid discharges, or may be due to tension of the nerves under the pressure of the growth. When the disease is situated above the levator ani and in the rectum proper, pain is rarely present because of the normal anesthesia of the rectum; however, when the growth attains sufficient magnitude to stretch the nerves, a distressing, aching pain is more or less constant; sciatic neuralgia is not uncommon. Probably the earliest symptom of malignant disease of the rectum is obstipation due to the encroachment of the tumor upon the lumen of the organ.

Diagnosis.—Proctoscopy, if practised on patients complaining of constipation or obstipation, will early discover the presence of such a tumor, if it exist, and afford an opportunity for its successful removal. It is my conviction that if proctoscopy were made the routine practice of the physician, malignant disease of the rectum would rarely be permitted the opportunity to become inoperable. It is to be regretted, however, that most cases when referred to the specialist have passed beyond the pale of justifiable surgical intervention. Ninety per cent. of the cases of malignant disease which have come under my observation have been brought to me with the ready-made diagnosis of bleeding piles or fistula; hemorrhoids, prolapsus recti, and fistula are the common sequels of malignant disease of the rectum. Under proctoscopy the physician may command such a view of the rectum and may have such access to the rectum that the tumor is not only seen distinctly, but is made accessible for the removal of a portion for microscopic examination. As the benign neoplasms of the rectum tend to pedunculation, all sessile growths should be suspected of malignancy and subjected to an expert microscopist's examination. Adenocarcinomata are usually multiple, and if discovered early have a grayish or straw-colored appearance. The colloid form of cancer is lead-colored or bluish, and in places is almost translucent. The melanotic form presents a peculiarly black complexion. All of these growths, a short time before they undergo degeneration, partake of a dark red color. Portions of these growths have a peculiarly glistening sheen; other portions undergoing superficial necrosis have a beef-red appearance. I have recently seen an adenocarcinoma lying in the second rectal chamber which presented an appearance not unlike a bunch of overripe currants; the mucosa of the noninvaded valve was pale.

Appearance through the Proctoscope Different from What is Felt by the Finger.—When the mass once begins to degenerate, it not infrequently sloughs rapidly, and the proctoscopy made later in such cases reveals instead of a contracted lumen due to the encroachment of the tumor, the rectum inflated and expanded to a normal degree, exposing a large ulcerated area apparently of great depth because of the infiltration and edema of its borders. Let the physician now place such a patient in a dorsal position and make a digital examination, and if the tumor be within reach, his finger will detect a mass which seems to his sense of touch not unlike the original growth. This fallacy is due to the collapse of the rectum and prolapse and invagination of the indurated structures. The anus is usually found much relaxed in cases of rectal tumor. The perineal and inguinal lymphatics sooner or later become involved in cases of malignant disease of the anus. Malignant disease of the rectum is accompanied by infiltration of the sacral lymphatic glands.

Treatment.—A malignant growth at the anus, when the inguinal lymphatics are not indurated, should be removed by a wide dissection of all the anal structures, and the rectum secured in the wound in some such manner as that described in the section on malformations of the rectum. Malignant growths at the rectum, when there is no involvement of an adjacent viscus, should be approached as is described in the chapter referred to. In cases of malignant disease of the rectum or anus, in which an adjacent viscus is invaded, removal of the growth does not promise much relief nor length of life. However, it should be remembered that removal of the rectum or anus, and vagina, uterus, and adnexa is surgery possible of achievement. When the disease is considered impossible of removal and the patient is suffering from obstruction or great pain, an artificial inguinal anus should be established and provision made for the patency of the lower bowel, that the rectum may be occasionally flushed from above. My experience teaches me that an artificial inguinal anus should never be made without first making the fullest explanation of what such an operation means. The wise physician will have a witness present when making this explanation. When such a patient declines operation for an artificial anus, temporary relief of the obstruction may be afforded by curettage of a channel through the growth. This operation may be painlessly performed through the proctoscope without the employment of any sort of anesthesia.

FOREIGN BODIES IN THE RECTUM.

The opportunities which proctoscopy by atmospheric inflation affords for the discovery and the removal of foreign bodies or im-

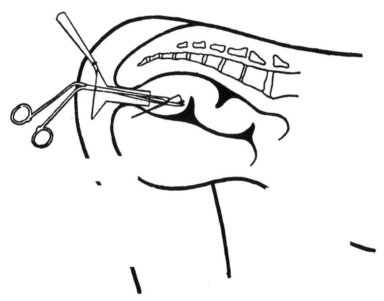

FIG. 64.—A METHOD FOR THE REMOVAL OF A FOREIGN BODY FROM A RECTAL CHAMBER.

pacted feces from the anus and rectum without anesthesia and without pain are obvious.

The Technic.—The patient should be placed on the chair in the horizontal semiprone-semiflexed posture, and that part of the rectum within the reach of the finger should be subjected to a careful digital exploration with the purpose of determining whether the object is situated above or below the levator ani, and whether its lower end penetrates the structures constituting the anus or the pelvic floor. Should the object penetrate the anus, the short ano-scope should be introduced as far as the point at which the object passes through the mucous membrane and the obturator then with-drawn. Now a pair of forceps, under the guidance of the eye, should be passed through the anoscope and made to seize the ob-

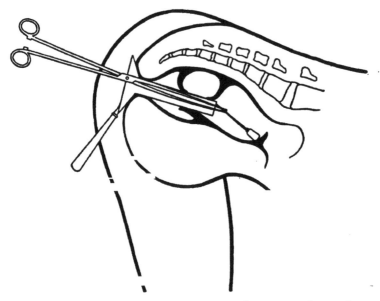

FIG. 65.—A METHOD FOR THE REMOVAL OF A FOREIGN BODY FROM A RECTAL CHAMBER.

ject (Fig. 64). This object should be carried by the forceps toward the promontory of the sacrum and thus removed from the tissue by making it retrace its course. When it is carried well up into the rectal chamber, it should be deposited there and the forceps and anoscope withdrawn. Foreign bodies in the rectal chambers may be discovered by placing the patient in Martin's posture and by the use of the means and methods described for proctoscopy. Should a foreign body transfix or penetrate a rectal valve or any other part of the rectal wall, it should be extracted in the same manner as is suggested for the extraction of foreign bodies from the anus—by making the foreign body retrace the course by which it entered the tissues.   Having dislodged it from the tissues and deposited it in the rectal chamber, it should be withdrawn under the grasp of the forceps through the proctoscope (Fig. 65).   Should it be too large to pass through this instrument, the patient should be anesthetized and the body removed by means of proctocolonoscopy, which I first described in the July, 1896, number of Mathews' "Quarterly Journal of Rectal and Gastro-intestinal Diseases," and which requires an expanding bivalve speculum.   Fish-bones, clyster-tube tips, coproliths, gall-stones, impacted scybala, and the stranger things sometimes lodged in this organ (see chapter on Obturation, vol. II, p. 238) may be removed by the proposed methods with practically no danger to the life or to the organs of the patient.

ARRESTED DEVELOPMENT OF THE ANUS AND RECTUM.

Atresia ani is the commonest form of congenital malformation of the lower intestine.   It is due to an imperfect coalescence of the proctodeum and the enteron.   In the course of embryonic development the rectum and anus are perfected before the third month. Occasionally there are met cases of imperforate anus in which not so much as an anal dimple is discernible.   In such cases the epiblast has not dipped to form the proctodeum.   In other cases of imperforate anus the proctodeum may have dipped into the mesoblastic layer to a normal degree and be surrounded by a perfectly developed external sphincter muscle, and the enteron or gut proper may be separated from the proctodeum by a narrow septum ; or there may be an absence of the lower portion of the rectum, of the entire rectum, or of a portion of the colon, or an absence of the large intestine ; in such cases a great interval exists between the terminal portion of the gut and the anus.   In a previous chapter (p. 258) an x-ray photograph is presented illustrating the distance to which the anus may be imperforate.

The symptoms of imperforate ani or recti are nonestablishment of defecation, flatulence, tympanites, and fecal vomiting, and if surgical intervention be not resorted to, death will result from shock or infection, which may be the sequel of intestinal perforation—occurrences unusual before the fifth day.

In cases of imperforate ani it is sometimes found that the rectum communicates with the vagina, the bladder, or the urethra ; and cases have been reported of its communication with the uterus.

Surgical intervention for the establishment of an artificial anus is demanded at the earliest possible moment. These patients often succumb to shock after the operation which is applied for their relief; hence it is imperative that whatever operation be undertaken there should be no procrastination. If the child be of apparently normal vitality, the radical operation for establishing an anus at its normal site should be undertaken at once. As it is difficult to determine prior to the operation at what state the development was arrested, it can not be determined how extensive a dissection may be necessary ; therefore a temporary artificial inguinal anus is to be preferred for the weakling. Under infiltration anesthesia an incision should be made in the inguinal region and a loop of the gut drawn out and supported on a glass rod, which should be made to transfix the mesentery. A few catgut sutures should be passed through the skin, the fasciæ, the parietal and intestinal peritoneum and muscular structure of the bowel, and tied to secure the gut in the wound for twenty-four hours, that the peritoneal cavity may be walled off by the organized exudate before the bowel is opened. If the operation is performed early and the little patient is not suffering from obstruction, the gut need not be opened until the expiration of the twenty-four hours. It scarcely matters what portion of the colon is anchored in the wound in cases of the kind under discussion. The two advantages which are afforded in choosing the ascending colon are that it is more easily found than the descending colon in the majority of these cases and that in the subsequent operation for the establishment of a permanent anus in the perineal region, the rectum and sigmoid flexure may be more easily drawn down.

The radical operation in cases of imperforate anus or congenital absence of the rectum requires an incision continuous with the raphe from a point approximately posterior to the transversus perinei muscle, or through the posterior quadrant of the proctodeum, backward to the tip of the coccyx. Tentatively the incision should be deepened in the direction of the upper sacral bodies. If the rectum should not now be discovered, the incision should be lengthened by a median incision through the bones of the coccyx by means of the cartilage knife or the scissors. The pelvic outlet in the newly born infant is scarcely more than ½ inch (1.27 cm.) in diameter, and hence the space made by the aforesaid incision may be too confined for intelligent manipulation of the finger in its endeavor to discover the bowel. It should be remembered that ossification of the pelvic bones is not far advanced at this period of development, and that therefore retractors may be successfully employed to enlarge the operation field. Manipulation of the intestine by means of a hand over the abdomen may carry the desired portion of the bowel within the reach of the searching finger. If the rectum should terminate in an adjacent pelvic viscus, a low loop should be drawn through the wound, double clamped and severed, and that part attached to the viscus closed with a purse-string suture and the desired portion anchored at the position in the wound where it will be least subjected to such traction as may tear it away.

Congenital stricture of the anus is situated in the zone between the external and internal sphincters. This condition may be relieved by a posterior proctotomy or by shallow bilateral incisions; the operation should be completed by suturing together the deep angles of the wounds, as is described in the section on valvotomy.

Congenital stricture of the rectum is due to hyperplasia of the mesoblastic layer of the rectal valves. Such congenital strictures are often multiple. These obstructions may be temporarily overcome and in some instances effectually cured by a method of interrupted dilation. The fingers constitute the best instruments for this purpose. At the beginning of the treatment in such a case the physician should use his little finger and direct its palmar surface toward the sacrum. When the patient shall have arrived at an appropriate age, if necessary, valvotomy should be resorted to under anesthesia.

ADDENDUM.

LITERATURE ON TUBERCULOUS CECAL TUMOR.

This literature belongs to the article on Tubercular Tumor of the Cecum, and should have been inserted on page 100, volume II.

1. Billroth, cited after Conrath, *l. c.*
2. Boas, Darmkrankheiten, S. 277.
3. Conrath, "Brun's Beiträge zur klin. Chir.," Bd. XXI, Heft 1, 1898.
4. Czerny, "Brun's Beiträge zur Chirurgie," Bd. VI u. IX.
5. Eisenhart, "Ueber Häufigkeit und Vorkommen der Darmtuberculose," Diss. inaug., München, 1891.
6. Hartmann und Pilliet, cited after Conrath, *l. c.*
7. Hofmeister, "Brun's Beiträge zur Chirurgie," Bd. XVII, 1896, S. 577.
8. König, "Deutsche Zeitschr. f. Chirurgie," Bd. XXXIV, 1892, S. 65.
9. Körte, *ibid.*, Bd. XL, 1895, S. 523.
10. Salzer, "v. Langenbeck's Arch.," Bd. XLIII.
11. Wittstock, "Zur Klinik des Ileus durch Darmtuberculose," Diss. inaug., Berlin, 1893.
12. Buttersack, "Zeitschr. f. Tuberculose u. Heilstätten Wesen," Nov., 1900.
13. Orth, "Spec. path. Anatomie," Bd. I, S. 839 to 842.
14. Cornet, G., "Die Tuberculose," in Nothnagel's "Specielle Pathologie und Therapie," Bd. XIV, 2te Hälfte.
15. Lartigan, August J., "A Study of Chronic Hyperplastic Tuberculosis of the Intestine," etc., "Journal of Experimental Medicine," vol. VI, p. 23.

INDEX OF AUTHORS.—VOL. II.

Compiled by Dr. Charles F. Conser, Instructor in the Clinical Laboratory of the University of Maryland.

INDEX OF SUBJECTS.—VOL. II.

Compiled by Dr. Wilbur F. Skillman, Assistant in the Clinical Laboratory of the University of Maryland.